Pediatric Radiology

Contributors

Rica G. Arnon, M.D.
Assistant Professor of Pediatrics
Section on Pediatric Cardiology
College of Medicine
University of Tennessee Center for the Health Sciences
Memphis, Tennessee

Barry Gerald, M.D.
Professor of Neuroradiology
Department of Diagnostic Radiology
College of Medicine
University of Tennessee Center for the Health Sciences
Memphis, Tennessee

Louis S. Parvey, M.D.
Assistant Professor, Department of Diagnostic Radiology
Director of Pediatric Radiology
College of Medicine
University of Tennessee Center for the Health Sciences;
Acting Director, Department of Radiology
LeBonheur Children's Hospital
Memphis, Tennessee

Jeno I. Sebes, M.D.
Associate Professor
Department of Diagnostic Radiology
College of Medicine
University of Tennessee Center for the Health Sciences
Memphis Tennessee

Robert L. Siegle, M.D.
Associate Professor
Department of Diagnostic Radiology
College of Medicine
University of Tennessee Center for the Health Sciences
Memphis, Tennessee

Daniel Kirk Westmoreland, M.D.
Assistant Professor
Department of Diagnostic Radiology
College of Medicine
University of Tennessee Center for the Health Sciences
Memphis, Tennessee

Pediatric Radiology

Jack G. Rabinowitz, M.D., F.A.C.R.
Professor and Chairman
Department of Diagnostic Radiology, College of Medicine
University of Tennessee Center for the Health Sciences;
Chief of Radiology, City of Memphis Hospitals
Memphis, Tennessee

With Six Contributors

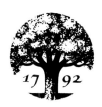

J. B. Lippincott Company
Philadelphia • Toronto

ISBN   0-397-50393-8

Library of Congress Catalog Card Number 78-7624

Printed in the United States of America
6 5 4 3 2 1

Library of Congress Cataloging in Publication Data

Rabinowitz, Jack G
    Pediatric radiology
    Includes bibliographies and index.
    1. Pediatric radiography.   I. Title.
RJ51.R3R3   618.9′2′007572   78-7624
    ISBN 0-397-50393-8

To my wife, children, and residents,
who have made my life and work pleasant and worthwhile

Preface

The prospect of writing a book on pediatric radiologic diagnosis appeared originally superfluous. A quick survey revealed a multitude of books available in this field of interest. Many of these are voluminous, and the reader is frequently besieged by countless pages of narration describing multiple diseases and radiologic findings. Despite many weeks of reading and digesting facts, the student of radiology is still unfortunately confronted with the realization that he has learned little relating to the approach and analysis of reading film. The introduction of the gamut concept has done much to diminish this problem. However, a book consisting only of gamuts is difficult and uninteresting reading, since it resembles a cookbook that is full of excellent recipes but lacks instructions. It assumes that the reader is versatile in film interpretation and has absorbed all the fundamentals of radiology and disease understanding. For many this is a frustrating experience. The present text was conceived to bridge the void that exists between the large textbook and the gamut. It presents a more direct approach to interpretation of radiographs by more closely aligning the text to the actual thought processes and discussion necessary for such interpretation. The basic format, therefore, deviates from the classical method of disease description and is constructed mainly with respect to the findings as they appear on the radiograph. The mechanisms and the differential diagnosis of each radiographic feature are described by areas of interest as well as age of presentation.

I believe that this format is a positive method for teaching radiology. Not only is it interesting reading, but it may be retained as a reference book during the course of daily film examination. Nevertheless, occasional redundancy is an inherent evil of the technique, despite the attempt to facilitate interpretation of radiographs. This failing does not detract from the overall purpose of providing the reader with a pleasurable perusal of general pediatrics by means of a description of radiologic features. Although this format can and should be utilized in any area of radiologic diagnosis, the author selected pediatrics because of his long-standing preference for this field.

I would like to thank my colleagues in the Department of Diagnostic Radiology at the University of Tennessee in Memphis, who collaborated and contributed their efforts and knowledge to some sections of this book.

In addition, I am deeply grateful to Linda Coad and Trish Franks for the enduring patience that they manifested during the innumerable hours required to retype the corrected manuscripts.

Above all, if it were not for the perpetual encouragement and support given by my wife, along with her contribution to Chapter 4, this book would not have been completed. For this, words cannot express by appreciation and gratitude.

JACK G. RABINOWITZ, M.D.

Contents

   Underlying Diseases** • *Louis S. Parvey, M.D.* 343

   General Comments 343
   Differential Diagnosis 343

10. **Systematic Radiographic Evaluation of the Skeleton**
    Louis S. Parvey, M.D., Jack G. Rabinowitz, M.D., F.A.C.R.,
    Jeno I. Sebes, M.D., and Daniel Kirk Westmoreland, M.D. 355

    Periosteal Reaction 355
    Solitary Osteolytic Lesions 368
    Solitary Sclerotic Lesions of Bone 374
    Multiple Osteolytic Lesions 386
    Multiple Sclerotic Lesions 398
    Osteopenia 412
    Metaphyseal Abnormalities 427
    Epiphyseal Abnormalities 452
    Short Bones and Dwarfism 474
    Radial Dysplasia 486
    Body Asymmetry 486
    Fractures in the Newborn 490

    Index 499

1

The Radiographic Features of Urinary Tract Disease in the Newborn, Infant, and Child

It is often difficult to evaluate the renal outline in the abdomen of newborns because of overlying intestinal gas and the relative paucity of perirenal fat. Adequate urographic evaluation using intravenous contrast material is also difficult to achieve during this period. The kidneys of newborns do not have the same capacity to concentrate urine as the kidneys of adults, and maximum concentration of urine may occur 3 to 4 hours after the initial intravenous injection. Consequently, the renal outline, pelvis, and ureters are not always completely visualized, and radiographs obtained in the early minutes of the examination may be unsatisfactory. The introduction of high doses of contrast material has improved the overall urographic visualization of the urinary system. It does, however, predispose to early diuresis and occasionally produces poor visualization of the kidneys. Dosages as high as 5 ml. per kg. have been utilized in newborn infants. However, we feel that a safe and adequate dose is 10 ml. for full-term infants and a somewhat smaller amount for the premature.

Enhanced demonstration of the renal structures can be obtained either by distending the stomach with air or with a carbonated beverage, or by positioning the patient in the prone position. In this position, the intestinal gas is displaced to either side of the abdomen, and the kidneys are better demonstrated.

The routine use of total body opacification is highly recommended, since it aids in detecting and identifying the presence of cystic structures. Total body opacification represents an increase in radiodensity of all vascularized soft tissues, and as a result cystic avascular masses appear radiolucent (Fig. 1-1). This phenomenon is radiographically apparent approximately 1 to 10 minutes after the injection and is most obvious in the first weeks of life because of the small volume of soft tissues in comparison to the relatively high doses of contrast medium used.

The overall appearance of the kidney in newborns is somewhat different from that of the adult kidney. The kidneys, in general, are much larger relative to overall body size. The kidney length may equal five or even six vertebral bodies (Fig. 1-2). This relative increase in length decreases proportionately as the infant grows older and as the lumbar vertebrae assume adult size and configuration. The kidneys in newborns also appear more spherical with both the upper and lower poles turned slightly inward toward the midline. The renal cortex is also comparatively thin. As the infant matures, the kidney becomes more elongated and the cortex increases in relative and absolute thickness. An interesting feature noted by Dunbar and Nogrady is the frequent appearance of nonobstructive dilatation of the collecting systems. In all these cases, follow-up examinations 3 to 6 months later were normal.

Transient herniation of the bladder wall

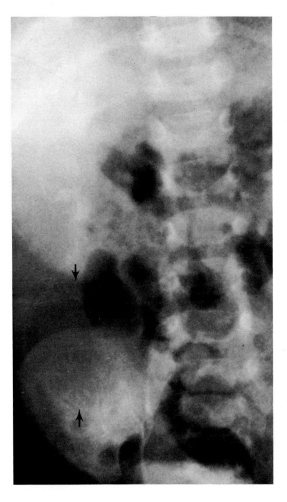

Fig. 1-1. Total body opacification. Duplication cyst. An intravenous urogram was performed because of a palpable mass in the right lower quadrant. The total body opacification phase delineates a sharply demarcated radiolucent mass within the right lower quadrant. At surgery this was found to be a duplication cyst of the cecum.

into the inguinal canal is frequently encountered up to the age of 6 months. This has been referred to as "bladder ears" and is a normal variation (Fig. 1-2B).

BILATERAL GENERALIZED RENAL ENLARGEMENT

The newborn with renal enlargement is usually referred for study because of palpable abdominal mass, increase in abdominal girth (this is particularly noted in the older child), or presence of other diseases or anomalies (e.g., malformed ears, widely spaced nipples) that are known to be associated with renal abnormalities. Since approximately 50 per cent of all abdominal masses discovered in newborns are retroperitoneal in origin, intravenous urography should be the initial procedure of choice. Bilaterally enlarged kidneys are usually smooth and fairly symmetrical.

Disease Entities

Normal kidneys
Duplication of pelvo-calyceal system
Bilateral hydronephrosis
Child of diabetic mother
Visceromegaly (e.g., storage disease, Beckwith-Wiedemann syndrome)
Renal vein thrombosis
Nephritis and nephrosis
Polycystic disease of the infant (Potter's Type I)

Differential Diagnosis

Occasionally one is presented with an infant with apparently normal but somewhat enlarged kidneys. This feature may represent one end of a spectrum of normal variants and is probably the most frequent cause of bilateral symmetrically enlarged kidneys. However, underlying abnormalities should be excluded before assuming this to be normal.

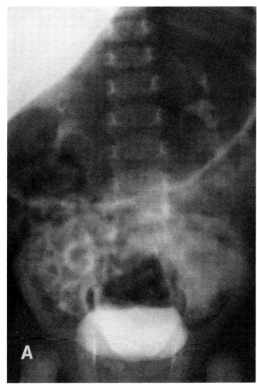
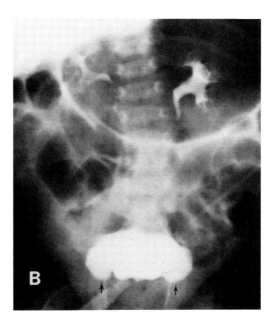

Fig. 1-2. Normal intravenous urogram. *(A)* The kidneys are seen through a distended stomach. The calyces, ureters, and bladder are fairly well demonstrated, although the renal outline cannot be completely evaluated. *(B)* "Bladder ears." The entire urogram is normal. The lateral walls of the bladder are displaced downward and project into the inguinal ring. This is a normal occurrence during this age.

As stated, normal kidneys may be as long as five or six vertebral bodies.

Duplication or triplication of the collecting systems results in a kidney larger than normal for any given patient. This embryologic variation may be unilateral or bilateral and is easily demonstrated during excretory urography. Two or more renal pelves associated with the additional collecting systems are noted. Multiple ureters, when present, facilitate the diagnosis.

Bilateral hydronephrosis is the result of obstruction involving both sides of the urinary tract. Hydronephrosis is suggested clinically when abdominal palpation reveals bilateral cystic masses that transilluminate. As far as the urographic studies are concerned, the abdominal film may reveal soft-tissue masses that represent large kidneys or a soft-tissue "Mickey mouse" configuration that represents the distended bladder and ureters (Fig. 1-3A). Renal function is often severely impaired but can be surprisingly preserved in some cases. Radiographs ob-

tained during the phase of total body opacification reveal large bilateral radiolucent structures (Figs. 1-3B, 1-4A). The earliest manifestation of functioning parenchyma is the appearance of a thin peripheral rim of opacification surrounding the dilated radiolucent calyces (Figs. 1-3B, 1-4A). This thin opacified cortical rim has been called the Dunbar crescent and is believed to be caused by compression of the residual cortical tissue with realignment of the compressed tubules into a more horizontal position. At times, small cystic collections of contrast medium will be seen within the renal papillae adjacent to the calyx. These are the dilated ducts of Bellini (Fig. 1-29). Delayed films are both necessary and valuable to determine the existence of residual functioning renal parenchyma. The markedly dilated calyces and pelvis, and eventually the ureters, may subsequently opacify. Angiography is probably unnecessary, although it is an excellent means of determining the amount of residual cortical tissue. During the vascular phase,

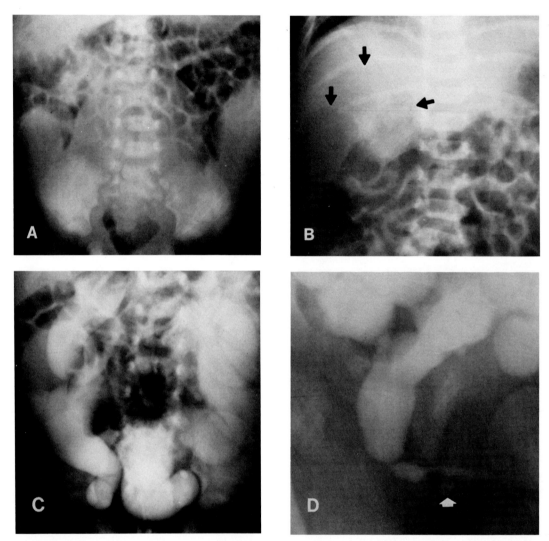

Fig. 1-3. Bilateral hydronephrosis and posterior urethral valves. *(A)* Abdominal film reveals soft-tissue masses presenting in a "mickey mouse" appearance. The central oval mass represents the dilated bladder; the two lateral ears represent distended and tortuous ureters. *(B)* During the intravenous urogram the severely dilated calyces appear as large, radiolucent, cystic structures *(arrows)*. The residual functioning parenchyma is rearranged as a crescent of radiodensity (Dunbar crescent) around the superior calyx *(upper and medial arrows)*. *(C)* Retrograde examination confirms these findings. The bladder is now decompressed, and the massively dilated ureters occupy almost the entire lateral abdominal flanks. *(D)* Posterior urethra is dilated by posterior urethral valves. Contrast medium is present within a cyst of the Cowper's gland *(arrow)*.

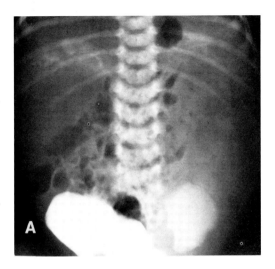
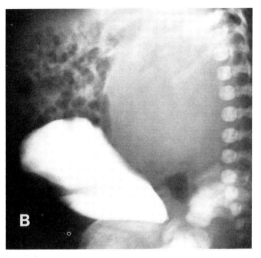
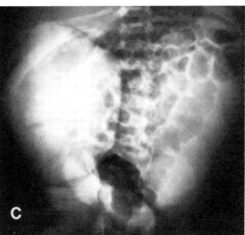

Fig. 1-4. Bilateral ureteropelvic obstruction. *(A)* Frontal and *(B)* lateral films demonstrate large, posteriorly located cystic structures that displace the bladder and the abdominal viscera anteriorly. Residual renal parenchyma opacifies superiorly. (Bladder remains opacified from previous cystogram.) *(C)* Delayed radiograph obtained hours after intravenous urography reveals bilaterally distended sack-like pelves. The ureters are not visualized. (The bladder is again seen in the pelvis.)

the intrarenal vessels are markedly stretched and thinned. Cortical thickness can be evaluated during the nephrogram phase.

Reversible hydronephrosis and hydroureter occur in neonates in association with *Escherichia coli* infection. This should be suspected in cases where evidence of vesicoureteral reflux or lower urinary tract obstruction is not apparent. Resolution of hydronephrosis and hydroureter generally follows successful antiobiotic therapy for the underlying sepsis. It is believed that mucosal edema and impeded ureteral peristalsis result in the transient distention.

Deposition of an abnormal substance within the renal parenchyma is responsible for the diffuse renal enlargement present in various storage diseases. The kidney in these lesions may resemble the normally enlarged kidney. Children of diabetic mothers and those with the Beckwith-Wiedemann syn-

drome also have enlarged kidneys as well as enlargement of other internal structures. The diagnosis is established by history and by observation of other clinical findings (e.g., macroglossia, omphalocele, hypoglycemia) in the Beckwith-Weidemann syndrome. The collecting systems in all of the diseases above present similarly. The calyces may be elongated and thinned due to an overall increase in the surrounding renal parenchyma.

Renal vein thrombosis rarely affects both kidneys. The kidney is diffusely swollen and overall function is quite variable. In some cases no contrast material will be apparent throughout the entire study, and in others a delayed and prolonged nephrogram occurs. With the latter some opacification of the more distal collecting system will eventually become visible.

Cystic disease in newborns occurs in a variety of forms. The rare infantile polycystic

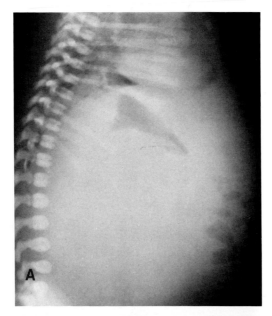

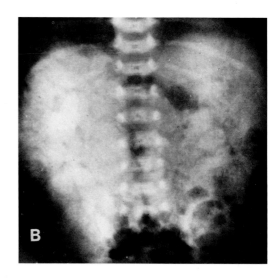

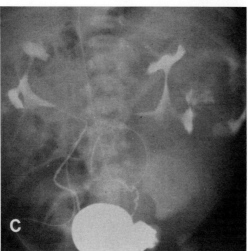

Fig. 1-5. Infantile polycystic kidneys (Potter's Type I). *(A)* The lateral abdomen reveals a huge mass occupying most of the abdomen. A small pneumomediastinum is also noted within the chest. (This is a frequent complication of severe renal disease.) *(B)* Nephrogram in another patient with infantile polycystic kidneys reveals a blotchy and streaky appearance. The contrast material, however, is beginning to accumulate centrally within dilated calyces. *(C)* Opacification of the collecting systems by means of retrograde pyelography reveals thin and elongated infundibula associated with enlarged and dilated calyces. Reflux of the contrast material into the left kidney substance and the surrounding perirenal structure is also encountered. The ureters are remarkably thin because of the diminished renal output. (*Continued on facing page.*)

disease, Potter's Type I, is characterized by huge masses that occupy almost the entire abdomen (Fig. 1-5A). Intravenous urography produces a characteristic irregular, mottled, and streaky nephrogram (Fig. 1-5B). Delayed studies may demonstrate contrast material within the calyces, although concentration is generally insufficient for adequate visualization. If performed, a retrograde examination reveals distorted collecting systems that manifest a bizarre elongated and splayed appearance (Fig. 1-5C). The infundibula are thin and stretched. Surprisingly, the calyces may be enlarged, dilated, and clubbed. Reflux of contrast material into dilated tubules occurs frequently (Fig. 1-5C). The infantile form of polycystic kidney is easily distinguished from the adult form, which rarely demonstrates gross abnormalities in this age group. Multicystic disease, Potter's Type II, which is probably the most common form of neonatal cystic disease, is rarely bilateral.

Nephritis and nephrosis should be suspected when the kidneys are enlarged and demonstrate delayed renal function. These entities may appear quite similar to many of those described above.

Discussion

Variation in the development of the renal pelvis is the end result of abnormal branching patterns of the developing ureter as it ex-

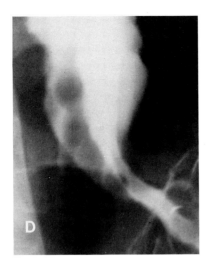

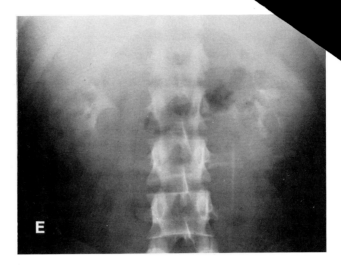

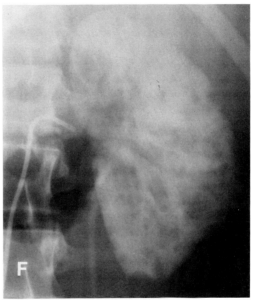

Fig. 1-5 (Continued). (D) Congenital hepatic fibrosis with renal cysts. A 17-year-old who presented with esophageal varices. Note the large, whirling esophageal varices in the distal esophagus. *(E)* Intravenous pyelogram reveals slightly enlarged, relatively well functioning kidneys. *(F)* Angiographic study reveals multiple, radiolucent cystic changes within the renal parenchyma. (Courtesy of Dr. Ed Mabry, Jr., Methodist Hospital, Memphis, Tennessee.)

tends from the Wolffian duct to meet the metanephric tissue, also called the nephrogenic blastema. When the ureteral bud bifurcates prematurely or multiple buds arise from the mesonephric duct, each undergoes normal dichotomous branching and nephron induction as if it were a single ureter. The resulting kidneys, which are "stacked" one atop the other, usually fuse, and the total kidney resembles an elongated but otherwise normal kidney.

Various processes that obstruct the urethra as well as other urinary tract structures can cause bilateral hydronephrosis; such processes are as follows: posterior urethral valves, bilateral ureteropelvic obstruction, bilateral ureterovesical obstruction, neurogenic abnormalities, Eagle-Barrett syndrome (prune belly), tumors of the bladder floor, and bladder neck contracture. The entities are discussed below in what may represent a decreasing order of significance and incidence. A specific diagnosis should be established as early as possible if an attempt is to be made to salvage the kidneys and the infant.

Posterior urethral valves occur almost exclusively in males and are by far the most common cause of bilateral obstructive renal disease in the pediatric age-group and of urinary ascites in newborns (Fig. 1-6A). The latter is the result of extravasation of urine, ini-

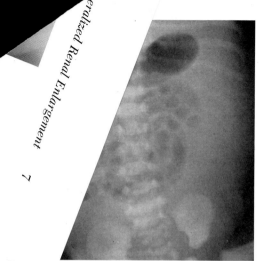

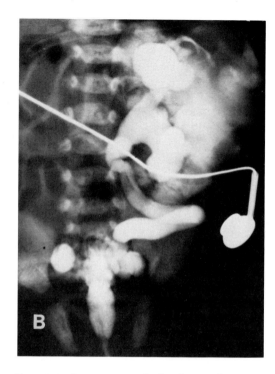

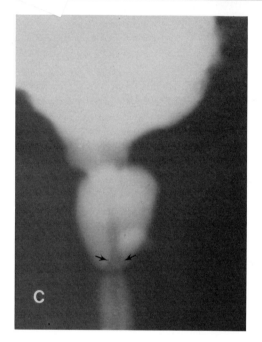

Fig. 1-6. Posterior urethral valve and urinary ascites. *(A)* The abdomen is markedly distended. The presence of ascites is suggested by an overall increase in radiodensity within the abdomen and the centrally located floating intestinal viscera. *(B)* A retrograde study was performed because of poor renal function. Massive reflux into a severely dilated left-sided collecting system is noted. Extravasation of contrast material into the kidney substance and the perirenal structures is apparent (pathway for urinary ascites). The bladder is contracted, but markedly trabeculated. There is obvious dilatation of the posterior urethra. *(C)* Close observation of the posterior urethra demonstrates the urethral valves *(arrows)* within a posterior urethra that resembles a uterine cervix.

tially into the perirenal tissues and then into the peritoneum (Fig. 1-6B). The absence of a strong urinary stream is an excellent clinical indicator for the presence of posterior urethral valves. However, this may be difficult to observe in the very young, and in general the symptoms may be nonspecific. Consequently, every newborn male presenting with bilateral hydronephrosis should have a voiding cystourethrogram performed to exclude this entity. Both the dilated bladder and the posterior urethra are visualized during the act of voiding (Figs. 1-3D, 1-6C). The urinary bladder is frequently large and severely trabeculated. Massive ureteral reflux into dilated and tortuous ureters is commonly noted (Fig. 1-6B). The valves appear as discrete and thin, radiolucent, linear defects that cross the lumen of the dilated posterior urethra. The terminal portion of the urethra looks like a uterine cervix or a spinnaker sail (Fig. 1-6C). The valves in all probability represent an exaggeration of the mucosal folds (plicae colliculi) normally seen in this area. Three types of valves have been described. Anterior or Type I have folds that extend anteriorly from the verumontanum. Posterior or Type II have folds that extend posteriorly from the verumontanum. Membranous or Type III have membranous folds. Type I is the most common. Recognizing the valve and not the type is all that is significant, since therapy is basically the same for all.

Bilateral hydronephrosis caused by obstruction at the ureteropelvic junction is easily recognized on urography. The

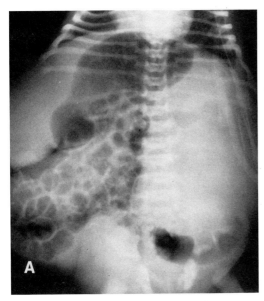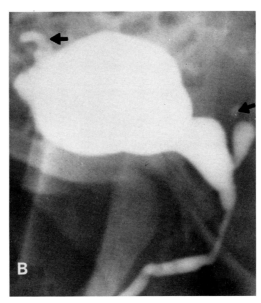

Fig. 1-7. Prune belly syndrome. *(A)* The abdomen is markedly flabby and projects to the right. The kidneys are well opacified and moderate dilatation of the pelvo-calyceal system is noted (the ureters were also slightly dilated). *(B)* The voiding cystourethrogram in this patient demonstrates some of the other anomalies described in the lower urinary system. A urachus *(upper arrow)* arises superiorly from the surface of the bladder. The posterior urethra is dilated because of absent prostatic tissue. A large utricle with a vestigial uterine appendage is also noted *(lower arrow).*

obstructed kidneys are frequently huge (Fig. 1-4). If viable renal parenchyma—and therefore some degree of function—are still present, intravenous urography with delayed examinations reveals severely dilated collecting structures that appear almost cystic (Fig. 1-4B). The ureters are rarely demonstrated during this examination, and they appear narrow and thin on retrograde pyelography. In advanced cases only a thin rim of functioning renal tissue persists, and the overall morphologic and radiologic appearance resembles that of the multicystic kidney. The cause of ureteropelvic stenosis is unknown. Various factors such as vascular ischemia and pressure atrophy have been suggested.

Obstruction at the ureterovesical junction is not common and differs radiographically from the above. The upper urinary tract, although distended, is far less involved, and the ureters by contrast are markedly dilated and tortuous. The bladder fills only slowly during the normal sequence of intravenous urography, and no reflux is noted on cystography. This lesion may be confused with the hydroureter and hydronephrosis associated with *Escherichia coli* sepsis. Consequently, a diagnosis of bilateral obstruction at the ureterovesical junction should not be seriously considered in a neonate with sepsis until enough time has passed to observe the progress of the kidneys and ureters following therapy for the sepsis.

A *neurogenic bladder* is easily recognized because of the associated abnormalities (e.g., meningoceles, hypoplasia or absence of the sacrum, tumors). Various classifications of neurogenic bladder, based upon the nature and the location of the abnormality, have been described. Basically, a dorsal root abnormality produces a dilated, atonic bladder whereas a cord lesion results in a trabeculated bladder. However, since more than one area is frequently involved, it is difficult to adhere to any rigid classification in describing the changes noted. In addition to the above radiologic findings, the external sphincter may be markedly spastic, causing marked impairment of bladder emptying.

The Eagle-Barrett syndrome (prune belly) presents with many abnormalities. The major clinical and radiologic features are hypoplasia or absence of the abdominal muscles and severe hydronephrosis and hydroureter (Fig. 1-7). Bladder and urethral anomalies have also been described. The condition is seen exclusively in males, and the diagnosis is aided by the presenting pot belly. Unde-

Table 1-1. **Bilateral Generalized Renal Enlargement in the Newborn**

Lesions	Size	Total Body Opacification	Function	Calyces
Normal	Upper limits	Normal	Normal	Normal
Duplication	Slightly enlarged	Normal	Normal	Two sets
Bilateral hydronephrosis	Mod. to severely enlarged	Lucent	Mod. to severely diminished	Dilated
Visceromegaly	High limits of normal	Normal	Normal	Slightly elongated
Renal vein thrombosis	Slightly enlarged	Normal	Mod. to severely diminished; Prolonged nephrogram	Stretched and thinned
Infantile polycystic disease	Huge	Non-revealing	Poor, blotchy nephrogram	Large, deformed and dilated

scended testes, clubfoot, and dislocated hips are other commonly associated anomalies. Systemic changes involving the gastrointestinal, cardiovascular, and respiratory systems also occur.

Tumors of the pelvic floor, such as a rhabdomyosarcoma or even a prostatic tumor such as sarcoma botryoides, secondarily invade the bladder floor and involve the posterior urethra as well. Elevation and displacement of the bladder with associated destruction of the bladder wall should suggest this diagnosis.

Bladder neck contracture is no longer considered a serious cause of obstruction, and there is increasing doubt about its validity as an entity. Prostatic median bar hypertrophy may rarely cause obstruction in the newborn.

When renal vein thrombosis occurs bilaterally the ultimate prognosis is decidedly poor. The disease far more frequently affects one kidney (see p. 13).

Deposition of various materials (e.g., mucopolysaccharides, glycogen) into the interstitium of the kidney is frequently an incidental part of an overall disease process. The clinical features are often apparent, and in some diseases bony changes may also be present in this early period. The Beckwith-Wiedemann syndrome is associated with diffuse visceromegaly in which the enlarged kidneys are part of the overall enlargement. In addition umbilical hernia, omphalocele, macroglossia, and hypoglycemia complete the remaining major features of this syndrome. A high incidence of neoplastic disease, such as Wilm's tumor, occurs in this syndrome; indeed, a propensity for neoplasia is encountered in many congenital syndromes.

Polycystic disease of the infant is an uncommon disease which is inherited as an autosomal recessive trait that effects both the kidneys and liver. According to Osathanondh and Potter, it is in many ways distinct from the adult form of polycystic kidneys. The renal abnormalities predominate in infancy and carry poor prognosis, and most infants succumb to the disease in a number of weeks or months. The liver assumes greater importance in later childhood. In patients presenting at adolescence or later only about 20 per cent of the nephrons are involved, and the renal lesion is usually an incidental finding. Radiologic examination reveals good renal function with tubular ectasia or mild cystic disease. The changes in the liver demonstrate proliferation of the bile ducts and fine periportal and subcapsular fibrosis. Progressive extension of periportal fibrosis results in portal hypertension with esophageal varices and splenomegaly (Fig. 1-5D,E,F). Early renal manifestations of the adult form of polycystic disease have been documented in infancy. In infants with a strong family history, the kidneys at this time are bilaterally large and the collecting system shows minor degrees of elongation, stretching, and distortion.

Nephritis and nephrosis are exceedingly rare in newborns, but may be seen in infants of diabetic mothers and in infants suffering from severe dehydration.

Table 1-2. **Hydronephrosis**

Lesions	Upper Collecting System	Ureters	Bladder	Urethra	Other
Posterior uretheral valve	Dilated	Dilated	Dilated and trabeculated	Posterior dilated	Reflux
U–P obstruction	Massive dilatation	Normal	Normal	Normal	
U–V obstruction	Dilated	Massive dilatation	Normal	Normal	
Nonspecific (Neonatal)	Dilated	Dilated	Normal	Normal	Disappears
Nonspecific with sepsis	Dilated	Dilated	Normal	Normal	No reflux; disappears if Rx for sepsis is successful
Neurogenic	Dilated	Dilated	Dilated a) Atonic b) Trabeculated	Sphincter dilated	Skeletal and other associated anomalies
Prune belly syndrome	Dilated	Dilated	Dilated	Dilated	Other associated anomalies

UNILATERAL DIFFUSE RENAL ENLARGEMENT IN THE NEWBORN

Unilateral renal enlargement is suggested clinically following palpation of an abdominal mass or the observation of asymmetrical enlargement of the abdomen. In this section, diseases causing diffuse enlargement of a kidney are discussed. Most of these entities may also occur bilaterally.

Disease Entities

Multicystic disease (Potter's Type II)
Hydronephrosis
Duplication
Renal vein thrombosis
Congenital mega-calyces
Compensatory hypertrophy

Differential Diagnosis

Multicystic kidney is in all probability the most common unilateral mass discovered within the first week of life. Palpation of the abdomen reveals a lobular cystic mass, which on transillumination easily transmits light. A routine radiographic examination of the abdomen reveals a mass within the renal area that increases the overall radiodensity of the abdomen and displaces abdominal viscera anteriorly and to the contralateral side (Figs.

1-8A, 1-9A). The pelvo-calyceal system is not visualized during intravenous urography, since this kidney is basically dysplastic. However, a cystic radiolucent appearance may be detected during the total body opacification phase (Fig. 1-8B). As in hydronephrosis, thin, faint, curvilinear crescents of opacification have been described. This feature is infrequent nevertheless. Retrograde pyleography reveals either an atretic ureter or absence of a ureteral orifice and a malformed trigone. In general, multicystic kidney should be differentiated from unilateral hydronephrosis. Both lesions appear strikingly similar and may be related in some ways. The hydronephrotic kidney in most patients, however, shows varying degrees of renal function (Fig. 1-10). This factor is most helpful in distinguishing the two, except in the occasionally encountered advanced stage of hydronephrosis with severe parenchymal destruction. The resulting marked dilatation of all the collecting structures produces an overall appearance resembling multicystic kidney. (The radiographic features of hydronephrosis and its causes are described on p. 3.) It is conceivable that arteriography might be helpful, but it is not indicated, since the ultimate therapy is probably the same in both cases. The renal artery in congenital multicystic kidney is hypoplastic or

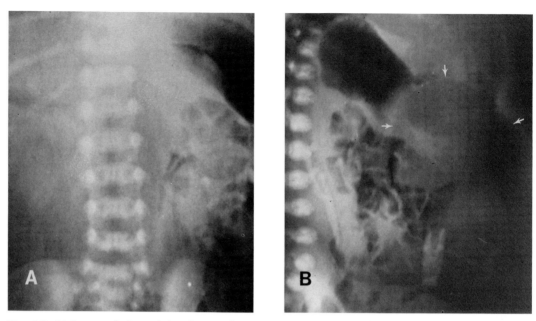

Fig. 1-8. Multicystic kidney. *(A)* A huge soft-tissue mass is present within the right abdomen and displaces all the abdominal viscera to the left. *(B)* A lateral film exposed during the total body opacification phase demonstrates a large radiolucent multicystic kidney *(arrows)* and a normally functioning kidney posteriorly.

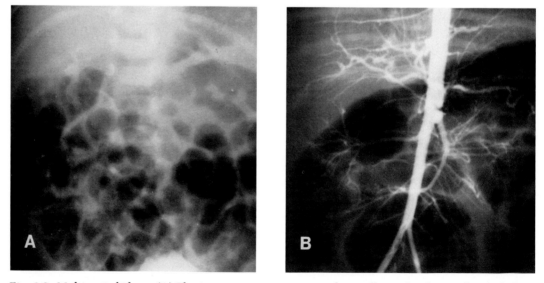

Fig. 1-9. Multicystic kidney. *(A)* The intravenous urogram reveals a well visualized normal right kidney and bladder and no opacification of the left. A mass was palpated on this side, and a corresponding area of increased radiodensity partially displacing some of the viscera is noted. *(B)* An aortogram suggests small irregular renal vessels supplying this mass.

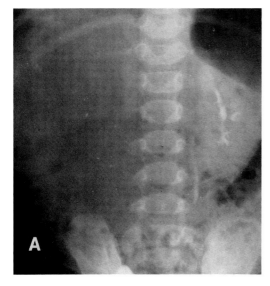

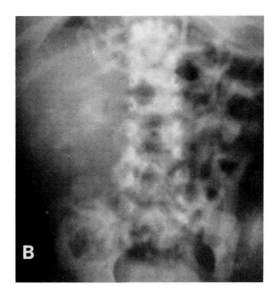

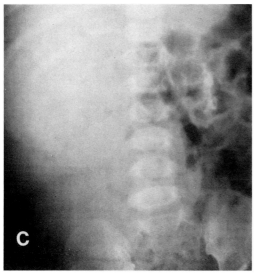

Fig. 1-10. Unilateral ureteropelvic obstruction. *(A)* Total body opacification phase. A large radiolucent structure occupies the right abdomen. A linear, opacifying radiodensity, the Dunbar crescent, surrounds the upper pole of the mass. The contralateral kidney is normal. *(B)* A film exposed approximately 0.5 hour later demonstrates beginning opacification of the collecting system. Several dilated calyces are now evident in the lower pole. *(C)* Several hours later the whole right abdomen is filled by the lobular, opacified renal pelvis that extends across the midline.

nonexistent (Fig. 1-9B), whereas in hydronephrosis it is still present. The intrarenal vessels are thin and envelop the dilated calyces.

Duplication of the collecting system as a cause of renal enlargement has been described and in general is recognized with little difficulty. However, prominent aberrant columns of Bertin that cause distortion and a mass impression upon the upper pole infundibulum have been associated with this anomaly (Fig. 1-11). For some reason this feature has not yet been described in newborns. The kidneys may require a minimal amount of growth before this anomaly becomes obvious. Nuclear scanning of the kidneys utilizing ^{99m}Tc-labeled pharmaceuticals may be useful in problematic cases. The columns of Bertin

represent normal renal tissue, and uptake is quite similar to the surrounding tissue. Angiographic studies of the kidney demonstrate similar normal features.

Renal vein thrombosis presents with a mildly expanding kidney, in contrast to other forms of renal enlargement discovered in the neonatal period. Hematuria, both macroscopic and microscopic, is also present. In general, the kidney is only slightly enlarged, and intravenous urography will demonstrate impaired renal function. Visualization of the collecting structures is variable and may occasionally be adequate. A persistent nephrogram is nevertheless the most frequent feature. Because of the diffuse parenchymal edema, the calyces are thin and stretched. The intrarenal vessels are similarly thinned

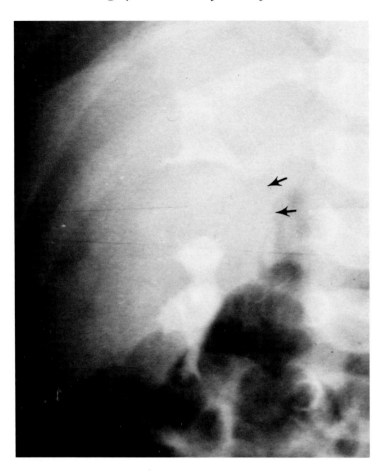

Fig. 1-11. Aberrant column of Bertin in duplication of the collecting system. There are two collecting systems on the right. The upper-pole infundilulum is displaced medially by an aberrant column of Bertin *(arrows)*.

and spread out on renal angiography, which is not an essential study. Inferior venacavography, by contrast, is an important diagnostic examination. Thrombi presenting as filling defects within the renal veins and multiple collateral venous channels are characteristic. Development of collateral routes and dissolution of the thrombus eventually take place, and renal function may return to normal. Varying degrees of atrophy do occur in severely affected kidneys.

An enlarged kidney presenting with a somewhat lobular surface resembling fetal lobulation can be the result of congenital mega-calyces. In this anomaly the calyces are not only dilated and markedly blunted but are seemingly more numerous than those present in a normal kidney. There is no impairment of renal function and the corresponding infundibula and renal pelvis are normal.

Discussion

Multicystic disease of the kidney is probably the most common cause of an abdominal mass discovered during the first week of life. Thereafter, hydronephrosis is more frequently encountered statistically. Osathanondh and Potter found that in this entity the ampullary portion of the collecting tubules fails to develop normally. This structure is essential for the normal inductive process of the metanephric blastema. Consequently, normal renal development does not occur. The final result is a kidney formed as a collection of cysts associated with immature glomeruli, foci of cartilage, and a decreased number of collecting ducts. About 25 per cent of the patients have important contralateral abnormalities; obstruction at the ureteropelvic junction is probably the most common. In fact, a hydronephrotic type of unilateral congenital multicystic disease has been described. In this entity, evidence of functioning glomeruli has been found intermingled with the remaining dyplastic tissue. This finding may explain why calyceal crescents have been observed during urography. It is conceivable that unilateral multicystic kidney actually represents the severest form of hydronephrosis occurring secondary to atresia of the ureter or pelvis, or both. This

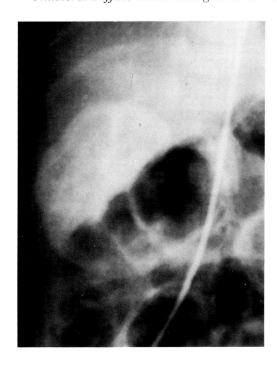

Fig. 1-12. Fetal lobulation. Right renal nephrogram closely demonstrates the lobular contour and thin cortex of a kidney in a newborn.

occurs during the metanephric stage of intrauterine development and may be a function of poor ureteral development or the result of a vascular insult to the budding ureter.

Here it may be worthwhile to briefly discuss the classifications of cystic disease as described by Osathanondh and Potter, since this classification is often referred to in the current literature. In general the branching ureteric bud consists of an interstitial or tubular segment that eventually makes up part of the outflow system and an ampullary portion which is the advancing end responsible for the induction process that results in the formation of definitive renal tissue from adjacent renal blastoma. Potter's Type I, infantile polycystic kidney, is apparently due to hyperplasia of the interstitial portions of the collecting tubules, and microdissection reveals hyperplasia and dilatation of the collecting tubules and ducts. Dysplasia is only minor. Biliary hyperplasia is seen in almost 100 per cent of cases. Type II, multicystic kidney, is due to marked inhibition of the ampullary activity of the tubules, and as a result normal renal differentiation is absent. Type III, adult polycystic kidney, is caused by multiple abnormalities of development involving both the ampullary and interstitial portions of the collecting tubules. This form is associated with cysts in other structures, such as the liver, pancreas, and lungs. Berry

aneurysms occur in 20 per cent of cases. Type IV results following a high degree of intrauterine obstruction with marked dilatation of the renal pelvis and calyces. This is commonly seen in cases of posterior urethral values.

Renal vein thrombosis is the most common vascular abnormality in newborns. It occurs following periods of dehydration and is commonly seen in infants of diabetic mothers.

Although the overall appearance of a kidney with congenital mega-calyces is disturbing, the disease is not progressive and the overall prognosis is good. Pathologically, the adjacent medullary tissue is thin, and the overall renal parenchyma appears reduced when compared to normal kidneys. Clinically, the patients are prone to infection and stone formation.

It should also be emphasized that unilateral hydronephrosis in infants and children is often associated with contralateral renal abnormalities, such as hydronephrosis, dysgenesis, and multicystic kidney. However, a hydronephrotic kidney may be large enough to protrude across the midline and affect the opposite kidney by compression.

Several pathologic findings have been noted in the obstructed ureteropelvic junction. These include hypertrophy of the musculature, varying degrees of ureteral stenosis, and fibrosis. A commonly associated finding in all is an aberrant vessel.

Table 1-3. **Unilateral Diffuse Renal Enlargement in the Newborn**

	Size	Total Body Opacification	Function	Calyces
Multicystic kidney	Large	Radiolucent	None	Not developed
Hydronephrosis	Large	Radiolucent	Moderately to severely impaired	Dilated
Duplication	Moderate enlargement	Normal	Good	Normal—2 sets
Renal vein thrombosis	Slightly enlarged		Moderate to severely impaired	Stretched
Congenital mega-calyces	Slightly enlarged	Normal	Normal	Increased in number; dilated

UNILATERAL ASYMMETRICAL ENLARGEMENT OF THE KIDNEY AND THE ENLARGED ADRENAL GLAND IN THE NEWBORN

Assymetrical enlargement of the kidney is caused by lesions producing single or multiple alterations along the surface of the kidney. Depending upon the nature and location of the lesion, the internal collecting systems are either elongated, displaced, or destroyed. A mass arising in the adrenal gland also causes alteration of the adjacent kidney. Therefore, certain abnormalities arising in this gland are included in this section.

Disease Entities

Developmental anomalies
    Fetal lobulation
    Horseshoe kidney
    Crossed ectopia
    Abnormal rotation
Duplication with localized hydronephrosis of the upper pole
Renal tumor
Renal cysts (single or multiple)
Abscesses (single or multiple)
Congenital neuroblastoma

Differential Diagnosis

Developmental anomalies are common and rarely cause diagnostic problems. The fetal kidney itself is characteristically lobular (Fig. 1-12). In general the kidney, is normal in size and the calyces demonstrate a normal distribution. As the kidney matures, the lobular character gradually diminishes, and the renal margin becomes smooth. The left kidney frequently retains a single bump along its lateral margin. This has been referred to as the dromedary bump.

In cases of renal agenesis, dysplasia, or severe hypoplasia, the contralateral kidney responds to its increased work demand by enlarging. A hypertrophied kidney is often clinically palpated and mistaken for an abnormal mass. The problem is easily resolved when the urogram demonstrates absent or poor renal function on one side and a normal but large kidney on the other.

The horseshoe kidney may pose some difficulty, since the kidney is easily palpated and the axis of the kidneys abnormally rotated. The lower poles are fused, and as a result the normal embryologic migration and rotation of the kidneys are interrupted. Radiographically, both kidneys are positioned close to the vertebral column with the inferior pole of the kidneys rotated medially (Fig. 1-13). The connecting soft-tissue mass is frequently seen superimposed across the midline of the abdomen. The calyces appear distorted and deformed because of the faulty rotation. This appearance has often resulted in the erroneous diagnosis of obstruction or a space-occupying mass.

Crossed renal ectopia is another positional anomaly that may be misinterpreted as an abnormal renal mass on palpation (Fig. 1-14). In this abnormality, one kidney embryologically shifts to the center and ascends on the contralateral side. Fusion with the other kidney may be incomplete (crossed renal ectopia) or so complete (crossed renal fused ec-

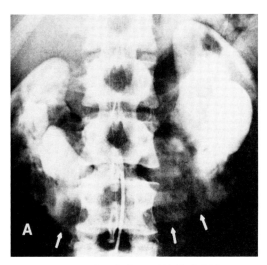

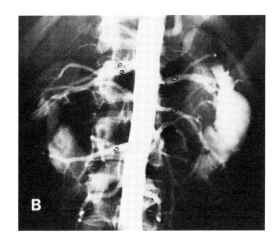

Fig. 1-13. Horseshoe kidney. *(A)* Both kidneys are positioned close to the vertebrae with the inferior poles rotated medially. A soft-tissue mass connecting both lower poles is well visualized as it crosses the vertebrae *(arrows).* *(B)* An aortogram reveals multiple vessels supplying this anomalous kidney.

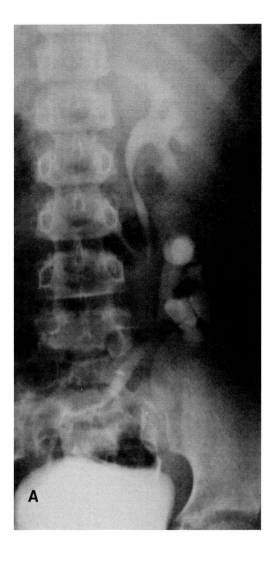

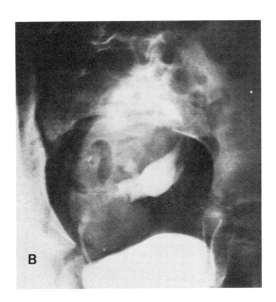

Fig. 1-14. Renal ectopia. *(A)* Crossed renal ectopia. Two normally developed kidneys are present on the left. The ureters insert normally into the bladder. *(B)* Ectopic pelvic kidney. A kidney of normal size and proportion is located in the pelvis. The pelvo-calyceal system is rotated and appears slightly distorted. The ureter is small because of the pelvic location.

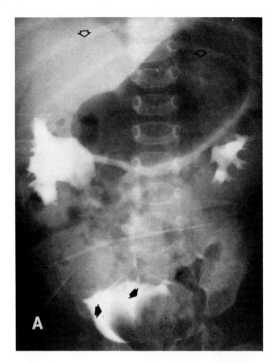

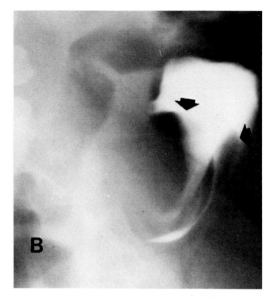

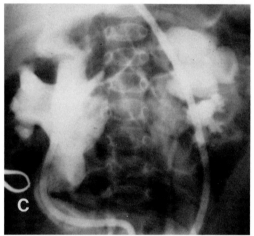

Fig. 1-15. Bilateral ureteroceles. *(A)* Intravenous urogram reveals bilaterally well visualized collecting systems that are displaced inferiorly, with a "drooping lily" appearance. In addition an excessive amount of renal tissue is located between the collecting systems and the upper pole of the kidneys *(open arrows)*. Within the bladder two large ureteroceles appear as sharply rounded radiolucent defects *(closed arrows)*. *(B)* Lateral film of the bladder better demonstrates the sharply demarcated oval radiolucent ureteroceles *(arrows)*. *(C)* The severely dilated obstructed upper collecting systems are opacified by means of a retrograde examination.

topia) as to form a single renal mass. During the urographic study the kidney is noticeably absent on one side, and two renal structures, each complete with a normal complement of calyces, pelves, and ureters, are present on the other side. The ureters, however, terminate on their proper side within the bladder trigone. Therefore the ureter draining the ectopic kidney crosses the midline to reach its respective kidney. The pelvic kidney is another form of ectopia that more often is mistaken for a pelvic tumor (Fig. 1-14B).

Malposition of the bowel has also been noted in cases with renal ectopia and agenesis. The anatomic splenic flexion occupies the renal fossa when the abnormality

is on the left. This is recognized on conventional radiography by the presence of air in the flexure lying medial and posterior to its expected location. Right-sided ectopia may be more difficult to identify, since the duodenum and jejunum now occupy the renal fossa.

Localized intrarenal hydronephrosis, or caliectasis, is a rare complication in newborns and is due to obstruction involving the infundibulum. This is more commonly noted in older children as a complication of inflammatory disease. Occasionally a vessel may cross and compress an upper pole infundibulum causing dilatation of the respective calyx.

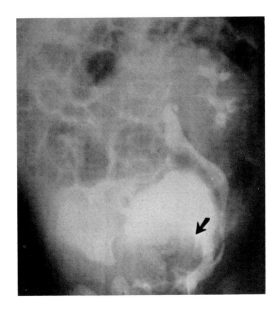

Fig. 1-16. Ureterocele. In a newborn with Eagle-Barret syndrome, a large well-defined radiolucent ureterocele obstructing the right kidney is noted within the bladder filled with contrast medium (*arrow*). The left ureter is dilated and tortuous.

When two complete collecting systems drain a single kidney, the ureter draining the upper pole terminates in an ectopic location. In the female this ureter inserts either in the vagina or perineum, while in the male it inserts most often in the posterior urethra. The ectopic ureter frequently terminates in a ureterocele. This structure obstructs the corresponding ureter and its collecting system. On the urographic studies an enlarged upper pole is present that appears radiolucent during the total body opacification phase. As in any severe hydronephrosis, the involved upper pole of the kidney, along with the calyceal structures, is not often visualized during intravenous urography (Fig. 1-15A). However, the existence of an obstructed calyx is suggested by the altered configuration of the lower calyceal system. The latter is depressed and rotated downward and outward and resembles a drooping lily. In addition an excessive amount of renal tissue is present above the depressed collecting system. If some viable renal tissue still remains, the obstructed calyces may eventually opacify. The ureterocele itself is recognized as a smooth, submucosal mass frequently located within the region of the trigone (Figs. 1-15, 1-16). During the early phases of the examination the ureterocele appears as a well-defined, radiolucent, oval, space-occupying mass that at times is large enough to fill the entire bladder lumen. The ureterocele also eventually fills with contrast material if the affected pole of the kidney is still function-

ing. Reflux of contrast material into a ureterocele is sometimes encountered, and the contraction of the bladder during evacuation reduces the size of a mass or even causes it to evert and appear as a diverticulum. A ureterocele may occasionally be large enough to obstruct the entire trigone and cause equal obstruction on the opposite side.

An enlarged asymmetrical mass within a well functioning kidney should suggest the diagnosis of a tumor or cyst. Urographic studies easily differentiate these entities; the total body opacification phase is quite important, since cysts have a radiolucent avascular appearance while neoplasms often manifest a mixture of both radiolucent and radiodense areas. In general the urogram is nonspecific and reveals displaced, elongated, and narrowed calyces in both entities. These features are of little help, except in identifying the size and location of the mass. Recently ultrasound has proven to be another useful and simple tool in differentiating these lesions. A true cyst is shown to be completely echo-free in contrast to the echo-filled neoplasm. Arteriography offers further diagnostic help but is often unnecessary. Although tumors and cysts both displace adjacent intrarenal vessels, most renal tumors are highly vascular, and the presence of abnormal tumor vessels within the mass is characteristic. No neovascularity is present in a cyst.

Statistically solid, mass-like kidney lesions are more common than kidney cysts in newborns. They are now considered to represent

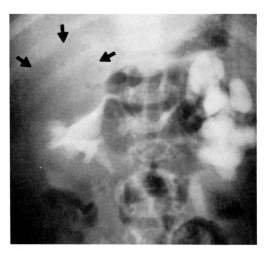

Fig. 1-17. Simple renal cyst. A large radiolucent mass surrounded by a thin rim of opacified renal parenchyma occupies the upper pole of the right kidney *(arrows)*. The upper calyceal group is smoothly depressed and elongated. Dilatation and irregularity of the collecting system is noted on the left. (Is there associated dysplasia?)

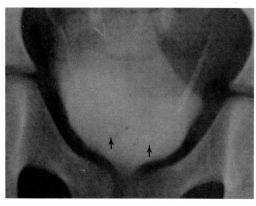

Fig. 1-18. Simple ureteroceles. A small collection of radiopaque material is retained within slightly dilated terminal ureters (simple ureteroceles; *arrows)*. The radiolucent halo surrounding the ureteroceles is caused by the invaginated bladder mucosa.

benign fetal renal hamartomas, mesenchymoma, and not Wilm's tumor. Both lesions, however, appear radiographically similar and can only be differentiated on pathologic criteria.

A suprarenal mass is often confused with a renal lesion. Congenital neuroblastoma is not common in this early period, but is still more frequent than Wilm's tumor. The tumor generally flattens and displaces the kidneys and the corresponding pelvo-calyceal system downward and laterally and causes only minimal intrarenal alteration (see p. 21). Adrenal cortical tumors are exceptionally rare. The radiologic features are the same although the accompanying hormonal effects are diagnostic.

Renal cysts, single or multiple, are rare in newborns. They are most often single, although multiple cysts do occur. Multiple cysts are not related to polycystic disease. The overall incidence of renal cysts increases as the patient ages. The kidney is normal and unaffected except for the calyces adjacent to the cyst. These are displaced and stretched but not destroyed (Fig. 1-17).

A localized abscess resembles a single cyst radiographically, although the cystic character may not be quite as apparent and at times may even be absent during the total body opacification study. In general, the overall function of the kidney is impaired either lo-

cally or diffusely. Local impairment is frequently not apparent, since it is generally difficult to opacify all the calyces equally.

Discussion

Until recently, benign fetal renal hamartoma has been confused with and identified as congenital Wilm's tumor. Recent histologic studies, however, indicate that these lesions arise from different cell types. Fetal hamartoma is basically of connective-tissue origin, while Wilm's tumor is of epithelial origin. The ultimate prognosis of a fetal hamartoma is excellent in contrast to Wilm's Tumor. Local recurrence is possible.

It is also conceivable that other tumors may be visualized in neonates, such as angiomyolipomas associated with tuberous sclerosis and angiomatous tumors associated with a variety of systemic vascular disorders.

The horseshoe kidney is a relatively uncommon phenomenon and occurs once in approximately 400 child autopsies. Its incidence in association with other anomalies (e.g., Trisomy 13, Turner's Syndrome) is high. The horsehoe kidney represents a form of arrested development of the renal blastema. In the early stages of embryologic development, the renal pelves are directed anteriorly, and the lower poles are approximated more closely than the upper poles. It requires only a slight shift of the lower poles

Table 1-4. **Unilateral Asymmetrical Enlargement of Kidney**

	Size	Position of Kidney	Total Body Opacification	Function	Calyces
Developmental	Varies	Varies	Normal	Normal	Distorted according to anomaly
Duplication with hydronephrosis of upper pole	Slightly enlarged	Normal	Radiolucent upper pole	Moderate to severely impaired in upper pole	Dilated upper pole calyces, depressed but well visualized lower pole calyces
Tumor	Enlarged	Altered	Mixture of radiolucent and radio-dense areas	Frequently normal	Distorted, elongated or destroyed
Cyst	Enlarged	Normal	Radiolucent	Normal	Distorted, stretched and elongated
Abscess	Enlarged	Normal	Radiolucent	Poor	Distorted and stretched
Nephroblastoma	Normal	Depressed	Normal	Normal	Displaced but not distorted

for them to touch and fuse. The degree of fusion varies from mere contact of the external surfaces to complete integration of the entire parenchyma. The subsequent abnormal upward development and migration of the renal blastema is probably caused by external factors, such as close approximation of umbilical vessels.

An obstructed duplex kidney is usually associated with an ectopic ureter and a ureterocele. This combination is more common in females. The ectopic ureter most often drains the upper pole of the kidney and inserts beneath the internal sphincter at the bladder neck or into the upper urethra. This relationship has been termed the "Weigert-Meyer" rule and results from the downward migration of the Wolffian duct as it gives rise to the ureter and participates in the growth of the trigone. A single ureter normally terminates laterally and superiorly to the duct. However, when a second ureteral bud is formed it continues to migrate downward with the Wolffian duct, and thus reaches a more medial and inferior site than the first. Ureteroceles frequently accompany the ectopic ureter and present as a cystic swelling of the intravesical ectopic ureter. Simple ureteroceles are related to stenosis of the ureter with dilation of the segment proximal to it (Fig. 1-18). These are rarely encountered in newborns and young infants, and are more often a problem of older children and adults.

Although congenital neuroblastoma and Wilm's tumor are rare, adrenal cortical tumors, benign or malignant, are even more unusual. These are often associated with excess production of androgenic hormone, the adrenogenital syndrome. In neonates this syndrome is most frequently the end result of one or more deficiences in enzyme activity and is characterized by adrenal cortical hyperplasia. Both sexes are affected. In males, excessive virilization produces enlargement of the external genitalia. In females, degrees of pseudohermaphroditism result that extend from simple hypertrophy of the clitoris to almost complete masculinization of the external genitalia. The adrenogenital syndrome may also be accompanied by severe adrenal insufficiency characterized by marked water and salt loss that leads to vascular collapse and death. Afflicted infants demonstrate the radiographic features of an airless abdomen and hyperaerated lung fields. Many of them also present with profound vomiting, and their clinical and radiographic findings have been mistaken for pyloric stenosis. However, pyloric stenosis is rare in the neonate, and the changes in the pylorus are probably related to spasm.

BILATERAL ASYMMETRICAL ENLARGEMENT OF THE KIDNEYS AND ENLARGED ADRENAL GLANDS IN THE NEWBORN

As with unilateral enlargement, bilateral asymmetrical enlargement of the kidneys must also be differentiated from lesions arising within the adrenal glands. Both kidneys are displaced inferiorly and laterally and the calyces are correspondingly depressed.

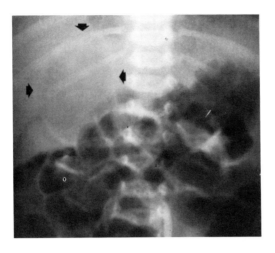

Fig. 1-19. Neonatal adrenal hemorrhage. A large avascular mass surrounded by a vascular rim is depressing the right kidney. A similar mass is present on the left but is poorly visualized because of overlying gas. However, note the depression of the left kidney. (Compare with Figs. 1-15A, 1-17; courtesy of Dr. P. Brill)

Localized calyceal changes that characterize an intrarenal mass, such as stretching and elongation, are rarely manifested.

Disease Entities

Duplication
Adrenal hemorrhage
Bilateral neuroblastoma
Bilateral renal tumors
Wolman's disease
Bilateral cysts

Differential Diagnosis

The diagnosis of bilateral duplication associated with localized hydronephrosis of the upper pole is similar to that for unilateral disease. Both lower collecting systems are depressed and therefore simulate the findings produced by adrenal lesions (Fig. 1-15A). It is important to note that with adrenal lesions the entire axis of the kidney is rotated and a normal amount of calyceal structures are present, as in bilateral adrenal hemorrhage (Fig. 1-19). Both bilateral adrenal hemorrhage and obstructed upper pole lesions appear as large, radiolucent lesions causing an overall depression of both kidneys during the total body opacification phase. In fact, Brill and colleagues have recently described an early vascular rim surrounding the radiolucent areas of adrenal hemorrhage that could be mistaken for an upper pole hydronephrotic renal duplication. However, in the latter the central radiolucency may fill with contrast medium on delayed films if there is adequate functioning parenchyma. The detection of an ectopic ureterocele within the bladder indicates renal rather than adrenal origin of the mass. It is also important to recognize the radiolucent character of hemorrhage in order not to confuse it with bilateral neonatal adrenal neuroblastoma. Fortunately, this condition is exceptionally rare and occurs mainly as single lesions. Only the more unusual bilateral necrotic tumors cause some confusion, since they too appear completely radiolucent during the total body opacification phase. Arteriography or ultrasonography may then be utilized to demonstrate the solid nature of the tumor. With time an adrenal hemorrhage eventually resolves, and calcium deposits in a rim-like fashion around the gland, which subsequently becomes smaller and denser.

Wolman's disease, a lipidosis resulting in abnormal deposition of neutral fats and triglycerides, may present with radiodense, ring-like calcifications in enlarged adrenal glands. Although these features may resemble adrenal hemorrhage, hepatosplenomegaly is also present and most afflicted children expire at an early age.

Bilateral, intrarenal, space-occupying lesions, such as tumors or cysts, are indeed rare in newborns. Radiologic recognition and differentiation between a mass and a cyst is nevertheless the same. It is conceivable that angiomyolipomas and cysts associated with systemic diseases may be apparent at this time.

Discussion

Obstruction associated with duplication is in all probability always associated with a ureterocele and dilated ureter, pelvis, and upper pole calyx.

The cause of adrenal hemorrhage in the neonate is unknown. Many cases of adrenal

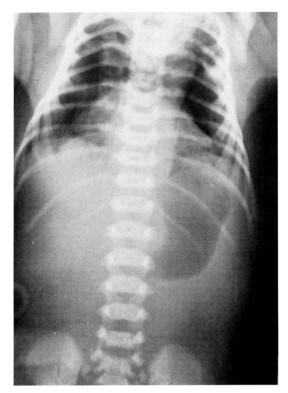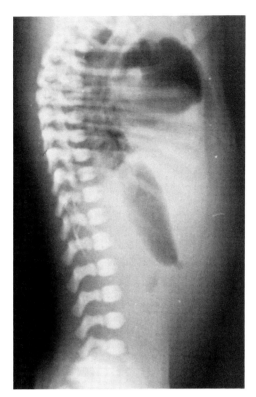

Fig. 1-20. Potter's syndrome. This patient was born with respiratory distress and the initial chest film revealed severe pneumomediastinum and pneumothorax. Despite the excessive accumulation of extra-pulmonary air, the thoracic volume is small and bell-shaped, suggesting hypoplastic lungs. This, as well as agenesis of the kidneys, was confirmed at autopsy.

hemorrhage are asymptomatic. However, massive hemorrhage occurs in cases with trauma, diabetes, and hypoxia. The clinical findings are prolonged jaundice and palpable abdominal masses. The jaundice is the result of hemorrhage within a closed space, coupled with the inability of the liver to conjugate the bilirubin due to transient deficiency of glucoronyl transferase in the neonates. The incidence of adrenal hemorrhage is probably quite high, and it is presently believed to be the most common cause of residual adrenal calcifications.

Polycystic disease (Potter's Type III) has also been found in tuberous sclerosis. Although angiomyolipomas have been described in older children with this disease, it is unusual to discover these tumors in infants. Occasionally, however, cystic lesions will be found in patients with Trisomy D or E, or the Zellweger (cerebro-hepato-renal) syndrome.

SMALL KIDNEYS IN THE NEWBORN

Fortunately, the incidence of congenitally small kidneys is low. In general, a small kidney is most commonly acquired following single or multiple insults to the kidney. Bilateral renal agenesis (congenitally poorly functioning kidneys), or Potter's syndrome, which represents the complete failure of renal blastemas to develop, is indeed rare. The condition is clinically suggested by the presentation of a characteristic facial appearance, the so called Potter facies. These infants present with large, low-set ears, prominent epicanthal folds, nasal flattening, and micrognathia. Most infants are stillborn. Pulmonary hypoplasia is another important feature that is associated with renal agenesis. This abnormality is characterized by respiratory problems, such as pneumothorax and pneumomediastinum, that are present almost always at the time of the first radiographic examination (Fig. 1-20). Pulmonary hypoplasia should be considered in all cases of air-block syndrome when other entities that may be responsible are unaccounted for. The extrarenal manifestations of Potter's syndrome (e.g., the facial appearance and pulmonary hypoplasia) are believed to be caused by the oligohydramnios that accompanies decreased renal function. This is substantiated by the fact that a number of lesions which re-

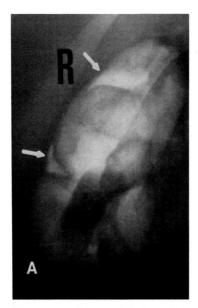 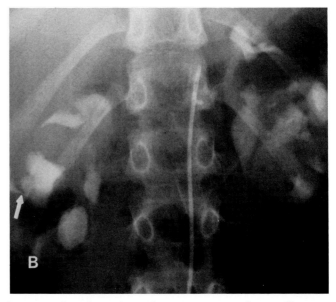

Fig. 1-21. Ask-Upmark kidney. *(A)* A nephrogram taken during a renal arteriogram reveals a small, irregularly lobular right kidney. The calyces *(arrows)* clearly approximate the outer margin of the kidney. *(B)* The calyces are severely distorted. A markedly stretched infundiulum *(arrow)* is noted on the right. This is a characteristic feature for this abnormality.

sult in nonfunctioning kidneys have produced similar findings, and Potter facies has been described in patients with normal kidneys and oligohydramnios. A small pelvis associated with a pneumomediastinum is another radiographic feature that should suggest renal agenesis.

Renal dysplasia and hypoplasia are two of the major developmental anomalies which produce small kidneys. Recently, dyplasia has been defined as a process that results in a very abnormal kidney, characterized by the absence of normal structures and the presence of cartilage and primitive ducts. At one time this term was only used to describe small kidneys, with or without the presence of cysts. However, enlarged cystic kidneys are now included in this category.

Disease Entities
Agenesis and aplasia
Dysplasia
Hypoplasia
Segmental hypoplasia (Ask-Upmark kidney)
Renal vein thrombosis (end-stage)

Differential Diagnosis

Unless there is clinical data which suggests the presence of a small kidney, most of the entities above pass unnoticed. Small kidneys are not easy to recognize on conventional abdominal films. A single kidney is more commonly affected and as a result the opposite renal structure is often hypertrophied and is clinically mistaken for a mass. Renal function is absent in cases of renal agenesis, aplasia, and most forms of dysplasia. An interesting radiologic feature noted in left-sided renal agenesis is the presence of the splenic flexure occupying the renal fossa (see p. 18).

Segmental hypoplasia or the Ask-Upmark Kidney is a variation of hypoplasia that is characterized by segments of poorly developed renal tissue surrounded by relatively normal renal parenchyma. The Ask-Upmark lesion can be local or diffuse, as well as unilateral or bilateral. As a result, the affected kidney is small and irregular in appearance. Deep notches or scars are present on the surface of the kidney that lies directly above the abnormal area (Fig. 1-21A). The underlying calyx is dilated and is separated from the indented notch on the surface by a thin rim of abnormal cortical tissue (Fig. 1-21A). As a result the corresponding infundilulum is elongated (Fig. 1-21B).

Arteriography is rarely required in this set of diseases. The renal artery is absent in renal agenesis or aplasia and very small and difficult to recognize in cases where renal tissue is poorly developed.

End-stage renal vein thrombosis is easily

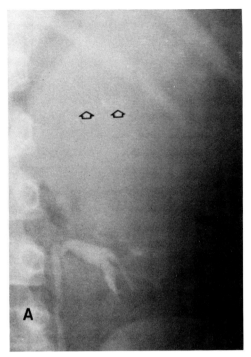 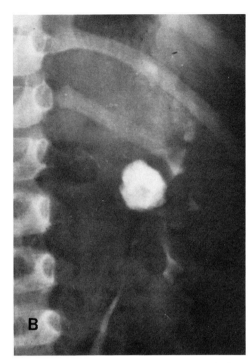

Fig. 1-22. Neuroblastoma. *(A)* A huge, well circumscribed neuroblastoma containing calcific deposits *(arrows)* within the center of the mass displaces the entire kidney downward, with no localized alteration of the pelvo-calyceal system. *(B)* Another neuroblastoma containing huge calcifications displaces the kidney symmetrically. Again note no distortion of the calyces.

diagnosed when correlated with previous clinical or radiographic features. Urographic studies performed at this stage reveal a small kidney with blunted calyces. Renal function may be quite adequate. Ureteral notching (extrinsic indentations) indicates the presence of venous, collateral vessels and should be noted. Both renal arteriography and venography must be performed to fully establish the diagnosis.

Discussion

Unilateral absence of a kidney is more common than bilateral absence, and affects males slightly more than females. It is conceivable that the pathogenesis may be different for each entity. In unilateral agenesis the fallopian tube on the same side is always absent. However, in bilateral agenesis the fallopian tubes are always present, but the uterus and vagina are absent or abnormal.

Aplastic kidneys are extremely small and rudimentary. They consist of either a tiny nubbin of grossly malformed tissue or a cluster of cysts. Multicystic and aplastic kidneys represent the most severe forms of renal dysplasia. Multicystic kidneys are generally large. Various ureteric abnormalities are found, the most severe being the atretic ureter. Stenosis, hydroureter, and ectopic ureter are other abnormalities that have been described.

Unilateral hypoplasia is a congenitally small kidney and resembles the small kidney associated with acquired renal disease. Differentiation is difficult, especially since the congenitally hypoplastic kidney is prone to infection. The reduced number of reniculi present in this kidney may be the only means of differentiating it from the small kidney associated with acquired disease. The cause of hypoplasia is unknown but may be the result of intrauterine blood loss or decreased blood supply.

The Ask-Upmark kidney is an interesting lesion and has been considered one of the most common causes of renovascular hypertension in childhood, which is curable when the disease is unilateral. Grossly, the Ask-Upmark kidney resembles that of chronic pyelonephritis. A careful examination is necessary to recognize the deep scar and the microscopic changes of undifferentiated renal tissue lying just beneath. Inflammatory changes may or may not be present.

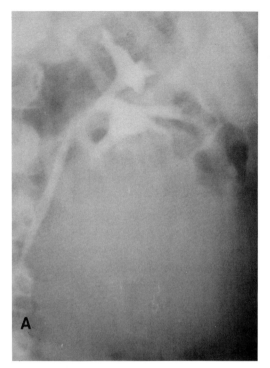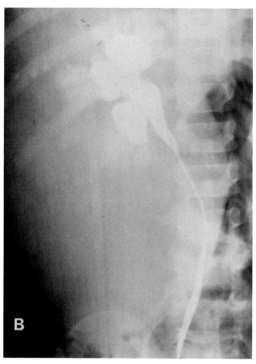

Fig. 1-23. Wilm's tumor. *(A)* A huge mass occupies the left lower pole. The tumor is well circumscribed and elongates and spreads the lower-pole calyces. There is almost no overall change of the renal position despite the size of the mass. *(B)* Another Wilm's tumor arising in the right kidney is demonstrated by means of retrograde pyelography. The tumor is mostly exophitic causing only minimal displacement of the lower pole. The ureter is deviated toward the midline.

UNILATERAL ASYMMETRICAL ENLARGEMENT OF THE KIDNEY AND ADRENAL GLAND IN THE INFANT AND CHILD

The lesions causing unilateral asymmetrical renal enlargement in infants include congenital lesions that are not evident in newborns. Radiographic visualization is enhanced in older children because of increased fat deposition around the internal structures. Conventional abdominal studies demonstrate a vague area of increased soft-tissue radiodensity that displaces adjacent viscera.

In addition to newborns, neuroblastoma is also common in infants and children. It is therefore imperative to determine the nature and site of origin of any suspected retroperitoneal mass. Differentiation between intrarenal and extrarenal lesions is often possible by means of intravenous urography. Intrarenal masses are confined by the renal capsule, and therefore pelvo-calyceal distortion is far more pronounced than actual displacement. This is quite different from the effects caused by adrenal lesions, in which the kidney as well as the internal calyceal structures are displaced almost uniformly, and localized calyceal distortion is less pronounced.

Disease Entities

Wilm's tumor
Neuroblastoma
Hydronephrotic upper pole with ureterocele
Duplication
Renal cyst
Abscess (xanthogranulomatosis pyelonephritis)
Adrenal carcinoma
Adrenal adenoma
Pheochromocytoma

Differential Diagnosis

The two most common lesions occurring in this group are Wilm's tumor and neuroblastoma. They occur with almost equal frequency, although the incidence of Wilm's tumor may be slightly higher. The resulting effect upon the kidney and the internal

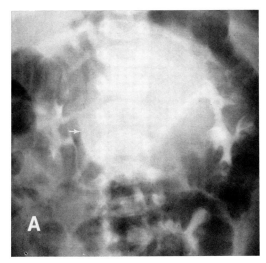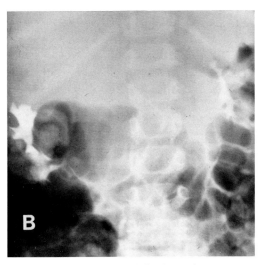

Fig. 1-24. Neuroblastoma. *(A)* A large neuroblastoma arising from the left adrenal displaces the viscera as well as the left kidney. The tumor extends across the midline to the opposite side *(arrow)* and contains calcifications throughout. These are not well reproduced. *(B)* Another patient with a huge neuroblastoma on the right. The right kidney is severely displaced downward and laterally, with only minimal distortion of the internal collecting systems.

calyceal structures enables physicians to differentiate the lesion in most cases. In some doubtful situations, additional radiographic features can be utilized. The presence of calcification strongly suggests neuroblastoma, since calcification occurs in approximately 50 per cent of neuroblastomas and is uncommon in Wilm's tumor (Fig. 1-22). The size of a lesion is of no significance, since both tumors can be enormous. Neuroblastoma, however, extends more frequently across the midline than Wilm's tumor, which is restrained for the most part by the renal capsule (Figs. 1-23, 1-24). Hydronephrosis and decreased renal function are more often associated with Wilm's tumor, which more readily compresses the renal pelvis and the remaining collecting system. Impaired renal function without obstruction also occurs when the tumor invades the kidney or extends into the renal veins. A neuroblastoma may cause similar manifestations when it completely invades the kidney, or when it arises medially and adjacent to the kidney pedicle. Arteriographic studies are probably not essential, but they are helpful in cases where a specific diagnosis is difficult to establish. The vascular changes themselves may not be specific since both tumors displace vessels and demonstrate varying degrees of neovascularity. However, identification of

the vessel supplying the tumor may establish its site of origin (Fig. 1-25). The use of inferior vena cavography has helped tremendously in the radiologic diagnosis and in the determination both of the extent of the tumor and the ultimate prognosis of the patient. Although the vessel is frequently displaced by adjacent mass, intraluminal extension indicates invasion, which must be diagnosed by the presence of a large filling defect. Collateral flow alone does not signify tumor invasion, since this may occur even in the presence of a patent vessel. Nevertheless, from a prognostic point of view, it has been shown that removal of all neuroblastoma tissue is difficult when the inferior vena cava is displaced.

In children under 1 year of age the association of nonfunctioning kidney and a patent inferior vena cava is suggestive of either multicystic kidney or another benign lesion.

Ectopic ureteroceles, in contrast to simple ureteroceles, are found exclusively in infants and children and are almost always associated with ureteral duplication. The upper pole ureter is most often obstructed, and asymmetrical renal hydronephrosis occurs (Fig. 1-26). Adrenal tumors other than neuroblastoma are quite rare and may simulate neuroblastoma radiographically. It is possible that adrenal venography may prove helpful when

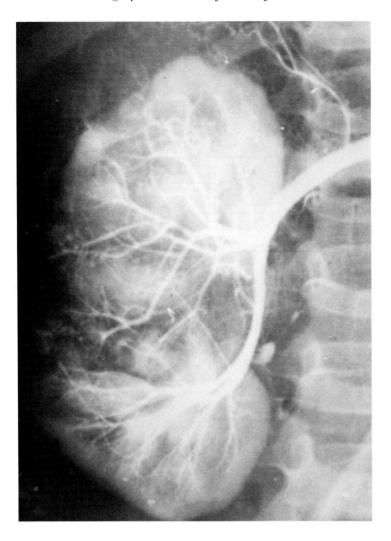

Fig. 1-25. Arteriogram: Wilm's tumor. Tumor tissue is present within the outer and superior lateral margin of the kidney. The central vessels are displaced and a fine neovascularity is noted within both lesions. The inferior adrenal artery is normal.

other studies do not give characteristic results. The presence of a pheochromocytoma is suggested by appropriate clinical and chemical evaluation, and the radiographic confirmation of a mass. Conventional radiographs and intravenous urography reveal a soft-tissue mass that displaces the kidney. Calcification occurs in only 5 per cent of the cases. Arteriography is necessary to further evaluate the presence of the extra-adrenal tumors. Occasionally, narrowing of the renal artery may be present.

An abscess appears as a local mass. Renal function depends upon the stage of the infection and varies from good to poor. When the abscess is walled off and localized, function is quite apparent and the calyceal structures are depressed and displaced by the space occupying lesion. Nephrotomography and angiography reveal a relatively hypolucent mass with some inflammatory

vascularity within the abscess wall. Xanthogranulomatosis pyelonephritis is an uncommon form of abscess characterized by the presence of lipoid laden foam cells and fibrogranulomas surrounding foci of renal suppuration. The radiographic findings are quite similar to a localized abscess. It is often difficult to differentiate xanthogranulomatosis pyelonephritis from a malignant tumor because of its tumefactive character. However, the presence of associated inflammatory disease within the kidney with or without calculi is highly suggestive of this process.

Discussion

Wilm's tumor is probably the most common malignant tumor in children and accounts for 30 per cent of all neoplasms in this age-group. It is most frequently seen in children under 5 years of age but surprisingly is

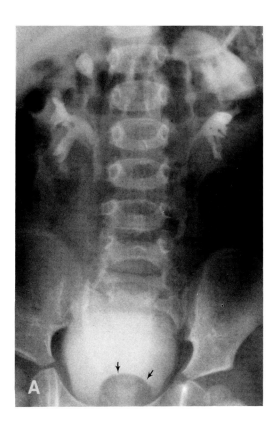

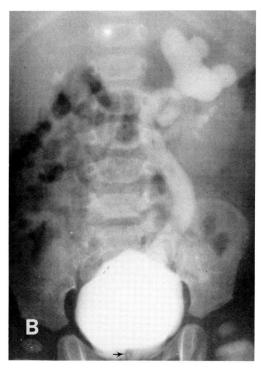

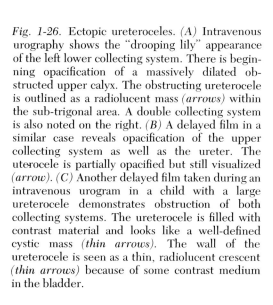

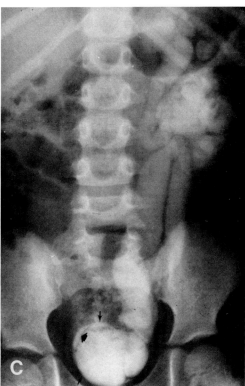

Fig. 1-26. Ectopic ureteroceles. *(A)* Intravenous urography shows the "drooping lily" appearance of the left lower collecting system. There is beginning opacification of a massively dilated obstructed upper calyx. The obstructing ureterocele is outlined as a radiolucent mass *(arrows)* within the sub-trigonal area. A double collecting system is also noted on the right. *(B)* A delayed film in a similar case reveals opacification of the upper collecting system as well as the ureter. The uterocele is partially opacified but still visualized *(arrow)*. *(C)* Another delayed film taken during an intravenous urogram in a child with a large ureterocele demonstrates obstruction of both collecting systems. The ureterocele is filled with contrast material and looks like a well-defined cystic mass *(thin arrows)*. The wall of the ureterocele is seen as a thin, radiolucent crescent *(thin arrows)* because of some contrast medium in the bladder.

Table 1-5. **Unilateral Asymmetrical Enlargement of the
Kidney and Adrenal Gland in the Infant and Child**

Characteristic	Wilm's Tumor	Neuroblastoma	Obstructed Double Collecting System
Calcium	Not common	Common	Absent
Position of kidney	Slight alteration	Displaced	Normal
Total body opacification	Mixture of radiodense and radiolucent areas	Mixture of radiodense and radiolucent areas	Radiolucent
Function	Normal to absent	Normal	Moderate to diminished in area involved
Calyces	Distorted, stretched, and destroyed	Displaced	Dilated calyx

rarely noted in infants under 6 months. The presenting symptom of Wilm's tumor is an abdominal swelling or mass. Hematuria is not a frequent symptom in children, in contrast to the hematuria seen in adults with tumors. Concommitant anomalies (e.g., aniridia, hemihypertrophy) are observed more often in children with Wilm's tumor than in the general population.

Wilm's tumor is a rapidly growing, solid tumor composed of cells derived from both nephrogenous and stromagenous blastema. Neonatal Wilm's tumor is no longer considered a disease entity, and tumors previously diagnosed as such are presently believed to have represented fetal hamartoma.

In contrast to Wilm's tumor, neuroblastoma has been encountered in younger infants. The lesion occurs anywhere along the sympathetic chain, although the majority are found within the adrenal gland. Extra-adrenal neuroblastomas have been observed in the Organ of Zuckerkhandl within the lower abdomen, the pelvis, and the upper thoracic area. Tumors occurring in the upper thoracic region are located in the posterior mediastinum and cause erosive changes in the adjacent vertebrae and ribs. In general, the tumor extends rapidly into the neighboring lymph nodes and causes widening of the paravertebral soft tissues. This feature has been noted in the lower thorax and occasionally is the earliest radiographic manifestation of the disease (Fig. 1-27). Calcific deposits similar to those noted in the primary tumor can also be detected in metastatic lesions within the liver. In addition, neuroblastoma commonly spreads to bones, whereas Wilm's Tumor affects the lungs (Fig. 1-28). Associated clinical symptoms referable to the systemic effects of catecholamines (e.g., fever, hypertension, diarrhea) may be the first indications of an occult lesion. Bizarre

myoclonic seizures and cerebellar symptoms have also been reported with neuroblastoma.

Ganglioneuroma is a benign lesion that mimics neuroblastoma in many ways except for its prognosis. Cases have been documented where biopsied, diagnosed neuroblastoma has been observed to mature into ganglioneuroma. Ganglioneuroma usually occurs in the posterior mediastinum, just as neuroblastoma, and the presence of calcification within the tumor is equally as common. However, it is usually more sharply demarcated and shows a more oval configuration.

Adrenal cortical tumors, benign or malignant, are rare and often associated with virilizing hormonal excretion and the adrenogenital syndrome. Bilateral adrenal hyperplasia and adenomas are more often the cause of this syndrome in infants, whereas Cushing's syndrome is more likely to be due to carcinoma. In adults this is reversed, and Cushing's syndrome is far more frequently associated with adrenal hyperplasia.

UNILATERAL SYMMETRICAL ENLARGEMENT OF THE KIDNEY IN THE INFANT AND CHILD

In estimating unilateral enlargement of a kidney, one must always keep in mind that the left kidney may normally be 1 cm. larger than the right. Moreover, the maximum length of a kidney is estimated to be equivalent to the length of four vertebral bodies including the intervertebral spaces comprised by them. This is a simple means of estimating renal size and is consistent throughout childhood except for the first to 1.5 years of life, during which time the length of the kidney is greater. Most often an enlarged kidney can be recognized visually without having to resort to actual measurement.

(Text continued on p. 34.)

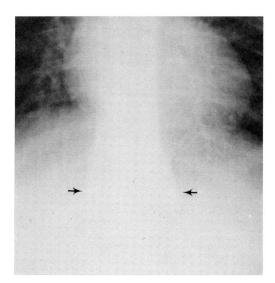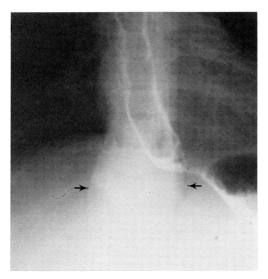

Fig. 1-27. Metastatic neuroblastoma diagnosed on chest examination. A routine chest film and barium swallow examination reveal a paravertebral soft-tissue mass of metastatic neuroblastoma within the lower thoracic region (arrows).

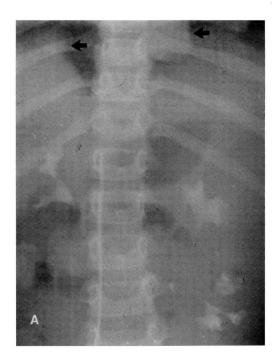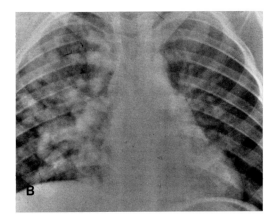

Fig. 1-28. Metastatic Wilm's tumor. (A) Intravenous urogram demonstrates a Wilm's tumor within the center of the left kidney. Two large pulmonary metastases (arrows) are also apparent. (B) Radiograph of the chest in another patient with diffuse pulmonary metastatic Wilm's tumor.

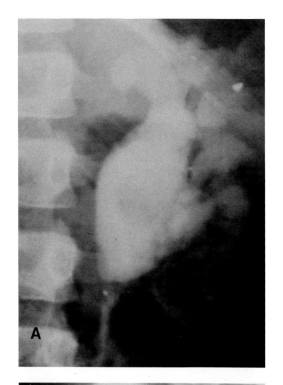

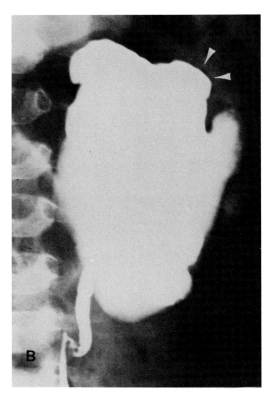

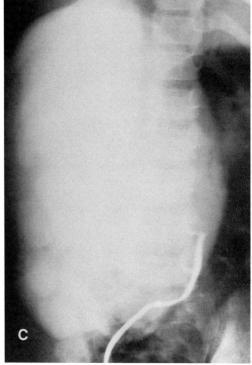

Fig. 1-29. Unilateral ureteropelvic obstruction. (A) A dilated pelvo-calyceal system is noted in a fairly well functioning kidney. The ureter is characteristically narrow. (B) A retrograde study was performed in a poorly functioning kidney and reveals a narrow ureter. The renal pelvis and the calyces are dilated. Reflux into small sack-like structures, the ducts of Bellini (arrows), is observed just above the calyces. (These ducts dilate because of the obstruction and are occasionally observed during intravenous urography.) (C) Retrograde examination in a nonfunctioning kidney reveals a huge sack-like pelvis and dilated calyces. The ureter is characteristically narrow.

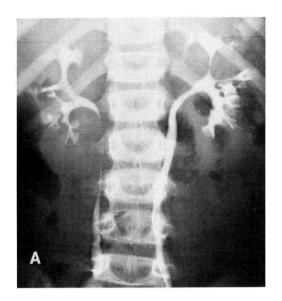

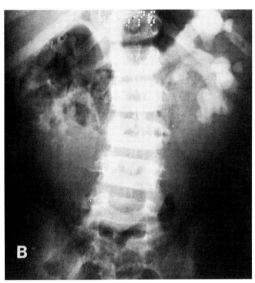

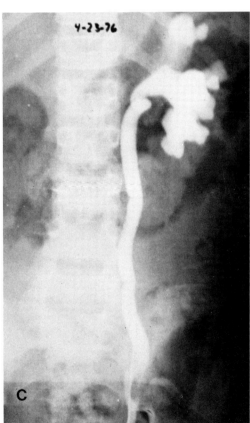

Fig. 1-30. Tuberculosis of the left ureter. *(A)* This 12-year-old male presented with fever and an enlarged left hilar node. An intravenous pyelogram was performed at the time that albuminuria was detected. Both kidneys are enlarged although the left ureter and associated calyces show early signs of obstruction. *(B)* Severe hydronephrosis of the left kidney is noted one month later. The ureter could not be adequately visualized. *(C)* Obstruction at the junction of the middle and distal third of the left ureter is depicted on retrograde pyelography. Resected section revealed tuberculosis.

Disease Entities

Hydronephrosis
  Ureteropelvic obstruction
  Stricture
  Tumor
  Ureterovesical obstruction
  Retro-caval ureter
  Calculus
  Extrinsic lesions
Infection
Compensatory hypertrophy
Duplication
Renal vein thrombosis
Diffuse neoplastic infiltration

Differential Diagnosis

Obstructive uropathy occurs anywhere within the ureter or the bladder and is caused by a variety of diseases. Hydronephrosis due to obstruction at the ureteropelvic junction is the most common cause of mass formation in the upper abdomin of a child. In fact, any abdominal mass in a child should suggest hydronephrosis until proven otherwise. When considering obstructing lesions, always keep in mind that the largest kidneys result from lesions located at the ureteropelvic junction. When the obstruction is located more distally, the ureter is affected early and more severely than the kidney. In general the radiographic findings depend greatly upon the severity of the obstruction. Opacification of the pelvo-calyceal system is often delayed in the initial phases of intravenous urography, and a prolonged nephrogram may be produced. Delayed studies are necessary in order to determine the status of the pelvo-calyceal structures. This may require anywhere from 30 minutes to 24 hours or more to complete. The dilated calyces eventually opacify if the renal parenchyma is still present and functioning (Fig. 1-29A). Obstructive hydronephrosis must be differentiated from other causes of renal enlargement. In general this is not difficult, although poor function and a delayed nephrogram are commonly encountered in renal vein thrombosis and diffuse interstitial pyogenic nephritis. However, delayed studies do not reveal dilated calyces. Instead, the calyceal system in these diseases may appear either normal or elongated and narrow.

Once the diagnosis of obstruction is established, specific attention is then given to localize and identify the lesion. In this respect, multiple delayed films in various positions (e.g., prone, oblique) should be attempted to outline the lesion. Retrograde pyelography may be required if renal function is inadequate (Fig. 1-29B, C). Obstruction at the ureteropelvic junction due to fibrosis or a crossing vessel occurs exactly within this anatomical location and is in the form of a short, segmental narrowing. Segmental lesions within other portions of the ureter may be the result of infectious disease, but in this age-group they are rare and unusual. These lesions have a characteristic appearance and are smooth, with manifest tapering margins at both ends of the lesion and no mucosal destruction (Fig. 1-30). Tuberculosis commonly involves the ureter but is almost always secondary to renal disease. Consequently, renal abnormalities, such as calyceal destruction and abscess formation, frequently accompany the ureteral problem. Extrinsic compression of the ureter by surrounding inflammatory disease results in transient or permanent hydroureter and hydronephrosis. For example, transient obstructions of the right ureter can be seen during an acute appendicitis or an acute exacerbation of Crohn's disease. Most frequently the right ureter is smoothly and symmetrically narrowed and may be displaced medially. Permanent obstructive changes occur when a chronic inflammatory process invades the retroperitoneum and envelops the ureter. Just such an occurrence occasionally arises in ilietis. Similar ureteral findings are also encountered in retroperitoneal fibrosis and lymphoma. A retro-caval ureter is an interesting congenital lesion which also causes obstruction of the right kidney. In this malformation, the interior vena cava lies in front of the right ureter causing partial or complete obstruction. The lesion is recognized radiographically by the medial deviation of the proximally dilated ureter and collapsed distal ureter (Fig. 1-31). Tumors as a cause of ureteral obstruction are uncommon and rarely malignant. Polypoid lesions are recognized by intraluminal filling defects that may dilate the nearby ureter. Obstruction at the ureterovesical junction can be diagnosed only if the lesion is so located. Calculi are uncommon but may occur

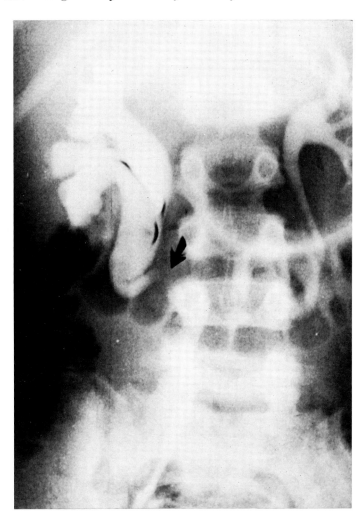

Fig. 1-31. Retro-caval ureter. Right-sided hydro-nephrosis is present. The proximal ureter is directed medially and is obstructed as it crosses the vertebrae by the inferior vena cava. The distal ureter is narrow and more medially positioned than normal.

secondary to infection, hyperparathyroidism, and tubular acidosis.

The radiographic features of interstitial disease associated with perinephric inflammation are diagnostic for an interstitial pyogenic infection. The outline of the kidney is therefore poorly defined on routine abdominal examinations. In addition, the overall radiodensity of the abdomen may appear increased because of the added inflammatory process. During the acute phase, function is severely diminished.

The compensatory hypertrophied kidney and a kidney with duplication of the collecting systems are unique in this discussion; the radiographic finding consists basically of a normal functioning but apparently enlarged kidney. The contralateral kidney often manifests pathologic changes when one kidney is hypertrophied. (Double collecting systems should offer no problems.)

Unilateral diffuse infiltrating neoplastic lesions are uncommon. Such lesions are more often bilateral, although greater involvement on one side may give the false impression of unilateral disease.

Extrinsic lesions producing obstruction may be caused by a number of disorders ranging from benign mass formation, such as a hematoma if the lesion is of recent origin, to a malignancy if the mass is long-standing. The diagnosis of an enlarged kidney, an associated abnormal mass, and displacement or direct involvement of the ureter indicates the nature of the lesion. A more specific diagnosis can be established by correlating the history with other radiologic features. For example, a recent history of trauma suggests

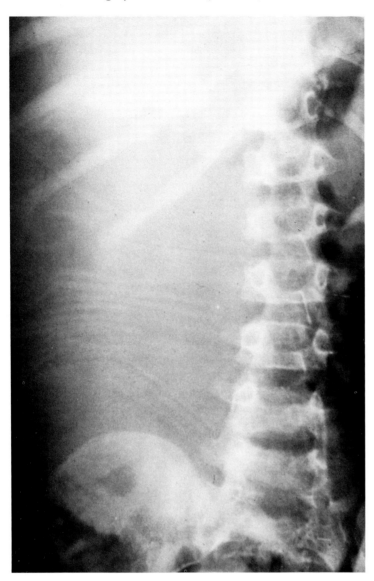

Fig. 1-32. Retroperitoneal hematoma. A large hematoma is present in the retroperitoneum following recent trauma. The right kidney is elevated and markedly dilated. The mass is not radiolucent and may look like a urinoma or other retroperitoneal tumors.

a hematoma (Fig. 1-32) or urinoma if extravasation is also encountered. A lipoma can be suspected if the lesion is radiolucent on the total body opacification phase (Fig. 1-33). The direction in which the ureter is displaced is also important. For example, lesions arising in the lymph nodes (e.g., lymphoma, metastasis) displace the ureters laterally. Soft-tissue tumors which arise retroperitoneally most likely cause medial displacement.

Further studies, such as arteriography, may be performed in situations where the diagnosis is not clear. With the exception of compensatory hypertrophy, the intrarenal vessels are stretched and narrowed. In hydronephrosis these vessels are also displaced around the dilated calyces. Perfusion throughout the kidney is dramatically delayed in infection and in renal vein thrombosis because of the interstitial filling by transudate, or exudate, and/or increased peripheral resistance. The nephrogram is interesting in both of these lesions, since the normal cortico-medullary junction is lost. In addition, streaky radiolucencies radiating toward the hilum of the kidney have been described in each during this phase. In acute interstitial nephritis, these radiolucencies are due mainly to tubules distended with pus; in renal vein thrombosis, they are due to interstitial edematous fluid. The remaining arteriographic and nephrographic features of stretching and poor perfusion are due to interstitial compression by the exudate or transudate. Renal venography is essential for an absolute diagnosis of renal vein throm-

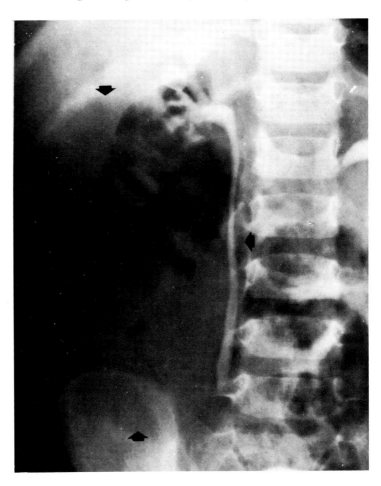

Fig. 1-33. Intraabdominal lipoma. A large radiolucent mass is visualized during the total body opacification phase *(arrows)*. Kidney and ureter are only minimally displaced and dilated since the mass was not in the retroperitoneum, but in the abdomen.

bosis. In this study the thrombus as well as developing collateral circulation become apparent.

Discussion

Many of the lesions causing obstructive hydronephrosis have already been discussed (see pp. 3, 11, 34). Infectious processes that involve the kidneys and the ureters are mainly acquired. Renal infection arises predominantly as an ascending infection from the lower urinary tract, but may also be transmitted to the kidney by way of the blood stream, as in tuberculosis which strikes the kidney before descending to affect the ureters. The initial infection localizes within the renal papillae and is basically a destructive process that affects the papillae and the adjacent calyx. The ureter can be involved by one or more diseased segments of various lengths. Extrinsic inflammatory lesions also smoothly narrow the ureter and simultaneously cause a certain degree of displacement. Most of these changes are transient and are due to local compression and paresis of the

ureteral muscle. Occasionally, chronic and extensive cases of Crohn's disease penetrate the retroperitoneum to engulf the ureters.

Acute pyogenic infection of the kidneys also arises secondarily from a distant primary lesion, such as a furuncle. The infection is commonly staphylococcal, and a diffuse interstitial pyogenic nephritis is established. The bacteria are transported by way of the lymphatics into the perinephritic tissues, and a reaction is also established in these tissues. The clinical symptoms are not always obvious, and the urine may be normal. Reliance on radiologic features, therefore, is quite important in order to establish an early diagnosis. Prompt and adequate therapy can result in resolution and a useful, functioning kidney. Otherwise, the infection can completely destroy the kidney or become walled-off into a subacute or chronic abscess.

The most common infection affecting the urinary system is acute pyelonephritis. This arises mainly from a lower urinary tract infection and as a result renal changes may be minimal. The most frequent radiographic ab-

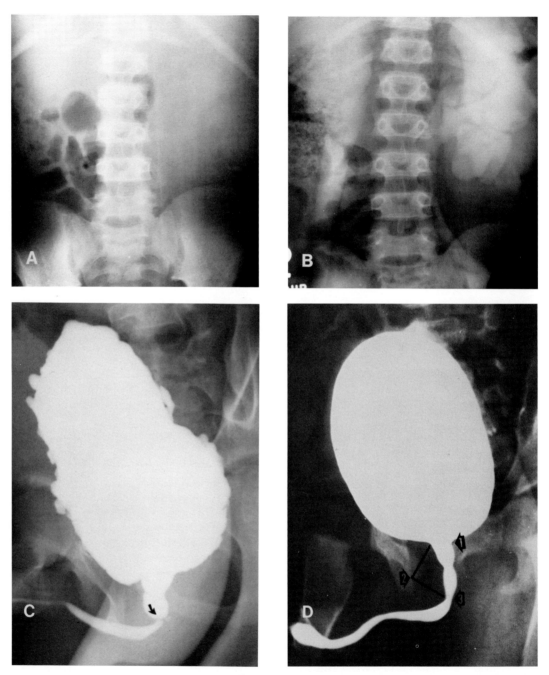

Fig. 1-34. Posterior urethral valve. *(A)* Enlarged kidneys are noted bilaterally. *(B)* Two hours later the obstructed calyces and dilated tortuous ureters are opacified. *(C)* Voiding cystourethrogram reveals a trabeculated distended bladder, a dilated posterior urethra, and an obstructing urethral valve *(arrow)*. *(D)* Normal cystourethrogram for comparison: *(1)* internal sphincter, *(2)* posterior urethra, *(3)* external sphincter.

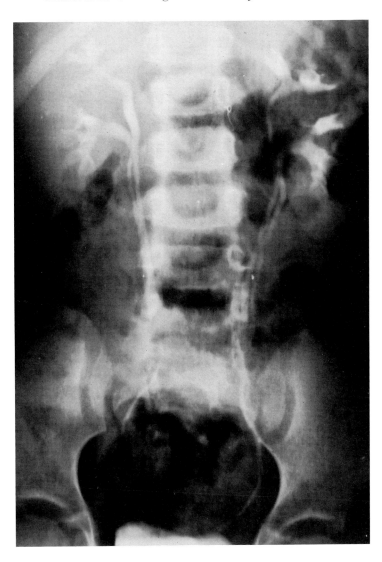

Fig. 1-35. Duplication. Both kidneys are enlarged and consist of two collecting systems and ureters. The ureters join before reaching the bladder.

normality may be slight dilatation and atony of the corresponding ureter and pelvocalyceal group. In the presence of severe infections, some alteration of renal function may be apparent. Persistent infection eventually destroy, the renal tissue in the region of the papillae, and obvious changes then occur within the adjacent calyx. Initially, this appears blunted but is eventually destroyed and scarred. Loss of adjacent cortical tissue causes scarring and an irregularly shaped kidney. Since the growth of the kidney is also affected, the overall result is a small and scarred structure.

BILATERAL RENAL ENLARGEMENT IN THE INFANT AND CHILD

As in unilateral disease of the kidney, many lesions in newborns that involve both kidneys can remain unrecognized for long periods of time. However, other acquired lesions may become evident at this age.

Disease Entities

Hydronephrosis
Hydronephotic upper poles and ureteroceles
Wilm's tumor
Neuroblastoma
Storage disease
Leukemia
Lymphoma
Angiomyolipomas (hamartomas)
Cystic disease
Glomerulonephritis
Nephrotic syndrome
Sickle cell disease
Duplication

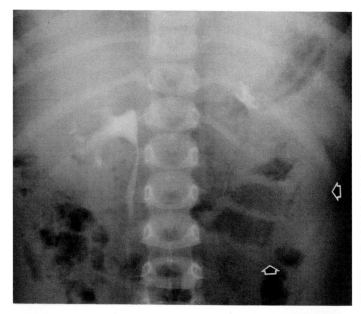

Fig. 1-36. Bilateral Wilm's tumor. A large soft-tissue mass representing a Wilm's tumor is present within the lower pole of the left kidney *(arrows)*. The lower pole calyces are not visualized. Another Wilm's tumor occupies the upper pole of the right kidney. The upper pole calyx is poorly seen, and the remaining collecting systems are displaced inferiorly.

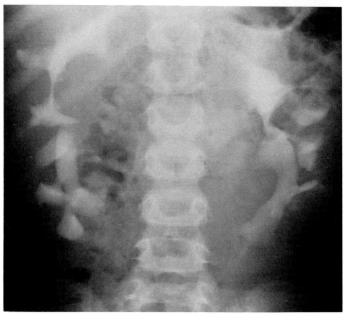

Fig. 1-37. Polycystic kidneys in tuberous sclerosis. The kidneys are markedly enlarged, and the calyces distorted by multiple intrarenal cysts.

Differential Diagnosis

Bilateral and unilateral hydronephrosis are etiologically identical. Ureteropelvic obstruction as a cause of hydronephrosis occurs commonly as a bilateral lesion and is the most frequently encountered anomaly within the urinary tract. The degree of obstruction may vary from one side to another. A posterior urethral valve is a common cause of distal urinary tract obstruction in infants and children and should always be considered in the presence of bilateral ureteropelvic dilatation associated with a trabeculated bladder. A voiding cystourethrogram is essential in demonstrating the dilated posterior urethra (Fig. 1-34). The differential diagnostic features of duplication, Wilm's tumor, neuroblastoma, and cystic disease (Figs. 1-35, 1-36, 1-37) have been discussed. The internal pelvocalyceal structures are displaced in both bilateral neuroblastoma and hydronephrosis of the upper poles. The position of the kidney is essentially unaltered in upper pole hydronephrosis, despite the downward displacement of the collecting systems. Bilateral Wilm's tumor should be differentiated from

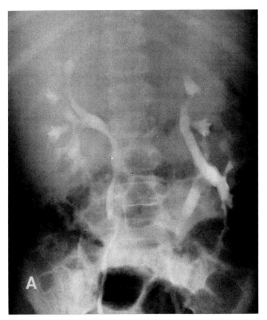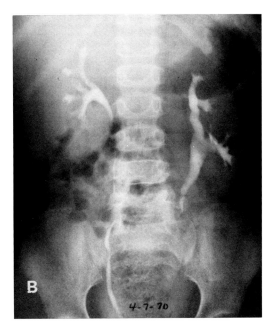

Fig. 1-38. Leukemic infiltration. *(A)* The kidneys are markedly enlarged in a patient with acute leukemia. The collecting systems are elongated but demonstrate no significant alteration. (The configuration on the left is congenital.) *(B)* Three months following remission of the acute process, the renal structures are reduced in size.

other lesions causing diffuse changes within the kidneys, such as leukemia, lymphoma, hamartomas, and cystic disease (Fig. 1-37). A bilateral angiomyolipoma (hamartoma) may look like a bilateral Wilm's tumor. However, the high fat component of the tumor may be recognized on the abdominal films by its radiolucent character, and the vascularity of hamartomas seen on angiography is in most cases characteristic.

Infiltrating processes, such as leukemia and lymphoma, cause stretching and elongation of the collecting system with little alteration and displacement of the calyceal orientation (Fig. 1-38). Distorted calyces branching in various directions indicate multiple cysts, a feature not commonly noted in Wilm's tumor (Fig. 1-37).

Familial cystic dysplasia also occurs in infants, and cystic involvement of the cortex and medulla predominates. The cysts are of varying sizes but are definitely smaller than those seen in the adult form of polycystic disease. The findings are similar to Wilm's tumor, although the infundilula in this form of cystic disease appear wide and short.

Acute glomerulonephritis may present with rapidly enlarging kidneys. Renal function is usually severely impaired in the early stages but returns to normal if the disease runs a benign course. The frequently associated chest findings of pleural effusion, cardiomegaly, and congestive failure help in establishing the diagnosis. In the nephrotic syndrome the kidneys are also enlarged and the calyces diffusely stretched. Renal function is often impaired.

Sickle cell disease has also been associated with enlarged kidneys that in many respects mimic an infiltrative process such as leukemia or lymphoma. However, the calyces are often quite dilated in sickle cell disease but remain unchanged in leukemia (Fig. 1-38). Although pyelonephritis is one of the major pathologic changes encountered in this disease, the dilated calyces are probably more often the result of vascular thrombosis and fibrosis. However, persistent and recurrent infection and infarction cause scarring, and ultimate loss of renal size ensues. In addition, it is not unusual to see enlarged kidneys without obstruction in hemophilia. These changes are usually noted as an incidental finding.

Discussion

Bilateral Wilm's tumor is fortunately not common and occurs in approximately 3 per

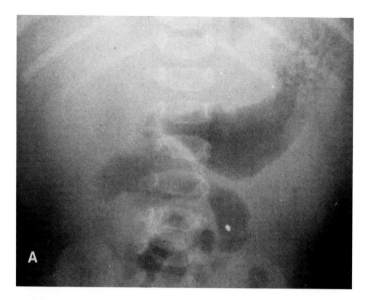

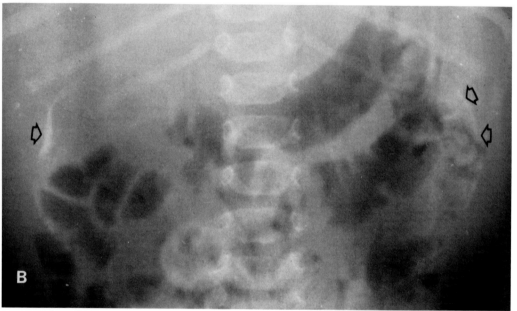

Fig. 1-39. Bilateral cortical necrosis. *(A)* Urography in a patient with massive hamaturia provided only a poor nephrogram. *(B)* Three weeks later linear calcifications *(arrows)* outlining the periphery of both kidneys are noted. (An incidental umbilical hernia is noted in the right lower quadrant.)

cent of cases. It is conceivable that the contralateral kidney may be affected by metastisis, particularly when a period of time has elapsed between discovery of the first and second tumor. However, there is no reason to doubt that the malformation may have affected both kidneys simultaneously, with one side growing more slowly. The extrarenal clinical manifestations of Wilm's tumor, such as aniridia and hemihypertrophy, are more commonly found with bilateral disease. Bilateral adrenal pheochromocytomas should be anticipated in familial lesions. Infiltrative lesions such as leukemia and lymphoma more often involve both kidneys. However, in-

volvement of the kidneys is overshadowed by the dominant systemic presentation of hepatosplenomegaly.

There is a high incidence of bilateral angiomyolipomas and occasionally cysts with tuberous sclerosis. Further radiographic evaluation demonstrates sclerotic and cystic changes within the bones, and cystic changes within the lungs.

The significance of renal enlargement in sickle cell disease is unclear and may be a manifestation of congestion. Dalinka noted that multiple transfusions were uniformly characteristic of hemophilia and sickle cell patients with bilaterally enlarged kidneys.

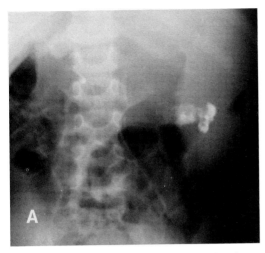

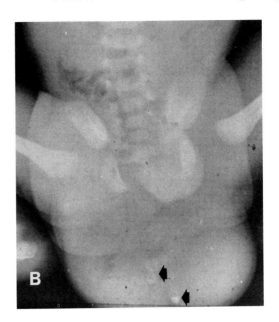

Fig. 1-40. Retroperitoneal teratoma. *(A)* A large retroperitoneal mass with irregular calcifications. The calcifications nevertheless have some structural form and suggest a teratoma. *(B)* A large sacrococcygeal teratoma extends down between both legs. Poorly seen but nevertheless well formed clacific masses are present within the tumor *(arrows).*

DISEASES ASSOCIATED WITH A PROLONGED NEPHROGRAM

A prolonged nephrogram is defined as a radiodense, persistent opacification of the entire renal parenchyma that arises late during the intravenous urogram. It is most often a manifestation of obstruction and appears as the contrast material accumulates and is retained within the collecting tubules. Occasionally, impairment of the tubules themselves may be responsible for the production of this phenomenon.

Disease Entities

Obstruction
Tamm-Horsfall proteinuria
Tubular necrosis
Renal medullary necrosis
Pyelonephritis
Renal vein thrombosis

Differential Diagnosis

The most common cause of a prolonged nephrogram in newborns, infants, and children is obstruction within the urinary tract. Although many lesions cause obstruction of the urinary tract, posterior urethral valve is the most common cause in newborns, and ureterovesical obstruction is the most common overall abnormality.

Obstruction by Tamm-Horsfall proteinuria occurs in all age-groups but is more commonly seen in infants. Under certain abnormal circumstances the proteinaceous casts precipitate and cause temporary tubular obstruction. The kidneys may be mildly enlarged during the urographic study, although a delayed and persistent radiodense nephrogram is the main radiographic feature. The collecting systems may also be visualized. In fact in some patients, an initial flash filling of these structures occurs on the early urograms prior to the development of the nephrogram. The collecting systems are generally normal, apart from a mild attenuation of the calyces.

Radiographic results similar to those noted in Tamm-Horsfall proteinuria may, be found in acute tubular necrosis. This abnormality, however, is encountered in older children. An equally radiodense nephrogram which appears early may also be seen in patients suffering from acute medullary necrosis due to leakage of the contrast material into the interstitial spaces of the kidney. This is a very severe pathologic situation and is usually associated with severe illness and shock.

Renal vein thrombosis occurs in all age-groups and because of the resulting renal

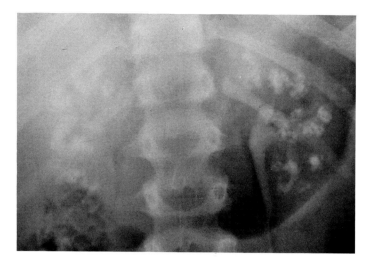

Fig. 1-41. Medullary sponge kidney. The presence of calcifications and dilated tubules located within the renal papillae immediately adjacent to the calyces is characteristic. This composite picture has been likened to a bouquet of flowers.

edema causes delayed excretion and a persistent nephrogram.

Discussion

Tamm-Horsfall protein is a urinary mucoprotein and is the main constituent of hyaline casts. It has been implicated as the cause of acute renal failure and renal tubular obstruction in dehydrated and oliguric patients. It has been suggested that the hypertonic contrast agents presently utilized are partially responsible for precipitating this protein. Consequently, for safety purposes all urographic studies should be performed only on well hydrated patients.

Renal cortical and medullary necrosis are serious complications that follow episodes of severe dehydration associated with neonatal sepsis or massive blood loss, which result in shock and poor renal perfusion. If the afflicted infant survives, the kidneys are often decreased in size and manifest changes that are characteristic for each condition. Rim-like calcifications outlining the cortex are noted in the kidneys previously affected by cortical necrosis (Fig. 1-39). Medullary necrosis eventually produces deformed calyces associated with collections of contrast material outside the calyx, representing the defects created by sloughed papillae.

KIDNEY CALCIFICATIONS

Calcifications are easily detected on the conventional abdominal film. The incidence, form, and location of calcifications vary from one lesion to the other and therefore represent vital radiographic clues in identifying the underlying lesion. The exact location of the calcification can be accomplished by utilizing multiple views or by noting the position of the mass or organ that contains the calcification. Urographic studies are obviously quite important in confirming the diagnosis when the kidney is suspected. The entities responsible for the deposition of calcium within the urinary tract can be classified according to the nature and form of the calcification. Three major categories exist.

Disease Entities

Amorphous calcification
   Neuroblastoma
   Wilm's tumor
   Teratoma
Nephrocalcinosis
   Hyperparathyroidism
   Medullary sponge kidney
   Renal tubular acidosis
   Idiopathic hypercalemia
Cortical calcification
   Renal cortical necrosis
   Dysplastic kidney
Adrenal calcification
   Adrenal hemorrhage
   Wolman's disease

Differential Diagnosis

Deposition of calcium within malignant tumors is frequently the result of dystrophic calcification within necrotic tissue and therefore assumes an amorphous appearance. In children, any retroperitoneal mass containing calcium should suggest neuroblastoma (Fig.

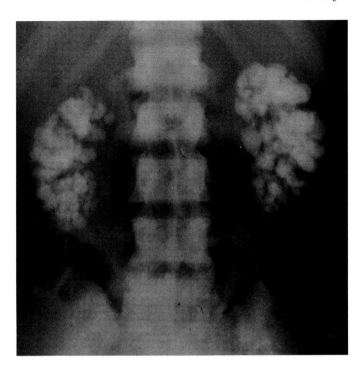

Fig. 1-42. Renal tubular acidosis. Both kidneys are outlined by clumps of calcifications that are apparently located to the renal papillae. The bones are diffusely sclerotic due to secondary hyperparathyroidism.

1-22). Neuroblastoma is common in this age group and presents with calcification in approximately 50 per cent of the cases. In contrast, the incidence of calcification in Wilm's tumor is relatively infrequent. The presence of calcification is thus a useful radiographic means of differentiating these two lesions.

Retroperitoneal teratomas are exceptionally rare tumors but commonly contain calcium, which may differentiate into primitive structures (e.g., bone, teeth) (Fig. 1-40). The sacrococcygeal teratoma is more common and presents as a huge mass originating from the presacral area extending down between the legs. Besides bone and calcium, the tumor may contain elements of other tissues (Fig. 1-40B).

Nephrocalcinosis is a term that is used to define calcium deposition within the parenchyma of the kidney, in contrast to deposition within the pelvo-calyceal system. The deposits are frequently restricted to the renal pyramids but can be scattered diffusely. Many renal lesions are responsible for this presentation. Histologically, the calcium may be located in either the basement membrane, cytoplasm, interstitium, or lumen of the collecting tubules.

Patients with hyperparathyroidism present with a stippled form of nephrocalcinosis. Radiographically, the associated bone changes of this disease are apparent. The majority of

cases of hyperparathyroidism in infants and children are secondary to chronic renal disease.

The calcifications noted in medullary sponge kidney are located within dilated tubules and assume a characteristic rosette appearance. The dilated tubules fill with contrast material during intravenous urography and are located adjacent to the calyces. The tubules are either linear or cystic in appearance (Fig. 1-41). Obviously, more dilated tubules are present than calcifications. The calyces may be slightly enlarged to accomodate the dilated tubules but in general are normal. This is a vital factor in distinguishing this entity from other lesions that produce small cystic collections in this area, such as tuberculous medullary necrosis and other infections.

Renal tubular acidosis is caused by the excessive loss of bicarbonate in the urine. As a result the basic radicals in the body are drained, along with calcium that is deposited in the tubules. The deposition can be massive and can outline an entire kidney (Fig. 1-42). Idiopathic hypercalcemia may also result in deposition of calcium and is probably due to a hypersensitivity to vitamin D, with excessive absorption of calcium through the gut wall.

Other lesions that produce nephrocalcinosis include chronic glomerulonephritis, sarcoidosis, and cretinism.

During the resolution of cortical necrosis, calcium deposits in a ring configuration around the entire kidney (Fig. 1-39). Multiple ring-like calcifications in a nonfunctioning kidney have also been found in multicystic disease. However, this feature is more commonly discovered in adults and is quite rare in children.

Calcifications within adrenal glands that appear to be normal are probably the result of previous neonatal adrenal hemorrhage. This was at one time believed to be caused by tuberculosis.

Wolman's disease is a rare, fatal lipidosis that is characterized by enlarged adrenal glands with ring-like calcifications.

REFERENCES

Bilateral Generalized Renal Enlargement in the Newborn

1. Baker, D. H., and Berdon, W. E.: The use and safety of high dosage pediatric urography. Radiology, *103:*371, 1972.
2. Berdon, W. E., Levitt, S. B., Baker, D. H., Becker, J. A., and Uson, A. E.: Hydronephrosis in infants and children. Value of high dosage excretory urography in predicting renal salvageability. Am. J. Roentgenol. Radium Ther. Nucl. Med., *109:*380, 1970.
3. Dunbar, J. S., and Nogrady, B.: The calyceal crescent-a roentgenographic sign of obstructive hydronephrosis. Am. J. Roentgenol. Radium Ther. Nucl. Med., *110:*520, 1970.
4. ———: Excretory urography in the first year of life. Radiol. Clin. North Am., *10:*367, 1972.
5. Froled, A., Ney, C., and Miller, H. L.: Unilateral hydronephrosis affecting the contralateral kidney and ureter. Radiology *104:*33, 1972.
6. Griesbach, W. A., Waterhouse, R. K., and Mellins, H. Z.: Voiding cystourethrography in the diagnosis of congenital posterior urethral valves. Am. J. Roentgenol. Radium Ther. Nucl. Med., *82:*52, 1959.
7. Griscom, N. T., and Krueker, M. A.: Visualization of individual papillary directs (directs of Bellini) by excretory urography in childhood hydronephrosis. Radiology, *106:*385, 1973.
8. Grossman, H., Winchester, P. H., and Colston, W. C.: Neurogenic bladder in childhood. Radiol. Clin. North Am., *6:*155, 1968.
9. Grossman, H., Winchester, P., and Waldbaum, R. S.: Syndrome of congenital deficiency of abdominal wall neuroculature and associated genitourinary anomalies. *In* Kaufman, H. (ed.): Progress in Pediatric Radiology. Vol. 3. p. 327. Chicago, Year Book Medical Publishers, 1970.
10. Gwinn, J. L., and Landing, B. H.: Cystic diseases of the kidneys in infants and children. Radiol. Clin. North Am., *6:*191, 1968.

11. Horag, B., and Hertz, M.: Congenital valves of the posterior urethra: radiological aspects. Clin. Radiol., *25:*445, 1974.
12. Osathanondh, V., and Potter, E. L.: Pathogenesis of polycystic kidneys . . . . Arch. Pathol., *77:*459, 1964.
13. Pais, V. M., and Retik, A. B.: Reversible hydronephrosis in the neonate with urinary sepsis, N. Engl. J. Med., *292:*465, 1975.

Unilateral Diffuse Renal Enlargement in the Newborn

14. Elkin, M., and Bernstein, J.: Cystic diseases of the kidney-radiologic and pathologic considerations. Clin. Radiol., *20:*65, 1969.
15. Felson, B., and Cussen, L. J.: The hydronephrosatic type of unilateral roentgenol, *10:*113, 1975.
16. King, M. C., Friedenberg, R. M., and Tena, L. B.: Normal Renal parenchyma simulating tumor. Radiology, *91:*217, 1968.
17. Lalli, A. F.: Multicystic kidney disease. Radiology, *89:*857, 1967.
18. Potter, E. L.: Normal and Abnormal Development of the Kidney. Chicago, Year Book Medical Publishers, Inc., 1972.
19. Spince, H. M., and Singleton, R.: Cystic and cystic disorders of the kidney: types, diagnosis, treatment. Urolog. Survey, *22:*131, 1972.
20. Talner, L. B., and Gittes, R. F.: Megacalyces: further observations and differentiation from obstructive renal disease. Am. J. Roentgenol. Radium Ther. Nucl. Med., *121:*473, 1974.
21. Uson, A. C., Cox, L. A., and Lattimer, J. K.: Hydronephrosis in infants and children. J.A.M.A., *205:*327, 1968,

Unilateral Asymmetrical Enlargement of the Kidney and the Enlarged Adrenal Gland in the Newborn

22. Berdon, W. E., Baker, D. H., Becker, J. A., and Uron, A. E.: Ectopic ureterocoele. Radiol. Clin. North Am., *6:*205, 1968.
23. Berdon, W. E., Wigger, J. J., and Baker, D. H.: Fetal renal hamartoma-a benign tumor to be distinguished from Wilm's tumor. Am. J. Roentgenol Radium Ther. Nucl. Med., *118:*18, 1973.
24. Meyers, M. A., Whalen, J. P., Evans, J. A., and Viamonte, M.: Malposition and displacement of the bowel in renal agenesis and ectopia.: new observations. Am. J. Roentgenol. Radium Ther. Nucl. Med., *117:*323, 1973.
25. Kurlander, G. J.: Roentgenology of the congenital adrenogenital syndrome. Am. J. Roentgenol. Radium Ther. Nucl. Med., *95:*189, 1965.

Bilateral Asymmetrical Enlargement of the Kidney and Enlarged Adrenal Glands in the Newborn

26. Brill, P. W., Krasna, I. H., and Aaron, H.: An early rim sign in neonatal adrenal hemor-

rhage. Am. J. Roentgenol. Radium Ther. Nucl. Med., *127:*289, 1976.

27. Rose, J., Berdon, W. E., Sullivan, T., and Baker, D. H.: Prolonged jaundice as presenting sign of massive adrenal hemmorrhage in newborn: radiographic diagnosis by intravenous pyelography with total body opacification. Radiology, *98:*263, 1971.

Small Kidneys in the Newborn

28. Ask-Upmark, E. Uber juvenile maligne nephrosklerose and ihr verhaltnis zu storungen in der nierenentwicklung. Acta Pathol. Microbiol. Scand., *6:*383, 1929.
29. Himmelfarb, E., Rabinowitz, J. G., Parvey, L., Gammill, S., and Arant, B.: Ask-Upmark kidney. Am. J. Dis. Child., *129:*1440, 1975.
30. Leonidas, J., Fellows, R. A., Hall, R. T., Rhodes, P. G., and Beatty E. C.: Value of chest radiography in the diagnosis of Potter's syndrome at birth. Am. J. Roentgenol. Radium Ther. Nucl. Med., *123:*716, 1975.
31. Potter, E. L.: Bilateral renal agenesis. J. Pediatr., *29:*68, 1946.
32. Rabinowitz, J. G., Pelzman, H., and Robinson, T.: Small pelvic outlet associated with underdevelopment of the urinary tract and other anomalies. Radiology, *101:*629, 1971.
33. Risdon, R. A., Young, L. W., and Chrispin, A. R.: Renal hypoplasia and dysplasia: a radiological and pathological correlation. Pediatr. Radiol., *3:*213, 1975.

Unilateral Asymmetrical Enlargement of the Kidney and Adrenal Gland in the Infant and Child

34. Hope, S. W.: Cancer of the urogenital tract: Wilm's Tumor and Neuroblastoma. J.A.M.A., *204:*125, 1968.
35. McDonald, P.: Genito-urinary tumors. *In* Progress in Pediatric Radiology. vol. 3. p. 271. Chicago, Year Book Medical Publishers, 1970.

Unilateral Symmetrical Enlargement of the Kidney in the Infant and Child

36. Lusted, L. B., and Keats, T. E.: Atlas of Roentgenographic Measurement. ed. 2. Chicago, Year Book Medical Publishers, 1967.
37. Rabinowitz, J. G., et al.: Acute renal carbuncle: the roentgenographic clarification of a medical enegma. Am. J. Roentgenol. Radium Ther. Nucl. Med., *116:*740, 1972.

Bilateral Renal Enlargement in the Infant and Child

38. Bar-Ziv, J., Hirsch, M. and Perlman, M.: Bilateral nephroblastomatasis. Pediatr. Radiol., *3:*85, 1975.
39. Dalinka, M. D., Lally, S. F., Rancier, L. F., and Mata, S.: Nephromegaly in hemophilia. Radiology, *115:*337, 1975.
40. Lalli, A. F.: Lymphoma and the urinary tract. Radiology, *93:*1051, 1969.
41. Marquis, J. R., and Khazem, B.: Sickle cell disease, renal roentgenographic changes in children. Radiology, *98:*47, 1971.
42. Potter, E. L.: Normal and Abnormal Development of the Kidney. Chicago, Year Book Medical Publishers, 1972.

Diseases Associated With a Prolonged Nephrogram

43. Fry, I. K., and Cattell, W. R.: The nephrographic pattern during intravenous urography. Br. Med. Bull., *28:*227, 1972.
44. Leonidas, J. C., Berdon, W. E., and Gribetz, D.: Bilateral renal cortical necrosis in the newborn infants: roentgenographic diagnosis. J. Pediatr., *79:*623, 1971.
45. Schwartz, R. H., Berdon, W. E., Wagner, J., Becker, J., and Baker, D.: Tamm-Horsfall urinary mucoprotein precipitation by urographic contrast agents: in vitro studies. Am. J. Roentgenol. Radium Ther. Nucl. Med., *108:*698, 1970.

Kidney Calcifications

46. Becker, J., and Robinson, T.: Congenital multi-cystic kidney in the adult. J. Can. Assoc. Radiol., *21:*165, 1970.
47. Hipona, F. A., and Park, W. M.: Calcific renal cortical necrosis. J. Urol., *97:*961, 1967.

2

Abnormal Abdominal
Radiographic Patterns
in the Newborn

Under normal circumstances, the entire gastrointestinal tract of a newborn infant contains air shortly after birth. Absence or even a paucity of gas after the first 24 hours is considered abnormal and may be related either to an obstruction or to a poor swallowing function. The latter may be associated with prematurity, heavy sedation, or respiratory difficulties requiring a respirator.

GASTRIC DISTENTION

Neonatal gastric distention signifies gastric outlet obstruction. A single distended viscus in the epigastrium associated with a corresponding single air fluid level on the upright position is the essential radiographic feature noted on abdominal examination. This has been termed the "single bubble" sign (Fig. 2-1). The stomach in most neonates is frequently distended by gas. However, little or no gas will be detected beyond the dilated stomach when it is obstructed. Vomiting is the main clinical presentation, and in some cases occurs within the first day of life.

Disease Entities

Gastric atresia
Antral spasm and peptic ulcer
Congenital antral membrane
Duplication
Congenital hypertrophic pyloric stenosis

Differential Diagnosis

Most of the entities listed above are quite rare except for hypertrophic pyloric stenosis, which has a significant incidence. This disease presents after the 2nd week of life and never in the immediate postnatal period. Consequently when signs of gastric obstruction occur within the 1st days of life, the abdomen, with the exception of the stomach, is gasless (Fig. 2-1). Small amounts of air detected beyond the stomach indicate an incomplete obstruction, and barium studies are then necessary to identify the obstructive lesion. The radiographic features are often characteristic although occasionally subtle. An antral membrane is only recognized after the barium has passed through the membranous opening. It appears as a thinly curved, radiolucent line that bulges toward the pylorus. If, however, only small amounts of barium pass distally beyond the membrane, the findings are inconclusive and resemble antral spasm. The stomach with antral spasm will relax and alter its configuration following an interval of 5 to 10 minutes. This is an important diagnostic feature of antral spasm, and is also helpful in distinguishing spasm from the persistent gastric deformity of pyloric stenosis. The administration of glucagon to relax and dilate the stomach in antral spasm may prove advantageous in some difficult cases. The incidence of peptic ulcer associated with antral spasm is considered to be unusually high. However, the ac-

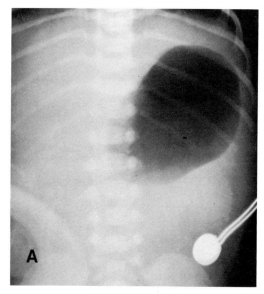
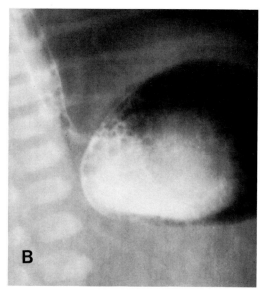

Fig. 2-1. Gastric atresia. "Single bubble" sign. (A) A large single gas-containing viscus is present in this 3-day-old infant. (The patient also had colonic atresia for which a recent colostomy had been installed. Note the linear strips of calcium that are deposited in the wall of the small bowel.) (B) Barium collected and remained within the gastric fundus. Complete atresia was encountered at surgery. This patient also had multiple areas of small bowel atresia. The intramural calcium within the normal bowel may be the result of intrauterine ischemia.

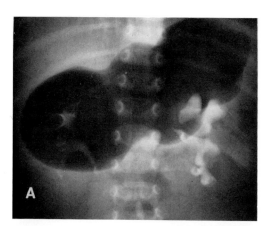

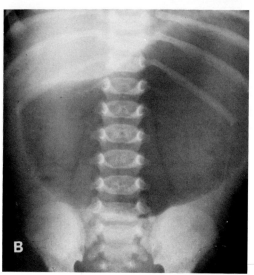

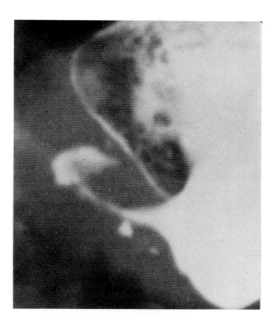

Fig. 2-3. Hypertrophic pyloric stenosis. The pyloric channel is narrow and elongated. The base of the bulb is indented by the hypertrophied muscle mass. (This indentation may also be noted within the proximal antrum.)

Fig. 2-2. Hypertrophic pyloric stenosis. (A) This film was exposed during an intravenous urogram. A markedly distended stomach with deep peristaltic contractions is present. Little gas within the colon and small bowel can be detected. (B) Another infant with severe pyloric stenosis demonstrates a massively dilated stomach with little peristalsis and almost no gas distally.

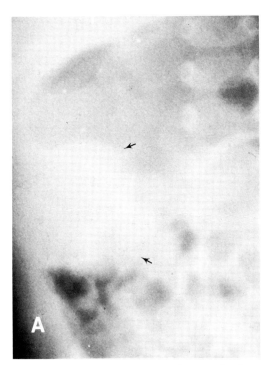 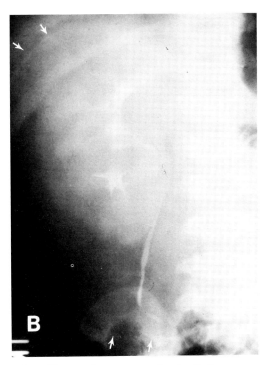

Fig. 2-4. Gastric duplication. *(A)* Gastric duplication manifested by a right upper quadrant soft-tissue mass that compresses and displaces the gastric antrum and the hepatic flexure *(arrows)*. (No barium studies were performed.) *(B)* Choledochal cyst. "Rim" sign. A huge cystic mass was palpated at birth. The intravenous pyelogram was intrinsically normal but produced a thin, opacified rim around the mass.

tual demonstration of the ulcerous niche is often impossible.

Hypertrophic pyloric stenosis must always be differentiated from antral spasm and gastric antral membrane, regardless of the time of onset. The clinical palpation of an olive-shaped mass is frequently sufficient to confirm the presence of hypertrophic pyloric stenosis. This is not always successful, and radiographic evaluation is then necessary. A markedly enlarged stomach demonstrating deep peristaltic contractions is usually seen on the abdominal radiograph (Fig. 2-2), although the stomach may be normal in caliber if the infant has just vomited. The barium study should be performed cautiously and with the infant maintained in a right lateral or exaggerated right posterior oblique position. These positions not only best demonstrate the posteriorly directed pylorus but also facilitate the passage of barium through the pylorus. The most characteristic feature is the narrow pyloric channel that appears most often as a thin, elongated tract of barium (Fig. 2-3), but occasionally as a double tract, the "railroad" sign. The following radiog-

raphic manifestations must be determined to substantiate the diagnosis when the pyloric tumor impedes any passage of barium into the channel: a dilated stomach with deep contractile waves; "shoulder" sign, produced by the proximal portion of the hypertrophied muscle mass impinging upon the barium column; and a "pyloric beak" sign, produced by the small amount of contrast material which enters the proximal portion of the pyloric canal. The duodenal bulb, when demonstrated, is frequently small and is indented at its base by the pyloric tumor (Fig. 2-3). Gastric retention alone is inadequate evidence for the determination of a diagnosis.

Gastric duplication may produce symptoms that resemble hypertrophic pyloric stenosis. The lesion is indeed rare and presents as a palpable mass associated with vomiting (Fig. 2-4). The commonly recognized radiographic appearance consists of an extrinsic mass compressing the adjacent viscera, since duplications rarely communicate with the parent structure. However, there have been several cases in which this compression resulted in an extreme elongation and narrowing of the

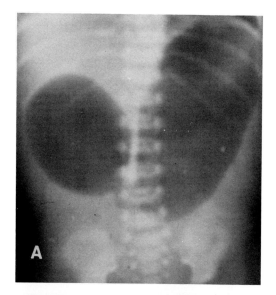

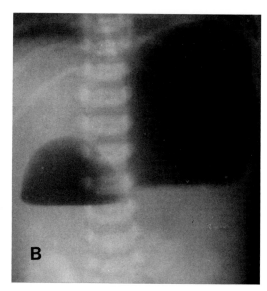

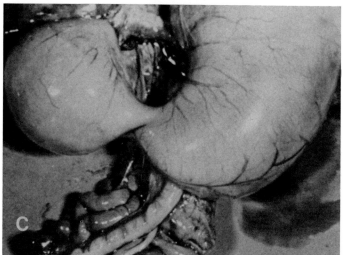

Fig. 2-5. Duodenal atresia. "Double bubble sign. *(A)* Note the large "double bubble" consisting of distended stomach and duodenum. *(B)* Two huge air fluid levels are produced on the upright film. *(C)* A surgical specimen correlating the "double bubble" with the stomach on the left and the duodenum on the right. The remaining viscera are collapsed.

canal that resembled pyloric stenosis. Occasionally, a cyst presenting in the right upper quadrant has been mistaken for a choledochal cyst, which is not necessarily associated with jaundice (Fig. 2-4B).

Although microgastria is certainly not related to gastric distention, it may be encountered in infants who present with vomiting. It is easily recognized on the gastrointestinal study. The normal stomach, when filled with barium, occupies a significant portion of the abdomen; in microgastrica, the stomach looks like a miniature of its normal counterpart.

Discussion

Pylorospasm is almost always associated with peptic ulcer disease. Neonatal hyperacidity and vagal stimulation may be respon-

sible for both. It should also be noted that patients with adrenogenital syndrome and adrenal insufficiency also present with antral spasm.

Hypertrophic pyloric stenosis is the most frequent cause of gastric obstruction. This entity often affects male infants and, for some strange reason, particulary firstborn males. The etiology of hypertrophic pyloric stenosis remains unknown. Not surprisingly, it may be related to preexisting antral spasm.

All cases of gastric atresia reported to date have involved the prepyloric area, and these cases were due to the formation of a septum covered by mucous membrane. An incomplete antral membrane probably represents a mild form of gastric atresia. These lesions are not common. The degree of

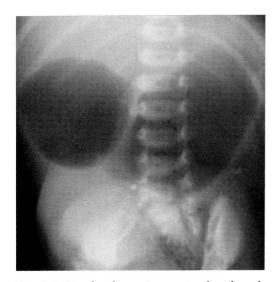

Fig. 2-6. Duodenal atresia associated with malrotation. Note the classic "double bubble" sign of duodenal atresia. However, a malrotation was also present. It is conceivable that the malrotation occurred early in fetal life and caused the duodenal atresia.

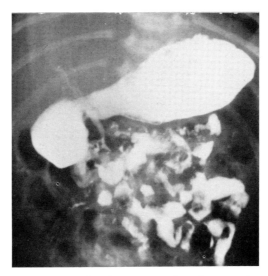

Fig. 2-7. Duodenal stenosis with reflux into the biliary tree. Gastrointestinal study reveals an incomplete obstruction in the mid-portion of the descending duodenum. Barium refluxes into the common bile duct and linear collections of air are seen within the liver. The remaining small bowel is collapsed.

obstruction and therefore the onset of symptoms is, no doubt, related to the size of the aperture within the diaphragm.

Duplication of the stomach is rarely encountered in the newborn period. The cyst may be spherical or tubular in configuration, and is generally contiguous with the greater curvature. The anomaly shares a common muscle layer and blood supply with the stomach. Surprisingly, the mucosa is not always gastric, but may consist of any form of the alimentary epithelium. Communication between the duplication and the stomach is unusual.

DUODENAL DISTENTION

Duodenal distention in newborns usually signifies duodenal obstruction and is characterized by marked gaseous distention of the stomach and the corresponding portion of duodenum proximal to the obstruction. When the obstructing lesion involves the second portion of the duodenum, a classic "double bubble" sign is formed (Fig. 2-5). Two dilated air-containing structures, the stomach and the duodenal bulb, form the major findings on the abdominal radiograph (Fig. 2-5A), and a corresponding pair of air fluid levels are encountered on the upright

position (Fig. 2-5B). These features frequently suffice. Nevertheless, subsequent contrast studies are occasionally needed for a more precise anatomic and pathologic correlation.

The clinical presentation of all duodenal lesions is similar and consists of a high obstruction, with vomiting as the main presenting symptom. Because of this, little abdominal distention is encountered. For reasons difficult to understand, hyperbilirubinemia is frequently encountered in these lesions.

Disease Entities

Duodenal atresia and stenosis
Annular pancreas
Abnormal mesenteric bands
Malrotation
Pre-duodenal portal vein
Intraluminal duodenal diaphragm

Differential Diagnosis

The radiographic differentiation between duodenal atresia and complete annular pancreas may be impossible in the immediate neonatal period, since the radiographic findings are similar. Moreover, complete annular pancreas may be associated with

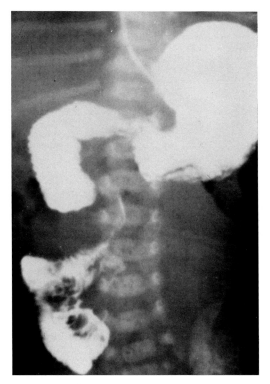

Fig. 2-8. Malrotation and obstruction by duodenal band. The duodenum is obstructed at the junction of its second and third portions by Ladd's band. The proximal jejunum decends on the right indicating malrotation.

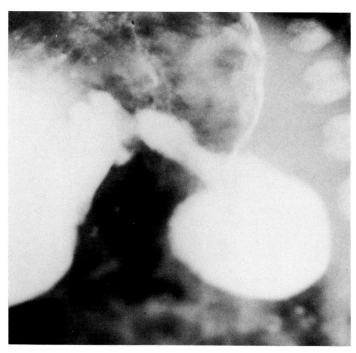

Fig. 2-9. Midgut volvulus with malrotation. The upper gastrointestinal study in an infant with vomiting reveals an obstruction within the third portion of the duodenum. The duodenal bulb is normal.

duodenal atresia. Isolated duodenal atresia, however, is far more common. It occurs early in fetal life and is therefore characterized by long-standing obstruction and *marked distention* of the duodenal bulb (Figs. 2-5, 2-6). This feature is important in differentiating duodenal atresia from duodenal obstructions of more recent origin (e.g., midgut volvulus). Stenosis indicates partial obliteration of the intestinal lumen, and as a result varying amounts of gas are visualized distal to the point of obstruction. Incomplete annular pancreas and duodenal stenosis fall into this category, and are both clinically and radiographically similar (Fig. 2-7). Both may exist for years before becoming clinically apparent. Some confusion may arise in duodenal atresia when a peculiar and rare anomaly of the common bile duct develops and allows for some air to pass distally beyond the atresia. The distal portion of the duct divides into two parts and forms an inverted Y configuration. The terminal ends insert both above and below the atretic segment.

Other forms of high obstruction of the duodenum occurring in the first day of life may be the result of abnormal mesenteric bands (Fig. 2-8) or, rarely, an anteriorly positioned portal vein. Both of these lesions cause distinct extrinsic impressions upon the second portion of the duodenum, and both may be associated with malrotation.

Malrotation with volvulus is frequently encountered in 3- or 4-day-old infants and is pathologically associated with obstruction and/or vascular compromise. The onset is acute. Although the stomach and duodenum are distended, the duodenum never obtains the size encountered in duodenal atresia. The actual level of obstruction depends upon the amount of twisted bowel and may extend anywhere near the ligament of Treitz proximally to the second portion of the duodenum (Fig. 2-9). Opacification of the gastrointestinal tract either from above or below should be done to confirm the diagnosis. Either route is satisfactory, although opacification from above is preferable. The latter is diag-

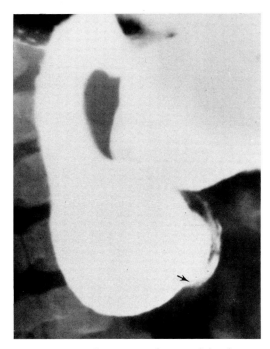

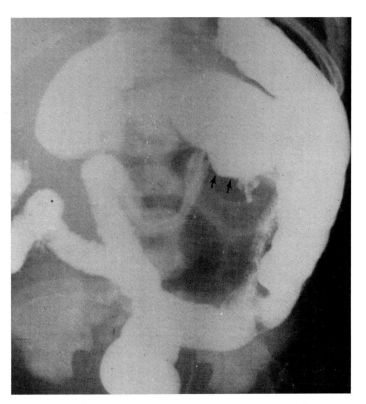

Fig. 2-10. Membranous occlusion of duodenum. Barium study reveals a distended duodenum that terminates in a balloon-like appearance resembling a wind sock. A small amount of barium passes through a narrow aperture in the membrane (*arrow*).

Fig. 2-11. Malrotation. Barium colon examination reveals the cecum within the left upper quadrant (*arrows*). This is a characteristic appearance of malrotation.

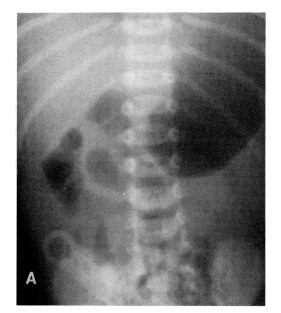

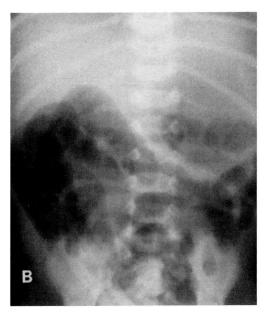

Fig. 2-12. Midgut volvulus. Progressive dilatation with infarction. (*A*) Abdominal film reveals distended loops of small bowel within the right upper quadrant. (*B*) Two days later there is progressive distention of small bowel in the right abdomen. The appearance resembles small bowel obstruction, although the accumulation of loops on the right side should suggest malrotation. At surgery, the entire small bowel was infarcted.

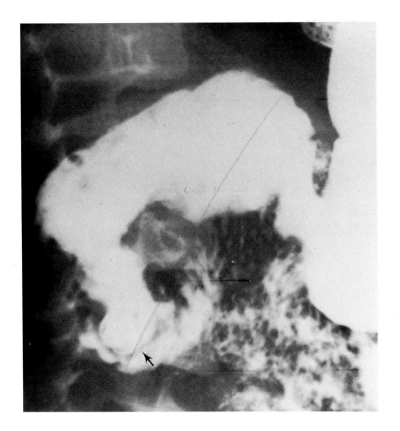

Fig. 2-13. Intraluminal diverticulum. Large intraluminal-like diverticulum that actually represents a stretched duodenal web. The wall of the web appears as a thin radiolucent structure outlined by barium on both sides of the lesion *(arrow)*.

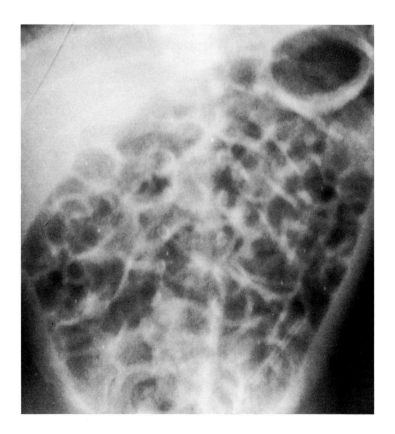

Fig. 2-14. Normal small bowel. Gas is distributed throughout the entire gastrointestinal tract. The small bowel loops manifest a polygonal configuration and the bowel diameter is equal in caliber throughout.

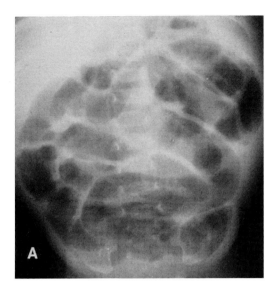

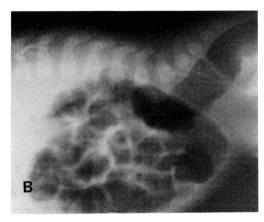

Fig. 2-15. Dilated small bowel. Pseudo-obstruction. *(A)* This infant was receiving assisted respiration by mouth, and an abdominal film was taken because of abdominal distention. The small bowel loops are markedly dilated and easily identified. A small bowel obstruction was suspected, since no obvious gas could be identified within the colon. *(B)* Prone cross-table projection easily identifies gas within the sigmoid and rectum and excludes the presence of small bowel obstruction.

nostic, easy to perform, and safe if done carefully. It has the additional advantage of excluding the presence of an intrinsic duodenal diaphragm, another anomaly frequently complicating malrotation (Fig. 2-10). This lesion causes further obstructive problems if it is not surgically removed (see p. 59). The barium enema examination is also helpful, and the demonstration of a malpositioned right colon is often diagnostic. The ascending colon and cecum in this entity, instead of descending normally into the right iliac fossa, are directed toward the left upper quadrant (Fig. 2-11). It is not uncommon to see some mobility of the cecum in newborns, and some caution must be taken when interpreting minimal positional changes of this structure. When vascular compromise occurs with volvulus, diffuse distention of the small bowel supervenes and becomes progressively worse. It may be difficult at this stage to distinguish this pattern from small bowel obstruction (Fig. 2-12). However, radiographic features suggesting peritonitis will be apparent, such as fluid in the abdomen and separation of loops of small bowel.

The presence of an intraluminal duodenal diverticulum can only be detected by means of a contrast examination of the upper gastrointestinal tract. Contrast material accumulates in a configuration resembling a wind sock. The wall of the diverticulum is visualized as a thin radiolucent structure when contrast material is present on both sides of the membrane (Fig. 2-13).

Discussion

The frequent association of duodenal atresia with other anomalies should be stressed. Duodenal atresia is noted in approximately 30 per cent of cases of Down's syndrome. This high incidence should always stimulate the search for other radiologic features of Down's syndrome (e.g., abnormal pelvis, vertebrae, and heart) whenever duodenal atresia is encountered. Duodenal atresia is also frequently associated with annular pancreas and atresia in other parts of the gastrointestinal tract, such as esophageal and anal atresia, as well as with other anomalies of the extremities and vertebral bodies.

In the annular pancreas, pancreatic tissue forms a partial or complete ring around the second portion of the duodenum. Embryologically, this arises when the free end of the ventral pancreatic bud becomes fixed and encircles the duodenum as this portion ro-

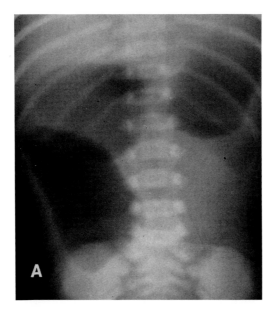

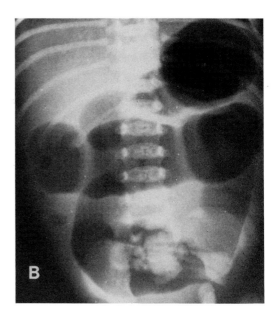

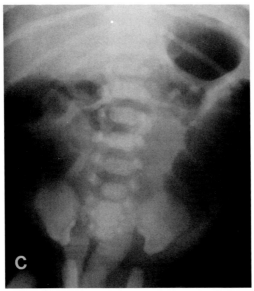

Fig. 2-16. Jejunal atresia in three patients. *(A)* The abdomen is scaphoid and only a few distended loops of bowel are present. *(B)* Mid-jejunal atresia. A longer loop of distended jejunum is present. Although the valvulae conniventes are not visualized, the minimal amount of bowel is indicative of a high obstruction. *(C)* The abdominal findings resemble the previous case although valvulae conniventes are apparent. Jejunal atresia in this patient was caused by agenesis of the dorsal mesentery. *(Continued on facing page.)*

tates to join the dorsal bud. A partial ring is responsible for incomplete duodenal obstruction and, depending upon the size of the stenosis, may or may not be clinically apparent during the neonatal period or even during the individual's lifetime. However, when a complete ring is formed or when it is associated with atresia, obstruction of the duodenal bulb and stomach appears early.

The failure of the intestines to undergo any form of normal rotation during fetal life results in abnormal position and fixation of the midgut. The midgut is that portion of the bowel that extends from the ligament of Treitz to the distal transverse colon. This portion of

the bowel herniates outside the abdomen in its early development. It begins its migration back inside the abdomen at approximately the 40-mm. stage, where it completes a 270 degree turn around the superior mesenteric artery. This rotation is usually performed by two basic segments, the duodenojejunal and the cecocolic. The return and rotation of each segment is sequential but independent of the other. Variations in rotation or fixation result in numerous abnormalities such as nonrotation, incomplete rotation, reverse rotation, and normal rotation with inadequate mesenteric peritoneal fusion. Volvulus or obstruction due to abnormal mesenteric bands may

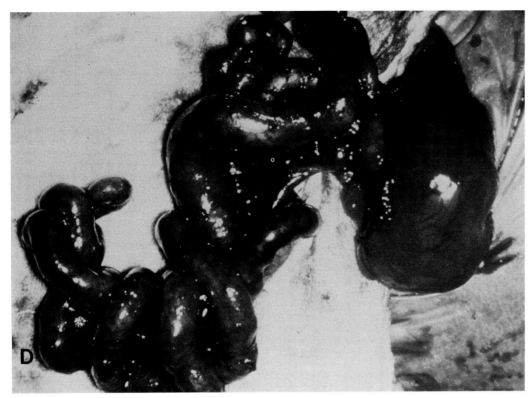

Fig. 2-16 (Continued). (D) Surgical specimen of patient with agenesis of the dorsal mesentery. Note the distal small bowel spiraled around the ileocecal vessel. This accounts for the terminology "apple peel" or "Christmas tree" deformity.

complicate any of these variations. Basically, obstruction at the level of the duodenum is due to nonrotation in which the entire midgut migrates back into the peritoneal cavity without completing its rotation around the superior mesenteric vessel. The small bowel then lies on the right side of the abdomen and the colon on the left. The mesenteric attachment of the right colon forms bands (Ladd's bands) that extend from this structure across the duodenum to the right upper quadrant. Moreover, the failure of the jejunum to rotate normally results in a narrow attachment of the small bowel mesentery to the posterior wall. This leads to excessive mobility of the small bowel and possible volvulus at the ligament of Treitz.

An intraluminal duodenal diaphragm and an anterior pre-duodenal vein are anomalies that may occur independently, but they are frequently associated with abnormal mesenteric bands and malrotation. In fact, the vein is frequently incorporated within such a band. It is important that this feature not be overlooked during surgery. This abnormally positioned vein is believed to be the result of faulty development of the portal vein, the right and left vitelline veins, and their anastomotic channels.

An intraluminal duodenal diverticulum is presently considered to represent a stretched duodenal diaphragm. The lesion most often becomes evident in the newborn period although symptoms are sometimes delayed. The diaphragm consists mainly of mucosa, and its main attachment is at the region of the ampulla of Vater. The diaphragm, when extended distally, produces a wind-sock appearance.

SMALL BOWEL DISTENTION

Normal small bowel appears on the abdominal radiograph as a conglomeration of polygonal gas structures (Fig. 2-14). Distended small bowel should be considered when this pyramidal presentation is no longer apparent and the gas filled viscera are easily identified as loops of bowel which are larger than normal in caliber (Fig. 2-15). In addition, no gas

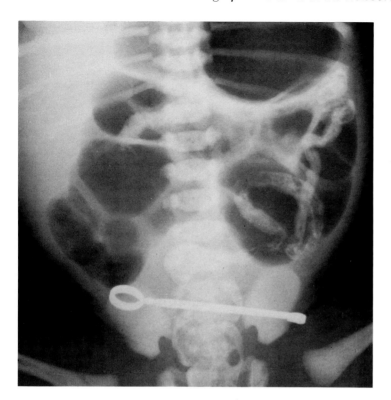

Fig. 2-17. Jejunal atresia. The abdomen is filled with distended loops of small bowel that occupy a large portion of the abdomen. The findings could be confused with ileal atresia. Residual barium is present within a narrow unused colon from a previous barium study. Note the presence of meconium within the rectum.

should be present in the colon or rectum. Distended small bowel can be distinguished from the colon by its more central location and the presence of multiple air fluid levels on an upright or cross-table study. Recently, Drs. Parvey and Seibert have recommended the use of a prone cross-table lateral projection to effectively demonstrate the distal colon. In this projection the sigmoid and rectum occupy the highest position and are easily recognized if patent (Fig. 2-15B). Nevertheless occasions do arise when it is difficult to differentiate small from large bowel, and a contrast examination of the colon is then indicated to identify this structure.

High jejunal lesions present with a clinical picture similar to duodenal obstruction (e.g., vomiting with little abdominal distention). The presence of bile within the vomitus localizes the lesion beyond the ampulla of Vater. The clinical onset of distal small bowel lesions differs; abdominal distention is more prominent and vomiting less frequent.

When the lesion involves the jejunum the gas filled loops of bowel are few in number and occupy the upper abdomen in both the supine and erect position (Fig. 2-16). The problem becomes more difficult when the

obstruction is located more distally and more of the abdomen is filled with distended bowel (Fig. 2-17).

In cases of congenital small bowel obstruction, a barium colon examination reveals a microcolon of varying caliber (Fig. 2-17). In general, the more distal the obstruction the smaller the colon, since little or no succus entericus can pass into the colon to distend it.

Disease Entities

Jejuno-ileal atresia and stenosis
    Agenesis of the dorsal mesentery
Meconium ileus
Duplication
Necrotizing enterocolitis (NEC)
Inspissated milk syndrome
Total aganglionosis of the colon
Malrotation and midgut volvulus

Differential Diagnosis

All of the lesions above are associated with small bowel dilatation. Jejuno-ileal atresia becomes evident clinically in the 1st day of life. A precise diagnosis is established only by determining the exact site of obstruction.

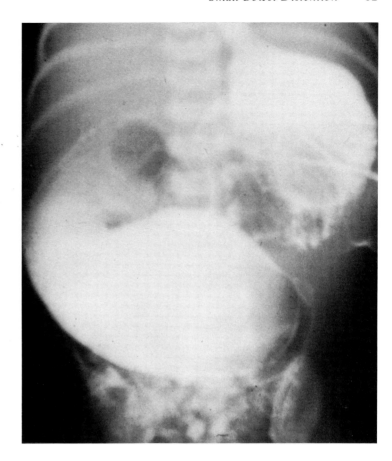

Fig. 2-18. Jejunal stenosis. Membranous occlusion. The stomach, duodenum, and proximal jejunum are markedly dilated and opacified with barium. Some barium is noted distally within collapsed bowel. This patient was originally operated upon for duodenal atresia. Persistent distention prompted the study.

This is accomplished by noting the amount, character, and position of the bowel loops on the abdominal film, or by subsequent contrast examination of the gastrointestinal tract, which may often be unnecessary and unwarranted. Complete or almost complete obstruction of the jejunum is located mainly within the upper quadrant, and only a few proximal loops of bowel are discernable (Figs. 2-16, 2-17, 2-18). Aside from atresia and stenosis, there are few other congenital obstructing lesions located so high in the bowel. Ileal obstruction is not difficult to recognize since the entire abdomen becomes filled with multiple loops of small bowel (Fig. 2-19). The pattern may be confusing if all the loops are filled with fluid. A gasless but distended abdomen should alert the physician to this possibility. A precise diagnosis of ileal atresia can only be presumed after meconium ileus, total colonic aganglionosis, necrotizing enterocolitis, and duplication have been excluded. The distended bowel encountered in uncomplicated obstructive lesions is intrin-sically normal. The bowel wall is smooth and regular, and distinct air fluid levels are apparent. This is not the situation in meconium ileus and necrotizing enterocolitis. Both of these lesions may present as small bowel obstructions, but are accompanied by specific and distinctive abnormalities within the bowel. The bowel wall in necrotizing enterocolitis is damaged and inflammatory, and ischemic changes manifested as thickened edematous bowel may occasionally be identified in the right lower quadrant (Fig. 2-20). The presence of intramural air is even more significant (see p. 77). An important radiographic feature that has become synonymous with meconium ileus is the absence of obvious and distinct air fluid levels within the distal small bowel in comparison to the remaining proximal bowel (Fig. 2-21). The meconium in this entity is abnormally thick and collects within the ileum. Fluid is trapped and contained within this abnormal meconium and does not easily become isolated to produce air fluid levels. The thick meconium also produces

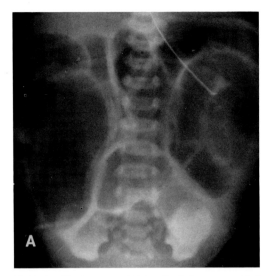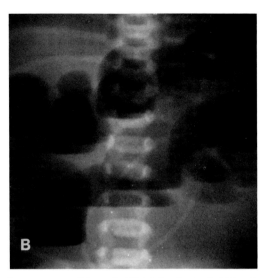

Fig 2-19. Ileal atresia. *(A)* Marked distention of almost the entire small bowel. *(B)* Multiple air fluid levels occupy most of the abdomen on the upright examination.

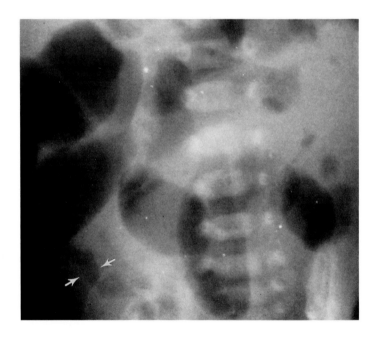

Fig. 2-20. Necrotizing enterocolitis. Small bowel distention. Abdominal distention in this patient is due to dilated loops of small bowel. However, the terminal ileum and cecum are narrowed and demonstrate mucosal thickening *(arrows).*

areas of increased radiodensity and a bubbly appearance within the right lower quadrant. The smallest microcolons have been associated with meconium ileus (Figs. 2-21, 2-22). Incidentally, carefully performed Gastrografin enemas with purposeful reflex into the small bowel have been proposed recently as a therapeutic means of relieving the obstruction in meconium ileus. The high osmolarity of Gastrografin stimulates a large outpouring of water that not only softens the meconium but functions as a lubricant.

The radiologic features of inspissated milk syndrome resemble meconium ileus, meconium plug syndrome, neonatal Hirschsprung's disease, and even necrotizing enterocolitis. Abdominal examination reveals a pattern of small bowel obstruction containing intraluminal masses surrounded by gas, with few or no fluid levels in the affected area. The patient is usually a premature infant who has passed a normal meconium stool, and in whom the obstructive findings become evident approximately 5 days after

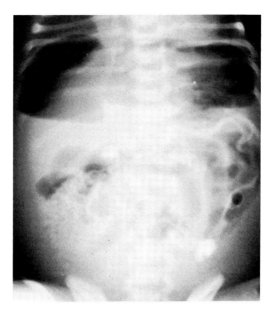

Fig. 2-21. Meconium ileus. Upright examination. A large pneumoperitoneum is present. The diagnosis of meconium ileus is indicated by the mottled, "soap bubble" appearance within the right lower quadrant. The small bowel is distended, and no air fluid levels are produced. Some minimal residual barium is visualized within a microcolon.

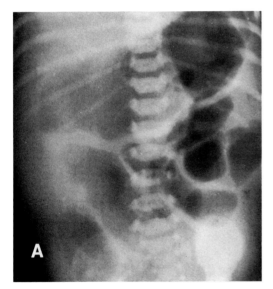

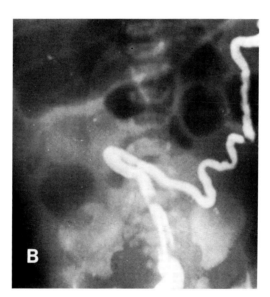

Fig. 2-22. Meconium ileus. *(A)* Note the increased radiodensity within the right lower quadrant. This is associated with a mottled appearance of inspissated meconium. *(B)* On the barium examination, a microcolon is obvious. Only the descending colon was filled.

the institution of artifical milk feedings. A carefully performed contrast study generally reveals a normal or slightly narrowed colon that contains multiple small filling defects.

Duplications are rarely symptomatic in newborns. However, when they obstruct, the findings resemble any uncomplicated small bowel obstruction. Duplications may occur anywhere throughout the entire gastrointestinal tract, but they are more frequently located in the ileocecal region. The diagnosis is suggested when a soft-tissue mass is found compressing and distorting bowel wall.

Small bowel obstruction is frequently the presenting feature of total aganglionosis of the colon. The aganglionic segment occasionally extends into the terminal ileum. Barium studies of the colon reveal a variety of changes. The colon may be normal in length and caliber, short in length but normal in caliber, short in both length and caliber, or "comma-shaped." The "comma-shaped" colon appears when the colon is small and

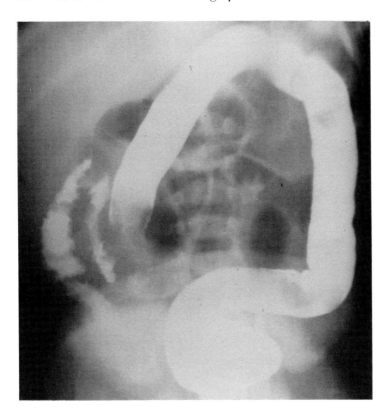

Fig. 2-23. Total aganglionosis of the colon with probable necrotizing enterocolitis. Barium studies in a patient with previous episodes of bloody diarrhea reveals a colon of normal caliber on the left. The sigmoid and splenic flexures, however, are foreshortened and a "comma-shaped" appearance is produced. The right colon is narrowed and edematous. This represents a healing stricture of necrotizing enterocolitis. At surgery, the entire colon was devoid of ganglion cells.

both the splenic and hepatic flexures are poorly developed (Fig. 2-23). Another radiographic pattern indicating the presence of total colonic aganglionosis is "jejunalization" of the colon. This implies that the normal haustral markings of the colon are replaced by circumferential markings resembling the plicae circulares of the small bowel. Both of these findings are strongly suggestive but not specific. Biopsy is required if a definitive clinical diagnosis cannot be established in the presence of the colonic findings above.

As mentioned in the section on Duodenal Distention (see p. 57), midgut volvulus with secondary vascular compromise presents with small bowel dilatation (Fig. 2-12). A symptom-free interval of approximately 3 days and the radiologic findings of peritonitis are strongly suggestive of its presence.

Discussion

Jejuno-ileal atresia, in contrast to duodenal atresia, is not associated with other important congenital anomalies. Multiple areas of involvement, however, are frequently present. The suggested etiology of atresia has shifted away from the embryologic consideration of faulty recanalization of the bowel to the pos-

sibility of a vascular insult occurring sometime during fetal life. In other words, atresia is now considered the end stage of intrauterine segmental bowel infarction that has undergone complete disintegration and resorption. This phenomemon has been reproduced in experimental animals and explains the presence of inflammatory changes encountered within and around the area of atresia. Incomplete recanalization, however, may be responsible for the development of some atresias (e.g., familial atresia and the duodenal atresia noted in Down's syndrome). Multiple gastrointestinal atresias resembling a string of pearls, with intraluminal calcifications and cystic dilatation of the bile ducts have recently been described. It has also been suggested that intrauterine vascular compromise may be responsible for gastrointestinal duplication. In one series of patients with gastrointestinal duplication, a large percentage of lesions were found intimately associated with areas of small bowel atresia.

An unusual abnormality associated with high jejunal atresia is agenesis of the dorsal mesentery (Fig 2-16C). In this anomaly the primary mesenteric branches supplying the ileum and jejunum are the ileocecal and mar-

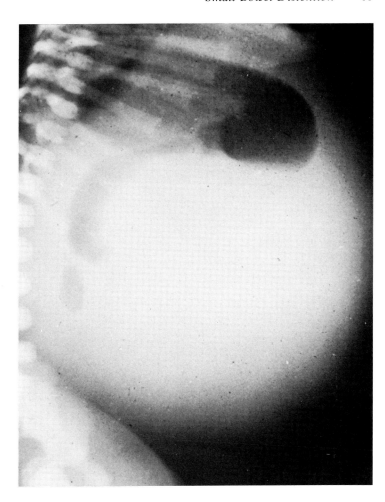

Fig. 2-24. "Pseudocyst." Meconium ileus. A huge soft-tissue mass occupies the entire abdomen and displaces and compresses all viscera.

ginal arteries. The remaining distal small bowel is spiraled around this vessel, and the term "apple peel" or "Christmas tree" deformity has been utilized to describe it.

Recent attempts to classify atresias on both a morphologic and prognostic basis may prove to be worthwhile. Type I, single atresia with a simple diaphragm, has a good prognosis. Type II, single atresia with discontinuity of the bowel, also has a good prognosis. Type III, multiple atresias, has a poor prognosis; there is no incidence of association with cystic fibrosis, and postoperative malabsorption occurs among treated patients. Type IV, the "apple peel" or Christmas tree" deformity, has a poor prognosis; there is no incidence of association with cystic fibrosis, and postoperative malabsorption occurs among all surviving patients treated.

The association of meconium ileus with cystic fibrosis is almost 100 per cent and occurs as the presenting manifestation in approximately 20 per cent of patients. The un-derlying cause of obstruction is the presence of abnormally thick meconium that accumulates within the ileum. This is the result of abnormal secretions produced by altered small intestinal glands. Abnormal pancreatic secretions also play a role but are only secondary in importance. Obstruction is only one event that may occur with meconium ileus, and at times other complications arise that further reduce the ultimate survival of the infant (e.g., perforation, atresia, volvulus, pseudocyst). Type I and Type II have been seen with meconium ileus, and result when the thick meconium not only obstructs but also interferes with local blood perfusion. Volvulus is another complication found with meconium ileus and may be associated with gangrene and peritonitis. Rarely, a large cystic mass or a "pseudocyst" is found. The mass may occupy the entire abdomen and contains necrotic intestinal tissue. The pseudocyst is a result of a relatively late-occurring intrauterine volvulus (Fig. 2-24).

Table 2-1. **Neonatal Small Bowel Distention**

Entity	Air Fluid Levels	Mass Appearance	Abnormal Gas Collections	Colon
Atresia	Yes			Microcolon. More pronounced with distal lesions.
Meconium ileus	None or few (RLQ)	Yes (RLQ)	Cystic bubbly appearance within mass	Severe microcolon
Duplication	Yes	Yes	None	Normal
Necrotizing enterocolitis	Yes		Pneumatosis intestinalis (cystic and linear)	Normal in calibre Mucosa ulcerated
Inspissated milk syndrome	None or few (RLQ)	Yes	Gas present around but not within mass	Normal
Total aganglionosis of the colon	Yes			Normal Reduced in calibre Reduced in length Comma shaped

Necrotizing enterocolitis frequently presents with small bowel distention that in many aspects simulates obstruction. Although the colon distends in necrotizing enterocolitis, the incidence of small bowel distention alone as the predominant radiographic feature is significant. In fact, we have begun to recognize small bowel dilatation, in association with acidosis and abdominal distention, as the earliest manifestation of the disease. In some patients the combination of these findings actually precedes the obvious clinical onset of the disease. However, gas-producing organisms eventually penetrate the necrotic bowel wall, and the classic features of pneumatosis soon become apparent.

Inspissated milk syndrome is a disease of premature infants who manifest a deficient capacity to absorb protein and amino acids. Rarely, high-calorie feeding overburdens their absorptive capacity and results in formation of putty-like milk masses which obstruct. Although the radiographic appearance may be confused with many of the other obstructing disease entities, the temporal onset of the disease following milk feedings and after the passage of normal meconium stool is characteristic. This relationship is rarely altered.

COLONIC DISTENTION

As in other parts of the gastrointestinal tract, a distended colon in the first days of life usually indicates obstruction. Identifying the colon may be difficult if the small bowel is correspondingly dilated and if the haustral pattern is not fully developed. However, the ascending and descending colons typically occupy a vertical position along the lateral abdominal walls and so are easily recognized (Fig. 2-25). A prone, cross-table examination is valuable in identifying distal colon (Fig. 2-15). In most situations, it is still necessary to resort to contrast examination of the colon to define the location and the nature of the obstructing lesion. The study should be done with barium using a straight catheter. Water-soluble contrast agents and the presence of a distended balloon catheter may distort some of the pathologic findings. Moreover, if water-soluble enemas are used initially, such as in the meconium plug syndrome, a repeat examination utilizing barium is always recommended to fully exclude underlying Hirschsprung's disease.

Disease Entities
Anorectal anomalies (imperforate anus, ectopic anus)
Hirschsprung's disease (aganglionosis, megacolon)
Meconium plug syndrome
Neonatal small-left-colon syndrome
Colonic atresia

Differential Diagnosis

Anorectal anomalies are the result of incomplete descent of the hindgut and are recognized in newborns by the presence of a rec-

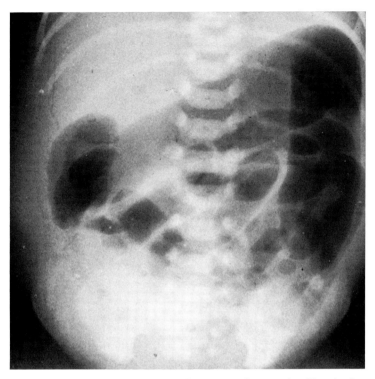

Fig. 2-25. Colonic distention. Membranous occlusion. The dilated colon is recognized by its anatomical position. The ascending and descending colons occupy vertical positions and the transverse colon extends horizontally across the abdomen.

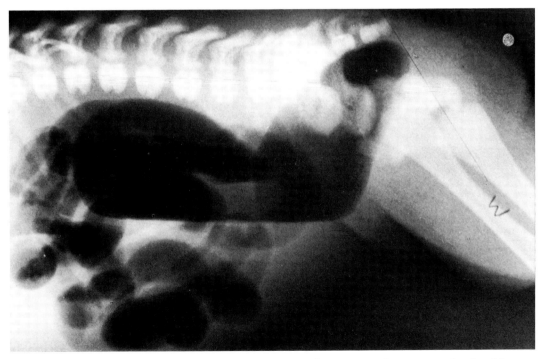

Fig. 2-26. Anal atresia. Cross-table, lateral, prone projection demonstrates the maximum height of the rectum as outlined by air. A metallic marker is placed at the region of the anal dimple. The soft-tissue space between the closed end of the rectum and the metallic tip is easily measured. Note the superior location of the rectum in comparison to the remaining bowel.

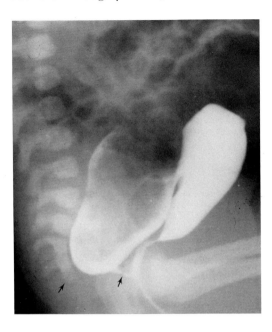

Fig. 2-27. Anal atresia. High lesion. Retrograde cystography reveals a fistulous communication between the posterior urethra and the dilated atretic rectum *(right arrow).* The lower sacral bodies are fused *(left arrow).* Both features indicate a high obstruction.

tal dimple and no anus. The level of the obstruction in this anomaly varies but is a significant feature in determining the ultimate prognosis of the patient and the type of surgery to be performed. Basically, the puborectalis muscle is intact in low lesions and disrupted when the obstruction is high. The development of this muscle sling is important, since it alone assumes the function of the anal sphincters which are always underdeveloped in these anomalies. Many radiologic studies have therefore been proposed to estimate the end point of the hindgut. Insertion of a thermometer or metallic markers into the region of the rectal dimple in conjunction with an upside down examination of the abdomen has been utilized for many years. This study is not always accurate because of the presence of impacted meconium and rectal spasm. A cross-table lateral prone projection is easier to perform but equally inaccurate (Fig. 2-26). Other studies to determine the anatomic level of the muscle sling have been recommended, such as the addition of the pubococcygeal line or more recently with the M line. These are approximations and therefore have certain inherent inaccuracies. The pubococcygeal line is drawn from the sacrococcygeal junction to the mid-pubic bone, and the M line is a horizontal line placed through the junction of the medial and lower third of the ischia (Fig 2-26). The M line more closely approximates the level of the puborectalis muscle,

and is perhaps more reliable. Certain anatomic abnormalities are associated with the descent of the hindgut and thus correspond best to the level of the lesion (e.g., high lesions are always associated with fistulas to the lower genitourinary tract). Linear air radiolucencies, directed toward or within the bladder or urethra in males or to the vagina in females, are therefore excellent radiographic criteria for such a lesion. Low lesions are always present when the fistula terminates externally. Contrast studies should always be performed in patients in whom no external opening has been found. This can be done by means of retrograde cystography or barium examination following construction of a colostomy (Figure 2-27). Anomalies of the spine and genitourinary system are frequently encountered and relatively specific. Abnormalities of the sacrum occur in approximately 60 per cent of patients with high obstructions (Fig. 2-27). For example, deformities of S3 and S4 indicate a high lesion and an underdeveloped puborectalis sling.

A properly performed barium colon examination frequently differentiates and identifies all diseases affecting the colon. Hirschsprung's disease is characterized by a relatively narrow aganglionic distal segment (Fig. 2-28). The colon proximal to the aganglionic segment is dilated. The *transition zone* is defined as that junction where abnormal and normal colon meet and is identified radiographically as the point where an

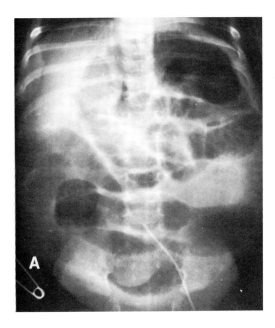

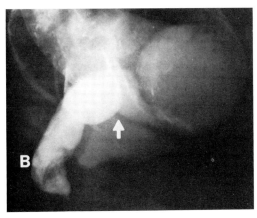

Fig. 2-28. Hirschsprung's disease. *(A)* Radiograph of the abdomen reveals distended large and small bowel. The colon may be difficult to identify. *(B)* Barium study of the same patient demonstrates a marked difference in the size of the lumen between the rectum and sigmoid. The junction represents the transition zone *(arrow).*

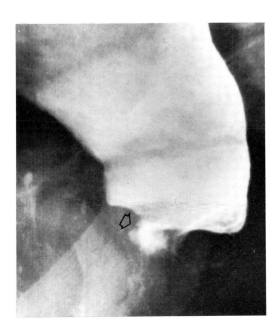

Fig. 2-29. Hirschsprung's disease. A lateral rectal film in a patient with Hirschsprung's disease demonstrates the relatively short aganglionic segment in the rectum *(arrow).*

immediate change in bowel width occurs. The transition zone in Hirschsprung's disease is frequently located at the rectosigmoid junction (Figs. 2-28B, 2-29). A similar reduction in caliber of the distal colon also characterizes the meconium plug syndrome . However, in this entity a large filling defect consisting of dry meconium is readily identified within the barium column at the site of dilatation (Fig. 2-30). Occasionally, the colon in Hirschsprung's disease is not obviously dis-

proportionate in width in the immediate neonatal period. However, close observation and measurement reveals a smaller transverse diameter in the rectum when compared to the sigmoid. Hirschsprung's disease must also be suspected when abnormal contractions or peristaltic activity of the distal colon are observed. These appear as serrations or thumb-print contractions and are helpful, but, nonetheless, are nonspecific findings. More important is the retention of

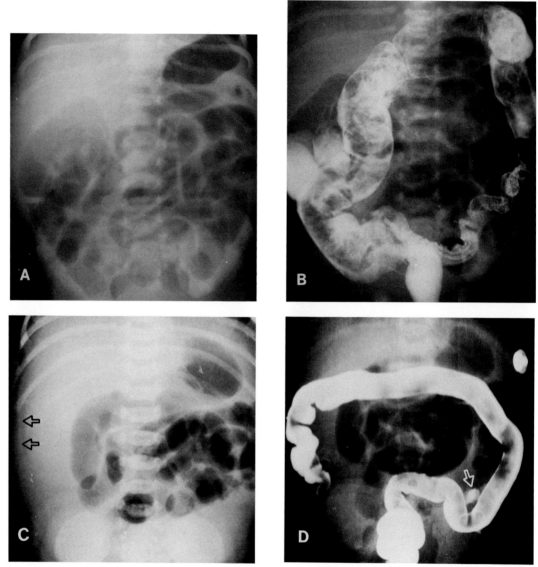

Fig. 2-30. Meconium plug syndrome. *(A)* Both small and large bowel are distended although the descending colon is not visualized. *(B)* Barium colon examination reveals a collapsed distal colon. Dilatation occurs abruptly in the middle of the descending colon, and large filling defects (meconium) fill the remaining colon. *(C)* A patient who presented with meconium peritonitis and meconium plug syndrome. Intraperitoneal calcification on the hapatic surface is poorly visualized *(arrows)*. *(D)* Note the perforation of the sigmoid colon *(arrow)*. This patient was eventually shown to have cystic fibrosis.

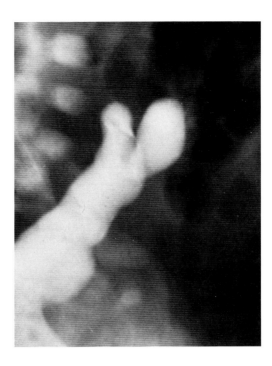

Fig. 2-31. Colonic atresia. Membranous obstruction. The barium colon terminates abruptly at the junction of the sigmoid and descending colon. The caliber of the distal colon is abnormally small in comparison to the dilated proximal colon. Obstruction was caused by a membrane (see Fig. 2-25).

barium within the proximal ganglionic colon on delayed abdominal radiographs exposed 24, 48, and even 72 hours after the original study. Barium studies performed at a later date in patients with meconium plug syndrome following the removal of the plug are always normal unless Hirschsprung's disease is also present.

Long-segment Hirschsprung's disease or aganglionosis involving the entire colon and perhaps the terminal ileum presents during the first 3 months of life as intermittent small bowel obstruction (see p. 63).

A recently described entity strikingly similar to the meconium plug syndrome is neonatal small-left-colon syndrome. The left colon is small and the proximal colon dilated. Differentiation on radiographic criteria alone may be difficult, and a biopsy of the bowel wall is often necessary. The disease occurs predominantly in infants of diabetic mothers, and careful observation has demonstrated an increased amount of subcutaneous fat in these infants.

Colonic atresia is a rare occurrence and is supected when the barium enema study reveals the presence of an obstructed microcolon (Fig. 2-31).

Discussion

The pathophysiology of Hirschsprung's disease is still unclear, and there is no ac-cepted explanation of why absence of ganglion cells in a segment of bowel wall results in contraction of that segment. Current interest has been directed toward the non-adrenergic inhibitory nervous system of the intestine, and recent experiments suggest that absence of this system in the aganglionic portion of bowel results in the pathophysiologic features of this disease. The disease frequently involves the distal colon beginning at the level of the rectosigmoid. It should be emphasized that the transition zone noted radiologically does not always correspond to the actual histologic junction of the aganglionic and ganglionic bowel. This junction is sometimes located more proximally in the colon, and biopsy of the bowel wall during surgery is necessary before a colostomy is performed. Furthermore, there is recent evidence to suggest that the colon above the aganglionic segment may be only hypoganglionic. (A true all-or-nothing relationship need not exist.) Colostomy performed in this area produces poor results. Hirschsprung's disease is rare in premature infants and affects males more commonly than females in a ratio of approximately 4 to 1. Total colonic aganglionosis or long-segment Hirschsprung's disease is slightly different. These lesions have a definite familial incidence and affect both sexes equally. It is often difficult to recognize aganglionosis of

222222222222222222

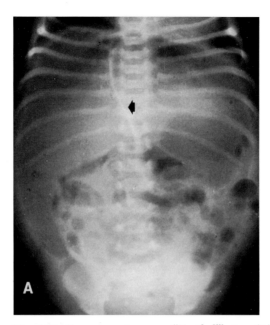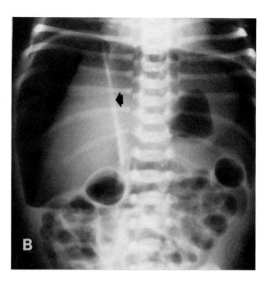

Fig. 2-32. Pneumoperitoneum. "Football" sign. *(A)* A massive, oval collection of air occupies the entire abdomen. The falciform ligament appears as an "S-shaped" line in the epigastrium *(arrow)*. *(B)* An upright examination in another patient with massive free air. A huge air fluid level is produced, and the air displaces the liver and spleen from the diaphragm. The falciform ligament is well outlined *(arrow)*.

an entire colon since the appearance of the colon is quite variable. It may be either normal in length and caliber, or short in length but of normal caliber, or small in both length and caliber (microcolon). Rectal biopsy is therefore highly recommended in patients presenting with any of these radiographic features, and in whom no diagnosis has been made. The etiology of Hirschsprung's disease is still unknown. Fetal arrest of the craniocaudad migration of neuroblasts has been suggested. This most frequently stops at the rectosigmoid junction. The failure of neuroblasts to mature and become ganglion cells may also be responsible. The last cells to mature are located in the distal colon.

Meconium plug syndrome is due to a basic functional disturbance of the colon that causes excessive water resorption and therefore a dry and hard meconium. Since the meconium plug syndrome has been associated with Hirschsprung's and fibrocystic disease, these two entities should always be excluded in patients presenting with this syndrome (Fig. 2-30).

The neonatal, small left-sided colon bears striking resemblance both clinically and radiographically to the meconium plug syndrome. However, biopsy studies reveal small cells of immature neuronal character in contrast to the normal structures described in the meconium plug syndrome. There is also a high incidence of maternal diabetes in this entity.

Anorectal anomalies have undergone considerable change in classification. More recently the high-ending hindgut with either a cutaneous or internal fistula has been called ectopic anus. Imperforate anus refers to the blind-ending bowel with no communication noted internally or externally (e.g., membranous imperforate anus, or anal atresia). Rectal and anal atresia are rare, and in both the anus is open and present.

PNEUMOPERITONEUM

Free air within the peritoneal cavity almost always indicates gastrointestinal perforation. Few other abnormalities account for its occurrence in newborns.

In the supine position free air accumulates beneath the anterior abdominal wall and projects as a vague, oval, radiolucency that may occupy the entire abdomen. This appearance has been termed the "football" sign (Fig.

Table 2-2. Neonatal Colonic Distention

Entity	Colon	Biopsy
Hirschsprung's disease	Transition zone at rectosigmoid. In newborns, altered peristalsis in aganglionic area. Delayed films demonstrate retention of contrast material.	No ganglion cells
Meconium plug syndrome	Transition zone also noted. Filling defect within proximally dilated colon. Distal colon narrow. Returns to normal after plug is removed.	Ganglion cells present
Neonatal small-left-colon syndrome	Similar to meconium plug when only left side is involved. Filling defect may not be visualized and changes do not revert back to normal.	Immature neuronal development
Colon atresia	Obstructed colon. Severe microcolon distal to atresia.	

2-32A). One must be aware of this subtle presentation since an abdominal supine examination may be the only study performed. Other structures located on the anterior abdominal wall are also outlined by air in this position. The falciform ligament extends upward from the umbilicus toward the liver and is projected as a linear radiodensity medially or at times just to the right of the midline in the upper abdomen (Fig. 2-32). The urachus occasionally produces a corresponding linear radiodensity that projects inferiorly from the umbilicus toward the bladder within the lower abdomen. The umbilical arteries are occasionally similarly identified.

Small amounts of free air are more difficult to detect in this position. However, air lying freely within the peritoneum adjacent to bowel wall produces an exquisitely sharp delineation of the bowel wall (Fig. 2-33). Normally only the internal mucosal surface of bowel, and not the entire wall thickness, is seen. Another feature, perhaps even more subtle, is an increase in radiolucency over the liver.

An additional projection (e.g., prone, upright, or cross-table lateral) not only helps confirm the presence of free air but, moreover, facilitates the detection of small amounts. Consequently, multiple projections are always recommended when examining an infant suspected of having abdominal disease. A distinct air fluid level within the abdominal cavity is easily demonstrated in the upright and the cross-table lateral examinations (Fig. 2-32B). In the prone position free air collects in the lateral peritoneal recesses and pushes the liver and spleen medially. Very small amounts of air can then be identified.

Disease Entities

Necrotizing enterocolitis
Gastrointestinal perforation—spontaneous or traumatic
Pneumomediastinum
Gastrointestinal atresia and other obstructions

Differential Diagnosis

Pneumoperitoneum is a common complication of necrotizing enterocolitis. It can occur at any time during the course of the disease and occasionally is the presenting manifestation. Concomitant air within the bowel wall or within the portal venous system pinpoints the diagnosis (Fig. 2-34; see pp. 77, 82).

Perforation of the stomach and colon together account for 75 per cent of all spontaneous perforations. Radiographic features that help locate the site and nature of the perforation are the amount of free air, the distribution of air within the bowel, and the time of onset. For example, gastric perforation occurring during the 1st day of life pro-
(Text continued on p. 76.)

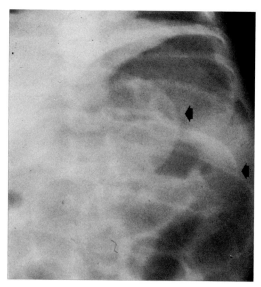

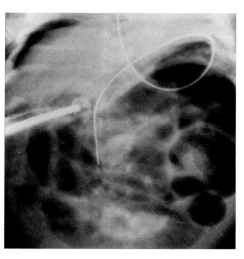

Fig. 2-33. Pneumoperitoneum. "Double wall" sign. The wall of the small bowel is sharply delineated (arrows). A small perforation of the distal ileum was discovered at surgery.

Fig. 2-34. Necrotizing enterocolitis and pneumoperitoneum. An abdominal radiograph demonstrates a crescent-shaped collection of free air beneath the right diaphragm. The entire small bowel is distended and intramural air (pneumatosis intestinalis) outlines the ascending colon.

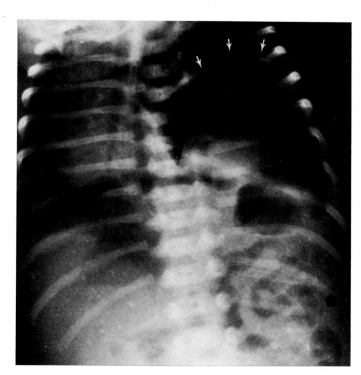

Fig. 2-35. Pneumoperitoneum. Perforated gastric fundus. The tip of the tube (black arrow) is well outside the stomach. Free air on the left outlines a severely elevated left hemidiaphragm (white arrows). Perforation of the greater curvature of the stomach and an eventration were simultaneously diagnosed and confirmed.

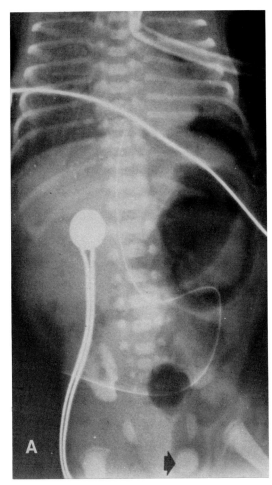

Fig. 2-36. Pneumoperitoneum, retroperitoneum and pulmonary disease. *(A)* This interesting radiograph was taken in a patient with respiratory distress syndrome. In addition to the pulmonary findings, interstitial emphysema and pneumomediastinum are also present. Air, however, had dissected retrograde into the retroperitoneum, peritoneum, and the scrotum outlining the left testicle *(arrow)*. *(B)* Pneumomediastinum is better defined on the lateral projection. The left kidney is surrounded by perirenal air. *(C)* Note the pneumoperitoneum in a patient with hyaline membrane disease and interstitial emphysema. The abdominal air disappeared 24 hours later.

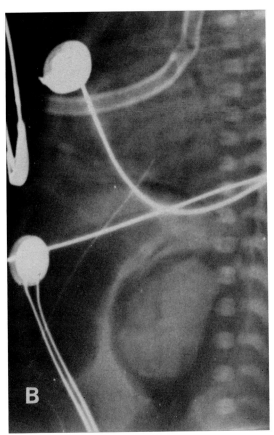

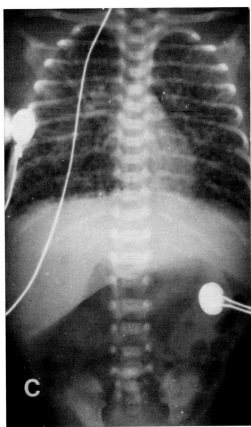

Table 2-3. Pneumoperitoneum

Entity	Amount of Gas	Stomach	Small Bowel	Colon	Other Characteristics
Spontaneous					
Stomach					
Early	Huge	None or little gas	No gas	No gas	
Delayed		No air fluid levels	Gas	Gas	
Colon	Huge	Gas and air fluid level	Gas	Gas	
Small bowel	Moderate	Gas and air fluid level	Gas	Gas	
Necrotizing enterocolitis	Moderate to huge	Gas and air fluid level	Dilated	Dilated	Pneumatosis
Obstruction	Moderate to huge	Gas and air fluid level	Dilated when atresia in small bowel or colon	Dilated when colon obstructed	
Traumatic	Huge	None if stomach perforated. Gas and air fluid levels when other viscus is involved.	Dilated	Dilated	History of tube insertion
Pneumo-mediastinum	Moderate to huge	Gas	Gas	Gas	Thoracic manifestations

duces a large pneumoperitoneum with little or no air present within the remaining gastrointestinal tract. However, a stomach that perforates sometime later (e.g., the 3rd or 4th day) still produces a large pneumoperitoneum but also results in air within the stomach and the remainder of the gastrointestinal tract. However, only small amounts of gastric contents remain within the stomach, and minimal or no air fluid levels are found in this structure on the upright examination (Fig. 2-32). The presence of a large air fluid level in the stomach should suggest another viscus, such as the colon, as the site of perforation. If a naso-gastric tube is inserted and the tip of the tube is identified outside the anticipated confines of the stomach, the perforation is always located along the greater curvature of the fundus (Fig. 2-35). However, the introduction of a tube or contrast material to determine the site of perforation is neither necessary nor recommended. Small amounts of free air are usually associated with small bowel perforation, since the amount of air present is inherently smaller (Fig. 2-34).

Traumatic perforations are frequently iatrogenic, and the temporal relationship between obvious trauma, such as tube insertion, and the occurrence of pneumoperitoneum is evidence enough. The incorrect placement of

a naso-jejunal tube within the duodenum for the purpose of hyperalimentation has recently been described as another cause of perforation of the duodenum. This occurs approximately 6 to 12 hours after the tube has been inserted. The tube, for reasons unknown, becomes hard and rigid when in the bowel.

An unusual cause of pneumoperitoneum is pneumomediastinum or pneumothorax secondary to pulmonary disease (Fig. 2-36). Air penetrates into the abdomen by way of normal diaphragmatic openings. This is probably the only pathologic event in the neonatal period that produces a pneumoperitoneum without bowel perforation. The findings of pulmonary disease, such as hyaline membrane disease and free air elsewhere within the thorax, are thus significant.

A bowel obstruction causing perforation, as in atresia or meconium ileus, produces distended or abnormal bowel in addition to pneumoperitoneum (Fig. 2-21). Bowel distention accompanying necrotizing enterocolitis takes the form of either a small bowel dilatation or an ileus (Fig. 2-34).

Discussion

The most common cause of pneumoperitoneum in the newborn is necrotizing enterocolitis. This occurs following the transmural

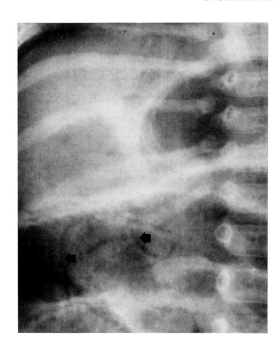

Fig. 2-37. Pneumatosis intestinalis with necrotizing enterocolitis. The entire radiographic spectrum of intramural air (e.g., bubbly, linear, and circular collections indicated by arrows) is depicted in this patient. In addition, air is present within the portal venous system.

dissection of air through the diseased bowel wall. Gastric perforation accounts for approximately 50 per cent of all idiopathic neonatal perforations. A number of theories have been proposed to explain the cause of idiopathic gastrointestinal perforation. The embryologic concept of poorly developed muscle fibers along the greater curvature of the stomach is no longer acceptable, and greater emphasis has been directed toward the "diving seal reflex" caused by perinatal hypoxia and stress. Forty-five per cent of infants with spontaneous perforation manifest some detectable asphyxia during the perinatal period. A similar pathogenesis is probably partially responsible for necrotizing enterocolitis. The "diving seal reflex" also occurs in infants in whom there is no obvious asphyxia or stress. However, minor asphyxia is probably induced as the umbilical cord is squeezed in the birth canal during the normal course of delivery. In most infants this episode is instantaneous and equilibrium is quickly restored. However, in some the reflex persists for longer periods, and a state of decreased perfusion of the gastrointestinal tract ensues. Additional stress such as distention is also a causative factor. Gastric fluid in the supine position produces an air lock mechanism within the fundus. This results in increased pressure within this structure and partially accounts for the high incidence of gastric perforation.

Traumatic perforation can occur at any time during the neonatal period and has been attributed to excessive pressure on the abdominal wall, improper or forced insertion of a rectal thermometer, therapeutic oxygen administration, and forceful resuscitation.

More recently hyperalimentation by means of naso-jejunal tubes has resulted in minute perforations of the duodenum. The tube is made from a polyvinyl plastic that undergoes considerable alteration in consistency after remaining in the bowel for 6 to 12 hours. The tube is transformed from a soft pliable structure into one that is hard and rigid. Consequently, if the tubes are malpositioned within the duodenum, they should never be manipulated externally or be allowed to move spontaneously as a result of peristalsis. The rigid tube poorly negotiates the sharp turns of the relatively fixed duodenum and should be removed before it perforates this viscus.

PNEUMATOSIS INTESTINALIS

Pneumatosis intestinalis (intramural gas) in newborns most often signifies severe disease of the bowel. Radiographically, it is characterized by localized bubbly collections of air, diffuse linear strips of air outlining the extent of the bowel wall, and double rings of gas radiolucencies when viewed on end (Fig. 2-37). The bubbly appearance is believed to be caused by gas located within the sub-

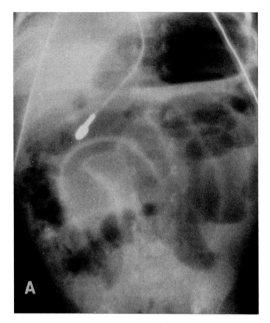
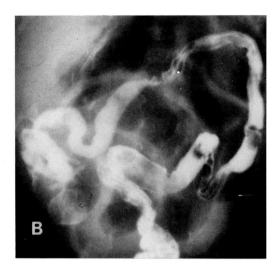

Fig. 2-38. Pneumatosis intestinalis. *(A)* A "soap bubble" appearance is present within the right lower quadrant. The small bowel is severely dilated suggesting obstruction. This pattern is not uncommon in necrotizing enterocolitis. *(B)* A barium examination was performed on this infant for undetermined reasons, and a narrow colon, possibly on the basis of stricture formation, is outlined. There is also perforation of the cecum with extravasation of contrast material.

mucosa and represents an early manifestation of the disease (Fig. 2-38). Subsequent penetration of gas into the bowel wall between the muscle layers and under the serosa results in a linear distribution (Fig. 2-39). Pneumatosis may affect any portion of the gastrointestinal tract although the duodenum is most often spared in necrotizing enterocolitis.

Disease Entities
Necrotizing enterocolitis in the premature
Hirschsprung's disease
Mesenteric vascular thrombosis
Obstructive bowel disease
Milk intolerance
Idiopathic pneumatosis

Differential Diagnosis

Intramural air simply represents a pathologic state and does not indicate a specific entity. Necrotizing enterocolitis in premature infants is by far the most common cause of pneumatosis in newborns. This is often accompanied by the clinical features of abdominal distention, acidosis, and bloody diarrhea. Occasionally, the radiographic appearance of pneumatosis appears prior to the onset of the clinical features of necrotizing enterocolitis. Recognition of pneumatosis is therefore quite important.

Enterocolitis accompanied by pneumatosis intestinalis is a severe complication that occurs in Hirschsprung's disease as well as other obstructive diseases. The age of the patient is important in distinguishing Hirschsprung's disease from necrotizing enterocolitis, since Hirschsprung's disease almost always occurs in older infants. Barium studies are not recommended unless Hirschsprung's disease is suspected. Extreme care should be exercised when the examination is performed, and specific attention must be given to identify the narrow distal aganglionic segment (Fig. 2-40). The mucosa in this segment may be normal whereas the proximal, ganglion-containing part of the colon is always severely ulcerated.

Bowel ischemia and the resulting necrosis that may follow malpositioning or prolonged use of an umbilical catheter is also manifested radiographically by pneumatosis. The diagnosis is easily suggested, since the entire

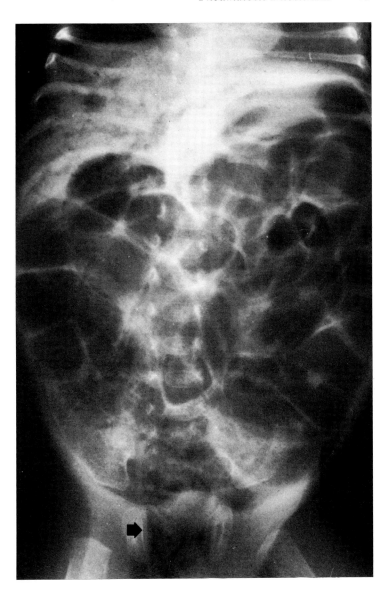

Fig. 2-39. Pneumatosis intestinalis with necrotizing enterocolitis. The small and large bowel are distended and diffusely outlined by linear collections of air. The air has dissected into the scrotum *(arrow)* as well as into the portal venous system.

process develops later in the neonatal period and always subsequent to recent placement of an intravascular catheter.

Pneumatosis *without* associated enterocolitis is a rare and benign complication of neonatal obstruction such as Hirschsprung's disease and atresias. Patients are rarely symptomatic. Barium studies, when performed, reveal non-ulcerated mucosa which is distorted and nodular due to the underlying air cysts.

Milk intolerance has been associated with pneumatosis. Some degree of mucosal damage probably exists, since bloody stools are known to occur. The temporal relationship between the presentation of the disease and the feeding of milk is diagnostic.

Idiopathic pneumatosis is decidely rare and is only presumed after all known causes are excluded (Fig. 2-41).

Discussion

Although pneumatosis intestinalis is a significant finding in necrotizing enterocolitis, Pochaczevsky and Kassner observed it in only 40 per cent of the patients they studied. The onset and appearance of pneumatosis during the course of this disease are unpredictable. Pneumatosis may occur in some individuals before the disease is clinically obvi-

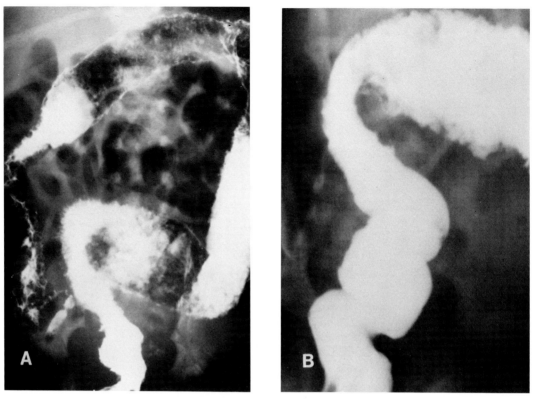

Fig. 2-40. Hirschsprung's disease with superimposed necrotizing enterocolitis. (A) The colonic mucosa is completely interrupted. Deep penetrating ulcers are present within the sigmoid. (B) A detailed view of the rectum reveals a classical transition zone at the rectosigmoid junction. The rectal mucosa is normal, whereas the mucosa within the dilated ganglion containing bowel manifests deep ulcerations.

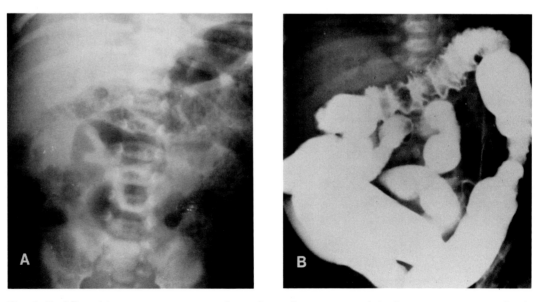

Fig. 2-41. Idiopathic pneumatosis intestinalis and portal venous gas. (A) This patient was completely asymptomatic. Cystic collections of gas are distributed throughout the entire colon. Note the presence of portal venous gas. (B) The mucosa is intact although deformed by the underlying cystic collections of air. The portal venous gas is still apparent.

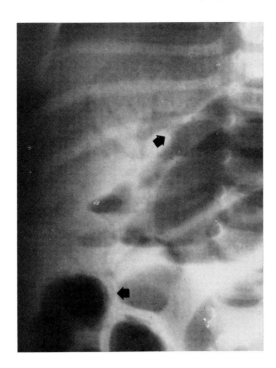

Fig. 2-42. Portal venous gas. Necrotizing entero-colitis. Note the massive accumulation of gas throughout the entire portal system. The portal vein *(upper arrow)* and its radiating branches are well filled with air. Intramural air *(lower arrow)* outlines the wall of colon and small bowel.

ous; in others it may actually disappear as the disease worsens; and finally in some it may not even appear at all. The ileocecal region is the most frequent site of involvement, and cystic, bubbly collections of air within this area represent an early manifestation of the disease.

Pneumatosis in necrotizing enterocolitis is probably the result of bowel wall invasion by gas-producing organisms. Recent experiments have shown a high percentage of hydrogen within the mural blebs suggesting that only certain hydrogen-forming bacteria, Klebsiella in particular, may be responsible for its production. Not surprisingly, in the absence of exogenous food the suspect bacteria do not produce hydrogen and pneumatosis does not occur. Pneumatosis once formed does not remain static. It may disappear, accumulate further and penetrate the bowel wall into the mesenteric venous system, or enter the peritoneal cavity (Fig. 2-34). Once in the mesenteric veins the gas is transported to the hepatic portal system (Figs. 2-37, 2-39). Portal venous gas and perforation are frequently associated with a deteriorating clinical situation. Although many factors may be responsible for the production of necrotizing enterocolitis, the main underlying pathologic event is mucosal destruction. Oral

feedings, and perhaps hyperosmolar formulas in particular, may be partially responsible for damaging the mucosal wall and allowing for bacterial overgrowth. Stress and hypoxia are other known important factors. Both can cause a physiological reflex that results in selective shunting of blood away from the gastrointestinal tract to areas of greater need, such as the heart and brain. The net result is poorly perfused and ischemic bowel. The natural protective mechanisms of the mucosa are altered and diminished, and mucosal damage with subsequent destruction ensues.

Enterocolitis is also a severe complication that occasionally arises in Hirschsprung's disease. The pathogenesis is unclear, but it appears that dilated bowel alone can sufficiently compromise the intramural vascular bed to produce ischemia. Pneumatosis has also been observed in Hirschsprung's disease and in other obstructing lesions, without underlying enterocolitis. Bowel distention causes diastasis of the mucosa with subsequent leakage of luminal air into the bowel wall. The bowel in this circumstance is normal, and the resulting clinical symptomatology is insignificant.

The recent use of umbilical feeding catheters has resulted in the undesirable complication of bowel ischemia. This has been attributed to thrombosis occurring along the

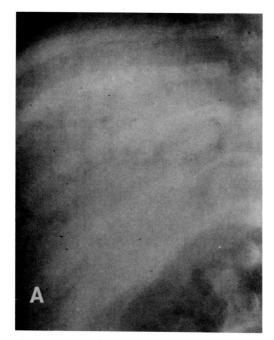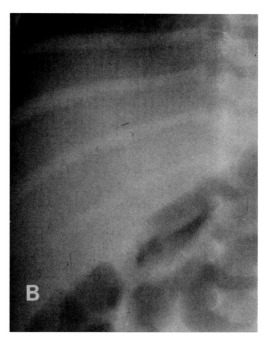

Fig. 2-43. Portal venous gas. *(A)* Obvious portal venous gas is present. *(B)* The gas disappeared 24 hours later despite the patient's continual deterioration. He expired 8 days later.

catheter or the faulty passage of the catheter into small vessels, causing occlusion. This entity is recognized by a precipitating clinical picture resembling necrotizing enterocolitis and by the presence of pneumatosis on the abdominal film.

Milk intolerance has been associated with pneumatosis and bloody diarrhea in newborns secondary to transient lactose intolerance. Pneumatosis in this situation is associated with a favorable outcome when the infant is fed a milk-free diet.

Idiopathic pneumatosis in the newborn period is distinctly rare. In the adult, this is associated with pulmonary disease, with passage of air into the mediastinum and then caudad into the retoperitoneal structures and mesentery. Although a similar course of events occurs in neonates, I have yet to encounter a case of pneumatosis intestinalis in an infant with hyaline membrane disease complicated by a pneumomediastinum.

PORTAL VENOUS GAS

Gas after it enters the mesenteric venous system is transported to the liver by the normal centrifugal flow of portal blood. It accumulates within the peripheral portal vessels and as a result produces the characteristic appearance of radiating tubular radiolucencies that branch from the porta hepatis to the edge of the liver (Figs. 2-37, 2-39, 2-42). This must be differentiated from gas within the biliary system which accumulates in the major biliary vessels and is located more or less centrally within the liver. Infrequently, gas within the biliary system has been seen with duodenal obstructions that dilate the ampulla of Vater (Fig. 2-7). The presence of gas within the portal system is not always obvious when minimal amounts are present. This has been confused with pneumatosis intestinalis or even intraluminal gas. However, patients with portal venous gas are critically ill, acidotic, and frequently in shock. They present with a distended abdomen, gastroenteritis, and bloody stools.

Disease Entities
Necrotizing enterocolitis
Sepsis
Umbilical vein catheterization
Peroxide enemas
Gastroenteritis

Differential Diagnosis

Portal venous gas is not peculiar to any of the entities above. Fortunately, peroxide enemas are no longer administered, and as a

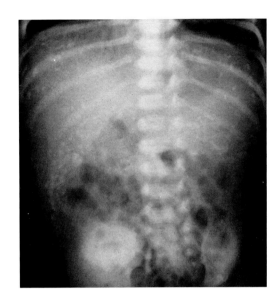

Fig. 2-44. Meconium peritonitis. Multiple amorphous collections of calcification are distributed throughout the entire peritoneum. Some are located on the surface of the liver and along the abdominal wall. The abdomen is not distended, and all studies of the gastrointestinal tract were normal.

result this complication is no longer a problem. The combination of pneumatosis intestinalis and portal venous gas is strong evidence for the presence of necrotizing enterocolitis (Fig. 2-42). However, portal venous gas can be observed without obvious pneumatosis intestinalis in some patients with sepsis and with necrotizing enterocolitis. The presence of an umbilical vein catheter associated with portal venous gas in a relatively asymptomatic patient excludes most of the serious illnesses.

Discussion

The pathogenesis of portal venous gas is not completely understood, except in those cases following introduction of an umbilical vein catheter or peroxide enemas. The majority of cases with portal venous gas are associated with necrotizing enterocolitis. The intestinal mucosa in this disease is severely ulcerated and damaged, and gas-producing organisms easily proliferate and penetrate the bowel wall. They eventually invade the mesenteric veins and are subsequently transported to the portal system. Pre- and postmortem cultures in patients with portal venous gas are often positive for gas-forming organisms. In some cases of sepsis, portal venous gas has been observed although the intestinal tract has appeared grossly normal. It is conceivable that distended bowel alone in the presence of sepsis can force gas into the submucosa without overt evidence of mucosal damage (Fig. 2-41).

The presence of portal venous gas often indicates a poor prognosis since it signifies severe underlying disease. However, the gas itself is not the cause of death. In fact, there are times when portal venous gas disappears despite the deterioration of the patient (Fig. 2-43). In addition intense medical therapy, as well as early surgical intervention directed at the primary causative factor, has greatly decreased the mortality.

ABNORMAL ABDOMINAL CALCIFICATIONS

The presence of abdominal calcification in newborns is indeed quite significant. Calcification is easily recognized by its greater radiodensity and its amorphous or linear appearance. The character and location of the calcification are often excellent clues to the site and nature of the lesion.

Disease Entities

Meconium Peritonitis
Adrenal hemorrhage
Hepatoblastoma
Dermoid tumor or teratoma
Neuroblastoma
Wilm's tumor
Splenic cyst
Intrahepatic calcification
Multiple gastrointestinal atresias with intraluminal calcifications

---

Differential Diagnosis

Meconium peritonitis indicates intrauterine perforation with the extrusion of me-

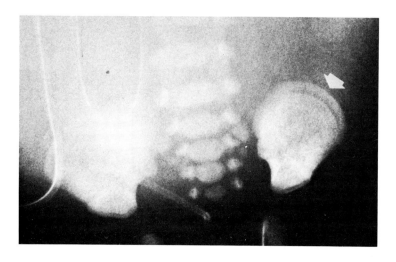

Fig. 2-45. Stress lines associated with meconium peritonitis. This newborn presented with meconium peritonitis, pseudocyst, and meconium ileus. The ilium demonstrates the bony changes commonly seen in patients with this disease, a radiopaque strip separated by an area of radiolucency *(arrow)*.

conium into the peritoneal cavity. Meconium calcifies quickly when in contact with peritoneal fluid and is thus easily recognized on the abdominal film. The calcifications appear radiographically as a single cluster, a few small scattered clusters, or long linear calcific radiodensities that collect along the abdominal wall (Fig. 2-44). Calcium may accumulate in the scrotum when meconium passes through the processus vaginalis. At times, calcium is deposited within the bowel wall itself, as well as within the lumen of the bowel. Both of these represent incomplete perforation and occur when meconium extends into the wall of the intestine through an ulceration. Bony stress lines seen at the ends of both long and flat bones have been described with meconium peritonitis. These are the result of bone growth interruption and are manifested as radiopaque strips that are separated from the epiphyses by a zone of radiolucency (Fig. 2-45).

A rim-like calcification within the adrenal gland indicates previous hemorrhage within this structure. Calcium does not precipitate immediately but only at the time the hematoma is being absorbed. Consequently, the early diagnosis of adrenal hemorrhage is established by observing the changes that occur during the total body opacification phase of intravenous urography (see p. 22). The deposition of calcium initially encircles the periphery of the structure, but eventually decreases in size and assumes the typical triangular or oval flocculent configuration of the normal adrenal gland.

Multiple mottled calcifications within the right upper quadrant in an enlarged liver indicate hepatoblastoma (Fig. 2-46). The calcifications are basically intrahepatic and not on the surface, as in meconium peritonitis. Other hepatic masses associated with calcifications are hemangiomas and atrioventricular malformations. These lesions are relatively uncommon in newborns. Hemangioma may be associated with platelet trapping and severe thrombocytopenia. Bleeding and congestive failure result if massive arterial shunting occurs in the atrioventricular malformation. The calcifications appearing in hemangiomas are multiple and small, resembling phleboliths. Arteriography may be helpful in distinguishing the lesions. Massive hypervascularity with early shunting into the venous system is apparent in hepatoblastoma. Hemangiomas are characterized by considerable vascular stasis. Non-neoplastic calcifications in the liver are seen with portal vein thrombosis. This has been described in premature infants and is located in the subcapsular segment of the left lobe. Calcifications within the liver also occasionally appear following the introduction of hypertonic solution into the liver parenchyma by means of poorly positioned indwelling umbilical feeding catheters. These solutions result in tissue necrosis.

Calcification can be seen within a dermoid tumor, neuroblastoma, and even a Wilm's tumor. Wilm's tumor and neuroblastoma are unusual in newborns. The location of the calcium deposit is important in identifying the

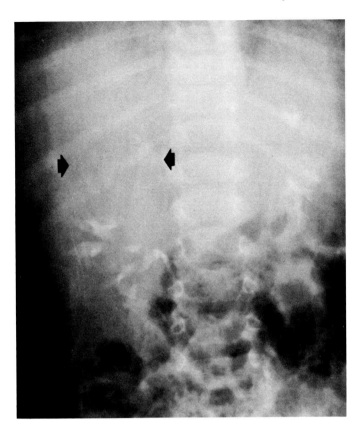

Fig. 2-46. Hepatoma. A mass containing multiple calcifications is present within the right upper quadrant *(arrows)*. The kidney is depressed. (A tumor within the adrenal gland could cause similar changes.)

lesion. Splenic cyst calcification is easily recognized by its characteristic ring-like configuration in the left upper quadrant.

Multiple, rounded collections of calcification lying in adjacent rows resembling "a string of pearls" have been recently described in newborns presenting with multiple atresias that can extend from the stomach to the rectum (Fig. 2-47). The pattern is quite typical. The calcifications are predominantly intraluminal, although intramural calcifications also occur. The lesions are usually enclosed by innumerable diaphagmatic atresias.

Discussion

Meconium peritonitis is a chemical peritonitis that occurs following intrauterine or early neonatal perforation of the gastrointestinal tract. A secondary bacterial peritonitis ensues if the perforation persists. In some cases the opening closes spontaneously in utero, and subsequent examination of the gastrointestinal tract is normal. The most

common cause of meconium peritonitis is intestinal obstruction associated with meconium ileus. This has been observed in approximately 40 per cent of cases. It has been less commonly associated with stenosis, volvulus, and abnormal mesenteric bands. In the uncomplicated cases of meconium peritonitis adhesions result only infrequently. The calcifications are usually slowly absorbed during the 1st few years of life.

Multiple gastrointestinal atresias with intraluminal calcifications is a newly recognized entity, originally noted in French Canadian families in the region of St. John Lake in Quebec. Cases described by Martin and colleagues were also traceable to that area. Our patients had French Canadian names, but they could not be traced to the same region. In addition to multiple gastrointestinal atresias, cystic dilatation of the bile ducts is also present, with bile stasis, due to the production and secretion of bile into a closed loop. The disease is probably transmitted as an autosomal recessive trait.

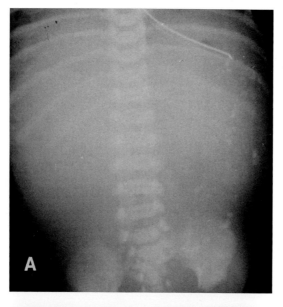

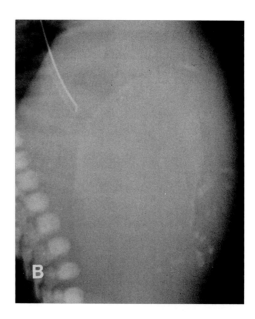

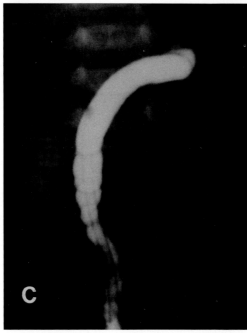

Fig. 2-47. Multiple gastrointestinal atresias.
(A) Intra-abdominal spherical calcifications are
present and resemble "a string of pearls." (B)
The lateral projection demonstrates a large
calcified cystic structure. At surgery a dilated
cecum with intramural calcification was found.
(C) Barium colon study manifests a small
unused distal colon with membranous atresia
in the sigmoid region. Other atresias of the
colon, stomach, and small bowel were also
present. Note the absence of gas in the
abdomen.

REFERENCES

Gastric Distention

1. Alochibaja, T., Putnam, T. C., Yablin, B. A. Duplication of the stomach simulating hypertrophic pyloric stenosis. Am. J. Dis. Child., *127*:120, 1974.
2. Riggs, W., Jr., and Long, L.: The value of the plain film roentgenogram in pyloric stenosis. Am. J. Roentgenol. Radium Ther. Nucl. Med., *112*:77, 1971.
3. Singleton, E. B., and King, B. A.: Localized lesions of the stomach in children. Semin. Roentgenol., *6*:220, 1971.
4. Swischuck, L.: Radiology of the newborn and young infant. Baltimore, Williams and Wilkins, 1974.

Duodenal Distention

5. Ashly, R.: Duodenal atresia with gas below the obstruction. Br. J. Radio., *42*:359, 1969.
6. Johnson, G. F.: Congenital preduodenal portal vein. Am. J. Roentgenol. Radium Ther. Nucl. Med., *112*:93, 1971.
7. Rabinowitz, J. G., and Moseley, J. E.: The small bowel in infants and children. *In* Marshak, R. H., and Lindner, A. E. (eds.): Radiology of the Small Intestine. ed. 2. Philadelphia, Saunders, 1976.
8. ———: The lateral lumbar spine in Down's syndrome". Radiology, *83*:74, 1964.

Small Bowel Distention

9. Favara, D. E., Franciosi, R. A., and Akers, D. R.: Enteric duplications: 37 Cases: vascular theory of pathogenesis. Am. J. Dis. Child., *122*:501, 1971.
10. Friedland, G. W., Rush, W. A., Jr., and Hill, A. J.: Smyth's "Inspissated milk syndrome." Radiology, *103*:159, 1972.
11. Gross, R. E., Holcomb, G. W., and Farber, S.: Duplications of the alimentary tract. Pediatrics, *9*:499, 1962.
12. Louw, J. H.: Jejuno-ileal atresia and stenosis. J. Pediatr. Surg., *1*:8, 1966.
13. Martin, L. W., and Zerella, J. T.: Small bowel atresia presented. J. Pediatr. Surg., *11*:399, 1976.
14. Neuhauser, E. B. D.: Roentgen changes associated with pancreatic insufficiency in early life. Radiology, *46*:319, 1946.
15. Parvey, L., and Seibert, J.: Personal communication.
16. Pochaczevsky, R., and Kassner, E. B.: Nectrotizing enterocolitis in infancy. Am. J. Roentgenol. Radium Ther. Nucl. Med., *113*:283, 1971.
17. Siegle, R. L. Rabinowitz, J. G., Karones, S. B., and Eyal, F. G.: Early changes of necrotizing enterocolitis. Am. J. Roentgenol. Radium Ther. Nucl. Med., *127*:629, 1976.
18. White, H.: Meconium ileus. New roentgen sign. Radiology, *66*:567, 1956.

Colonic Distention

19. Berdon, W. E., and Baker, D. H.: The roentgenographic diagnosis of Hirschsprung's disease in infancy. Am. J. Roentgenol. Radium Ther. Nucl. Med., *93*:432, 1965.
20. Berdon, W. E., Hochberg, B., Baker, D. H., Grossman, H., and Santulli, T. V.: The association of lumbosacral and genitourinary anomalies with imperforate anus. Am. J. Roentgenol. Radium Ther. Nucl. Med., *98*:680, 1964.
21. Berdon, W. E., Koontz, P., and Baker, D. H.: The diagnosis of colonic and terminal ileal aganglionosis. Am. J. Roentgenol. Radium Ther. Nucl. Med., *91*:680, 1964.
22. Clatworthy, H. W., Jr., Howard, W. H. R., and Loyd, R.: Meconium plug syndrome. Surgery, *39*:131, 1956.
23. Gans, S. L.: Classification of ano-rectal anomalies: a critical analysis. J. Pediatr. Surg., *5*:111, 1970.
24. Hope, J. W., Borns, P. F., and Berg, P. K.: Roentgenologic manifestations of Hirschsprung's disease. Am. J. Roentgenol. Radium Ther. Nucl. Med., *95*:217, 1965.

Pneumoperitoneum

25. Coopersmith, H., and Rabinowitz, J. G.: A specific sign for neonatal gastric perforation. J. Can. Assoc. Radiol., *24*:141, 1973.
26. James, A. E., Heller, R. M., White, J. H., Schaeffer, S. A., Shaker, I. J., Haller, J. A., and Dorst, J. P.: Spontaneous rupture of the stomach in the newborn: clinical and experimental evaluation. Pediatr. Res., *10*:79, 1976.
27. Kiesewetter, W. D.: Spontaneous rupture of the stomach in the newborn. Am. J. Dis. Child., *91*:162, 1956.
28. Lloyd, S. R.: The etiology of gastrointestinal perforation in the newborn. J. Pediatr. Surg., *4*:77, 1969.
29. Pochaczevsky, R., and Byrk, D.: New roentgenographic signs of neonatal gastric perforation. Radiology, *102*:145, 1972.
30. Siegle, R., Rabinowitz, J. G., and Sarasohn, C.: Intestinal perforation secondary to nasojejunal feeding. Am. J. Roentgenol. Radium Ther. Nucl. Med., *126*:1229, 1976.

Pneumatosis Intestinalis

31. Pochaszevsky, R., and Kassner, E. G.: Necrotizing enterocolitis in infancy. Am. J. Roentgenol. Radium Ther. Nucl. Med., *113*:283, 1971.
32. Rabinowitz, J. G., and Siegle, R. L.: Changing clinical and roentgenographic patterns of necrotizing enterocolitis. Am. J. Roentgenol. Radium Ther. Nucl. Med., *126*:560, 1976.

33. Siegle, R. L., Rabinowitz, J. G. Karones, S. B., and Eyal, F. G.: Early diagnosis of necrotizing enterocolitis. Am. J. Roentgenol. Radium Ther. Nucl. Med., *127:*629, 1976.

Portal Venous Gas

34. Arnon, R. G., and Fishbein, J. F.: Portal venous gas in the pediatric age group. J. Pediatr., *79:*255, 1971.
35. Susman, N., and Senturia, H. R.: Gas embolization of the portal venous system. Am. J. Roentgenol. Radium Ther. Nucl. Med., *83:*847, 1960.
36. Wiot, J. F., and Felson, B.: Gas in the portal venous system. Am. J. Roentgenol. Radium Ther. Nucl. Med., *86:*920, 1961.

Abnormal Abdominal Calcifications

37. Martin, C. E., Leonidas, J. C., and Amoury, R. A.: Multiple gastro-intestinal atresias with intraluminal calcifications and cystic dilatation of bile ducts: a newly recognized entity resembling "a string of pearls." Pediatrics, *57:*268, 1976.
38. Rabinowitz, J. G., and Moseley, J. E.: The small bowel in infants and children. *In* Marshak, R. H., and Linden, A. E. (editors): Radiology of the Small Intestine. edition 2. Philadelphia, Saunders. 1976.
39. Wolfson, J. J., and Engel, R. R.: Anticipating meconium peritonitis from metaphyseal bands. Radiology *92:*1055, 1969.

3

Abnormal Abdominal Radiographic Patterns in the Infant and Child

GASTRIC OUTLET OBSTRUCTION (GASTRIC DISTENTION)

Gastric outlet obstruction in infants and children is most often caused by a narrowed antrum. Many of the lesions responsible for the narrowing are unusual and uncommon. The onset and severity of the symptoms depend upon the nature and the degree of prevailing stenosis, and they are usually nondescript in mild cases. Repeated episodes of abilious vomiting are common. The routine abdominal radiograph reveals varying degrees of gastric distention but can be surprisingly normal. The use of contrast material to evaluate the gastrointestinal tract in any suspicious case of obstruction cannot be overemphasized.

Disease Entities

Short Segment Narrowing
    Pyloric stenosis ("burned out")
    Pylorospasm
    Stricture (post-peptic ulcer or post-corrosion)
    Antral web
Long Segment Narrowing
    Duplication
    Gastric ulcer
    Lymphoma and leukemia
    Eosinophilic gastritis
    Chronic granulomatous disease of childhood
    Crohn's disease
Foreign Body

Differential Diagnosis

The classic features of hypertrophic pyloric stenosis are well known. They appear in male infants of approximately 3 weeks of age who present with projectile vomiting, and whose radiographs manifest a markedly dilated stomach with deep peristaltic waves, a narrow and elongated pyloric channel, a "shoulder" sign, and a "teat" sign. A few patients with this abnormality present late in infancy with none of the obvious clinical or radiographic features. In these patients the only radiographic finding is a short nondescript segment of narrowed antrum with intact mucosa. Peristalsis is not particularly prominent or altered, and gastric emptying may be entirely normal.

Other short, segmental, stenotic lesions that occur in the antrum consist of gastric mucosal diaphgram and pylorospasm. Pylorospasm is usually associated with active peptic ulcer disease and in contrast to the other lesions is a dynamic process. Varying degrees of constriction may be observed during the course of a single study. In some instances, the spasm may be so severe and persistent that distinction from an organic lesion is impossible. Antispasmodics relax the spastic segment and will not affect the anatomic findings encountered in pyloric stenosis.

A gastric mucosal diaphragm may be difficult to recognize when it is located close to the pylorus. The diaphragm consists of a thin, membranous septum that is directed perpendicularly to the long axis of the an-

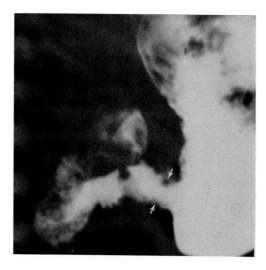

Fig. 3-1. Gastric antral diaphragm. The entire diaphragm is not visualized because of previous surgery. The area of antral narrowing *(arrows)* represents the diaphragm. Note the partial "double bubble" appearance formed by the duodenum and the antrum distal to the membrane.

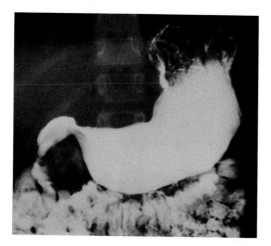
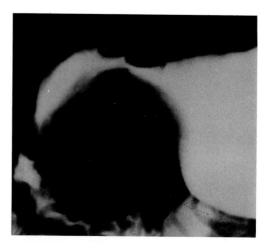

Fig. 3-2. Gastric duplication. Well-defined intramural mass is present within the antrum of the stomach and narrows both the antrum and duodenum in a smooth, uniform fashion.

trum. Radiographically it looks like a thin, radiolucent line measuring 1 to 4 mm. in thickness when both the duodenal bulb and stomach are distended with contrast material. The gastric segment located between the diaphragm and the pyloric channel then produces a "double bubble" effect with the duodenum. This appearance is quite characteristic and may be the only feature demonstrable when the diaphgram is relatively short (Fig. 3-1).

Duplication cysts and post-corrosion or peptic ulcer stricture also cause antral narrowing but are more often associated with longer stenotic segments. A stricture that develops following peptic ulcer disease is due to multiple, recurrent episodes; it is there-

fore rare in neonates and is more commonly found in the older child. A narrowed fibrotic antrum also occurs as the result of corrosion following ingestion of alkaline or acidic agents. A duplication cyst may be recognized by an extrinsic or intramural location which causes a smooth asymmetrical narrowing of the antrum (Fig. 3-2).

Gastric antral narrowing has recently been recognized as an important manifestation of chronic granulomatous disease of childhood. The lesion is nondistinctive in appearance and may involve a single curvature or the entire antral circumference. Occasionally a sharp proximal margin is produced which, when present, distinguishes this lesion from other antral lesions.

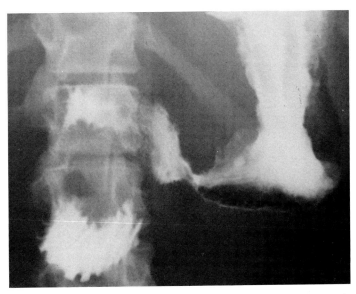

Fig. 3-3. Gastric and duodenal Crohn's disease. The antrum, body of stomach, and duodenum are involved. The antrum gradually tapers toward the pylorus and manifests an irregular, thickened, and ulcerated mucosa. The mucosa of the duodenal bulb and descending portion of the duodenum is serrated and irregular.

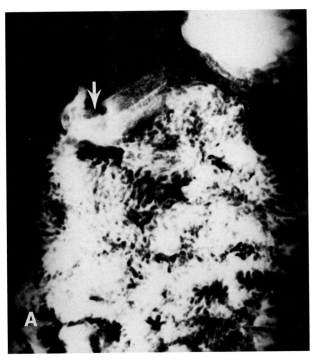
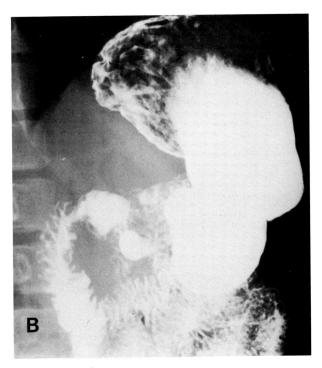

Fig. 3-4. Eosinophilic gastroenteritis. *(A)* Small polypoid lesions are noted along the greater curvature of the antrum *(arrow).* The entire small bowel is infiltrated, and the wall is thick and nodular. Eosinophils were isolated from the stool. *(B)* The stomach and small bowel appear normal following treatment with steroids.

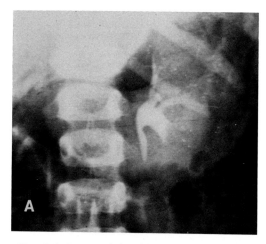 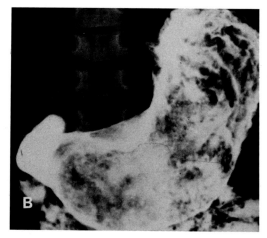

Fig. 3-5. Bezoar. *(A)* A large soft-tissue mass is present within a dilated stomach. This was detected during intravenous pyelography. *(B)* Barium surrounds an irregular intraluminal defect. The configuration of the stomach as well as the mucosal folds remains intact.

Crohn's disease of the stomach is unusual in the pediatric age-group, but it should be considered when the antrum is not only narrow but also nodular and thickened (Fig. 3-3). The deformity is somewhat characteristic and consists of tubular narrowing and poor distensibility. This combination of findings resembles the sacramental "ram's horn." Involvement of the duodenum and small bowel is almost always present.

Another unusual cause of diffuse antral narrowing is an eosinophilic infiltration that, in addition, contains numerous plasma cells. The narrowing may be diffuse and severe and can simulate linitis plastica. A circumscribed, localized infiltration that assumes the appearance of a discrete polypoid lesion also exists (Fig. 3-4). This form is not restricted to the gastric antrum and can be found anywhere within the gastrointestinal tract.

Gastric lymphoma and leukemia also produce polypoid lesions. However, mucosal ulcerations are frequently present in lymphoma.

The formation of a gastric bezoar is distinctly unusual in the pediatric age-group, but occurs frequently in mentally retarded or disturbed children. The abdominal radiograph demonstrates a soft-tissue mass surrounded by air within the body of the stomach. Barium studies reveal an intraluminal, freely mobile, irregular mass that is not associated with any alterations of the mucosal folds, wall, or contractility (Fig. 3-5). Gastric obstruction occurs as the bezoar impacts within the pylorus. The mass then continues to grow by accretion.

Discussion

The pathogenesis of "burned out" pyloric stenosis is interesting. Patients with this disease are older than the usual patient with pyloric stenosis, and they present with a prolonged history of abilious vomiting, failure to thrive, and a barely palpable or more often non-palpable pyloric muscle. Two possible mechanisms have been proposed. The more acceptable relates to a "burned out," involuting smooth-muscle tumor that is replaced by a diffuse and overabundant production of fibrous tissue. This sequence probably represents the natural healing pattern of the muscle mass in most cases of pyloric stenosis. An alternate but less acceptable explanation suggests an atypical, smouldering variant of the disease. Therapy is the same regardless of the underlying nature of the disease; a pyloroplasty or pyloromyotomy is required.

A number of theories, such as fetal vascular accident, failure of canalization, inadequate entodermal proliferation, and excess local entodermal proliferation, have been suggested to explain the occurence of gastric atresias, including membranous atresia (of which the gastric antral web may be the most benign form). None appear entirely

Table 3-1. **Lesions Causing Gastric Outlet Obstruction**

Type of Obstruction	Radiographic Features
Short Segment Narrowing	
Pyloric stenosis ("burned out")	Nondescript
Pylorospasm	Changeable—relaxes with antispasmodics
Stricture	Associated with peptic ulcer history
Antral web	"Double bubble" appearance, radiolucent perpendicular line
Long Segment Narrowing	
Duplication	Extrinsic or intramural mass effect
Gastric ulcer	Long stricture with ulcer
Lymphoma	Mass with ulceration
Eosinophilic gastritis	May be polypoid or infiltrative (linitis-plastica-like)
Chronic granulomatous disease	Sharp proximal margin
Crohn's disease	Tubular narrowed antrum ("ram's horn")

acceptable. It is interesting that in one series of gastric webs significant concomitant abnormalities were noted, such as coarctation of the aorta, duodenal stenosis, and patent ductus arteriosus.

Peptic ulcer disease is rare in children, and the fibrosis that ultimately produces a stricture requires repeated episodes of ulceration to develop. Infants swallowing corrosive materials, such as lye, are likely to experience strictures within the esophagus, since this material is neutralized by the gastric acid juices. Ingestion of acidic material is more injurious to the stomach.

The gastric involvement caused by chronic granulomatous disease of childhood has recently been shown to be due to local granuloma formation. The granulomas are located within the submucosal tissues and cause diffuse thickening of the antral wall. Necrotic focal areas are predominant. Edematous tissue, some granulomas, eosinophils, and histiocytes are found in other areas. In four of the five cases recently described, the gastric manifestations represented the only features of the disease. Consequently, any patient, particularly males with the antral abnormalities and histologic findings described, should have a nitroblue tetrazolium dye test to exclude this disease.

Only a few cases of eosinophilic infiltration of the bowel have been described in childhood. The etiology still remains obscure, and it is conceivable that the diffuse and circumscribed forms may be separate and unrelated entities. Several physicians suggest that the diffuse form may have an allergic origin. The character of the infiltration and the dramatic response following administration of corticosteroids support this contention.

Two kinds of bezoars exist; phytobezoars are composed of vegetable fibers, and trichobezoars are composed of hair. Bezoars are not completely benign entities, since a number of complications arise secondary to their development. These include extension into the jejunum, intussusception, hypoproteinemia secondary to malnutrition, and gastric perforation. About 10 per cent of patients have a gastric ulcer, and almost all manifest a hypochromic microcytic anemia. There is also a high incidence of gastritis. Lactobezoar is an unusual form of bezoar that may develop in infants receiving undiluted formula.

DUODENAL DISTENTION

Duodenal dilatation in infants and children is the result of either obstructive or nonobstructive disease. The latter usually reflects an underlying generalized disease process. A dilated duodenum is recognized on routine abdominal films as a large gas collection just to the right of the stomach. Duodenal obstruction should be strongly suspected when a foreign body remains localized within the right upper quadrant over a prolonged period of time (Fig. 3-6).

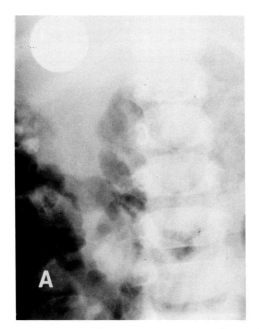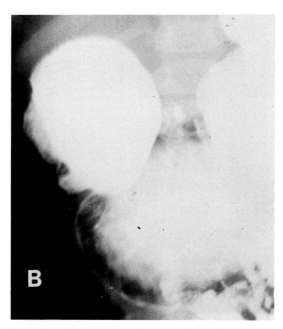

Fig. 3-6. Annular pancreas. Persistent foreign body in the right upper quadrant. *(A)* Metallic coin is located in the right upper quadrant. *(B)* Barium study demonstrates markedly dilated stomach and duodenum. Note the collapsed small bowel distal to the obstruction.

Disease Entities

Obstructive
  Stenosis
  Annular pancreas
  Intraluminal diverticulum (duodenal web)
  Peritoneal band
  Superior mesenteric artery syndrome
  Pre-duodenal portal vein
  Malrotation
  Acute hematoma
  Neoplasm
Nonobstructive
  Normal duodenum
    Zollinger-Ellison syndrome
    Scleroderma
    Crohn's disease
  Abnormal duodenum
    Duodenal ulcer
    Parasite infestation
    Crohn's disease
    Zollinger-Ellison syndrome
    Cystic fibrosis
    Adjacent inflammatory disease

Differential Diagnosis

A short stenotic lesion in the mid-portion of the duodenum indicates either a congenital stenosis or an incomplete annular pancreas. The proximal duodenal segment is dis- tended in both lesions. An annular pancreas is a circumferential lesion with gradually tapering margins that causes concentric narrowing of the duodenum (Figs. 3-6, 3-7). Duodenal stenosis is probably similar. However, extrinsic lesions such as a peritoneal band or a pre-duodenal portal vein produce sharp linear defects upon the duodenum and are frequently associated with malrotation. A tightly overlying superior mesenteric artery is another abnormality that under certain conditions causes extrinsic linear compression of the duodenum (Fig. 3-8). The superior mesenteric artery syndrome occurs in asthenic individuals who have recently grown or lost too much weight. The presenting symptoms are bloating, eructation, and epigastric pain. The proximal duodenum is dilated and the flow of barium stops just to the right of the vertebral column (Fig. 3-8). The superior mesenteric artery produces a vertically oriented, linear defect that is anatomically located at the level where the duodenum passes between the angle of the aorta and the superior mesenteric artery.

Duodenal web and intraluminal diverticulum are terms that actually refer to the same entity in different stages of development. When the web is not distended and when contrast material is located on both

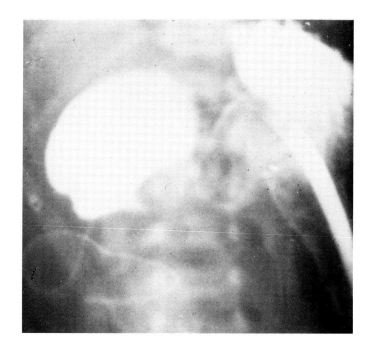

Fig. 3-7. Annular pancreas. Injection of contrast was done by means of gastrostomy. The duodenum is severely dilated. The stenotic channel is concentrically narrowed with tapering margins. This finding is not well manifested often.

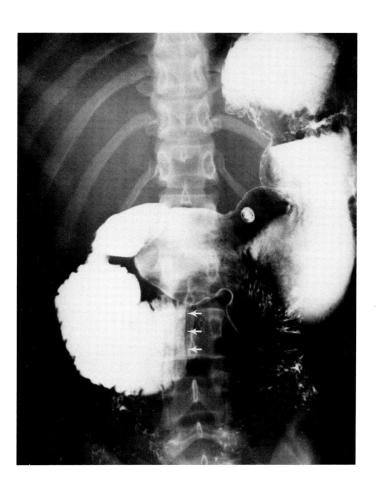

Fig. 3-8. Superior mesenteric artery syndrome. The duodenum is dilated and stops just to the right of the vertebral midline (arrows). The defect is sharp and vertically oriented.

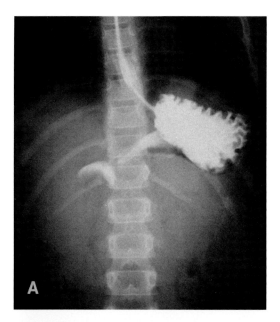
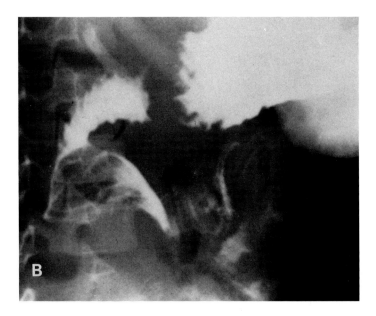
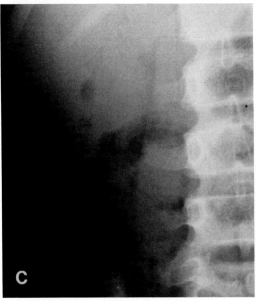

Fig. 3-9. Duodenal hematoma. *(A)* A huge hematoma occupies the epigastrium and displaces the stomach, duodenum, and transverse colon. Complete obstruction is encountered in the immediate postbulbar region although the bulb is small and uninvolved. *(B)* A large hematoma that begins in the proximal duodenum and extends distally into the proximal jejunum. The mucosa in the first part of the duodenum is thickened. However, the remaining portion of the descending duodenum and the distal duodenum are dilated and demonstrate a classic "coil spring" appearance. *(C)* Abdominal radiograph of the right upper quadrant in the same patient demonstrates the "coil spring" appearance as a mass of radiodensity without the use of barium.

sides, it appears as a thin convex radiolucency that extends transversely across the duodenum. If the duodenum only fills proximal to the web, it may balloon out, producing a wind-sock configuration (Figs. 2-10, 2-13). However, the ballooned-out structure appears to project within the duodenal lumen when barium fills the duodenum distal to the stretched web, thereby surrounding it. The term intraluminal diverticulum was used previously to describe this presentation.

Intramural hematoma is one of a few noncongenital lesions that causes duodenal obstruction after the neonatal period. The clinical and radiographic features of this disorder are characteristic. The patient usually presents with a rapid onset of nausea and vomiting following a recent episode of blunt trauma to the abdomen. A distended duodenum associated with a few loops of distended bowel within the epigastrium is the main radiographic feature on the abdominal film. This is frequently accompanied by an ill-defined mass that displaces the stomach and adjacent viscera (Fig. 3-9A). The radiographic features of this lesion on the upper gastrointestinal study are distinctive. However, an upper gastrointestinal study is not

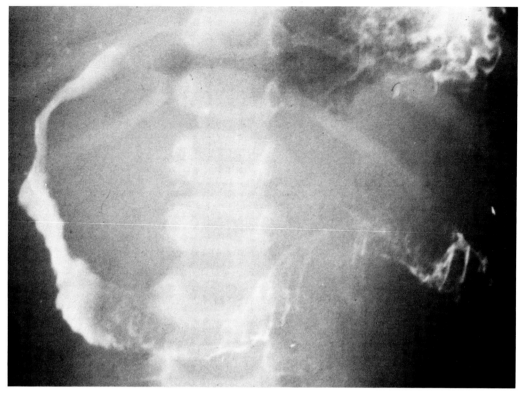

Fig. 3-10. Retroperitoneal lymphosarcoma. A large mass in the region of the pancreas displaces the entire duodenum, producing nodular, irregular, mass-like impressions on the loop. Note the fixation and thickening of the mucosal folds despite the displacement of the ligament of Treitz.

altogether necessary. The hematoma usually spares the duodenal bulb but involves a long segment of bowel immediately distal to the bulb that measures approximately 10 to 20 cms. in length. It rarely causes complete obstruction (Fig. 3-9A). The proximal portion of the hematoma causes only thickening of the mucosal folds. However, as it spreads distally it forms a more well-defined mass that compresses the bowel wall and by so doing may either narrow or widen the bowel lumen (Fig. 3-9B). This appearance is in all likelihood produced by an asymmetrically located hematoma that stretches the valvulae conniventes over and around it. As a result, the mucosa is thinned and elongated, producing a "coil spring" appearance (Figs. 3-9B, 3-9C). Most duodenal hematomas resolve spontaneously.

Duodenal hematomas must be distinguished from lesions that originate in the retroperitoneum and secondarily involve the duodenum. Retroperitoneal sarcoma can both displace and invade the duodenum. Therefore the radiographic findings consist principally of extrinsic nodular masses that

displace this structure, causing little ulceration of the mucosa in the early phases of the disease (Fig. 3-10). Primary duodenal lymphosarcoma is most unusual and is radiographically associated with a mass and ulceration.

A pancreatic pseudocyst is also uncommon, but is easily recognized as a well-defined retro-gastric mass that produces a smooth, well rounded, and uniform indentation upon the adjacent duodenal loop and stomach (Fig. 3-11). This is quite different from the irregular impressions caused by neoplastic disease.

When the duodenum is diffusely dilated and no obstruction or intrinsic abnormality is present, a variety of conditions such as scleroderma, Zollinger-Ellison syndrome, and occasionally Crohn's disease should be considered. This finding is non-distinctive and only when other radiographic features are recognized can a diagnosis be established. For example, dilated esophagus and small bowel suggests scleroderma; multiple gastric, duodenal, or small bowel ulcerations are indicative of Zollinger-Ellison syndrome;

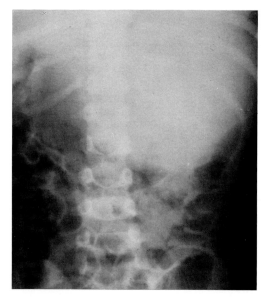
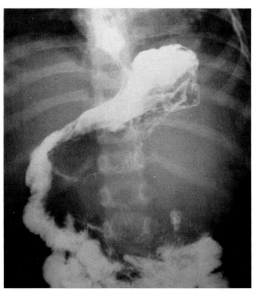

Fig. 3-11. Pancreatic pseudocyst. A large, well rounded, cystic epigastric mass that displaces the stomach upwards and the third and fourth portions of the duodenum downward.

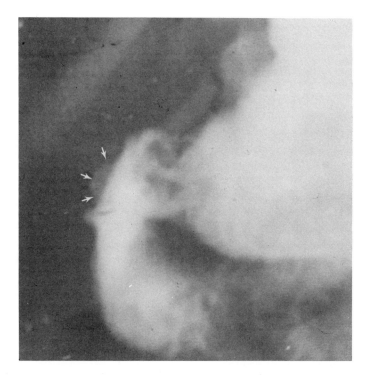

Fig. 3-12. Duodenal ulcer. A 6-year-old with a large ulcer (*arrows*) arising in the apex of the duodenal bulb. The surrounding mucosa is edematous.

and distal small bowel abnormalities suggest Crohn's disease.

Although nonspecific dilatation may accompany both Crohn's disease and the Zollinger-Ellison syndrome, it is not unusual to observe specific mucosal or mural abnormalities involving the duodenum in either lesion. Other lesions, such as peptic ulcer disease, parasitic infestation, and adjacent inflammatory reactions, also produce duodenal dilatation and associated deformities.

Peptic ulcer disease occurs most frequently in the duodenal bulb, and various abnormalities that vary from thickened edematous folds to an obvious ulcerous niche are encountered (Fig. 3-12). An ulcerous niche is identified by a collection of barium distinct and separate from the remaining

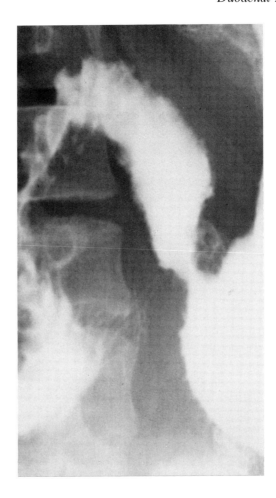

Fig. 3-13. Crohn's disease of the duodenum and stomach. This is the same patient as in Fig. 3-2. Here there is better detail of the duodenum. The entire descending duodenum is nodular. Superficial ulcerations are seen along the surfaces of both the duodenum and stomach.

barium contained within the bowel lumen. When viewed in profile, it is seen penetrating away from the lumen into the bowel wall and surrounding tissues (Fig. 3-12). The inflammatory reaction that accompanies an ulcer produces varying degrees of spasm that modify the usual cone-shaped bulb. Occasionally, thickened edematous folds radiate to the base of the ulcer. The duodenum just proximal to the ampulla may be dilated and edematous. At this level, the elevated acid contents are neutralized by the alkaline pancreatic secretions.

The incidence of peptic ulceration in the Zollinger-Ellison syndrome can be as high as 90 per cent. These ulcers resemble other forms of peptic ulcers, but they are characteristically multiple, ectopic, and recurrent. The disease is caused by markedly elevated gastrin levels that stimulate the stomach to secrete huge amounts of gastric fluid and acid. As a result, the gastric folds are thick and the stomach contains large amounts of fluid. The entire duodenum is dilated and edematous, since the pancreatic secretions are incapable of neutralizing the abnormally excessive gastric juices.

Crohn's disease affecting the duodenum is rare and is almost always associated with distal involvement of the small bowel. The radiologic and pathologic changes produced are similar; nodular alterations, mucosal ulceration, and even stenosis may be encountered (Fig. 3-13).

Dilatation of the duodenum is also encountered as a result of parasitic infestation. *Ancylostoma duodenale* (hookworm) and *Stronglyoides stercoralis* are two parasites that mainly affect the duodenum. Giardia affects only the distal portion of the bowel, as well as the proximal jejunum. The hookworm attaches itself to the mucosal surface, where it produces superficial inflammatory and ulcerative changes that are manifested radiographically by mucosal swelling and irregularity. The early infestation of the adult Strongyloides worm is also on the mucosal surface, and the initial pathologic response is therefore superficial, resembling that produced by the hookworm. The adult parasite eventually

Table 3-2. **Lesions Causing Duodenal Obstruction**

Type of Obstruction	Radiographic Features
Circumferential	
Stenosis	Tapering margins—2nd portion of the duodenum
Annular pancreas	Tapering margins—2nd portion of the duodenum
Linear	
Peritoneal band	Most often located in 2nd portion of duodenum.
Pre-duodenal vein	Commonly associated with malrotation
Malrotation	Obstruction in 2nd or 3rd portion of duodenum
Superior mesenteric artery syndrome	Junction at 2nd and 3rd portions of duodenum just to right of vertebral column
Duodenal web	Intraluminal radiolucent membrane or wind-sock configuration
Intrinsic	
Hematoma	Mucosal thickening, "coil spring" appearance, obstruction
Neoplasm	Obstruction, mass, and ulceration

burrows into the bowel wall where it excites a more profound inflammatory reaction. The radiographic findings are then more irregular and nodular, and are accompanied by obvious mucosal ulcerations. Granuloma followed by fibrosis constitutes the late findings and strikingly resembles Crohn's disease.

The duodenum in cystic fibrosis is occasionally dilated and is accompanied by thick mucosal folds and nodular indentations. The cause of these changes is uncertain.

Discussion

Intramural hematomas occur as a result of abdominal trauma and occasionally in patients with blood dyscrasias. The duodenum, because of its fixed position anterior to the spine, is particularly susceptible to blunt trauma that compresses it between the anterior abdominal wall and the vertebral column. The remaining small bowel, because of its loose mesenteric attachment, moves freely away and thus escapes injury. The clinical symptoms are distinctive and require only a few hours or days to develop. Although the duodenum appears obstructed radiographically, surgery is seldom required since the hematoma resolves spontaneously in the majority of cases and disappears during the course of a few days or weeks with conservative therapy.

Peptic ulcer disease is 7 times more common in the duodenum than in the stomach. The character of the disease as well as the causative factors depend upon the age of the patient. As the child grows older, duodenal ulcer disease becomes more frequent and more significant. In addition, psychological stress becomes increasingly more important as an inciting factor in comparison to physical stress, which is believed to be responsible in the very young. In the first 6 months of life the presenting symptoms of peptic ulcer disease are usually catastrophic events, such as hemorrhage or perforation. Pain and discomfort similar to that of adult disease eventually become the predominant clinical features.

There has been considerable discussion regarding the existence of the superior mesenteric artery syndrome. Substantiating factors include its presentation under certain conditions, its manifestation of specific radiographic features, and its cure following correction of the anatomic abnormality. Normally, the superior mesenteric artery and the mesentery are displaced from the aorta and the spine by retroperitoneal fat. If this fat padding is lost or absent, or if the individual is placed in a hyperextension body cast, the duodenum is compressed against the spine as it passes between the aorta and the superior mesenteric artery. Some immobilized children presenting with hypercalcemia produce similar clinical and radiographic findings.

The Zollinger-Ellison syndrome is rarely found in childhood. It is caused by islet cell tumors or hyperplasia of the pancreas, which result in the production of a gastrin-like substance.

Cysts of the pancreas are either congenital or acquired. Congenital cysts are usually multiple, asymptomatic, and associated with

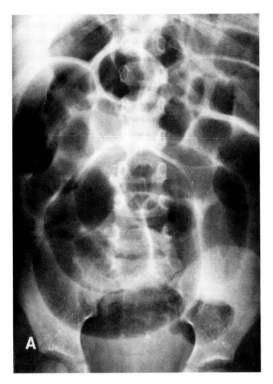

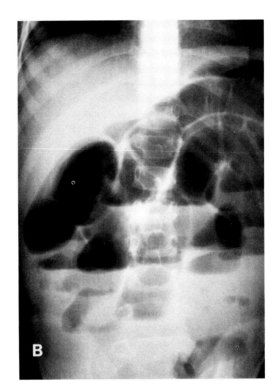

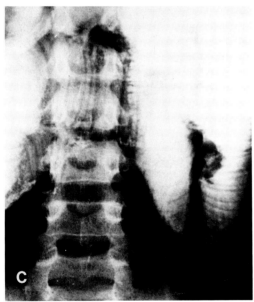

Fig. 3-14. Small bowel obstruction. *(A,B)* Henoch-Schönlein purpura. The entire small bowel is dilated. In the left upper quadrant the valvulae conniventes appear as multiple, thin, circular rings that outline the entire circumference of the bowel. No gas is identifiable within the colon. Note the "stepladder" appearance in the upright position. *(C)* Lymphosarcoma. Barium fills an obstructed jejunum. The valvulae conniventes are remarkably well outlined. An irregular, nodular, neoplastic lesion with central ulceration ("bull's eye") is present on the left.

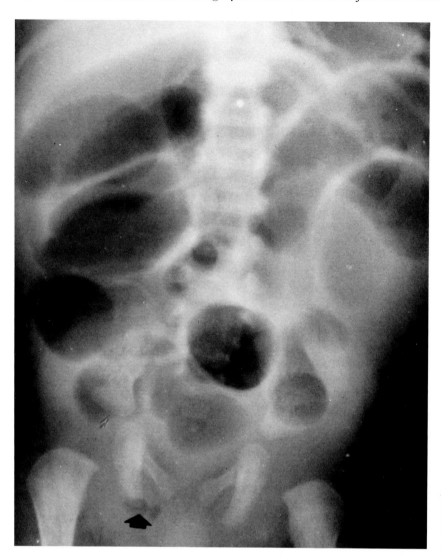

Fig. 3-15. External inguinal hernia. Acute small bowel obstruction in a young infant with a right inguinal hernia. Note the collection of air projected over the right obturator foramen *(arrow).*

generalized polycystic disease. Pseudocysts are acquired and therefore contain no true cyst wall. They occur as a complication of pancreatitis, mumps, and trauma. Purposeful trauma should be considered in any child under the age of 5 years who enters with pancreatitis and its sequelae.

SMALL BOWEL DISTENTION

Small bowel dilatation reflects acute or chronic disease. The amount of distention is not related to the nature of the underlying lesion and can consist of a single segment, multiple segments, or the entire small bowel. The anatomical features that characterize each segment of bowel are usually recognizable on the abdominal radiograph. The jejunal folds, when distended, appear as multiple circular rings that outline the entire lumen of bowel (Fig. 3-14). The folds gradually decrease in size and are practically flat in the distal ileum. As a result, when the distal bowel is dilated, it appears as a smooth-walled structure. In the presence of an acute small bowel obstruction, the small bowel alone is distended, and little or no gas is identified in the colon (Figs. 3-14, 3-15). Gas is noted in the colon when the obstructive process is intermittent or chronic. A dynamic ileus is usually characterized by dilatation of both small and large bowel (Fig. 3-21). Occasionally only a few loops of bowel are dilated, and some difficulty then arises in differentiating this presentation from a chronic intermittent obstruction.

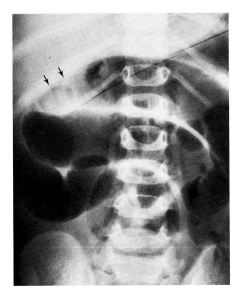 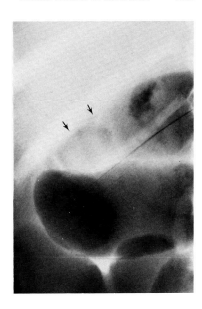

Fig. 3-16. Intussusception. Small bowel obstruction. Dilated small bowel occupies the major portion of the abdomen. Note the "coil spring" appearance within an area of increased radiodensity in the right upper quadrant *(arrows)*.

Disease Entities

Acute
  Obstruction
    Hernia
    Intussusception
    Neoplasm
    Mecomium ileus equivalent
    Adhesions
    Appendiceal Abcess
  Ileus
    Infection
    Postoperative dilatation
    Food allergy
Chronic
  Obstructive
    Jejunal and ileal stenosis
    Crohn's disease
    Tuberculosis
    Neoplasm
    Duplication
    Parasitic infestation
    Postoperative obstruction
    Blind loop obstruction
    Total aganglionosis of colon and terminal
      ileum
  Nonobstructive
    Malabsorption—celiac disease
    Parastic infestation
    Allergy
    Disaccharide intolerance
    Immunoglobulin abnormalities
    Malrotation of bowel
    Abetalipoproteinemia
    Eosinophilic gastroenteritis

Differential Diagnosis

An acute small bowel obstruction clinically presents with abdominal distention and vomiting; the higher the obstruction, the earlier and more severe is the vomiting. The radiographic findings in the early stages of obstruction are characteristic. The small bowel is dilated, and differential air fluid levels, forming an inverted but incomplete C or U configuration, are produced within the same loop of bowel on the upright or cross-table lateral projection. This important feature is the result of existing hyperperistalsis and in its most exaggerated form produces a "stepladder" appearance (Fig. 3-14A). Bowel obstruction is a dynamic affair, and the radiographic features gradually change as bowel contractility diminishes in intensity. The height of the air fluid levels flatten, and intraluminal fluid continues to accumulate. In the most severe forms, enough fluid may be present to displace most or all of the air. The abdomen at this time appears gasless in the supine projection. Careful observation reveals multiple, oval, soft-tissue masses (pseudotumors) that may demonstrate small, discrete, air fluid levels in the erect position.

Acute small bowel obstruction is caused by a variety of lesions, and surgical intervention is required in most cases. Although a precise diagnosis may appear academic, it does aid the surgeon and decreases the morbidity of the procedure.

Small bowel hernias are easily recognized and common enough in the older infant to

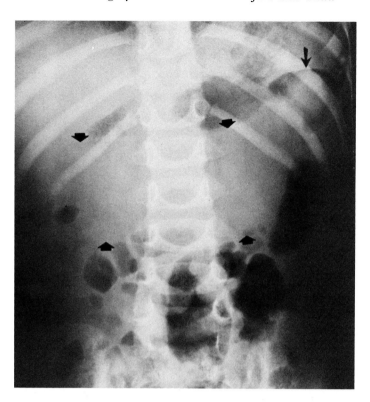

Fig. 3-17. Intussusception. Abdominal film in young infant with crampy abdominal pain reveals a large soft-tissue mass in the epigastrium *(lower arrows)*. The leading edge of the mass *(upper arrow)* is located in the left upper quadrant and is surrounded by a halo of air within the colon.

warrant primary consideration in all acute obstructions. An external hernia frequently produces a soft-tissue radiodensity that overlies the normally radiolucent obturator foramen. This may be subtle, but it is important nevertheless. Occasionally small collections of air within the soft-tissue mass better define the lesion (Fig. 3-15).

Once the possibility of an inguinal hernia is excluded, attention should be directed to the abdomen itself. A soft-tissue mass, abnormal gas collections, and air fluid levels not related to distended bowel are important additional radiographic features. If none of these are present, intussusception, internal hernia, or a simple obstruction caused by a congenital band or adhesion are the likely diagnostic possibilities. However, an adhesion in the absence of previous surgery or infection would be unusual.

A soft-tissue mass associated with small bowel obstruction is often found in intussusception, neoplasm, closed loop obstruction (pseudotumor), acute appendicitis with abscess formation, or the meconium ileus equivalent.

Intussusception is probably the most frequent cause of acute small bowel obstruction in infants under 2 years of age. The clinical presentation is distinctive and consists of crampy, recurrent, abdominal pain that gradually increases in severity and is eventually accompanied by currant-jelly stools. The radiographic findings encountered on the routine abdominal film are often non-distinctive, and the findings of small bowel obstruction and/or a soft-tissue mass are the only reliable signs (Fig. 3-16). The soft-tissue mass represents the intussuscepting bowel and often appears as poorly defined radiodensity with a forward edge that occasionally protrudes into the distal gas column (Fig. 3-17). This finding is most often noted on the right side of the abdomen but can be seen in the epigastrium and occasionally within the distal colon. Since the right colon forms a major portion of the intussuscepting mass, the right lower quadrant is frequently devoid of gas or viscera. The barium colon examination plays a vital role in intussusception. It not only confirms the diagnosis, but in most instances it is a safe and effective means of reducing the lesion. Hydrostatic reduction should always be the initial therapeutic modality if and when clinical or radiographic evidence of small bowel obstruction or peritonitis is absent. Some physicians still advocate reduction even in the presence of

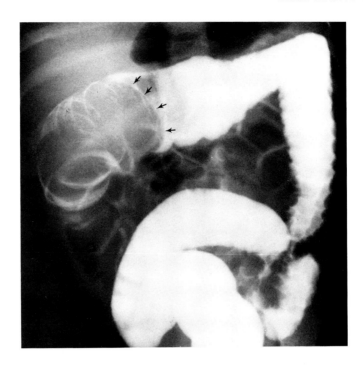

Fig. 3-18. Instussusception. "Coil spring". The barium column stops abruptly at the hepatic flexure forming a concave configuration around the edge of the mass *(arrows)*. As the barium slowly progresses between both loops of bowel, the classic "coil spring" appearance is produced. Note the edematous mucosa in the descending colon. This indicates the original extent of the mass.

small bowel obstruction. However, small bowel obstruction in intussusception is probably the best radiographic indication of an already existing irreducable or gangrenous lesion. Peritonitis is even more serious, since it is always associated with gangrenous bowel or perforation. Attempted reduction in these two situations is dangerous, and immediate surgical intervention is necessary. The duration of symptoms is not important unless they are the result of obstruction or peritonitis.

Certain considerations should be adhered to rigidly when reducing an intussusception. Extreme caution should be exercised and the abdomen never manipulated. It is best to sedate the infant in order to avoid any unnecessary increase in abdominal pressure. The buttocks are tightly held or strapped to prevent leakage of barium around the tube. The height of the barium source is important and should not be maintained much higher than 36 ins. from the table top.

During the procedure barium will flow readily into the colon until it reaches the leading point of the intussusception. It then stops abruptly and forms a concave configuration around the edge of the mass (Fig. 3-18). The barium passes slowly in a spiral, ring-like fashion around the main body of the lesion and produces the characteristic "coil spring" appearance (Fig. 3-18). Continual pressure must be applied by the barium column in order to push the intussuscepted colon back. This occurs at an uneven rate until it reaches the ileocecal valve, where again a temporary and at times considerable delay is caused by the edematous ileocecal valve. It is important at this stage to maintain constant pressure if the bowel is to be squeezed through the valve (Fig 3-19). More recently, the use of glucagon has been advocated to dilate and relax the ileocecal valve. Once the bowel has been successfully reduced beyond the ileocecal valve, the small bowel must be flooded to exclude concomitant small bowel intussusception (Fig. 3-20). The colonic mucosa often shows evidence of edematous changes distal to the point where the intussuscepted mass was encountered initially. This is probably not the result of the procedure but of the continual to-and-fro movement of the intussuscepting lesion prior to its incarceration.

A major decision that must be made during the procedure is when to terminate an unsuccessful reduction. It is difficult to establish absolute guidelines, since these are often modified by subjective and emotional reactions that may develop as the procedure progresses. Basically, enough time must be given to insure that the bowel will move under pressure. A 5-minute delay in any one location is usually considered adequate. After such a delay the child is allowed to evacuate

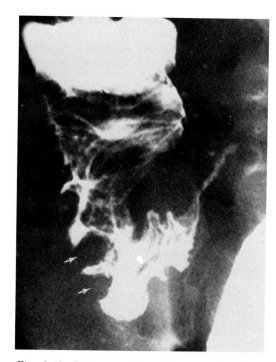

Fig. 3-19. Intussusception. The mass has been reduced to the ileocecal valve and appears as a large filling defect. Note the "coil spring" appearance around its superior surface. Two juvenile polyps are attached to the lateral wall of the cecum (arrows).

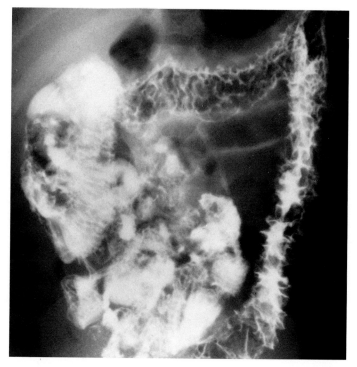

Fig. 3-20. Reduced intussusception. Most of the small bowel is flooded with barium following a successful reduction. The entire colonic mucosa is edematous, emphasizing again the distance that the lesion can migrate within the colon.

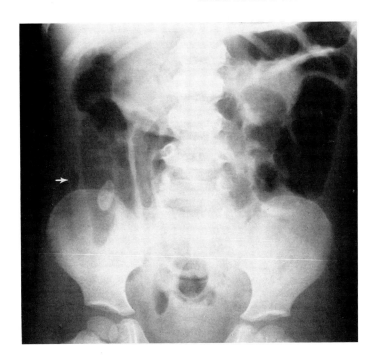

Fig. 3-21. Appendicitis. Note the abnormal collection of gas in the right flank alongside the ascending colon *(arrow)*. A large appendicolith is projected over the right iliac crest. Small and large bowel distention indicate the presence of an ileus.

the barium, and the reduction is reattempted. In most instances the simple mechanics of evacuation alone result in a successful reduction. A repeat failure should be sufficient, and the procedure is then terminated. However, some physicians recommend a third attempt. Surgery is the obvious treatment of choice following unsuccessful reduction. The following recommendations cannot be over-emphasized: *Do not* attempt hydrostatic reduction in the presence of small bowel obstruction or peritonitis; *do not* raise the barium column too high from the table (36 ins. is recommended); *do not* palpate the abdomen unnecessarily.

In patients over 2 years of age it becomes imperative to exclude a lesion as the leading cause of intussusception (Fig. 3-19). This can be attempted during or following the initial reduction procedure.

A closed loop obstruction is produced when a segment of bowel is obstructed at two points, as in volvulus. The prognosis in this type of obstruction is worse than in a simple obstruction, since the vascular supply is easily compromised, and infarction promptly ensues. The obstructed loop fills quickly with fluid. In the early stages, however, gas is still confined within the lumen, yielding a configuration resembling a "coffee bean." The two thickened edematous bowel walls lying in close approximation to each other

comprise the central radiodensity of the "coffee bean." When the air is completely replaced by fluid, a soft-tissue mass results (pseudotumor).

Meconium ileus equivalent is a late manifestation of fibrocystic disease and can present as an acute obstruction anytime after the neonatal period. The radiographic features are similar to neonatal meconium ileus and consist of a pattern of acute small bowel obstruction, associated with increased radiodensity and a "soap bubble" appearance in the right lower quadrant, which are due to inspissated fecal material. Barium studies are rarely required but will confirm the diagnosis if refluxed into the terminal ileum to demonstrate the thickened intraluminal material.

Amorphous gas collections lying outside the gastrointestinal tract suggest the presence of an abscess or perforated viscus. When grouped together, they are contained within an abscess and may displace adjacent viscera (Fig. 3-21).

Although the radiographic features of an ileus generally differ from small bowel obstruction, the amount of bowel affected, and the type and location of the dilated bowel are variable. Frequently a single distended loop, "the sentinel loop," or simply a few distended loops of bowel are present. This presentation is due to an adjacent inflammatory process, and as a result the loops can be con-

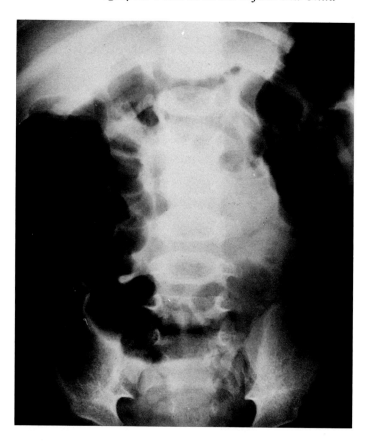

Fig. 3-22. Celiac disease. This addominal film shows the unevenly distended, fluid filled loops of small bowel.

sidered as "marker loops." For example, dilated small bowel located in the right lower quadrant signifies the possibility of an acute appendicitis or ileitis. The diagnosis is substantiated when other radiographic features such as an appendicolith or a soft-tissue mass are evident (Fig. 3-21). Ileitis is suggested when a vague soft-tissue mass containing irregularly thickened bowel is apparent. Distended loops of small bowel localized in other portions of the abdomen suggest adjacent inflammatory disease (e.g., right upper quadrant—cholecystitis, midepigastrium—pancreatitis).

A diffuse pattern that consists of dilated small and large bowel is non-distinctive and can reflect either localized or diffuse inflammatory disease, peritonitis, blood in the peritoneum, or recent surgery. The radiographic finding is usually universal or selective dilatation of the small and large intestine, with long air fluid levels at similar levels within the same loop of bowel.

Chronic small bowel dilatation is caused by lesions that either organically produce stenosis of the bowel or cause intermittent alterations of bowel function or motility.

Most of these cannot be differentiated on routine abdominal examinations, and the use of contrast medium to opacify the gastrointestinal tract is almost always necessary. A nonflocculating barium suspension is recommended in order to avoid producing confusing features.

Malabsorption is suspected when a pattern of unevenly distended loops of bowel containing varying amounts of fluid is encountered on the abdominal film (Fig. 3-22). Celiac disease is the most common mucosal disease producing this disorder and in many ways represents the prototype of malabsorption. The clinical presentation of celiac disease is rather insidious but begins soon after an infant has been exposed to wheat cereal in his diet. The child fails to thrive and presents with bulky, foul-smelling, pale stools. The single most characteristic radiologic manifestation in malabsorption is dilatation of the small bowel and, more specifically, the jejunum. The mucosal folds become straightened and less prominent (Fig. 3-23). Segmentation, flocculation, and hypersecretion are common findings associated with malabsorption but are probably less specific.

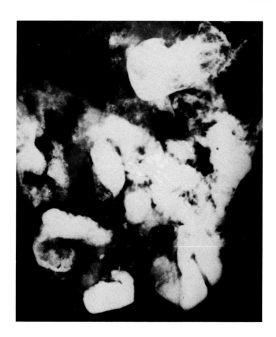

Fig. 3-23. Celiac disease. Barium is unevenly distributed throughout the gastrointestinal tract. The jejunum is dilated, and some barium is apparent within the ileum.

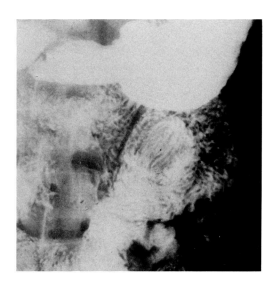

Fig. 3-24. Celiac disease. Intussusception. The "coil spring" appearance of intussusception is present within the jejunum. Aside from slight distention of bowel, no other changes of malabsorption are obvious.

Segmentation occurs when dilated loops of small bowel that are separated from one another by strands of barium present in collapsed intestinal loops. Flocculation represents broken and coarse collections of barium. The "moulage" sign is a term reserved for dilated loops of small bowel that appear to be amorphous. This occurs mostly in the jejunum and is a further expression of hypersecretion and segmentation. Bowel motility is also altered, causing intermittent intussusception and diminished transit time (the time required for barium to traverse the small bowel). Orthograde small bowel intussusception is, however, rarely demonstrated during the course of a single examination (Fig. 3-24). Despite the many radiologic signs associated with celiac disease, the diagnosis is still best established by small bowel biopsy.

Malabsorption in general is the result of a single or combination of multiple abnormal physiologic mechanisms. Some show specific organic findings and others present with radiographic features that are indistinguishable from celiac disease.

Cystic fibrosis is perhaps the most common disorder associated with malabsorption. Ten per cent of the patients present with meconium ileus in the neonatal period. The majority also manifest pulmonary disease in

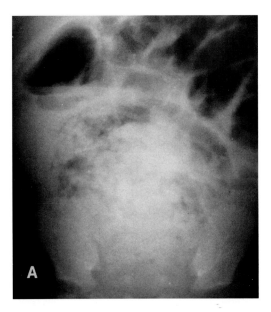

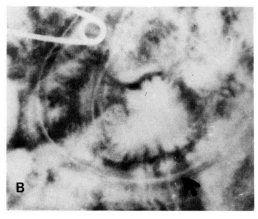

Fig. 3-25. Ascariasis. *(A)* A routine abdominal film manifests the worms as large, irregular, whirling radiodensities. *(B)* The worms appear as long, linear, radiolucent filling defects within the barium column. The gastrointestinal tract of the parasite is also seen as a thin, elongated, barium-containing structure *(arrow)*.

varying degrees of severity at the time the diagnosis is established. Although the small bowel changes of malabsorption are identical to those of celiac disease, certain mucosal alterations encountered in the duodenum and colon are quite distinctive.

Congenital hypoplasia of the exocrine pancreas with neutropenia is another cause of pancreatic insufficiency. Metaphyseal dysostosis is also a regular feature of this syndrome (the Schwachman-Diamond syndrome).

Abetalipoproteinemia, although rare, is quite distinct. In some patients mild to moderate thickening of the mucosal folds of the duodenum and jejunum are present in addition to malabsorption. Neuromuscular disease, retinal abnormalities, acanthocytosis, and absence of serum beta-lipoprotein complete the clinical spectrum. Serum beta-lipoprotein is essential for the transport of fat from the gut, and its absence accounts for the development of the malabsorptive disorder.

Other lesions resulting in malabsorption are parasitic infestations, immunodeficiency states, inflammatory disease, the blind loop syndrome, malrotation, and the short loop syndrome. Most of these demonstrate characteristic radiographic findings.

Parasitic infestations are commonly associated with malabsorption and dilated small bowel. *Ascaris lumbricoides* is a roundworm,

responsible for infestation that presents with vague gastrointestinal complaints, and it is almost always associated with malnutrition and obstruction. Roundworm infestation is recognized on the routine abdominal radiograph by multiple, whirling masses of radiodensity that appear when the worms are outlined by air within the lumen (Fig. 3-25A). During the barium examination the parasites themselves look like linear filling defects within the bowel lumen. The Ascaris worm occasionally ingests the barium, and the alimentary canal of the worm is then seen as a thin, thread-like collection of barium (Fig. 3-25B). Obstruction results when a mass of worms becomes large enough to impact and occlude the bowel lumen. Frequently, the worms migrate and obstruct other structures such as the bile duct, pancreas, stomach, and occasionally the esophagus.

Giardiasis is caused by *Giardia lamblia*, a harmless protozoon that occupies the duodenum and upper jejunum. Heavy infestation results in absorptive and inflammatory abnormalities. The radiographic findings consist of thickening and distortion of the mucosal folds within the duodenum and proximal jejunum, as well as generalized dilatation of the bowel itself. *Giardia lamblia* has been noted in approximately 20 per cent of

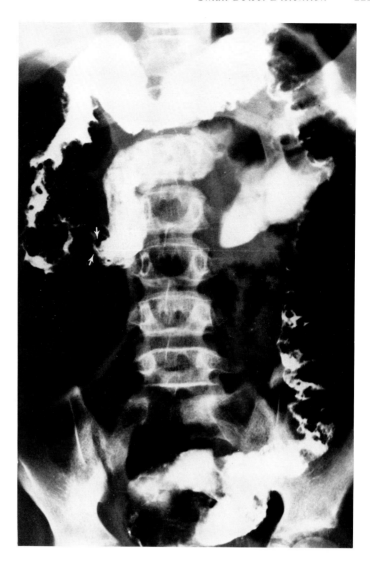

Fig. 3-26. Aganglionosis of the colon and terminal ileium. A 12-year-old female with a history of constipation since the neonatal period. Evacuation film shows a somewhat fore-shortened right colon. Reflux occurs into a narrow terminal ileum. Note the zone of transition *(arrows).*

patients with immunoglobulin disorders and is often accompanied by nodular lymphoid hyperplasia (Fig. 3-38; see p. 121).

Malabsorption identical to that of celiac disease, but non-gluten responsive, has been described in patients with immunoglobulin abnormalities. Other characteristics of these abnormalities, in addition to malabsorption, resemble those of nodular lymphoid hyperplasia and nodular intestinal lymphangiectasia.

Food allergy produces clinical features of diarrhea, failure to thrive, and edema. Radiographs taken at the time of reaction demonstrate dilated and edematous mucosa. Most infants respond to the withdrawal of the antagonistic agent.

The presence of lactase deficiency is suggested when recurrent diarrhea is correlated with the ingestion of milk products. The radiologic investigation consists of challenging the patient with a barium preparation containing the suspected milk product. If the small bowel examination shows dilatation, barium flocculation, and rapid transit, a confirmation is obtained when a repeat study performed without the addition of the challenging material is normal. One must be certain, however, that significant quantities of sugar are not present in the flavoring or coloring agent.

Malabsorptive states also result following congenital or surgically created anatomical alterations of the bowel. This has been ob-

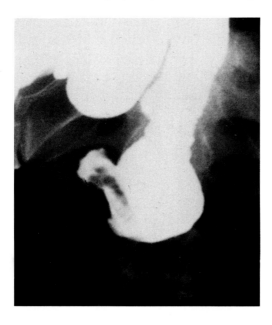

Fig. 3-27. Meckel's diverticulum. A large diverticulum projects from the ileum into the pelvis. The filling defect at the base of the lesion is composed of gastric mucosa and contains a central ulcer *(arrows)*.

served in malrotation, and the short bowel and blind loop syndromes. These abnormalities are easily recognized during contrast studies. A blind loop is created following an end-to-side or side-to-side anastomosis. Segments of bowel are partially excluded from the direct current of the intestinal stream, and as a result bolus collects within these segments, causing dilatation. A similar pathologic state results when bowel proximal to any severely stenotic surgical anastomosis dilates and collects stagnant bolus. A blind loop is occasionally identified on the abdominal study as a persistently dilated air-containing viscus. Contrast material remains within this dilated loop well after the completion of an upper gastrointestinal study. The other two abnormalities, short bowel and malabsorption, are easily recognized.

Chronic obstruction caused by a lesion that produces stenosis can be excluded only if the entire small bowel is carefully evaluated. This is important, since many obstructing stenotic lesions are known to cause secondary malabsorptive changes in the bowel. One common lesion is Crohn's disease (see p. 125). This is most frequently encountered within the right lower quadrant, although "skip lesions" may be found throughout the small bowel. The bowel between the stenotic segments often distends. There are other inflammatory lesions that present as stenotic lesions. Most have a characteristic appearance or are associated with mucosal changes. When obstruction is caused by an adhesion,

the narrowed segment is abrupt, well-defined, and demonstrates intact mucosa.

Rarely, a patient with colonic and terminal ileal aganglionosis survives beyond the neonatal period and is detected in early childhood with a history of constant constipation. The radiographic findings are the same: a somewhat foreshortened colon with prompt reflux into a narrow terminal ileum. If an adequate amount of barium is refluxed, a transition zone in the small bowel may be detected (Fig. 3-26).

Discussion

→ Intussusception and incarcerated hernia are the most common causes of acquired small bowel obstruction in childhood. Intussusception occurs most often during the 1st 3 years of life, with a peak incidence between the 3rd and 12th month of the 1st year. In approximately 95 per cent of the infants below the age of 2, the most likely mechanism is a functional disturbance resulting from an increased deposition of fat and lymphoid tissue within the bowel. Diet change with subsequent increased peristaltic activity may be another precipitating factor. Specific causative lesions are encountered in approximately 50 per cent of cases of intussusception in children over 2 years of age. Peyer's patches, lymphoma, large mesenteric nodes, duplications, Meckel's diverticulum, and polyps are well known causes. Meckel's diverticulum accounted for nearly half of the lesions in a recent study of lesions causing

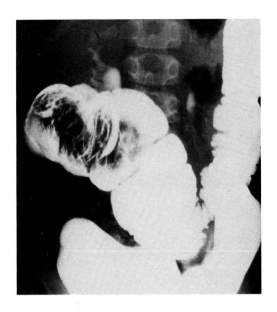

Fig. 3-28. Burkitt's lymphoma. A large, bulky mass forms the leading point in this intussusception. Note the "coil spring" appearance of the barium surrounding the tumor.

intussusception. Meckel's diverticulum is a frequent cause of recurrent bleeding, abdominal pain, and inflammatory disease simulating appendicitis (Fig. 3-62). The lesion is difficult to demonstrate radiographically, since it commonly contains muscle in its wall and empties its contents as easily as the surrounding bowel (Fig. 3-27). Nuclear imaging with sodium pertechnetate ^{99m}Tc has proved helpful, since it is positive when gastric mucosa is present within the lesion. The agent is concentrated and secreted by the parietal cells in the gastric mucosa. Lymphosarcoma is a common cause of intussusception and obstruction in children over the age of 6 years. Large, bulky, cecal masses due to Burkitt's lymphoma of the American type are being described with increasing frequency (Fig. 3-28). In general, intussusception occurs in three major pathologic forms: *Ileocolic* consists of invagination of the ileum into the colon and comprises 90 per cent of cases; *ileal-ileal-colic* consists of invagination of small bowel into small bowel and then into colon; *colo-colic,* as the term implies, consists of invagination of colon into colon. The major complication that arises in any intussusception is compression and angulation of the mesentery between the layers of the bowel. This causes partial inhibition of venous drainage and eventually impedes arterial flow, resulting in gangrene.

Although it is difficult to conceive of an acute appendicitis with abscess formation resulting in small bowel obstruction, the abscess in all probabilities causes a localized functional ileus that in effect produces the same results. It is also possible that the abscess itself behaves as a mass lesion and actually compresses adjacent bowel.

Intestinal malabsorption results when the transfer of one or more nutrients from the intestinal lumen into the circulation is impeded. This may be the result of an abnormal bowel wall, inappropriate intraluminal enzymes, or dysfunction of absorptive mechanisms in the small bowel mucosa. Celiac disease is caused by specific intolerance of the gut to gluten present in ingested wheat and rye cereal protein. The diagnosis is established when a normal bowel response is obtained following removal of gluten from the patient's diet. Small bowel biopsy reveals flattened epithelial cells and atrophied villi. The intermittent forms of malabsorption relating to disaccharide intolerance are due to absence of one or more intestinal disaccharidases. The most common of the inborn errors of metabolism is lactase deficiency. In general, the complex starches are reduced initially by pancreatic enzymes to disaccharades and are then absorbed intact into the small bowel mucosa, where they are split by specific enzymes into monophasic sugars. The absence of these enzymes results in vomiting and diarrhea due to osmotic effects of the unabsorbed sugars.

Malabsorption which arises in spontaneously occurring or surgically created small bowel diverticula is the result of hypomotility, stasis, and overgrowth of intestinal anerobic organisms. The mechanism by

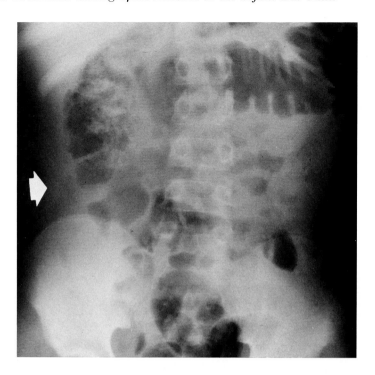

Fig. 3-29. Acute appendicitis. The colon is dilated because of an acute appendicitis. Note the well developed haustra. The ascending colon is displaced medially by a gas-containing mass *(arrow).* Small bowel dilatation is also apparent.

which bacterial overgrowth induces malabsorption is not entirely clear. Intestinal bacteria deconjugate bile salts, which can result in irritation of the mucosa. In addition, a lesser amount of bile salts is then available to aid in the digestion of fat. A macrocytic anemia is also produced, since the bacteria compete with the mucosal-absorbing cells for vitamin B.

DILATATION OF THE COLON

The dilated colon is easy to recognize in infants and children. The haustra are well developed, and the configuration of the colon is now mature. Although some confusion may arise in distinguishing haustra from the valvulae conniventes of small bowel, the haustra are thicker and larger and rarely extend across the entire width of the bowel (Fig. 3-29).

The colon dilates when affected directly by an obstructive process or by an ileus, or in conjunction with a non-colonic disease process.

When the colon is obstructed it is frequently the only viscus evident radiographically. The location and occasionally the nature of the obstructing lesion may be demonstrated by maximally positioning air at the point of obstruction. This may require the use of multiple projections. Gas may be found in the small bowel if the ileocecal valve is incompetent. If large amounts of gas are present the radiographic presentation may be confusing, since gas in both the small bowel and colon is also noted with an ileus. However, the viscera are usually proportionally dilated when an ileus is present.

Disease Entities
Acute Obstruction
  Neoplasm
    Benign
    Malignant
  Trauma
Chronic Obstruction
  Hirschsprung's disease
  Psychogenic megacolon
  Stricture
  Adhesion
Ileus
  Toxic megacolon
  Inflammation
    Infectious
    Non-infectious
Nonspecific Dilatation
  Hypothyroidism
  Bedridden patients
  Celiac sprue
  Neuromuscular disorders

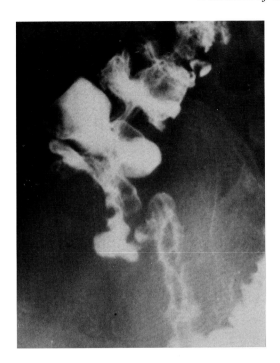

Fig. 3-30. Carcinoma of the cecum. A large polypoid mass replaces the cecum with extension into the terminal ileum that resembles Crohn's disease.

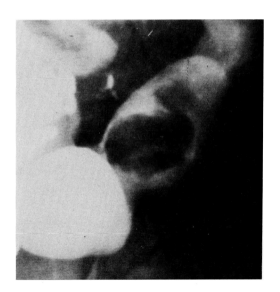

Fig. 3-31. Juvenile polyp. Large well circumscribed polyp is present in the sigmoid colon. Note the large stalk.

Differential Diagnosis

Distinguishing an acute from a chronic obstruction on a radiographic basis alone is often feasible, since the configuration of the colon frequently differs. In an early acute obstruction the haustra are prominent and well defined. In chronic obstruction they appear fewer in number and may be prominent in some areas of the colon and absent in others. The inner contour of the bowel is also irregular, and the entire colon appears flaccid and thickened (Fig. 3-33A). A barium enema examination is always necessary to defini-

tively identify the obstructing lesion, regardless of the type of obstruction.

Obstructing neoplasms are more often polypoid in nature. Sarcoma and adenocarcinoma comprise the majority of these masses. The surface of the mass is nodular and irregular (Fig. 3-30). Burkitt's tumor is a particular form of lymphoma that frequently presents as a large bulky lesion within the cecum (Fig. 3-28). The annular constricting carcinoma with overhanging margins so commonly seen in the adult is rare in infants and children. Most polypoid lesions originate from the mucosa or submucosa. Benign le-

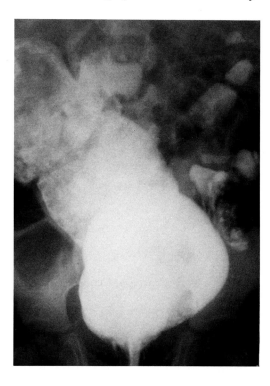

Fig. 3-32. Psychogenic megacolon. The rectum and sigmoid are dilated and contain most of the barium. The remaining colon is normal in caliber.

sions are recognized by their characteristic smooth and regular surface (Fig. 3-31), although they can occasionally be lobular. The presence of a stalk attaching the lesion to the mucosal surface is an important radiographic feature, since it almost always signifies a benign process. Some submucosal lesions (e.g., lipomas, fibromas) are known to prolapse into the lumen of the bowel and simulate mucosal lesions. Abdominal trauma may be associated with a dilated colon because of obstruction due to hematoma within the bowel, because of a generalized ileus, or because of a combination of both. In any event, the colon is almost always intrinsically normal, since any mass encountered is either an extrinsic or an intramural hematoma. Perforation of the colon is more often associated with free abdominal air and decompressed colon.

Acute colonic obstruction is not common in infants and children. The dilated colon most frequently reflects a chronic abnormality, mainly Hirschsprung's disease and psychogenic megacolon. Hirschsprung's disease usually begins in the neonatal period, and although some patients with this disease go undetected and are treated only for minor chronic constipation, the onset of the patient's symptoms can almost always be traced back to the neonatal period. Psychogenic

megacolon begins somewhat later, during the 1st or 2nd year of life, and is a result of poor or forced toilet training. The barium study in either disease is characteristic. The entire colon in psychogenic megacolon is diffusely and equally dilated. In some cases, only the rectum and sigmoid colon are enlarged, forming a pear-shaped chamber (Fig. 3-32), with the remaining colon only slightly dilated. The presence of a transition zone is pathognomonic for Hirschsprung's disease and is never seen is psychogenic megacolon. As a result, the caliber of the distal aganglionic colon is narrow in comparison to the proximally dilated normal colon (see Chapter 2, p. 68, and Fig. 3-33). Chagas' disease and plexiform neurofibromatosis within the pelvis are two disorders that have a similar radiographic presentation.

Anal strictures or anal fissures also cause diffuse dilatation of the colon, producing radiographic findings similar to psychogenic megacolon. However, the presence of a tight stenotic anus and the knowledge of previous surgery are distinctive features.

Hypothroidism, the immobilization in institutionalized, bedridden children, spinal cord lesions, celiac sprue, and certain neuromuscular disorders are rare causes of chronic constipation and a dilated colon.

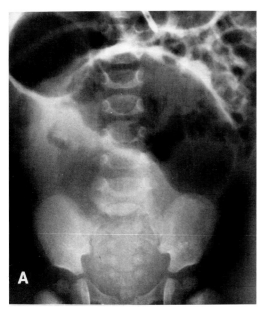
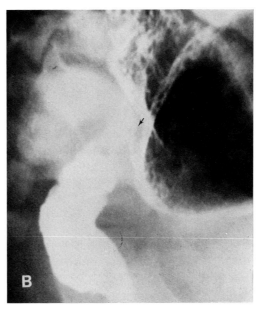

Fig. 3-33. Hirschsprung's disease. (A) Abdominal film demonstrates a markedly distended colon. No air is detected in the rectum. Note the flaccid configuration of the colon and the lack of any haustral pattern. (B) Barium is present in a narrow rectum. The remaining colon is markedly dilated and a well-defined transition zone is present at the rectosigmoid junction (arrow).

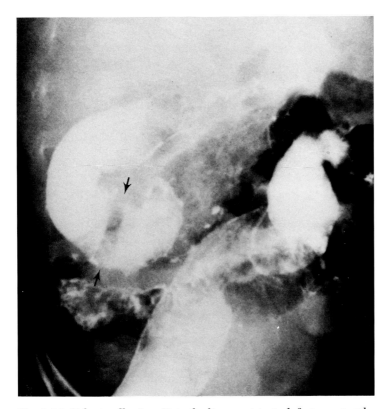

Fig. 3-34. Colonic adhesion. Note the linear extrinsic defect crossing the cecum (arrows).

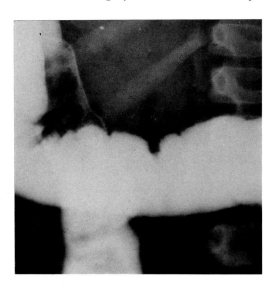

Fig. 3-35. Early granulomatous colitis. Detailed study of the proximal transverse colon demonstrates a roughened irregular mucosa caused by multiple irregular ulcerations along the superior border. The haustral pattern is also poorly recognizable.

Colonic adhesions are uncommon and in the absence of previous surgery almost nonexistant. The radiographic finding, as with adhesions in the small bowel, is a linear, extrinsic, obstructing defect (Fig. 3-34).

Acute infectious or noninfectious inflammatory disease of the colon may also present with a dilated colon on the abdominal radiograph. Barium studies are often performed to evaluate the disease and its extent. However, in the presence of acute inflammation this should be performed with caution to avoid any unwanted complications. Ulcerative colitis in its early stages may be limited only to the distal colon, although in some cases the entire colon can be involved. The ulcerations produced are superficial and sometimes difficult to demonstrate. They are best observed on the evacuation and air contrast studies. During the evacuation phase, the mucosa is no longer lace-like but appears coarse, irregular, and spotty. Small punctate ulcerations are the major findings on the air contrast study. Similarly shaped, small barium collections, projecting from the colonic surface as V-shaped notches, are usually normal. These notches were believed to represent the crypts of Lieberkühn but are more likely the innominate grooves on the mucosal surface. The notches are anatomically positioned in a regular row-like fashion along the entire intestinal tract and disappear when the colon is completely filled and distended with barium. Ulcerations are more irregular in shape, size, and location and persist when the colon is completely filled. The bowel wall in ulcerative colitis appears blurred and abnormal.

Early granulomatous colitis may be even more difficult to detect, since in general the disease begins within the submucosa and is frequently segmental and asymmetrical. Apthous ulcerations represent early manifestations of this disease and should be noted carefully (Fig. 3-35). The asymmetric involvement of the bowel wall eventually produces abnormal out-pouchings, such as pseudo-diverticula, on the opposing uninvolved side. This is another important radiographic finding, although it is not absolutely characteristic.

Other forms of acute inflammatory disease that dilate the colon consist of toxic megacolon, acute salmonellosis, shigellosis, and amebiasis. These lesions are uncommon, but must be recognized early so that proper therapy can be instituted. The radiographic findings on the abdominal study alone are often diagnostic for toxic megacolon (Fig. 3-36). As a result, the use of contrast medium is contraindicated. The transverse and sigmoid colons are almost always the principal structures affected, although it is not unusual for an entire colon to be involved. The contour of the colon is severely altered since the haustral pattern is no longer apparent, and the diseased bowel appears as a dilated irregular tube. The inner margin of the bowel is markedly irregular due to the universal presence of ulcers and swollen mucosa (pseudopolyps).

Barium studies performed on patients with

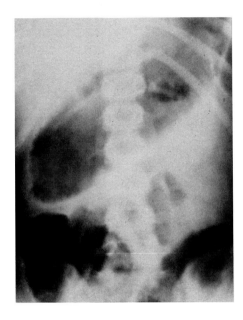

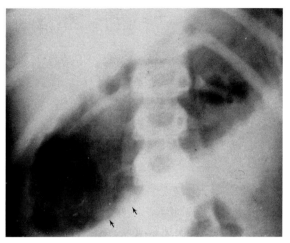

Fig. 3-36. Toxic megacolon. The transverse colon is severely dilated and is completely devoid of any normal configuration. The haustral pattern is no longer visible, and the bowel wall is ulcerated and nodular *(arrows).*

infectious colitis demonstrate mucosal edema and ulcerations that vary in size and configuration. The radiographic features in many ways resemble ulcerative or granulomatous colitis. However, the radiologic and pathologic changes encountered in infectious colitis are probably far more extensive than those in a patient with nonspecific colitis of equal duration.

An unusual form of an acute evanescent segmental colitis has recently been described. The lesion is reversible and does not appear to be characteristic of any major form of viral, bacterial, or parasitic colitis. This condition can be mistaken for Crohn's disease.

Discussion

Hirschsprung's disease in the older child is benign and is therefore diagnosed late, during the 2nd and 3rd year of life. Abdominal distention and chronic constipation are the main clinical problems, although some children present with failure to thrive, malnutrition, and anemia. The severe complication of enterocolitis which occurs in newborns is rarely encountered in the older child.

Colonic trauma is unusual. The force required to damage the colon is considerable, and in most cases additional intra-abdominal injuries are present. The splenic and hepatic flexures are the most frequent sites of rupture. Rectal damage is the result of pelvic fractures.

The dilatation of the colon in celiac sprue is probably related to the size of the stool and the rate of elimination from the rectum. Although cellular and ultrastructural abnormalities probably exist, the colon is less frequently involved than the small bowel, since it is exposed to a lesser concentration of gluten.

Surprisingly, carcinoma of the colon is the most common cancer of the gastrointestinal tract, despite its overall rarity. The lesions are most frequently located in the rectum and sigmoid colon and consist of a colloid-producing adenocarcinoma. Bulky, large lesions are also seen in lymphosarcoma but are more commonly found in the ileocecal region.

Toxic megacolon is a major and often catastrophic complication of ulcerative colitis. The onset is rapid and the patients are clinically toxic. The lesion can occur at any time during the course of the disease, but it is encountered more frequently in individuals with a known history of ulcerative colitis. Toxic megacolon is not restricted to ulcerative colitis and has been found in Crohn's disease and amebiasis.

NODULAR ALTERATIONS OF THE SMALL BOWEL

Normally, the small bowel mucosa produces a feathery, lace-like contour along the wall of the bowel. These folds are numerous

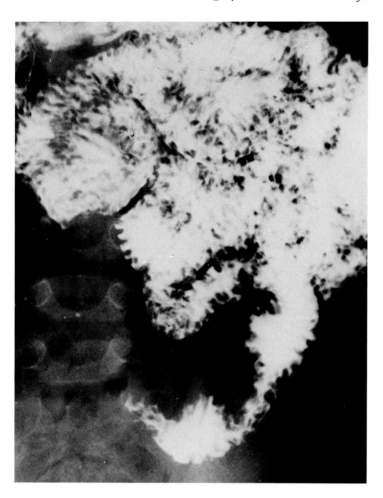

Fig. 3-37. Nodular lymphoid hyperplasia. Note the well-defined nodular pattern that has replaced the normal lacy appearance of the small bowel.

and feathery in the jejunum and gradually become shallower and fewer in the distal portions of bowel. When the mucosal folds are thickened or replaced by well-defined circular or oval lesions, the mucosal surface assumes a nodular appearance. In children, the distal ileum contains prominent lymph follicles and is normally nodular. However, similar nodular changes detected more proximally always indicate an abnormal disease process.

Bowel edema uniformly thickens the mucosal folds and occasionally simulates nodular disease. However, the thickened folds, when closely examined, are not well-defined or truly nodular (see p. 129). Differentation between the two is further complicated, since some of the lesions producing nodular alterations of the small bowel are also associated with a degree of intramural edema, which partially accounts for the ultimate radiologic presentation.

Disease Entities

Diffuse
 Lymphoid hyperplasia
 Intestinal lymphangiectasia
 Lymphosarcoma
 Amyloidosis
  Edema
  Vasculitis
Local
 Tumor metastasis
 Lymphosarcoma
 Alpha-chain disease
 Whipple's disease
 Mastocytosis
 Eosinophilic gastroenteritis
 Crohn's disease
 Yersinia ileitis
 Tuberculosis
  Edema
  Vasculitis

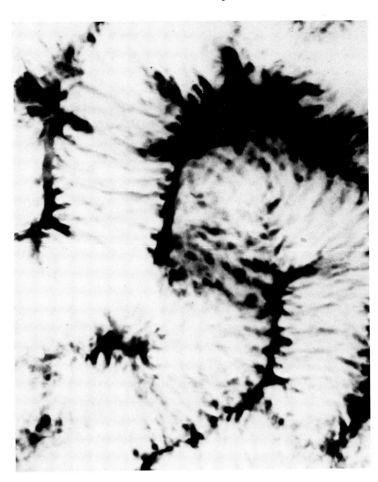

Fig. 3-38. Nodular lymphoid hyperplasia.Giardiasis. Spot film of the jejunum in a patient with giardiasis and lymphoid hyperplasia demonstrates well-defined, rounded nodules.

Differential Diagnosis

Nodular lymphoid hyperplasia is distributed uniformly throughout the entire small bowel as innumerable, tiny, smooth, nodular filling defects measuring 2 to 3 mm. in diameter (Figs. 3-37, 3-38). The nodules are round and regular and not associated with mucosal alteration. A nodular pattern is also encountered occasionally in intestinal lymphangiectasia (Fig. 3-39). However, the changes in this disease more often consist of redundant and excessive folds with increased secretions. As a result, the barium study appears irregular and dilute, and the mucosa is coarse. In fact, in some cases the combination of edema and increased secretions may cause severe blunting and fragmentation of the folds to produce a pattern resembling malabsorption.

Amyloidosis is a rare infiltrative bowel disease in children that causes a pseudo-nodular appearance. When the ileum is involved the entire small bowel appears similar in appearance. This has been referred to as "jejunalization."

A pattern simulating intestinal lymphangiectasia and amyloid disease is also produced in Whipple's disease. It is questionable whether this disease occurs in the pediatric age-group. In this entity, the valvulae conniventes are thickened and sometimes nodular. However, Whipple's disease is mainly limited to the jejunum and more often produces a wild, redundant configuration.

Distinct nodular masses are characteristic for lymphosarcoma. The nodules, however, vary in size and configuration and may be irregular in contour as well as ulcerated (Fig. 3-40). Lymphosarcoma is more often localized in only portions of the bowel, although the entire bowel can be involved diffusely. This neoplasm is primarily cellular and submucosal in origin and can also infiltrate the bowel wall diffusely, causing a smooth thickening of the intestinal folds with-

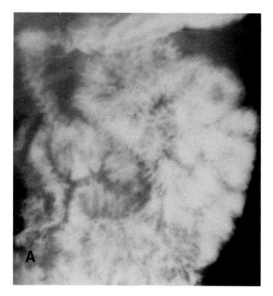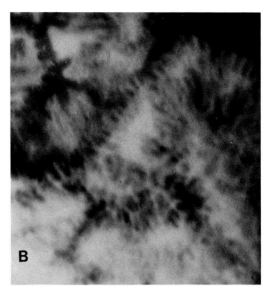

Fig. 3-39. Intestinal lymphangiectasia. *(A)* The mucosa demonstrates a somewhat nodular appearance. The barium is diluted and the mucosal folds are irregular and redundant due to the excess amount of fluid. *(B)* A more detailed view of a section of small bowel better reveals the findings above.

out evidence of hypersecretion. The features above are often accompanied by extra-visceral lesions within the neighboring mesentery (Fig. 3-40).

Metastatic disease and the rare alpha-chain disease (heavy-chain disease) in many aspects are radiologically similar. Alpha-chain disease frequently involves the small bowel, with a nodular pattern that is accompanied by a spiky and scalloped contour. A sprue-like pattern with segmental dilatation, as well as enlarged mesenteric lymph nodes that produce extrinsic compression or dislocation of the small bowel, also occurs.

Mucosal thickening and mucosal nodularity, or both, have been described in mastocytosis, an uncommon disorder characterized by mast cell proliferation in the skin, bone, lymph nodes, and other parenchymal structures. The lesions occur mainly in the jejunum but have also been noted in the ileum. They present as nodules that vary in size and, when small, may be ill-defined. The precise nature of the changes have not been completely elucidated. The thickened folds are believed to be caused by an underlying cellular infiltrate, whereas the edema and the nodules are believed to be caused by urticarial infiltrations.

Eosinophilic gastroenteritis affects not only the stomach and small bowel, but the colon as well. At times only the small intestine is involved diffusely or segmentally. The mucosa becomes thickened and blunted, and a "cobblestone" or nodular appearance results (Fig. 3-3). The radiologic changes reflect the presence of underlying edema as well as a chronic inflammatory infiltration composed mainly of eosinophils. Occasionally, the edema and cellular infiltrations are extensive and completely efface the mucosa, resulting in a narrowed lumen. When the muscularis becomes infiltrated, paradoxical dilatation of the involved segment has also been noted. Eosinophilic gastroenteritis can be confused with regional ileitis and tuberculosis. The characteristic location of regional ileitis and tuberculosis (within the distal ileum) and the high eosinophil count of eosinophilic gastroenteritis are important distinguishing attributes.

Localized areas of nodularity, or what has been termed a "cobblestone" appearance, is an important radiographic feature of ileitis (Crohn's disease; Fig. 3-41). A "cobblestone" appearance is the result of a number of factors: edema of the mucosa and submucosa, in which the swollen folds that are unattached

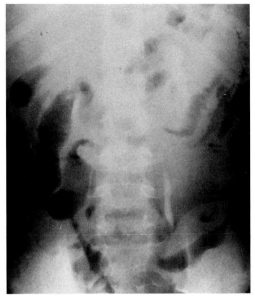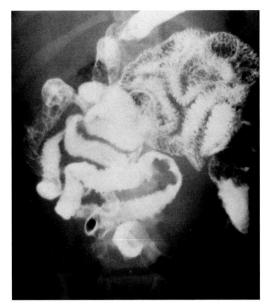

Fig. 3-40. Lymphosarcoma. Extensive disease involving both the bowel and mesentery. The ileum is involved with an irregular nodular process. A section of the bowel is also infiltrated diffusely causing complete mucosal effacement. Large adjacent mesenteric masses also displace this loop. The same changes can be recognized on the abdominal film.

to the muscularis bulge up into the lumen; a network of longitudinal and transverse ulcerations, leaving the intervening portions of the mucosa intact; and marked fibrosis that produces traction on the overlying mucosa in a compartmentalized fashion. Ileitis frequently extends into the surrounding tissues. The bowel wall and the intervening mesentery become quite thickened. As a result the involved loops of bowel are displaced away from the normal viscera.

Yersinia ileitis is an acute enteritis that undergoes a number of radiographic changes during its development and simulates acute Crohn's disease in the early and late phases. The initial stage lasts for 3 weeks. The main pattern consists of numerous, round, uniform, mural nodules in the distal ileum. These findings are also associated with a thickened wall and a narrow lumen. During the 4th and 5th week, the radiographic and pathologic picture consists of diffuse edema. As a result the mucosa is flattened and effaced. A stage of resolution then commences and lasts for approximately 3 to 5 more weeks. During this time, the nodules described reappear and slowly regress. Needless to say, the transition between the various stages is not often distinct, and the duration of each stage can vary from individual to individual.

Discussion

Localized lymphoid hyperplasia normally occurs in the lamina propria of the terminal ileum and has been referred to as "nonsclerosing ileitis." When the process extends outside the confines of this structure it must be considered abnormal. Lymphoid hyperplasia is prevalent during early and midchildhood and is twice as frequent in males as in females. It may present clinically in both an acute and chronic form, and commonly arises following an upper respiratory tract infection. Adenovirus has been implicated as the causative agent in some acute cases. Certain disabling symptoms such as weight loss, diarrhea, anemia, and intussusception have been associated with this disorder.

Dysgammaglobulinemia associated with nodular lymphoid hyperplasia of the small bowel has also been reported. These morphologic changes are associated with decreased gamma globulin, decreased or absent IgM and IgA, increased susceptibility

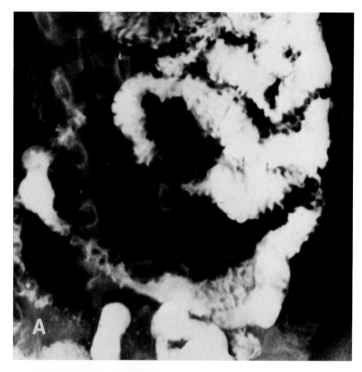

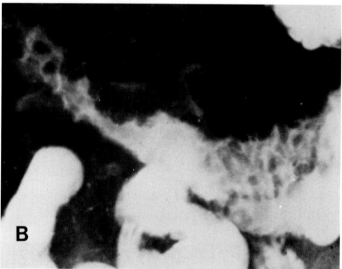

Fig. 3-41. Crohn's disease in a 13-year-old male. *(A)* A diffuse and irregular nodular pattern involves a large portion of the small bowel. The effected loops are widely separated by intervening thickened mesentery. *(B)* Close observation of a single diseased segment of bowel better demonstrates the nodular "cobblestone" appearance. The wall of the bowel is also asymmetrically thickened.

to infestation with *Giardia lamblia*, sinopulmonary infections, diarrhea, and steatorrhea. In many patients, the gamma globulin levels have been found to be normal, with only moderate deficiency in IgA and IgM noted on immunoelectrophoreses. Microscopically, conglomerates of hyperplastic lymphoid tissue containing mitotic activity within the germinal centers of the lymphoid follicles are present throughout the small bowel, as well as the colon. The cause of the hyperplasia is still undetermined but may represent a compensatory reaction to functionally inadequate lymphoid tissue. Patients with hypogammaglobulinemia have an 8 per cent risk of developing a malignancy. This is usually of the lymphoreticular variety, although three of the nine patients first described developed carcinoma of the gastrointestinal tract, two in the stomach and one in the colon.

Whipple's disease is associated with a syndrome of intermittent arthralgia, abdominal pain, steatorrhea, and weight loss. Thus

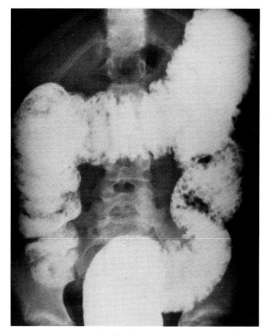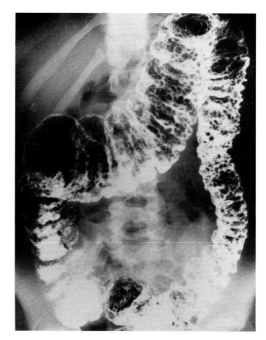

Fig. 3-42. Familial polyposis. Barium and air contrast studies of the colon demonstrate polypoid lesions throughout the entire colon. The lesions are round, well-defined, and almost equal in diameter.

there is a strong clinical and biochemical resemblance to sprue. However, the presence of sudan-negative and PAS-positive macrophages within the lamina propria and lymph nodes is distinctive of Whipple's disease. The PAS-positive material, as well as certain gram-positive granules identified within the macrophages, have been shown by means of electronic microscopy and histochemistry to represent bacteria and bacterial substances. This accounts for the positive clinical response following antibiotic therapy.

Classification of amyloidosis into a primary and secondary form is no longer valid. Although the entity is indeed unusual in children, it does occur in familial Mediterranean fever, and familial amyloidosis. Amyloidosis associated with chronic bronchiectasis, regional ilietis, and tuberculosis was more common in the past when antibiotic therapy was not available.

Alpha-chain disease is characterized by diarrhea, abdominal pain, loss of weight, and finger clubbing. It occurs among Non-Europeans living in the Mediterranean region and is related closely to Mediterranean lymphoma. Histological examination of small bowel reveals a diffuse plasmocytosis. These plasma cells, however, produce only a part of the two alpha chains and no light chains.

Most patients also demonstrate elevated plasma levels of intestinal alkaline phosphatase.

Urticaria pigmentosa is the cutaneous and often the first manifestation of mastocytosis. Infiltration within the dermis, reticuloendothelial system, and within other organs is distinctive. The mast cell contains a myriad of biochemically active substances such as histamine, heparin, and hyaluronic acid. The cells also stimulate fibrosis and other cellular infiltrations. As a result myelofibrosis, periportal fibrosis, and systemic fibrosis are often found in the late stages of the disease. Systemic mastocytosis can occur without cutaneous manifestations in an occasional case. However, sclerotic bone lesions and an enlarged liver and spleen are found in 50 per cent of cases.

Regional enteritis is the most common inflammatory disease of the small bowel that produces radiographic changes. The early acute manifestations are strongly mimicked by acute Yersinia ileitis. Crohn's disease is not restricted to the terminal ileum and has been found in any portion of the gastrointestinal tract. The early symptomatology is usually vague and misleading, and in a high proportion of cases it does not conform to the symptomatology typical of Crohn's disease in adults. While most children complain of some sort of abdominal pain, it is not uncommon for many to present with arthralgia, fever, and poor growth and development. Two main forms exist, the stenotic and non-stenotic. It requires at least 4 to 6 years for stenosis to develop in granulomatous enteritis. Therefore, it is understandable why the majority of children present with the non-stenotic form, in which the mucosal change of "cobblestoning" is an important feature.

Considerable disagreement exists regarding the relationship between acute ileitis and Crohn's disease. Acute ileitis probably represents one of several entities. In a recent study it was shown that in patients with acute ileitis the course of the disease proceeded in one of two directions; either Yersinia organisms were isolated and the patient never developed Crohn's disease, or no evidence of Yersinia was demonstrated and the patient developed Crohn's disease. The pathologic changes in Yersinia ileitis are caused by edema, hyperplasia of lymphoid tissue, and enlargement of regional lymph nodes.

POLYPOID LESIONS

Basically, polypoid lesions differ from nodular defects by their ultimate appearance within the bowel lumen. The lesions appear as nodular filling defects within the barium column and as well-defined soft-tissue masses during an air contrast examination. Most polypoid masses originate from the mucosal surface.

Disease Entities

Small Bowel
    Peutz-Jeghers syndrome
    Juvenile gastrointestinal polyposis
    Adenomatous polyp
    Submucosal masses (lipoma, fibroma, neurofibroma)
Colon
    Juvenile polyps
    Adenomatous polyp
        Familial polyposis
        Gardner's syndrome
        Turcot syndrome
    Peutz-Jegher's syndrome
    Nodular lymphoid hyperplasia
    Peudopolyposis
    Juvenile gastrointestional polyposis
    Lymphoma

However, some lesions do arise within the submucosal layers, such as a lipoma, but occasionally develop large enough and prolapse into the lumen. Consequently, the origin and the exact nature of the lesion may not be obvious in some cases without benefit of histologic examination.

Differential Diagnosis

In general, gastrointestinal polyps are divided into three major histologic categories: juvenile polyps, adenomatous polyp, and hamartomatous polyp. The radiographic features of each are basically the same, although the size of the lesions may vary. All demonstrate a round configuration and a smooth surface. The nature of each lesion is ascertained by correlating the overall pathologic, clinical, and radiologic findings.

The routine abdominal features in most polyposis syndromes are frequently insignificant, although the polyps in the Peutz-Jeghers syndrome can be large enough to cause small bowel intussusception and/or obstruction. Peutz-Jeghers polyps are encountered mainly in the small bowel but may be found in all portions of the gastrointestinal tract. The polyps vary in size and are either sessile or pedunculated. It is not unusual to demonstrate multiple lesions 2 to 3 cm. in diameter on compression spot films. Multiple lesions 1 to 2 mm. in diameter are common but rarely visualized on the radiographs.

Juvenile polyps, by contrast, occur essentially in the colon. These polyps are most often solitary and it is unusual to find more than three in a single patient. (Figs. 3-19, 3-31). The polyp is believed to be inflammatory in origin and histologically consists of an epithelial component surrounded by abundant connective tissue with dilated intestinal glands.

Adenomatous polyp is also found in the colon but, in contrast to juvenile polyps, is almost always multiple and diffuse in infants and children.

The distribution and the number of polyps present often determine the type of disorder. For example, a single polyp in the colon represents a benign juvenile polyp. Multiple small polyps of almost uniform size that carpet the entire mucosal surface of the colon indicate familial polyposis (Fig. 3-42). Multiple polyps which vary in size and are found in

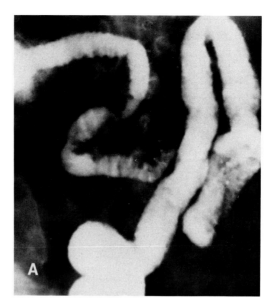

Fig. 3-43. Nodular lymphoid hyperplasia of the colon. *(A)* Nodular defects are present throughout the entire colon simulating diffuse polyposis. *(B)* Biopsy of a polypoid lesion within the rectum reveals large accumulations of lymphocytes.

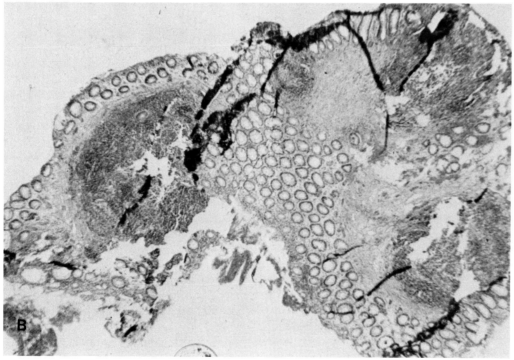

the colon and in the small bowel are the hallmark of Peutz-Jeghers syndrome.

Diffuse polyposis of the colon is also associated with other syndromes. The additional presence of facial and cranial osteomas and soft-tissue desmoids indicates Gardner's syndrome; Turcot syndrome is associated with tumors of the central nervous system, usually supratentorial gliomas. The Canada-Cronkite syndrome is seen in older patients and has yet to be encountered in the pediatric age-group.

The guidelines above are not foolproof; a syndrome consisting of diffuse *juvenile* gastrointestinal polyposis also exists. The disorder radiographically resembles familial colonic polyposis, although histologically it is more closely related to the Canada-Cronkite syndrome. When it occurs in infancy it may result in the rapid demise of the infant by virtue of protein loss, hemorrhage, or gastrointestinal obstruction.

Benign nodular lymphoid hyperplasia may further complicate the differential diagnosis

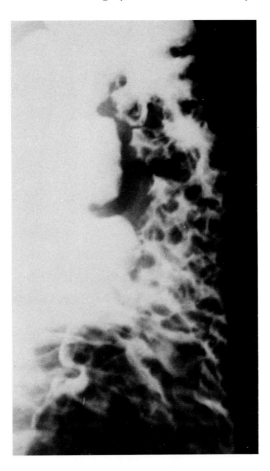

Fig. 3-44. Lymphosarcoma of the colon. Air contrast examination demonstrates well-defined nodules within the descending colon. The majority appear smooth and equal in diameter. However, a few are large and irregular, demonstrating its neoplastic character.

when the nodules enlarge and simulate intraluminal filling defects (Fig. 3-43). More often they consists of diffuse nodular defects that demonstrate central umbilications upon compression.

The pseudopolyposis that develops in association with ulcerative colitis is the result of an intense inflammatory reaction and can be diffuse. The underlying disease is recognized by the surrounding mucosal ulcerations and the loss of the normal colonic haustral configuration. Large or small irregular polypoid masses that produce contour defects along the margins of the bowel wall are characteristic of neoplastic disease (Figs. 3-14B, 3-44). Neoplasia as such is fortunately not a common primary presentation. Carcinoma is an undesirable complication in familial polyposis and ulcerative colitis.

Discussion

Peutz-Jeghers syndrome is an unusual condition that is characterized by autosomal dominant inheritance, mucocutaneous melanotic pigmentation, and gastrointestinal polyposis. Polyposis can be found throughout the gastrointestinal tract, and radiologic examination not only confirms the diagnosis but determines the extent and severity of the lesions. The pigmented lesions in this syndrome are usually evident during infancy and early childhood. Normally, they occur around the lips, particularly along the mucosal surface of the lower lip, and appear as brown or black macules ranging from 1 to 5 mm. in diameter. The next most common site is the buccal mucosa. Frequently, the presenting symptoms are intussusception and rectal bleeding; rarely, massive gastrointestinal bleeding occurs. Although gastrointestinal polyps are present in infancy or early childhood, they seldom cause symptoms until adolescence or young adult life. Most physicians regard the polyps as benign, nonproliferating hamartomas in which normal epithelium covers strands of smooth muscle. They are not considered precancerous, although an increased incidence of carcinoma of the colon, stomach, and duodenum has been described in this syndrome.

Table 3-3. **Characteristics of Polyposis Syndromes**

Disease	Location	Histology	Age of Onset	Malignancy Potential	Other Features
Familial polyposis	Colon	Adenomas	Childhood and adolescence	High	Dominant
Peutz-Jeghers	Mainly small bowel	Hamartomas	Childhood and adolescence	Increased	Pigmentation
Gardner's	Colon	Adenomas	30 years	High	Osteomas Desmoid
Juvenile polyps	Colon	Inflammatory	2-4 years	None	None
Juvenile gastrointestinal polyposis	Mainly colon	Inflammatory	1-2 years or later when familial	None in early lesions increased in familial cases	
Turcot	Colon	Adenomas	2nd decade	Brain tumor	Recessive
Canada-Cronkite	Mainly stomach and colon	Inflammatory	40 years and above	1-3%	Ectodermal changes

(Schwartz, A. M., McCauley, R. G.: Juvenile gastrointestinal polyposis. Radiology, *121:*441, 1976.)

The presence of multiple adenomatous polyps within the colon is significant, since it is associated with a high incidence of family involvement and intestinal malignancies. A recently described entity, diffuse juvenile polyposis, simulates the radiographic appearance of familial polyposis, although the gross histologic appearance and etiological background are distinctly different. The occurrence of mixed forms, consisting of a conglomeration of juvenile and adenomatous polyps, has also been reported. Morrison believes that the juvenile polyp is basically a hamartoma, while other physicians believe that its origin is inflammatory, secondary to blockage of the mucosal gland duct by inflammation accompanying mucosal ulceration. The familial occurrence of juvenile polyps would favor a hamartomatous origin. Unlike familial adenomatous polyposis, the malignant potential of multiple juvenile polyposis is thought to be low, although an increased incidence of intestinal malignancy has been found in some families.

Lymphoid tissue is normally present throughout the small and large intestine and may form discrete nodules, lymph follicles, in the large bowel within the submucosa. The term lymphoid hyperplasia has been applied to some cases where the lymph follicles enlarge and cause visible indentations within the mucosa (Fig. 3-43B). Although nodular lymphoid hyperplasia associated with dysgammaglobulinemia was described originally as occurring within the small bowel, it has now been found in the colon. Nodular lymphoid hyperplasia following necrotizing enterocolitis *per se*, or with Hirschsprung's disease, is a not an uncommon complication.

EDEMA OF THE SMALL BOWEL

The radiographic pattern of bowel edema is best observed in the jejunum. The early changes are uniformly and symmetrically thickened mucosal folds that eventually resemble a stack of coins (Fig. 3-45). This presentation is also a well known feature of intramural hemorrhage. Mild dilatation of the bowel is almost always present. The edematous bowel wall and intervening soft tissues cause the loops of bowel to separate from

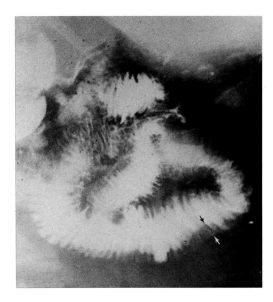

Fig. 3-45. Small bowel edema. A young child with nephrotic syndrome demonstrates thickened mucosal jejunal folds that have a "stacked coin" appearance. The thickness of the mucosal fold can be evaluated by measuring the inner and outer margin of the folds *(black and white arrows).* The bowel is also dilated.

each other, or uncoil. The motor activity of the bowel is also altered, resulting in abnormal bowel contractility and decreased peristalsis. In differentiating edema from other patterns that thicken bowel wall, careful observation reveals a lack of nodularity and mucosal ulceration. The presence of fluid within the lumen dilutes and coarsens the appearance of the barium.

Disease Entities

Diffuse
  Primary protein loss: protein-losing
      enteropathy
    Intestinal lymphangiectasia
    Whipple's disease
    Regional enteritis
    Menetrier's disease
    Ulcerative colitis
    Chronic congestive heart failure (constrictive pericarditis)
  Secondary protein loss: hypoproteinemia
    Liver disease
    Nephrotic syndrome
    Burn
    Exudative skin lesions
Localized
  Zollinger-Ellison syndrome
  Giardiasis
  Vasculitis
    Henoch-Schönlein purpura
    Connective-tissue disorders
  Acute inflammatory reactions

Differential Diagnosis

Edematous fluid may collect either diffusely or locally within bowel. The main cause of diffuse edema is hypoproteinemia. The fluid in this situation is essentially a transudate and is cell-free, in comparison to the majority of localized collections that occur in conjunction with intrinsic or extrinsic inflammatory disease. Since protein can be lost from the bowel or other structures in the body, diffuse bowel edema is subdivided into primary and secondary forms. The primary form indicates direct loss of protein from the bowel (protein-losing enteropathy), and the secondary form indicates protein loss from structures other than bowel (e.g., burns, liver disease).

Protein-losing enteropathy does not represent a single disease entity but describes a composite of conditions that include intestinal lymphangiectasia, Menetrier's disease, regional enteritis, and Whipple's disease. The radiographic features of intestinal lymphangiectasia consist of redundant folds, a small nodular pattern, or fragmentation and an excessive accumulation of fluid within the bowel wall and the intestinal lumen. In many ways, the entire presentation resembles Menetrier's disease. However, in Menetrier's disease the stomach is the principal site of protein loss, and marked rugosity of the folds and excessive fluid are noted within that organ (Fig. 3-46). The features of Whipple's disease and regional ileitis are quite distinct but may be somewhat disturbed when associated with diffuse bowel edema.

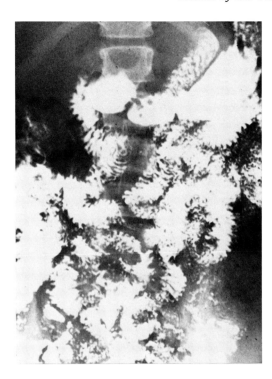

Fig. 3-46. Menetrier's disease. The entire small bowel and the gastric folds are thickened. This distinguishes the disease from most other enteropathies.

The radiographic analysis of localized bowel edema is an intriguing diagnostic problem. The Zollinger-Ellison syndrome is often associated with dilatation and edema of the duodenum and proximal small bowel. Giardiasis also affects the duodenum and proximal jejunum, but the changes usually begin within the distal duodenum. Henoch-Schönlein purpura may involve the entire bowel, but more often one or more localized areas are involved. The altered fold pattern that results is the most characteristic radiographic feature in the syndrome and is due to edema and/or hemorrhage. The folds become thickened and blurred because of the marked edema and increased secretions. In fact, the underlying changes may be so pronounced that the entire fold pattern is obliterated. The secretions also cause segmentation and fragmentation of the barium column. The effects of hemorrhage are more prominent, and irregular thumbprint impressions are produced along the contour of the wall (Fig. 3-47). Similar patterns have been encountered in certain systemic connective-tissue disorders, such as rheumatoid arthritis, polyarteritis, systemic lupus erythematosus, and dermatomyositis (Fig. 3-48). The underlying pathogenic mechanism in all of these disorders consists of a small-vessel, necrotizing vasculitis; superimposed changes of seg-

mental infarction can and do occur. The end result is a narrowed rigid segment of bowel with hazy and blunted mucosal folds.

Hereditary angioneurotic edema also presents as an area of focal submucosal edema. The diagnosis is facilitated by the presence of a positive family history and current past episodes. Otherwise, the lesion is not radiographically distinguishable from focal edema or hemorrhage cuased by any of the abnormalities above. The changes, however, are transitory. They are found only when the patient is symptomatic and disappear as the symptoms resolve.

Discussion

The most common cause of noninflammatory intestinal edema is hypoproteinemia resulting from either kidney or liver disease, or from protein loss through body tissues (e.g., the gastrointestinal tract or the skin). Intestinal edema occurs when the serum albumin level is 1.9 gms./100 ml. or lower.

Intestinal lymphangiectasia is a specific lesion that results in the loss of protein into the gastrointestinal tract. The clinical presentation varies in severity, and findings ranging from chronic diarrhea to gross anasarca have been described. The nodular fold changes represent a combination of mucosal and submucosal edema, as well as dilatation of

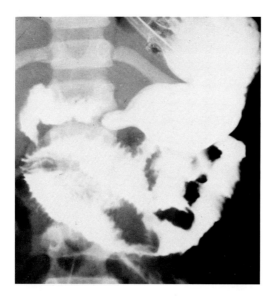

Fig. 3-47. Henoch-Schönlein purpura. The pathologic changes are mainly in the jejunum in this patient. On the right the folds are edematous and present a "stacked coin" appearance. Thumbprint impressions associated with mucosal effacement are present more proximally on the left and probably represent intramural hemorrhage.

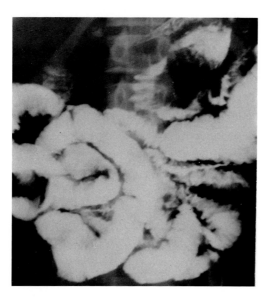

Fig. 3-48. Periarteritis nodosa. Note that the radiographic features are somewhat similar to those of Fig. 3-47. The folds are markedly edematous and thickened.

the lymphatics within the mucosa and submucosa. Protein is released through the bowel wall as a result of a tear occurring in the dilated lymphatic vessels or through an intact epithelium secondary to obstruction. Symptomatic improvement occurs when patients are placed on a low fat diet. This decreases lymph production and, consequently, the pressure within the lymphatics. The addition of medium-chain triglycerides to the diet has also been helpful, since these substances are transported directly to the liver by way of the portal system and bypass the lymphatics. The exact etiology of this disease is unknown, although a congenital disorder of the lymphatic system seems probable.

It appears that not only is albumin lost in

protein-losing enteropathy, but that in some instances there is also an excessive loss of lymphocytes and immunoglobulins. In one patient with constricitve pericarditis the entire deficiency was reversed following pericardectomy.

The necrotizing vasculitis which occurs in connective-tissue disorders and in Henoch-Schönlein purpura may compromise the vascular supply to segments of bowel, causing ischemic or hemorrhagic changes within the intestinal wall. Therefore, occasional complications such as perforation, massive bleeding, and multiple infarctions are known to result. Henoch-Schönlein purpura is common in males between the ages of 2 to 8 years. It is a self-limiting disease that may develop sev-

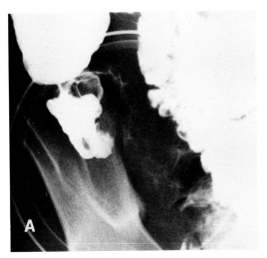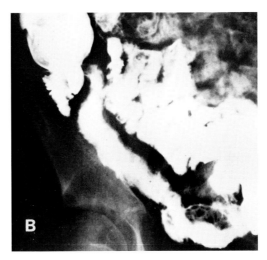

Fig. 3-49. Crohn's disease *(A)* The terminal ileum is spastic and poorly visualized. *(B)* This film was exposed during the same examination after the terminal ileum relaxed and re-expanded. Note the mucosal ulcerations and early nodularity.

eral weeks after a streptococcal infection. It is characterized by the onset of a slowly developing skin rash that is quite variable in its presentation. Abdominal and joint pain, as well as a form of glomerulonephritis, also appear. The abdominal pain and tenderness often simulate an acute abdominal catastrophe. However, the renal disease is potentially the more serious problem, since it can evolve into a chronic process.

Hereditary angioneurotic edema is a distinct clinical problem. It is a rare familial disease that is transmitted by an autosomal gene. The syndrome consists mainly of recurrent attacks of circumscribed subepithelial edema of the skin and mucous membranes of the respiratory and gastrointestinal tracts. In contrast to most episodes of angioneurotic edema, there is no response to epinephrine and antihistamines. The basic biochemical defect in hereditary angioneurotic edema is a deficiency of or a defect in alpha gamma globulin, which is an inhibitor of the activated first component of the complement esterase. The reason for periodic activitation is unknown, and the onset of disease can occur anywhere between infancy and the 4th decade of life.

NARROWED BOWEL

Lesions which cause acute or chronic stenosis of the bowel may be single or multiple, or may be diffuse and involve the entire small and large bowel. Some lesions prefer-

entially affect either the small or large bowel, whereas others affect both equally. The bowel proximal to the stenotic lesion is usually dilated.

Disease Entities
Localized
   Crohn's disease
   Tuberculosis
   Yersinia ileitis
   Chronic granulomatous disease of childhood
   Post-inflammatory strictures
   Neoplasm
Diffuse
   Ulcerative colitis
   Crohn's disease
   Hemolytic uremic syndrome
   Infectious colitis

Differential Diagnosis

Crohn's disease consists of two phases, an early, non-stenotic phase and a later stenotic phase. It is not unusual to observe transient narrowing of bowel during an acute episode (Fig. 3-49). This is a physiologic phenomenon caused by local ulceration and spasm and has occasionally been confused with the "string" sign, a term that originally described chronically thickened bowel. The bowel usually re-expands when the acute episode abates or when the spasm disappears. It is not possible, therefore, to estimate chronicity or activ-

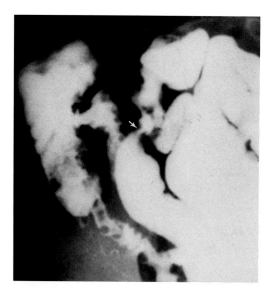

Fig. 3-50. Crohn's disease (stenotic phase). Stenotic changes are present in this patient. The terminal ileum has a "cobblestone" appearance and is somewhat narrow. A smaller but more stenotic area is present proximally within the ileum *(arrow).* The bowel proximal to this lesion is dilated.

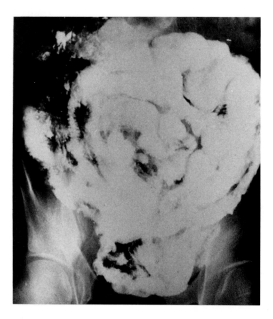

Fig. 3-51. Tuberculous enteritis and peritonitis. The bowel is contained within a densely fibrotic peritoneum. The ileum is narrowed by intrinsic disease.

ity on the basis of a stenotic segment alone. Chronic disease is more often accompanied by other pathologic changes such as rigidity, separation of loops, fistulas, and distended proximal bowel. A rigid narrow loop resembles a pipe-stem and is the result of mucosal thickening and contraction of the involved bowel wall. The mucosa in this segment is frequently effaced and ulcerated. The length of such a lesion is variable and may be as small as 1 to 2 cm. (Fig. 3-50). Multiple, diseased segments are commonly present, and bowel located proximal to the diseased segment and between the multiple, diseased segments is often normal but dilated. Fistulas

are also encountered in this state. These extend into the bowel wall, the mesentery, and the abdomen. The involved loops are frequently separated from one another and appear to surround a mass. The mass most often represents an indurated mesentery, although it is occasionally caused by an abscess that results from perforation.

Gastrointestinal tuberculosis in many ways mimics ileitis. Both are granulomatous diseases and both normally occur in the terminal ileum. Tuberculosis is uncommon, although it is still found in individuals from Africa or the Far East. The infection in the bowel begins with a primary reaction similar to that in

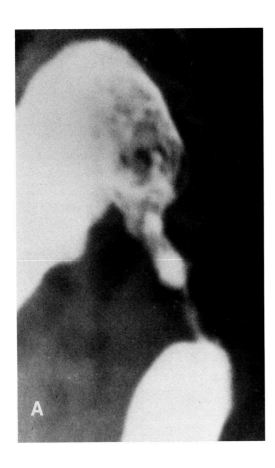

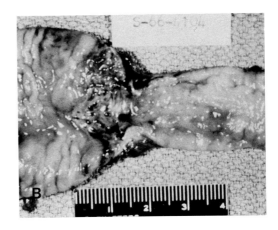

Fig. 3-52. Stricture complicating necrotizing enterocolitis. *(A)* Barium study performed 3 weeks after diagnosis of necrotizing enterocolitis reveals a developing stricture in the descending colon. *(B)* Pathologic specimen demonstrates the diseased segment. The mucosa is denuded and ulcerated. Note the difference in diameter between the distal and proximal lumen.

the lung. The bowel wall is affected initially with mucosal ulceration and edema. Tubercle bacilli are transported to the regional lymph nodes which subsequently become enlarged. The cecum is exceedingly spastic and contractile when active disease is present; this is known as the Sterlin sign. Similar reactive changes occur in the presence of adjacent inflammatory reactions (e.g., Crohn's disease or appendicitis). The tuberculous ulceration is somewhat unique in appearance, since it encircles the bowel wall and initially produces a circumferential stricture as it heals. As the disease progresses, further fibrosis develops producing greater bowel deformities (Fig. 3-51). During this stage, it may be difficult to differentiate the disorder from Crohn's disease on radiographic criteria alone. In the past, it was believed that tuberculosis affected both sides of the ileocecal valve, and that Crohn's disease affected only the small bowel; presently, ileocolic involvement by Crohn's disease is a well known occurrence.

Acute inflammatory bowel infections caused by *Yersinia enterocolitica* are becoming more common. The clinical, radiograph-

ic, and pathologic presentations simulate acute Crohn's disease and have been described previously. The diagnosis is established by the laboratory isolation of the organism from the stool or operatively removed appendix, or by serologic testing for specific antibodies. The radiologic findings have been divided into three stages, in which a narrow bowel associated with mural nodularity is noted in the early phase of the disease.

As in the stomach, granulomatous disease of childhood should be a consideration in some infants presenting with narrow but irregularly nodular defects in the bowel.

Strictures developing as a complication of necrotizing enterocolitis are being seen more frequently as the survival rate in this disease continues to improve. The strictures occur in either the small bowel or colon, although the latter is more frequently affected (Fig. 3-52).

Diffuse involvement of the colon by inflammatory disease is quite unusual in the pediatric age-group. Crohn's disease affects the colon, but in asymmetrical alternating segments, and is commonly associated with small bowel disease. Universal involvement of the large intestine does occur, but again

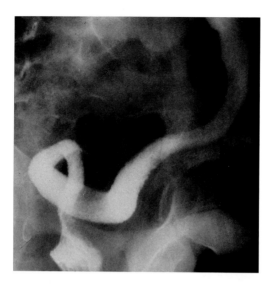

Fig. 3-53. Ulcerative colitis. A section of the colon demonstrates the classic picture of chronic ulcerative colitis. The colon is narrow and tube-like. The mucosa is distinctly ulcerated.

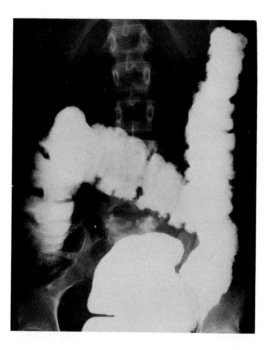

Fig. 3-54. Ulcerative colitis. The colon retains some semblance of a normal configuration. However, ulcerations and evidence of pseudopolyposis are noted along the contour of the bowel.

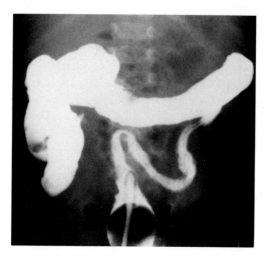

Fig. 3-55. Salmonella colitis. The entire left side of the colon is narrow and involved with a diffuse ulcerative process.

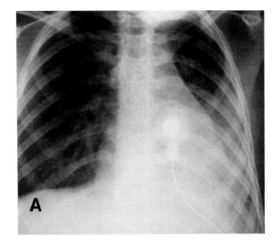

Fig. 3-56. Hemolytic uremic syndrome. *(A)* Chest film reveals left lower lobe pneumonia with pleural effusion. *(B)* Abdominal film exposed at the time that the patient developed bloody diarrhea reveals severe distention of the small bowel and sigmoid colon. *(C)* The rectum is narrowed, and an irregular nodular and ulcerated mucosa is seen.

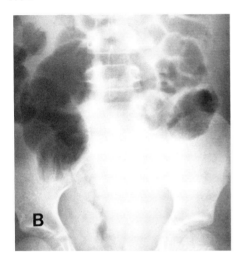

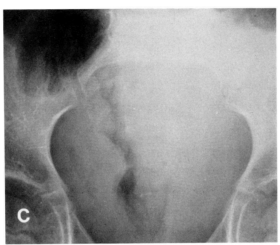

the ileum is commonly affected. There are some cases where no small bowel disease can be detected, and radiographic differentiation from ulcerative colitis may be difficult. However, fistulas and multiple deep ulcerations of varying sizes typify granulomatous disease. The bowel in chronic ulcerative colitis is usually foreshortened, the flexures depressed, and the lumen narrowed. The entire colon appears rigid and tubular (Fig. 3-53), and the mucosa may be ulcerated or may show evidence of re-epitheliazation. In earlier stages the mucosa is irregular, nodular, and ulcerated (Fig. 3-54). Pseudopolyposis, which represents the acutely swollen mucosa, eventually becomes more and more prominent.

Acute infectious colitis may be accompanied by diffuse or localized changes of the colon. These consist of loss of haustral configuration, edema, and ulcerations that vary in size and configuration. The pattern resembles a combination of ulcerative and granulomatous disease (Fig. 3-55).

Hemolytic uremic syndrome usually follows an episode of gastroenteritis or pulmonary disease (Fig. 3-56A) and is associated with intestinal lesions that in most cases preclude the onset of renal failure. The colon is generally narrow and demonstrates focal mural thickening or thumbprinting due to edema and hemorrhage (Figs. 3-56B). Pseudomembranous colitis can be superimposed with this syndrome.

Discussion

The early diagnosis of regional enteritis in children, particularly between the age of 10 to 15 years, requires a certain awareness of the condition. The high incidence of nonstenotic lesions encountered in children of this age-group in comparison to adults is understandable since it requires 4 to 6 years for

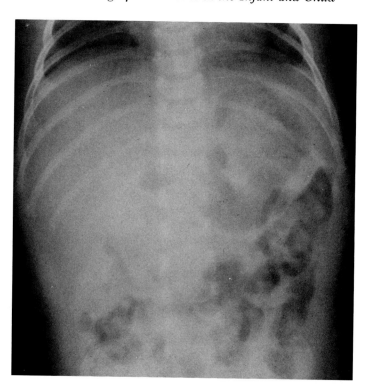

Fig. 3-57. Fatty liver. Cystic fibrosis. The entire right upper quadrant is radiolucent when compared to the normal radiodensity of the surrounding abdomen. The difference in radiodensity assumes the exact position and configuration of the liver.

the disease to progress from a non-stenotic to a stenotic phase. Stricture formation in Crohn's disease is due to a combination of edema and fibrosis. The strictures formed may be single or multiple and of varying length. "Skip areas" are characteristic, and between the lesions the dilated bowel contains normal mucosa. Proximal and distal extention of the disease has not been observed yet. The radiologic similarity between tuberculosis and Crohn's disease is understandable. Both are basically a granulomatous process. In this hemisphere tuberculosis of the gastrointestinal tract is quite reare, and any nodular stenotic or non-stenotic process should always be regarded initially as nonspecific granulomatous disease of the Crohn's variety. Hyperplastic tuberculosis is not a bulky polypoid mass but is the result of thickening of the intestinal wall due mainly to fibrosis. Multiple "skip areas" also occur in tuberculosis. Tuberculosis involves the lymphatics, and lymphatic obstruction may result in malabsorption, which further complicates the features caused by fibrosis and adhesions (Fig. 3-51).

Acute gastroenteritis, ileitis, or enterocolitis are common disorders caused by *Yersina enterocolitica*. However, a spectrum of other entities outside the gastrointestinal tract have also been reported. These include erythema nodosum, Reiter's syndrome, migratory polyarthritis, myocarditis, and hepatosplenomegaly. Most of the cases are short and self-limiting, however, when septicemia occurs the overall mortality can be as high as 50 per cent.

The hemolytic uremic syndrome consists of hemolytic anemia, renal failure, and the thrombocytopenia that frequently occurs in a healthy child following an upper respiratory disease or gastroenteritis. All the radiographic features reflect an underlying process of ischemia, presumably due to occlusion of the microvasculature by fibrin deposits. A similar process is found in the kidney. This syndrome must be recognized early or the correct diagnosis may be obscured.

FATTY LIVER

A fatty liver is recognized by the presence of an overall radiolucency that occupies the exact position and configuration of the liver within the right upper quadrant (Fig. 3-57). A total body opacification study utilizing intravenous contrast material increases the overall tissue radiodensity of the body and therefore better demonstrates the radiolucent character of the liver.

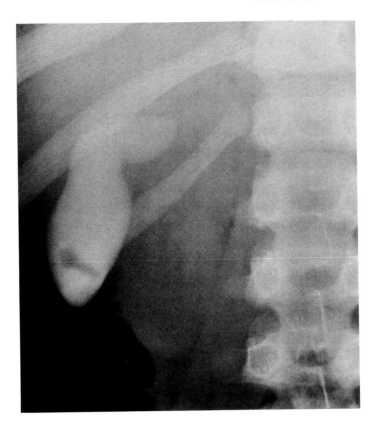

Fig. 3-58. Gallbladder calculi. Sickle cell disease. Oral cholecystography reveals a well functioning gallbladder with a large, oblong, filling defect. This represents bile sludge. Note the vertebral body changes of sickle cell disease.

Disease Entities

Cystic fibrosis
Reye's syndrome
Malnutrition
Kwashiorkor
Hepatitis
Hepatic toxicity: high-dose corticosteroids

Differential Diagnosis

A fatty liver alone is not a specific finding, although cystic fibrosis is probably the most frequent cause. The clinical presentation as well as additional radiographic findings are necessary to distinguish each lesion. In most cases the duration of the underlying disease is important. Chronic lesions associated with fatty livers include cystic fibrosis, and kwashiorkor; fatty livers also occur as a result of long-term high-dose corticosteroid therapy. The diagnosis in each case is usually well known before the fatty liver becomes apparent. The acute lesions which cause fatty radiolucent livers include Reye's syndrome and acute starvation; fatty livers also occur in association with the administration of drugs which cause acute hepatic toxicity. The cause

of fatty infiltration in many of these diseases in unclear but is apparently related to protein depletion with fat substitution.

INTRA-ABDOMINAL CALCIFICATION

Calcifications are easily recognized by their consistency and increased radiodensity. The configuration, location, and radiodensity of the calcium deposit depend upon the underlying disease process.

Disease Entities

Biliary calculi
Renal calculi
Appendiceal calculus
Amorphous intrahepatic calcification (chronic granulomatous disease of childhood)
Intra-abdominal calcification
Neoplasia

Differential Diagnosis

Biliary calculi are quite uncommon in young patients and the symptoms are not always distinctive. As a result the diagnosis is often delayed or erroneous. The identifica-

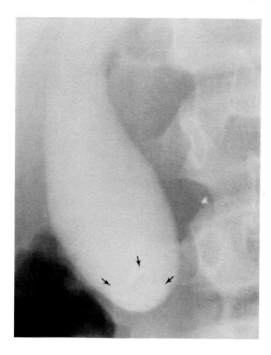

Fig. 3-59. Gallbladder calculi. Multiple calculi are seen within this well functioning gallbladder. They appear to be bordered by a ring of increased radiodensity. Note that the calculi group together within the fundus of the gallbladder *(arrows)*.

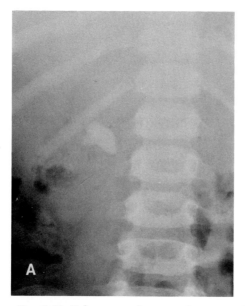

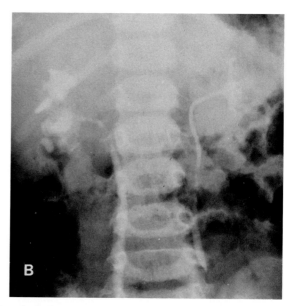

Fig. 3-60. Pelvo-ureteral stones. Cystinosis. *(A)* A fairly large-sized calculus having the configuration of a collecting system is present at the pelvo-ureteral junction. Smaller calculi are noted peripherally within the kidney. *(B)* The intravenous pyelogram contains a distorted collecting system on the right.

tion of gallstones on routine abdominal radiographs has been quoted to be as high as 50 per cent in some studies. With oral cholecystography, the accuracy increases to approximately 75 per cent (Fig. 3-58). The stones are located anteriorly within the right upper quadrant and are therefore readily differentiated from the posteriorly located renal calculi, with which they are often confused

initially. Multiple biliary calculi group closely together (Fig. 3-59). Renal calculi more often are restricted to renal calyces and often assume the configuration of a calyx (Fig. 3-60, 3-61).

The radiographic demonstration of an appendicolith is the single most important finding indicating an acute appendicitis (Fig. 3-21). Appendiceal calculi are located pre-

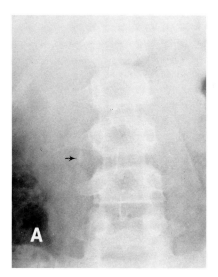 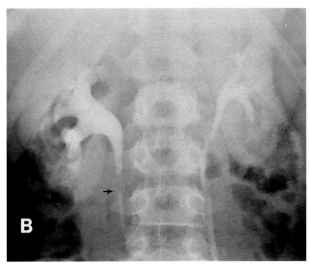

Fig. 3-61. Ureteral calculus. *(A)* A small oval-shaped calculus is present in the right mid-abdomen adjacent to the third vertebral body *(arrow).* This is easily distinguished from a stone within the gall bladder by its medial position. *(B)* Intravenous pyelogram reveals a partially obstructed ureter on the right *(arrow).*

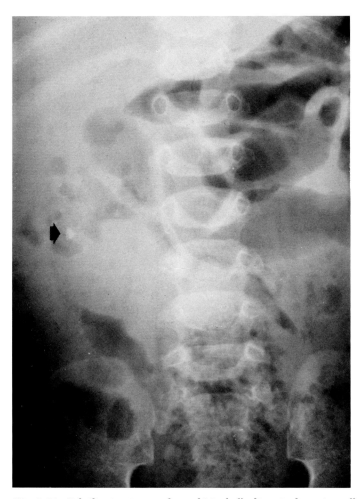

Fig. 3-62. Calcification in a perforated Meckel's diverticulum. A small calcification is present within the right upper quadrant *(arrow).* This is associated with a surrounding inflammatory process and small bowel distention. Although this presentation could easily be caused by an appendiceal abscess, the underlying lesion was a Meckel's diverticulum.

141

dominantly in the right lower quadrant. The exact position depends mainly upon the location and direction that the appendix assumes. The configuration of the calculus is frequently multilaminated since the stone grows by accretion of mucous containing calcium phosphate crystals that form concentric rings of calcium. Rarely, a Meckel's diverticulum produces a similar calculus (Fig. 3-62).

Calcifications also appear within tumors and metastases. This form demonstrates no specific configuration and is often amorphous in appearance (see p. 84). Since calcification occurs in necrotic tissue, a similar type of deposit is also encountered in an abscess. This is a well known complication of chronic granulomatous disease of childhood. This disease should be strongly suspected in an infant with chronic recurrent infections in the lung, soft tissues, and bones.

Discussion

A number of theories have been given for the development of biliary lithiasis. These can be grouped into two categories: those based on modification of the composition of bile ("lithogenic"), and those based on modification of the gallbladder itself. Hemolytic disease is often associated with cholelithiasis. In one series of patients, spherocytosis and sickle cell disease were the most commonly reported hemolytic anemias associated with cholelithiasis and were noted in 19 per cent of the cases. In our experience, sickle cell disease is the most common anemia associated with biliary calculi in infants and children. Calcifications may be seen in patients with renal infections. Bacterial accumulation causes alteration of the composition of the urine.

Tissue necrosis with dystrophic calcification is the main cause of calcification in both neoplasm and abscess. Absence of certain intracellular enzymes accounts for the inability of the neutrophil to phagocytize certain bacteria such as *Serratia marcescens*. As a result, the patient is prone to repeated chronic infections. Pyogenic liver abscess *per se* is an uncommon problem in children and is generally encountered in the compromised pediatric host. The patients usually present with fever and hepatomegaly. The most common causative agent is *Staphyloccocus aureus*.

REFERENCES

Gastric Outlet Obstruction (Gastric Distention)

1. Bell, M. J., Ternberg, J. L., McAlister, W., Keating, J. P., and Tedisco, F. J.: Gastric diaphragm—a cause of gastric outlet obstruction in infants and children. Pediatrics, 90:196, 1977.
2. Farman, J., Faegenburg, D., Dallemand, S., and Chen, C. K.: Crohn's disease of the stomach: the ram's horn sign. Am. J. Roentgenol. Radium Ther. Nucl. Med., 123:242, 1975. 123:242, 1975.
3. Felson, B., Berkman, Y. M., and Hoyumpa, A.: Gastric mucosal diaphragm. Radiology, 92:513, 1969.
4. Griscom, T. N., Kirkpatrick, J. A., Girdany, B. R., Berdon, W. E., Grand, R. J., and Mackie, G. G.: Gastric antral narrowing in chronic granulomatous disease of childhood. Pediatrics, 54:456, 1974.
5. Harris, V. J., and Hanley, G: Unusual features and complications of bezoars in children. Am. J. Roentgenol. Radium Ther. Nucl. Med., 123:742, 1975.
6. Jona, J. Z., Belin, R. P., and Burke, J. A.: Eosinophilic infiltration of the gastrointestinal tract in children. Am. J. Dis. Child., 130:1136, 1976.
7. Swischuk, L. E., and Tyson, K. R.: Burned out pyloric stenosis: an elusive gastric outlet obstruction. Radiology, 117:373, 1975.

Duodenal Distention

8. Berkman, Y. M., and Rabinowitz, J. G.: Gastro-intestinal manifestations of strongyloidiasis. Am. J. Roentgenol. Radium Ther. Nucl. Med., 115:306, 1972.
9. Burrington, J. D., and Wayne, E. R.: Obstruction of duodenum by superior mesenteric artery: does it exist in children? J. Pediatr. Surg., 9:733, 1974.
10. Curci, M. R., Little K., Sieber W. K., and Kiesewetter, W. B.: Peptic ulcer disease in childhood re-examined. J. Pediatr. Surg., 11:329, 1976.
11. Slouis, T. L., Berdon, W. E., Holler, J. E., Baker, D. H., and Rosen, L.: Pancreatitis and the battered child syndrome: report of two cases with skeletal involvement. Am. J. Roentgenol. Radium Ther. Nucl. Med., 125:456, 1975.

Small Bowel Distention

12. Ein, S.: Leading Points in childhood intussusception. J. Pediatr. Surg., 11:209, 1976.
13. Gerald, B.: Aganglionosis of the colon and terminal ileum; long term survival. Am. J. Roentgenol. Radium Ther. Nucl. Med., 95:230, 1965.
14. Khilnani, M. T., and Keller, R. J.: Roentgen

alterations in the gastrointestinal tract in immunoglobulin abnormalities. Am. J. Gastroenterol., 56:512, 1971.

15. LeVine, M., Schwartz, S., Katz, I., Burko, H., and Rabinowitz, J. G.: Plain film findings in intussusception. Br. J. Radiol., 37:678, 1964.
16. Marshak, R. H., and Lindner, A. E.: Malabsorption syndrome. Semin. Roentgenol., 1:138, 1966.
17. Schwachman, H., Diamond, L. K., Oski F. A., and Khaw, K. T.: The syndrome of pancreatic insufficiency and bone marrow dysfunction. J. Pediatr., 65:645, 1964.

Dilatation of the Colon

18. Bryk, D.: The altered colon in colonic obstruction. Am. J. Roentgen, 115:360, 1972.
19. Friedland, G. W., and Filly, R.: Evanescent colitis in a child. Pediatr. Radiol., 2:73, 1974.
20. Kappelman, N. B., Burrell, M., and Taffler, R.: Megacolon associated with coeliac sprue. Am. J. Roentgenol. Radium Ther. Nucl. Med., 128:65, 1977.
21. Williams, I.: Innominate grooves in the surface of mucosa. Radiology, 84:877, 1965.
22. Zwad, H. D.: Filling of Leiberkuhn's crypts of the colon during contrast examination: contribution to differential diagnosis of colitis. Fortschr. Geb. Roentgenstr. Nuklearmed., 120:278, 1974.

Nodular Alterations of the Small Bowel

23. Cohen, A. S.: Amyloidosis. N. Engl. J. Med., 277:522, 1967.
24. Doe, W. F., Henry, K., and Doyle, F. H.: Radiological and histological findings in 6 patients with alpha-chain disease. Br. J. Radiol., 49:3, 1976.
25. Ekberg, O., Sjostrom, B., and Brahme, F.: Radiological findings in Yersinia ileitis. Radiology, 123:15, 1977.
26. Hermans, P. E., Heizenga, K. A., Hoffman, H. N., Brown, A. L. and, Markowitz, H.: Dysgammaglobulinemia associated with nodular lymphoid hyperplasia of the small bowel. Am. J. Med., 40:78, 1966.
27. Jona, J., Belin, R. P., and Burke, J. A.: Lymphoid hyperplasia of the bowel and its surgical significance in children. J. Ped, Surg., 11:997, 1976.
28. Marshak, R. H.: Granulomatous disease of the intestinal tract (Crohn's disease). Radiology, 114:3, 1975.
29. Mosely, J., Marshak, R. H., and Wolf, B. S.: Regional enteritis in children. Am. J. Roentgenol. Radium Ther. Nucl. Med., 84:532, 1960.
30. Shackelford, G. D., and McAlister, W. H.: Primary immunodeficiency diseases and malignancy. Am. J. Roentgenol. Radium Ther. Nucl. Med., 123:144, 1975.

31. Vardy, P. A., Lebenthal, E., and Schwachmann, H.: Intestinal lymphangiectasia; a reappraisal. Pediatrics, 55:842, 1975.

Polypoid Lesions

32. Jodard, J. E., Dobbs, W. J., Phillips, J. C., and Scanlon, G. T.: Peutz-Jeghers syndrome: clinical and roentgenographic features. Am. J. Roentgenol. Radium Ther. Nucl. Med., 113:316, 1971.
33. Rabinowitz, J. G., Wolf, B. S., Feller, M. R., Krasna, I.: Colonic changes following necrotizing enterocolitis in the newborn. Am. J. Roentgenol. Radium Ther. Nucl. Med. 103:359, 1968.
34. Schwartz, A. M., and McCauley, R. G.: Juvenile gastrointestinal polyposis. Radiology, 121:441, 1976.
35. Stemper, T. J., Kent, T. H., and Summers, R. W.: Juvenile polyposis and gastrointestinal carcinoma. Ann. Intern. Med. 83:639, 1975.
36. Velcek, F. T., Coopersmith, I. S., Chen, C. K., Kassner, E. G., Klotz, D. H., and Kottmeir, P. K.: Familial juvenile adenomatous polyposis. J. Pediatr. Surg., 11:781, 1976.

Edema of the Small Bowel

37. Khilnani, T. T., Marshak, R. H., Eliasoph, J., and Wolf, B. S.: Intramural intestinal hemorrhage. Am. J. Roentgenol. Radium Ther. Nucl. Med., 92:1061, 1964.
38. Marshak, R. H., Khilnani, M. T., Eliosoph, J., and Wolf, B. S.: Intestinal edema Am. J. Roentgenol. Radium Ther. Nucl. Med., 101:379, 1967.
39. Marshak, R. H., Wolf, B. S., Cohen, N., and Janowitz, H. D.: Protein losing disorders of the gastro-intestinal tract: roentgen features. radiology, 77:893, 1961.
40. Nelson D. L., Blease, M., et al.: Constrictive pericarditis, intestinal lymphangiectasia and reversible immunologic deficiency. J. Pediatr., 86:548, 1975.

Narrowed Bowel

41. Hardt, H., Wirth, K., and Hoffgen, K. U.: Radiologic findings in infections by Yersinia pseudotuberculosis and Yersinia enterocolitica. Fortschr. Geb. Roentgenstr. Nuklearmed., 119:26, 1973.
42. Marshak, R. H.: Granulomatous disease of the intestinal tract (Crohn's disease). Radiology, 114:3, 1975.
43. Peterson, R. B., Meserall, W. P., Strago, G. G., and Gooding, C. A.: Radio-graphic features of colitis associated with the hemolytic uremic syndrome. Radiology, 118:667, 1976.
44. Sebes, J. I., Mabry, E. H., Jr., and Rabinowitz, J. G.: Lung abscess and osteomyelitis of rib due to Yersinia enterocolitica. Chest, 69:546, 1976.

45. Tochen, M. D., and Campbell, J. R.: Colitis in children with the hemolytic-uremic syndrome. J. Pediatr. Surg., *12*:213, 1977.
46. Werbeloff, L., et al.: The radiology of tuberculosis of the gastro-intestinal tract. Br. J. Radiol., *46*:329, 1973.

Fatty Liver

47. Griscom, N. T., Capitanio, N. A., Wagnor, N. L., Culham, G., and Morris, L.: Visible liver. Radiology, *117*:385, 1975.

Intra-abdominal Calcification

48. Harned, R. K., and Babbit, B. P.: Cholelithiasis in children. Radiology, *117*:391, 1975.
49. Joffe, N.: Radiology of acute appendicitis and its complications. CRC Crit. Rev. Clin. Radiol. Nucl. Med., 7:97, 1975.
50. Phillips, J. C., and Gerald, B. E.: The Incidence of cholelithiasis in sickle cell disease. Am. J. Roentgenol. Radium Ther. Nucl. Med., *113*:27, 1971.

4

Rica G. Arnon, M.D.

General Guidelines and the Systematic Approach for the Radiographic Evaluation of Cardiac Disease

CARDIAC STATUS

Cardiac Size

The evaluation of the size of the heart is helpful in the diagnosis of congenital heart disease. Although significant heart disease may be associated with cardiomegaly, a normal heart size never excludes severe cardiac involvement.

The determination of the cardiothoracic ratio is an acceptable and simple method for evaluating cardiac size. This is accomplished by relating the largest transverse diameter of the heart to the widest internal diameter of the chest (Fig. 4-1). A cardiothoracic ratio of 0.5 or less is considered within normal limits. In newborns, however, a cardiothoracic ratio of 0.55 on a supine inspiratory film exposed at 40 ins. focal film distance is quite acceptable. These measurements are also influenced by the phase of the cardiac cycle (systole or diastole) and by the phase of respiration.

Cardiac Silhouette: Chamber Enlargement

Since the majority of chest radiographs are exposed in the anteroposterior and lateral projections, the structures that form the cardiac borders in these positions are important (Fig. 4-2A). The left border consists of the curve of the aortic arch, the main pulmonary artery, the left atrial appendage, (this is not always visualized), and the sweeping long curve of the left ventricle, which also forms the cardiac apex. The right border consists of the superior vena cava, which presents as a vertical shadow, and the right atrium.

The right atrium forms the entire curve that begins below the superior vena cava and extends to the diaphragm. The right ventricle is located anteriorly and is not border-forming in a posteroanterior radiograph. The aortic knob is usually inconspicuous in children. However, the position of the arch can be determined by the displacement of the trachea. The trachea is always positioned opposite the aortic arch. In the presence of a normal left aortic arch, the tracheal air column deviates to the right. The descending aorta may be seen alongside the left paraspinal area.

In a lateral projection of the chest (Fig. 4-2B), the right ventricle is the anterior border-forming structure. It lies adjacent to the lower third of the sternum and is surrounded superiorly by the retrosternal clear space. In infants, however, the thymus is still enlarged and normally occupies and obliterates this space. The posteroinferior cardiac border of the heart is formed by the left ventricle, above which lies the border of the left atrium. As it reaches the right atrium the inferior vena cava is easily identified as a vertical, curvilinear radiodensity, extending posteriorly through the diaphragm. The posterior cardiac border normally does not protrude significantly beyond it.

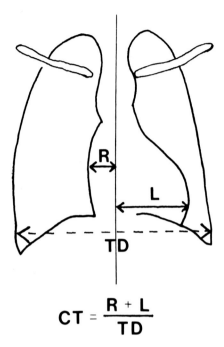

$$CT = \frac{R + L}{TD}$$

Fig. 4-1. Determination of the cardiothoracic ratio. *R*—Maximal cardiac dimension to the right of the midline. *L*—Maximal cardiac dimension to the left of the midline. *TD*—Transverse dimension at the widest expansion of the bony chest. The cardiothoracic ratio is obtained by entering these parameters in the above formula.

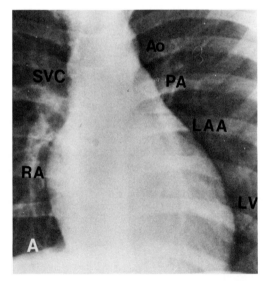
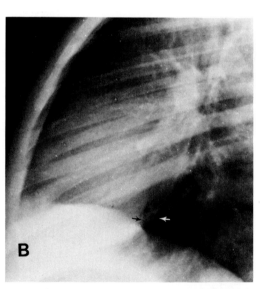

Fig. 4-2. (*A*) Posteroanterior view of the chest of a normal 6-year-old. *Ao*—aorta, *PA*—pulmonary artery, *LAA*—left atrial appendage, *LV*—left ventricle, *SVC*—superior vena cava, *RA*—right atrium. (*B*) Lateral projection of the same patient. The posterior border of the heart *(LV; white arrow)* is clearly seen just beyond the inferior vena cava *(black arrow)*. The right ventricle is contiguous with the lower third of the sternum.

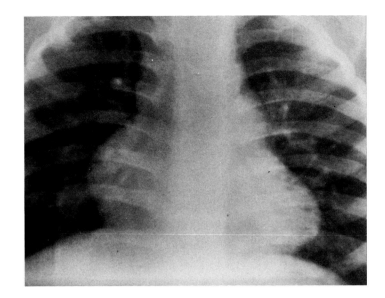

Fig. 4-3. Right atrial enlargement. Pulmonary valvular stenosis. Note the prominent right atrium extending to the right. Additional findings which suggest pulmonary valvular stenosis include an elevated apex, indicating right ventricular enlargement, and a prominent main pulmonary artery segment.

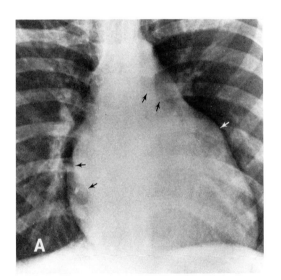

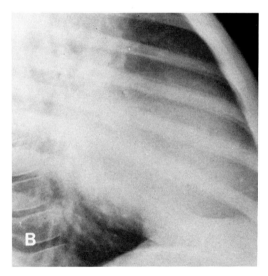

Fig. 4-4. Left atrial enlargement. Mitral insufficiency. *(A)* Chest radiograph showing moderate cardiomegaly, with massive left atrial enlargement as evidenced by an enlarged left atrial appendage *(white arrow)*, elevated left main stem bronchus, *(upper black arrows)* and a double radiodensity *(lower black arrows)*. Also note the left ventricle dilatation as manifested by downward displacement of the cardiac apex. *(B)* The enlarged left atrium is seen pushing the left bronchus as it expands posteriorly.

Specific chamber enlargement can be recognized as an exaggeration of the normal cardiac contours. Figures 4-3, 4-4, 4-5, 4-6, and 4-7 illustrate certain criteria that can be utilized to evaluate each chamber.

Enlargement of the right atrium (Fig. 4-3) is indicated by further prominence to the right of the right cardiac or right atrial border on the frontal projection. Enlargement of the left atrium (Fig. 4-4) occurs in several directions, posteriorly, superiorly, and to the right

and left. As a result, it causes many alterations within the cardiac contour, as well as alterations of a number of adjacent structures. The left atrial appendage becomes more prominent and bulges selectively on the frontal projection, shown in Figure 4-4A. A double radiodensity outline is observed on the right side of the heart. The inner, linear radiodensity is usually the border of the left atrium as it expands to the right. The outer radiodensity represents the right atrium.

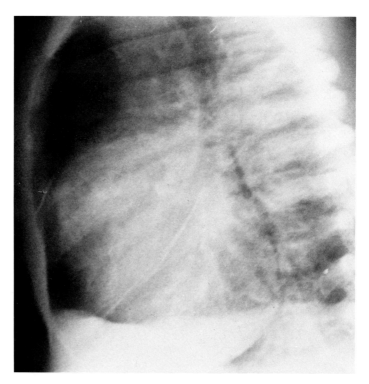

Fig. 4-5. Left ventricle enlargement. Tricuspid atresia with transposition of the great vessels. In this lateral film of a 2-month-old the greatly enlarged left ventricle extends posteriorly to reach the vertebral bodies.

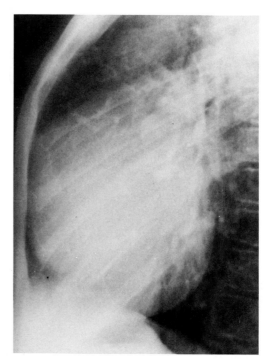

Fig. 4-6. Lateral film of a patient with both left and right ventricular enlargement. The retrosternal space is occupied by the anteriorly enlarged right ventricle, and the left ventricle is expanding posteriorly.

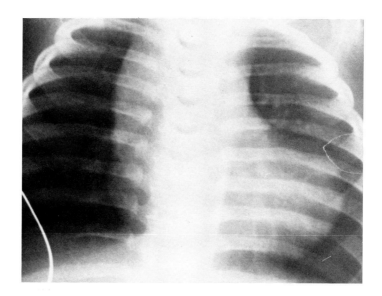

Fig. 4-7. Right ventricular enlargement and pseudotruncus arteriosus. A 3-month-old shows cardiomegaly and marked right ventricular enlargement, manifested by a definite elevation of the cardiac apex. The right atrium is slightly prominent and the main pulmonary artery segment is absent. Decreased pulmonary blood flow is apparent.

Superior expansion widens the carinal angle and elevates the left main bronchus. In the lateral projection shown in Figure 4-4B, the left atrium enlarges posteriorly. This displaces the left main bronchus superiorly and indents the anterior margin of the adjacent esophagus, best demonstrated when the esophagus is filled with barium.

With left ventricular enlargement (Figs. 4-5, 4-6) the cardiac apex enlarges downward and laterally ("down and out") on the frontal projection. On the lateral projection there is significant posterior displacement of the left ventricular border beyond the shadow of the inferior vena cava. The border of the heart approaches the vertebral column. When the right ventricle is enlarged the apex of the heart is elevated on the frontal projection (Fig. 4-7). Anteriorly, the border of the right ventricle impinges upon and fills in the retrosternal clear space (Fig. 4-6). It is important to remember that the right ventricle has no visible borders on the frontal projection. It is an anterior structure and enlarges anteriorly and to the left, pushing the left ventricle and the apex "up and out." It is a common error to mistake a prominent right atrial border for the right ventricle.

Pulmonary Vessels

The pulmonary vasculature consists of arteries, veins, and lymphatics, with the arteries, and to some extent the veins, forming the major part of the hilum (Figs. 4-8, 4-9).

As the pulmonary arteries branch from the main pulmonary artery segment, they can be seen both longitudinally and on end. If one divides the pulmonary lung field vertically into three sections, central, medial, and lateral, the pulmonary arteries are best seen in the medial and central lung fields (Figs. 4-8A, 4-9A). They taper progressively toward the periphery and are normally not apparent in the more lateral lung fields. The pulmonary veins are less well-defined than the arteries and in the region of the hilum are lower in position and more horizontally directed than the arteries. Under normal circumstances, the lymphatics are not seen.

In congenital heart disease one deals with increased, normal, or decreased pulmonary arterial flow. Increased arterial flow is recognized when the arteries appear enlarged and extend into the lateral third of the lung field (Figs. 4-8B, 4-9B). More vessels are seen on end and are often larger than the bronchus they accompany. In older patients in an erect position, there is also evidence of redistribution of flow. Ordinarily, because of the hydrostatic pressure the pulmonary arteries are more distended in the lung bases than in the apices. If there is increased pulmonary arterial flow, the partially collapsed vessels of the lung apices offer the least resistance to additional flow. Thus a small shunt produces the greatest change in the lung apices.

Decreased arterial blood flow is suspected when the hilum appears small, and the re-

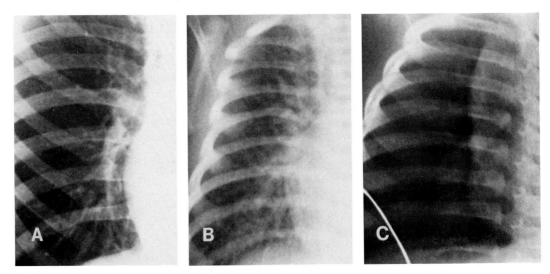

Fig. 4-8. Hilar vessels. *(A)* Normal vessels. The hilum is composed of branching pulmonary arteries, veins, and bronchi that taper gradually toward the periphery. *(B)* Shunt vasculature (ventricular septal defect). The lung fields demonstrate increased pulmonary blood flow. The central vessels are large and tortuous and are well seen throughout the lung fields. Note the many vessels seen on end. The borders of the vessels are hazy and fuzzy because of superimposed interstitial edema caused by heart failure. *(C)* Decreased pulmonary blood flow. This film of pulmonary atresia shows few, if any, identifiable vessels.

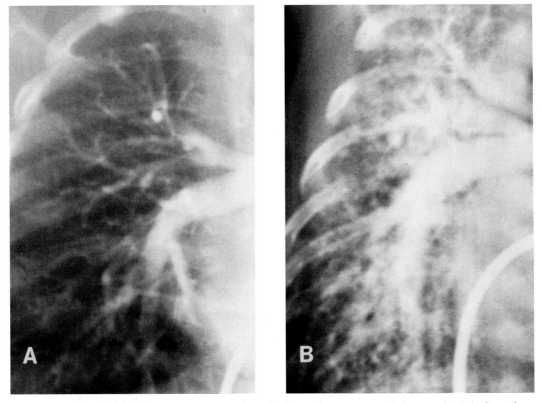

Fig. 4-9. (A) Normal pulmonary angiogram with gradual branching pattern of the vessels. *(B)* The pulmonary arteries of a patient with shunt vascularity demonstrate numerous tortuous vessels extending within the peripheral lung fields.

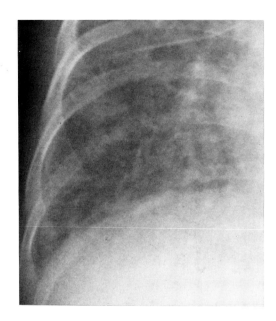

Fig. 4-10. Right lower lung field in a patient with pulmonary venous obstruction. The lung fields are hazy and the fissures are wet. Kerley's B lines are quite prominent within the outer lower lung field.

maining lung fields appear empty and devoid of pulmonary vessels (Fig. 4-8C). The vessels themselves are small and thin, and the lung fields appear hyperlucent because of this.

Venous and lymphatic engorgement are associated with pulmonary venous hypertension. Left ventricular failure, obstruction to the pulmonary venous return (e.g., mitral atresia, pulmonary venous stenosis, atresia), and obstruction associated with total anomalous pulmonary venous return are some of the many causes of pulmonary venous hypertension. In this state the margins of the pulmonary vessels are hazy and indistinct. The haziness often involves the entire lung field (Fig. 4-10). Dilated lymphatics appear as short, horizontal, linear radiodensities within the outer inferior lung fields. These are the classic Kerley's B lines (Fig. 4-10). The central lymphatics, Kerley's A lines, are thin, linear, and fuzzy radiodensities that radiate toward the hilum. Pleural effusion associated with wet fissures is another feature. The classical, fluffy, butterfly distribution of pulmonary edema seen in adults is rarely encountered in the pediatric age-group.

When the pulmonary arterial blood flow is obstructed or when there are no pulmonary arteries, bronchial arteries provide an alternate route for the pulmonary blood supply. These vessels produce a lacy pattern throughout the lung fields. An additional important radiologic feature is the empty hilum that results from small pulmonary arteries or

when there are no pulmonary arteries. The bronchial vessels arise from the descending aorta, and therefore present higher in the hilum than the pulmonary vessels (Fig. 4-11).

Severe pulmonary arterial hypertension associated with increased vascular resistance is recognized by extreme dilated central pulmonary arteries that narrow abruptly beyond the central subdivision (Fig. 4-12). This discrepancy is often referred to as pruning of the vessels. Pulmonary arterial hypertension usually develops as a result of longstanding, large left-to-right shunts with dynamic pulmonary hypertension, or secondary to severe lung disease such as cystic fibrosis.

Cardiac Situs

When a malpositioned heart is encountered, it is also necessary to determine the abdominal situs.

Abdominal situs solitus is the term used when the liver is on the right, and the stomach is on the left.

Abdominal situs inversus is used when the liver is on the left, and the stomach is on the right.

Abdominal situs indeterminate usually refers to a midline stomach and liver.

Reporting the cardiac situs (dextrocardia, levocardia) and the abdominal situs avoids use of cumbersome and confusing classifications, such as dextroversion and dextroposition.

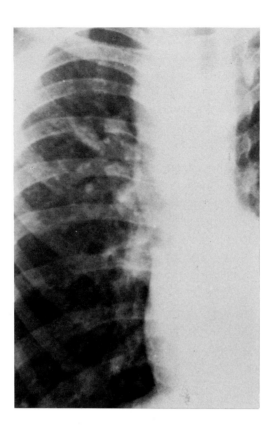

Fig. 4-11. Truncus arteriosus Type IV. There are no identifiable pulmonary arteries. The vessels around the right hilar area are large, tortuous, bronchial arteries that arise high from the aorta.

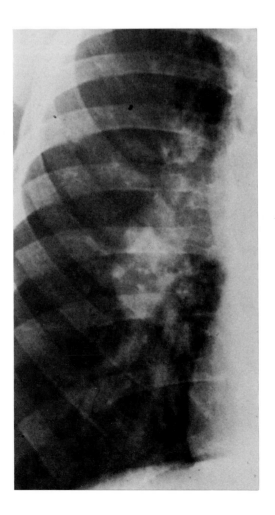

Fig. 4-12. Pulmonary arterial hypertension associated with irreversible histologic changes. The right pulmonary artery is markedly dilated. Note the discrepancy in caliber between the central vessel and its immediate branches. This abrupt change is called pruning.

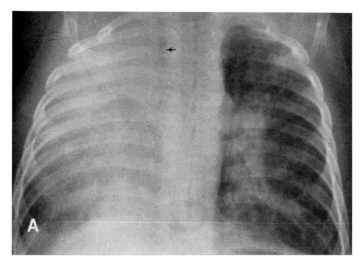

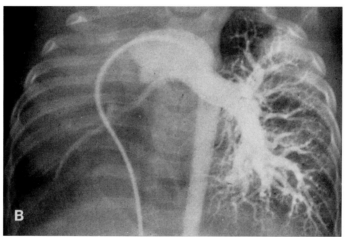

Fig. 4-13. Hypoplastic right lung. *(A)* A 3-month-old cyanotic infant with dextrocardia. Note the small intercostal spaces on the right and the hyperinflated lung on the left. The trachea is pulled to the right *(arrow)*. The heart borders cannot be distinguished from the adjacent hypoplastic lung. *(B)* The pulmonary angiogram reveals an absent right pulmonary artery, and essentially the entire pulmonary flow is directed to the left. There is an associated patent ductus arteriosus and a small artery supplying the right lower lung field.

Dextrocardia can be either primary or secondary to volume changes which may occur in association with a hypoplastic right lung or mass displacement. The secondary form is easily distinguished from the primary form. Dextrocardia secondary to a hypoplastic right lung (Fig. 4-13) manifests smaller intercostal spaces and increased radiodensity in the right hemithorax due to the mediastinal shift and hypoplastic lung. The opposite lung field, by contrast, is hyperinflated.

Dextrocardia associated with *situs inversus totalis* occurs without congenital heart disease in 90 to 95 per cent of patients. Kartagener's syndrome (dextrocardia, situs inversus, sinusitis, and bronchiectasis) belongs to this category. When any other combination of cardiac malposition and abdominal situs exists, a spectrum of anomalies ranging from mild to severe congenital heart disease may be present (Fig. 4-14). These anomalies

are usually associated with dextrocardia and an indeterminate abdominal situs that is the result of asplenia or polysplenia syndromes. They are also accompanied by severe abnormalities of the great vessels (conotruncal) and anomalous systemic venous return (e.g., azygos continuation of the inferior vena cava and anomalous pulmonary venous connections). The pattern of the bronchial tree is a helpful feature in distinguishing polysplenia from asplenia. Asplenia is usually associated with bilateral right-sidedness (right bronchial configuration on both sides); bilateral left-sidedness indicates the possibility of polysplenia.

Bony Thorax

Any structural abnormality that may shed light on a probable diagnosis should be noted. For example, severe pectus excavatum, straight back syndrome, and severe

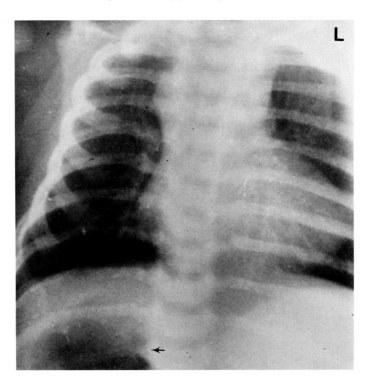

Fig. 4-14. Chest radiograph in a newborn with single ventricle and pulmonary atresia, manifesting levocardia and abdominal *situs inversus*. The stomach is on the right *(arrow)*. The elevated apex on the left indicates right ventricular hypertrophy. The pulmonary artery segment appears empty and is associated with decreased pulmonary blood flow.

scoliosis can modify the observed cardiac silhouette in both size and shape. Moreover, abnormalities of the ribs, vertebra, and sternum are associated with a number of cardiac diseases. For example, vertebral anomalies are associated with the Vater syndrome. Increased vertical diameter of the lumbar vertebra associated with a bifid manubrium is strongly suggestive of Down's syndrome, and the cardiac diagnosis of a common atrioventricular canal should be considered.

Notching of the fourth to eighth ribs is associated with coarctation of the aorta in patients beyond infancy. This is due to the dilated intercostal arteries that function as a collateral supply to the lower aorta (see p. 175). Unilateral notching has also been observed following a Blalock-Taussig procedure.

Abnormality of the ribs related to previous cardiac surgery should be noted. A left thoracotomy is usually performed for ductal ligation, banding of the main pulmonary artery, and coarctectomy. Occasionally a Blalock-Taussig shunt (subclavian artery to pulmonary artery) is also performed on the left. Right-sided thoracotomies are performed for creation of aorticopulmonary shunts, and atrial septectomy for transposition of the great vessels.

The main points in the evaluation of a chest radiograph for congenital heart disease deserve reiteration. The initial step is to determine the presence or absence of cardiomegaly, remembering that a normal heart size does not exclude severe disease. Once the possibility of cardiac disease has been established, specific chamber enlargement should be noted; a correct evaluation is greatly dependent upon the experience of the physician. Particular attention must then be given to the pulmonary vessels (arterial, venous) and lymphatics; are they increased or decreased in number and size, or are they normal?

In addition to cardiac size and shape, it is also imperative to observe the position of the heart in relation to the abdominal organs, such as the stomach and liver, and the location of the aortic arch. For example, a right-sided aortic arch is frequently encountered in tetralogy of fallot, truncus arteriosus and transposition of the great vessels.

In general, congenital heart disease is divided into two major categories, acyanotic and cyanotic. Cyanotic heart disease is further subdivided into two groups, one associated with increased pulmonary arterial vascularity and the other with decreased pulmonary arterial vascularity. Acyanotic congenital heart disease is often associated with a left-to-right shunt, and as a result the lung fields are either normal or hypervascular.

Since both cyanotic and acyanotic congenital heart disease can be associated with increased pulmonary arterial vessels, the presence or absence of clinical cyanosis must be known in order to even begin consideration of a proper differential diagnosis.

The outline below provides the reader with basic guidelines for evaluating the cardiac status from a chest radiograph. After analyzing the features in a systematic manner, it becomes possible to further categorize the cardiac disease into two major groups, cyanotic or acyanotic. For example, the radiographic finding of cardiomegaly with increased pulmonary arterial blood flow in an acyanotic patient belongs in Group IIa. Specific chamber enlargement and other features discussed in the following sections help to establish a diagnosis.

Steps in Evaluating the Chest Radiograph in Relation to Heart Disease
A Heart size
B Specific chamber enlargement
C Pulmonary vascularity
    Type: arterial, venous, lymphatic
    Status: increased, normal, decreased
D Location of the aortic arch (right, left)
E Cardiac and abdominal situs
F Presence or absence of cyanosis
    I Cyanotic heart disease
        a. With increased pulmonary blood flow
        b. With decreased pulmonary blood flow
    II Acyanotic heart disease
        a. With increased pulmonary blood flow
        b. With normal pulmonary blood flow

CYANOTIC CONGENITAL HEART DISEASE

There are many disease entities to consider when a physician is confronted with a cyanotic child with congenital heart disease. Several of these begin with the letter *T*: transposition of the great vessels, tetralogy of Fallot, tricuspid atresia, truncus arteriosus, and total anomalous pulmonary venous drainage (TAPVD). Others include single ventricle, double outlet right ventricle, pulmonary atresia with intact ventricular septum or with ventricular septal defect, and hypoplastic left heart syndrome.

Cyanotic heart disease is divided into two groups, based on association with *increased pulmonary blood flow*, or with *decreased pulmonary blood flow*. Excluding tetralogy of Fallot and pulmonary atresia with intact ventricular septum, all of the diseases listed may present with increased, normal, or decreased pulmonary blood flow. In this section, each is classified according to the most common presentation. An understanding of the anatomy and hemodynamics associated with cyanotic congenital heart disease is mandatory in order to fully evaluate the features of each disease and to arrive at a presumptive diagnosis.

CYANOTIC CONGENITAL HEART DISEASE WITH INCREASED PULMONARY BLOOD FLOW

The cyanotic lesions associated with increased pulmonary blood flow usually present with cardiomegaly that is often proportional to the increase in pulmonary blood flow. There are certain outstanding features in each lesion that facilitate recognition.

Disease Entities
Transposition of the great vessels
Truncus arteriosus
Total anomalous pulmonary venous drainage
Double outlet and common ventricle
Hypoplastic left heart
Tricuspid atresia

Differential Diagnosis

Transposition of the great vessels is presently the most common and most important of all the cyanotic lesions. Afflicted infants are surprisingly large, and, apart from the marked cyanosis, they appear relatively healthy. During the neonatal period, the size and configuration of the heart may be entirely within normal limits. Only as the child matures do the characteristic features of this disease become evident. In this anomaly the aorta arises from the right ventricle and the pulmonary artery from the left ventricle (Fig. 4-15). Consequently, both circulations run a parallel course that is incompatible with life unless an adequate inter-circulatory communication or mixing exists, such as an atrial or ventricular septal defect or a patent ductus arteriosus. Balloon atrial septotomy is rou-

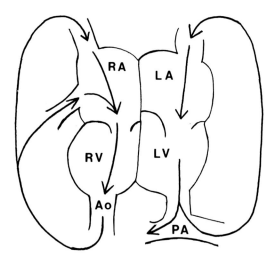

Fig. 4-15. Schematic illustration of a heart with transposition of the great vessels. The aorta arises from the right ventricle and the pulmonary artery from the left ventricle. Without any inter-circulatory communication, this combination is incompatible with life.

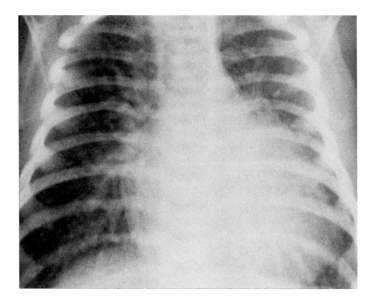

Fig. 4-16. Transposition of great vessels. A radiograph of a 2-day-old, suggesting an "egg on the side" configuration, with cardiomegaly, prominent right atrium, narrow mediastinal pedicle, and increased pulmonary blood flow.

tinely performed during cardiac catheterization in order to facilitate an adequate interatrial communication.

With this disorder the right ventricle is the systemic ventricle, and right ventricular enlargement associated with mild cardiomegaly is present. The transposed great vessels are anatomically positioned one behind the other, with the aorta anterior to the pulmonary artery. When associated with an involuted thymus this feature accounts for the narrow mediastinal pedicle and explains why the pulmonary artery is not visible in its usual location. As a result, the cardiac configuration assumes the so called "egg on the side" appearance, a term that has become almost synomonous with transposition of the great

vessels (Figs. 4-16, 4-17). The vascularity is almost always increased, except in those cases associated with pulmonary stenosis. Ventricular septal defects and sub-valvular pulmonary stenosis are frequently present. The severity of these lesions determines the amount of pulmonary blood flow.

Truncus arteriosus is a rare form of cyanotic heart disease in which the fetal common arterial trunk persists. It comprises approximately 0.4 per cent of all congenital heart disease. There is always an associated membranous ventricular septal defect, and both ventricles, therefore, eject blood into this common vessel. Truncus arteriosus is classified as follows (Colette and Edwards):[3]

Type I has a single trunk that divides into

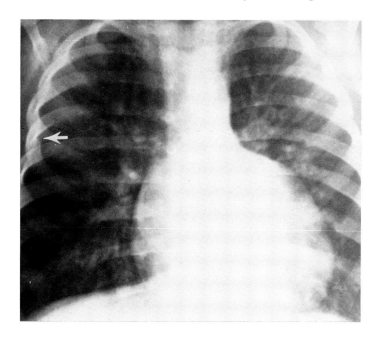

Fig. 4-17. Transposition of great vessels. The same features are noted as in the patient of Fig. 4-16. Minimal deformity of the right fifth rib *(arrow)* is present as a result of previous surgical intervention for the creation of an atrial communication (Blalock-Hanlon procedure).

TRUNCUS ARTERIOSUS

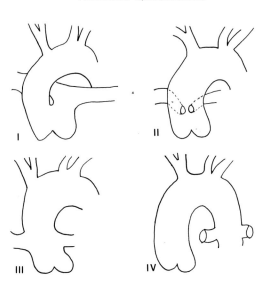

Fig. 4-18. Truncus arteriosus. This schema demonstrates the various types of truncus.

the main pulmonary artery and aorta (Fig. 4-18); Type II has pulmonary arteries that originate separately from the posterior aspect of the ascending aorta; Type III has pulmonary arteries that originate separately from each side of the ascending aorta; Type IV has no pulmonary arteries; the lungs are supplied by bronchial vessels that originate from the descending aorta.

All of the above except for Type IV present with increased pulmonary blood flow, providing that no associated obstruction impeding

the pulmonary blood flow is present. The excess pulmonary venous return causes the heart to dilate, and the patients present with cardiomegaly, increased vascularity, and biventricular enlargement. The presenting features in truncus arteriosus Type I are usually characteristic (Fig. 4-19). The mediastinal vascular shadow is often quite large because of the large trunk. The pulmonary artery causes considerable widening on the left, and the entire trunk also displaces the superior vena cava laterally, causing a further bulge on

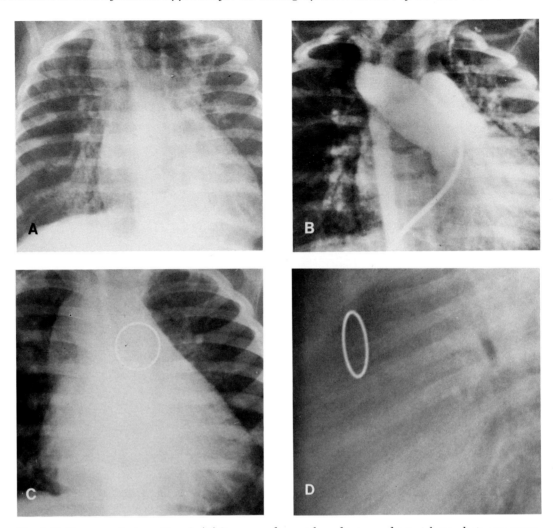

Fig. 4-19. Truncus arteriosus Type I. *(A)* Severe cardiomegaly and increased arterial vascularity are apparent. The enlarged vascular structure within the mediastium is the actual common arterial trunk that gives rise to a right aortic arch and main pulmonary artery. *(B)* Angiogram confirms these findings and demonstrates the common trunk dividing into the pulmonary artery and aorta which descends on the right. *(C)* Frontal and *(D)* lateral projections of the same patient following surgical correction in which a valved conduit was used to reconstruct a right ventricular outflow and a main pulmonary artery. The metallic ring projecting over the cardiac shadow is the stent supporting the porcine valve that is functioning as the pulmonary valve.

the right. In Types II, III, and IV (Figs. 4-20, 4-21) in which there is no main pulmonary artery, the truncal size is usually smaller. The cardiac configuration in these three types in some way resembles transposition of the great vessels, although the overall size of the heart in all forms of truncus arteriosus is far larger than that encountered in transposition of the great vessels. An important feature is the presence of a right aortic arch in 36 per cent of patients with truncus arteriosus (Figs. 4-20, 4-21).

Total anomalous pulmonary venous drainage is unusual and occurs in 1 per cent of patients with congenital heart disease. In this anomaly there is no direct communication between the pulmonary veins and the left atrium. Instead, the pulmonary veins return to the right heart by way of patent embryonic channels. The various anomalies encountered can be classified on either an anatomic or embryologic basis. An embryological classification is useful, since it describes not only the site of the anomalous drainage but adds to

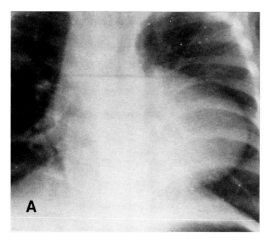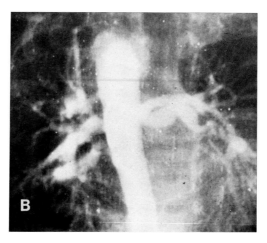

Fig. 4-20. Truncus arteriosus Type IV. *(A)* This lesion strongly resembles tetralogy of Fallot. Note the "coeur en sabot" configuration, a right aortic arch, no main pulmonary artery segment, and decreased pulmonary perfusion. The trachea is deviated to the left because of the anomalous aortic position. *(B)* Aortic injection demonstrates the large bronchial vessels arising from the descending aorta.

the knowledge of its origin based on preexisting embryonic channels. This classification consists of total anomalous pulmonary venous drainage (A) into the common cardinal vein (coronary sinus, innominate vein), (B) into the right cardinal system (right superior vena cava, azygous vein), (C) directly into the right atrium, and (D) into the umbilico-vitteline system (portal vein, ductus venosus).

The pulmonary venous blood, therefore, returns to the right atrium by way of these circuitous routes, producing volume overload in the right atrium, right ventricle, and pulmonary arteries. As a result these structures are enlarged and the lungs over-circulated. Right heart failure with evidence of pulmonary edema is often present.

Most often the pulmonary veins form a single trunk behind the heart before joining a systemic venous channel. The most common systemic channel encountered is the common cardinal system. The common pulmonary vein drains into a vertical vein that communicates subsequently with the innominate vein and superior vena cava before entering the right atrium. The pathognomonic appearance of a "snowman" or a "figure eight" is produced (Fig. 4-22). The head of the "snowman" is formed by the draining veins, and the body is formed by the enlarged heart. If venous drainage is unobstructed, the right heart is enlarged and there is increased pulmonary blood flow. However, if the anomalous vein is obstructed, impeding venous re-

turn, the heart will be small and the features of pulmonary venous obstruction with associated dilated lymphatics, wet fissures, and interstital edema predominate (Fig. 4-23). This presentation is almost always found in Form D, where the common pulmonary vein drains by way of a long channel through the diaphragm into the portal vein or the ductus venosus (Fig. 4-23C). The long route and the subsequent passage through the liver produce increased resistance to pulmonary venous return.

Double outlet right ventricle and single ventricle have no distinct appearance on the routine chest radiograph. The magnitude of the cardiac enlargement is proportional to the increase in pulmonary blood flow in both lesions, which depends upon the presence or absence of pulmonary stenosis and other associated cardiac abnormalities. Double outlet right ventricle is present when both vessels arise side by side from the right ventricle. The only outlet to the left ventricle is through a ventricular septal defect. This can be subcristal, usually associated with less cyanosis, or supra-cristal, where oxygenated blood is directed into the pulmonary artery and desaturated blood into the aorta. A single ventricle or a common ventricle functions basically as a large ventricular septal defect unless there are other associated anomalies. Aside from catheterization there may be no way to distinguish one lesion from the other.

Hypoplastic left heart syndrome is a rare

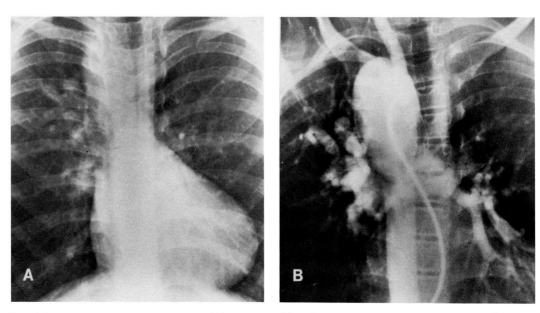

Fig. 4-21. Truncus arteriosus Type IV. *(A)* A 6-year-old with truncus arteriosus Type IV. A right aortic arch is quite apparent and dilated. The main pulmonary artery segment is absent. The vessels on the right arise high in the hilum, suggesting bronchial vessels. *(B)* The aortogram confirms the abnormality and clearly outlines the origin of the vessels from the descending aorta.

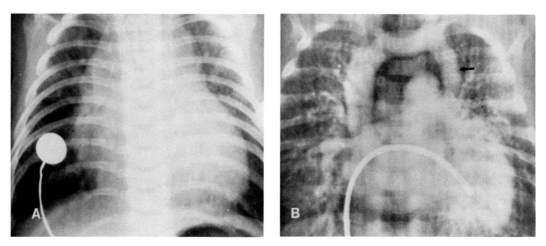

Fig. 4-22. Total anomalous pulmonary venous return. Form A. The cardiac structure is enlarged and presents a "snowman" configuration. Pulmonary vascularity is slightly increased. *(B)* Injection into the right ventricle reveals a patent ductus arteriosus. The entire pulmonary venous return connects to a large vertical vein arising on the left *(arrow).* The abnormal venous pathway forms a large inverted U as it reaches the right atrium.

Fig. 4-23. Total anomalous pulmonary venous return. Form C. *(A,B)* Diffuse congested changes are present throughout the lung fields producing a somewhat hazy and fuzzy picture. In both lateral lower lung fields Kerley's B lines are present. The horizontal and oblique fissures are thickened due to the presence of pleural effusion. *(C)* Venous phase following contrast injection into the pulmonary artery demonstrates the pulmonary veins joining a common channel *(arrows)* that distends below the diaphragm into the portal vein. No anatomic obstruction is visualized.

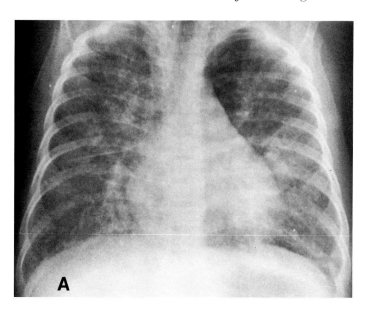

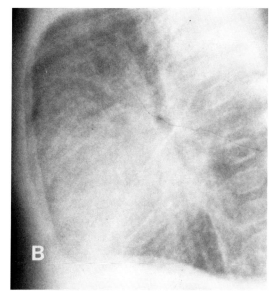

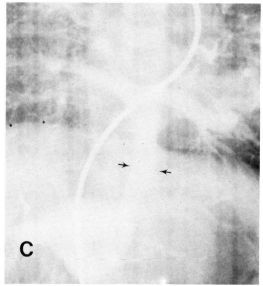

anomaly. It does, however, account for a significant number of deaths in the neonatal period. The term itself, hypoplastic left heart syndrome, describes a clinical presentation related to a spectrum of anomalies associated with obstructive lesions to the left side of the heart. The patients usually present with a sudden onset of profound cardiovascular collapse that is associated with gray color and an absent pulse. Anatomically the size of the left ventricle varies from a nonexistent, slit-like chamber to a small but, nevertheless, functioning ventricle. The size of this chamber is related to the obstructing anomaly (e.g., mitral and aortic atresia). In its severest form,

where both mitral and aortic atresia exist, the pulmonary venous return is shunted through the atrial septum into the right atrium, resulting in an admixture and a single functioning right ventricle. The degree of cyanosis usually depends on the amount of pulmonary blood flow.

The cardiac silhouette is enlarged and globular with a large main pulmonary artery, increased pulmonary blood flow, and findings of congestive heart failure. The radiographic appearance of this lesion is not distinctive. However, the clinical presentation, sudden onset of profound shock in a previously healthy neonate, suggests the diagnosis.

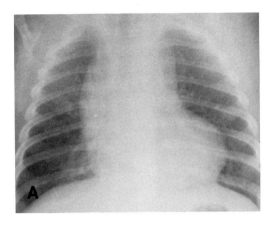

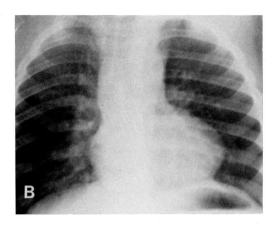

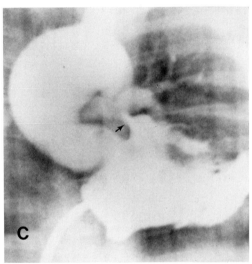

Fig. 4-24. Tetralogy of Fallot. *(A)* Chest radiograph of a newborn with tetralogy of Fallot. The cardiac size is normal, although the apex is elevated indicating right ventricular enlargement. The pulmonary vessels appear normal. *(B)* The same patient at 1 year of age demonstrates the more classical "coeur en sabot" appearance. The enlarged aorta and the empty main pulmonary artery segment are now evident. *(C)* Right ventricular angiogram shows opacification of both the aorta and the main pulmonary artery. The aorta is extremely dilated. The pulmonary valve is atretic *(arrow)* and the small pulmonary artery fills retrograde from the aorta by way of a patent ductus.

Tricuspid atresia, although usually associated with decreased pulmonary blood flow, can occasionally present with cardiomegaly and increased pulmonary blood flow. This is usually associated with transportation of the great vessels (see p. 164).

Discussion

Most cyanotic congenital heart diseases present in infancy. The more severe the lesion, the earlier it becomes apparent. In general, the degree of cyanosis is inversely proportional to the rate of pulmonary blood flow (e.g., with increased pulmonary blood flow, cyanosis may not be obvious). Transposition of the great vessels, because of the possibly poor inter-circulatory mixing, is an exception to the rule. In this lesion, inspite of a large pulmonary blood flow, the cyanosis can be most intense.

Physicians must also be aware that the presence of either a large patent ductus arteriosus or a ventricular septal defect is imperative for survival in many of the cyanotic lesions. Both may close unexpectedly, producing clinical deterioration and a definite decrease in the pulmonary circulation.

CYANOTIC CONGENITAL HEART DISEASE WITH DECREASED PULMONARY BLOOD FLOW

Decreased pulmonary blood flow indicates obstruction somewhere within the right heart or the pulmonary arteries. The diameter of the pulmonary arteries and, therefore, their radiographic appearance depends upon the severity of the obstruction. In general the vessels appear thin and sparse as they extend into the periphery of the lung. The hilar regions on both the frontal and lateral projections are also small or empty, and the lung fields are hyperlucent.

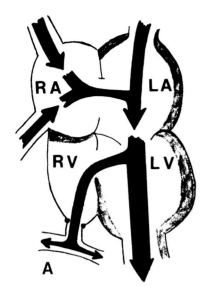

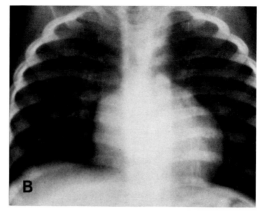

Fig. 4-25. Tricuspid atresia. *(A)* Schematic drawing demonstrating the classic flow pattern in tricuspid atresia. *(B)* A 2-day-old with cyanosis and dyspnea. The heart and right atrium are not markedly enlarged. However, the left atrium is prominent. There is a double radiodensity behind the heart. The lung fields are poorly perfused and the pulmonary artery segment is almost completely absent.

Disease Entities

Tetralogy of Fallot

Tricuspid atresia

Pulmonary atresia with intact ventricular septum

Ebstein's anomaly

Severe pulmonary valvular stenosis with intact ventricular septum

The following entities when associated with pulmonary blood flow obstruction:

    Truncus arteriosus

    Total anomalous pulmonary venous drainage

    Double outlet and common ventricle

    Hypoplastic left heart

    Tricuspid atresia

Differential Diagnosis

At times it may be difficult to distinguish one anomaly from the other, since the majority are associated with a small pulmonary artery. However, certain changes in the cardiac configuration and specific chamber size may be helpful in differentiating one lesion from the other.

Tetralogy of Fallot, as described by Fallot, consists of a ventricular septal defect, right ventricular outflow obstruction, an overriding aorta, and resultant right ventricular hyper-

trophy. This lesion, following transposition of the great vessels, is the second most common cyanotic lesion. Tetralogy of Fallot usually presents with a normal-sized but nevertheless characteristic appearance, the so called "boot-shaped" or "coeur en sabot" heart (Figs. 4-7, 4-24B). This configuration is the result of right ventricular enlargement and its associated uplifted apex, a large ascending aorta, and a small main pulmonary artery segment, or none (Fig. 4-24B). The aorta is always large since it receives all the blood from the left ventricle and most of the blood from the right ventricle. The pulmonary vascularity may be normal or decreased, depending upon the degree of right ventricular outflow obstruction. The most severe form is associated with pulmonary atresia and has been termed pseudotruncus arteriosus. Since only one major vessel arises from the heart it strongly resembles truncus arteriosus Type IV. However, in this entity the lungs are perfused by way of the pulmonary arteries supplied by a ductus, in contrast to the bronchial artery supply associated with arteriosus truncus Type IV. Tetralogy has also been confused with tricuspid atresia with severe pulmonary outflow obstruction.

In the neonatal period, the cardiac configuration may be non-distinctive (Fig. 4-24A). Right ventricular obstruction, how-

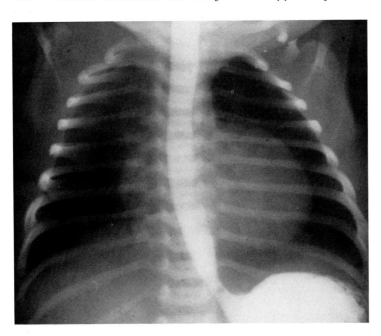

Fig. 4-26. Pulmonary atresia with intact ventricular septum in a newborn with severe dyspnea and cyanosis. The heart is markedly enlarged and the lungs almost non-perfused. The right atrium is also enlarged. A small right ventricle was demonstrated by angiography.

ever, is often progressive, and changes occur eventually that produce the classic appearance. The presence of a right aortic arch is important, since this anomaly, with mirror image branching, is present in 25 per cent of patients with tetralogy.

Tricuspid atresia is a rare anomaly which comprises only 1 per cent of all congestive heart diseases. The pathologic changes consist of no tricuspid valve and therefore no direct communication between the right atrium and the right ventricle. The entire systemic venous return is shunted across the atrial septum into the left side of the heart. The left atrium and ventricle dilate in order to accomodate the volume of both the pulmonary and systemic venous return. Blood flow to the lungs is directed from the left ventricle into the right ventricle and pulmonary artery by way of a ventricular septal defect (Fig. 4-25). The size of the septal defect determines the size of the right ventricle and the amount of pulmonary blood flow. Transposition of the great vessels is a commonly associated finding. Consequently, tricuspid atresia is classified according to this anatomic variation and its hemodynamic and functional status. Type I, tricuspid atresia with normally related great vessels, occurs (a) with pulmonary atresia and no ventricular septal defect, (b) with pulmonary stenosis and a small ventricular septal defect, and (c) with no pulmonary stenosis and a large ventricular septal defect; Type II,

tricuspid atresia with transposition of the great vessels, occurs (a) with pulmonary atresia and no ventricular septal defect, (b) with pulmonary stenosis and a small ventricular septal defect, and (c) with no pulmonary stenosis and a large ventricular septal defect. Type Ib and IIc are the most common. There is always some degree of cardiomegaly due to left atrial and left ventricular enlargement. The right atrium and ventricle are not prominent (Fig. 4-25B). This is an important differential feature, since both tetralogy of Fallot and transposition of the great vessels are associated with enlarged right ventricles. The presence of the main pulmonary artery segment on the chest film will depend on the rate of pulmonary blood flow and whether there is transposition. It is important to remember that when increased pulmonary perfusion is noted in tricuspid atresia, a large ventricular septal defect, with little or no pulmonary stenosis, is present, or there is associated transposition. However, only 20 per cent of tricuspid atresias present with increased pulmonary blood flow.

Pulmonary valve atresia with intact ventricular septum is associated with replacement of the pulmonary valve by a diaphragm consisting of fused cusps that seal the pulmonary artery from the right ventricle. The right ventricle is usually hypoplastic, although in one form a large right ventricle with tricuspid insufficiency is also encountered. A con-

Table 4-1. **Radiographic Features of Cyanotic Heart Disease With Decreased Pulmonary Blood Flow**

Disease	Right Atrium	Right Ventricle	Pulmonary Artery	Left Atrium	Left Ventricle	Aorta
Tetralogy of Fallot	Normal	Enlarged	Small	Normal	Normal	Enlarged
Tricuspid atresia	Normal	Small	Small to normal	Enlarged	Enlarged	Enlarged
Pulmonary atresia	Enlarged	Small or enlarged	Absent	Enlarged	Enlarged	Enlarged
Ebstein's anomaly	Normal to huge	Small	Small	Large	Large	Large

comitant atrial septal defect and a patent ductus arteriosus are necessary to sustain life. Consequently, there is a right-to-left shunt at the atrial level, with resulting left atrial and left ventricular enlargement. Physiologically, this lesion behaves like tricuspid atresia; differentiation between the two is impossible unless the right ventricle is entered upon catheterization.

In the immediate neonatal period the chest radiograph may be normal, although it often exhibits cardiomegaly and decreased pulmonary blood flow within a few days, unless significant patent ductus arteriosus is also present. The cardiac size and configuration are variable and depend upon the size of the right ventricle. The right atrium is almost always large (Fig. 4-26). The lesion is distinguished from pulmonary valvular stenosis by the presence of a concave or flat main pulmonary artery segment. With pulmonary valvular stenosis, the pulmonary artery segment is often dilated (poststenotic dilatation).

Ebstein's anomaly is a rare entity in which the posterior and often the medial leaflet of the tricuspid valve are not attached normally to the annulus. The annulus appears to be displaced downward. A large part of the right ventricle is incorporated into the right atrium and only a small portion of the right ventricle remains. This has been termed "atrialization" of the right ventricle. The deformity is believed to be due to incomplete undermining of tricuspid valve tissue by the endocardium. This accounts for the supposed downward displacement of the tricuspid valve ring and the associated redundant tricuspid valve tissue. The anomaly varies in severity, and lesions extending from the most severe to the mildest form (*forme fruste*) can be seen.

The severe malformation can present early in the neonatal period with decreased pulmonary blood flow due to massive tricuspid regurgitation and a right-to-left shunt at the atrial level. The cardiac silhouette is enlarged with a prominent right atrium and decreased pulmonary blood flow. Sometimes this radiographic presentation is indistinguishable from severe pulmonary stenosis in right ventricular failure.

Severe pulmonary valvular stenosis with intact ventricular septum is not cyanotic heart disease *per se*. However, with severe stenosis patients present with right ventricular failure and a right-to-left shunt at the atrial level. Therefore, they manifest clinical cyanosis and a decreased pulmonary blood flow. In the presence of mild to moderate stenosis, the cardiac size will be normal or mildly increased. The cardiac output is normal, and therefore the pulmonary blood flow will be normal. When the pulmonary blood flow is reduced because of critical stenosis, the cardiac silhouette is large, with marked prominence of the right atrium and ventricle. The cardiac apex is elevated and a the main pulmonary artery is enlarged due to poststenotic dilatation. This feature may not be observed in infants and small children. Occasionally main pulmonary artery dilatation is directed in an anteroposterior dimension and is, therefore, not recognized on the frontal projection (Fig. 4-37B). Severe pulmonary stenosis may occasionally mimic Ebstein's anomaly.

Truncus arteriosus, total anomalous pulmonary venous drainage, double outlet and common ventricle, hypoplastic left heart, and tricuspid atresia, all of which are classified as cyanotic congenital heart diseases with

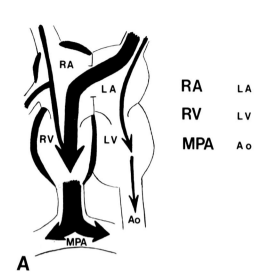
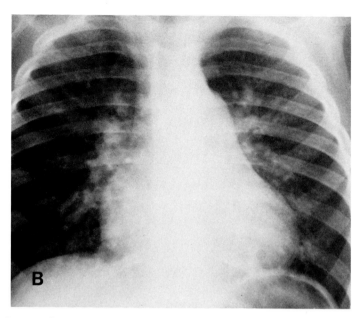

Fig. 4-27. Atrial septal defect. (A) Schematic drawing indicating the direction of blood flow and respective chamber and vessel enlargement. The large arrows represent the increased shunt volume, and the large letters on the side indicate the enlarged structures. (B) Corresponding chest radiograph demonstrates right atrial and right ventricular enlargement (elevated apex). The main pulmonary artery segment and pulmonary vessels are prominent. Note the vessels on end surrounding both hila.

increased pulmonary blood flow, may sometimes be accompanied by *decreased pulmonary blood flow* when an obstruction that impedes the pulmonary blood flow is also present.

Discussion

In general, patients with cyanotic heart disease associated with severe pulmonary stenosis or atresia must have an alternate route to perfuse the lungs. This is accomplished either through a patent ductus arteriosus or through bronchial arteries. Obviously the time of presentation and the severity of cyanosis is related to the efficiency of an alternate route of lung perfusion. Other factors may be involved, as in patients with tricuspid atresia, in whom the pulmonary blood flow is essentially dependent on a left-to-right shunt through a ventricular septal defect.

Again it is important to emphasize that although structures such as a patent ductus arteriosus in pulmonary atresia or severe tetralogy and a large ventricular septal defect in tricuspid atresia are life supporting, they can close spontaneously, causing the death of the patient if no other means for pulmonary blood flow is established.

It is also helpful to note the location of the aortic arch, since 28 per cent of patients with tetralogy of Fallot, 36 per cent of patients with truncus arteriosis, and 2 to 5 per cent of patients with transposition of the great vessels exhibit a right aortic arch, usually with mirror image branching.

ACYANTOIC CARDIOMEGALY WITH INCREASED PULMONARY BLOOD FLOW

In this category of heart disease an abnormal communication exists between the left and right side of the circulation. Since pressure on the left side of the heart is higher than on the right, blood is shunted from left to right except in the presence of pulmonary hypertension. The size of the heart and the pulmonary arteries are related to the size and location of the defect, as well as to the size of the shunt. A pulmonary-to-systemic flow ratio greater than 2 to 1 is required before any variations in pulmonary circulation are detected. The cardiac chambers accomodating the increased shunt volumes dilate. This is reflected on the chest radiograph as cardiomegaly with increased pulmonary vascular markings.

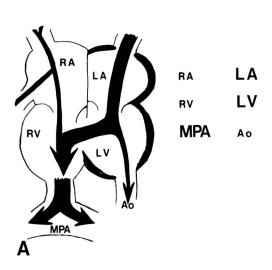 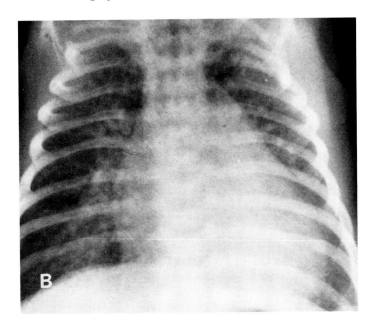

Fig. 4-28. Ventricular septal defect. *(A)* A schematic drawing demonstrating direction of shunt and chamber enlargement. *(B)* A 3-month-old with a large ventricular septal defect. There is marked cardiomegaly consisting of a prominent left ventricle, left atrium, and main pulmonary artery. Pulmonary arterial vascularity is markedly increased. The vessels are somewhat fuzzy and indistinct, suggesting congestive failure and pulmonary edema.

It is important to recognize that congenital heart disease with a potential left-to-right shunt may not be apparent in neonates during the first few days of life. The pulmonary vascular resistance in neonates is normally high and allows for only minimal shunting from left to right. As a result, the pulmonary vasculature appears normal, despite the presence of an intracardiac defect. As the pulmonary resistance decreases toward the adult level, the left-to-right shunt becomes clinically and radiographically obvious, producing changes in the overall size of the cardiovascular silhouette and the pulmonary vessels. In general, enlarged pulmonary arteries are recognized by the presence of clear and well-defined vessels surrounding the hilar area. When seen on end they look like a bunch of grapes. These vessels also appear to be more numerous and occupy more of the peripheral lung fields than normal vessels.

Disease Entities

Atrial septal defect (ASD)
Ventricular septal defect (VSD)
Patent ductus arteriosus (PDA)
Partial anomalous pulmonary venous drainage
Endocardial cushion defects

Differential Diagnosis

The following discussion is based on specific cardiac chamber enlargement. The radiographic features described may not be present before the pulmonary vascular resistance decreases and the shunt is established.

An atrial septal defect can be the result of abnormalities of the septum primum or the septum secundum. It is the eighth most common congenital heart disease. With a defect of the septum secundum a portion of the blood returning to the left atrium is shunted across the defect into the right atrium (Fig. 4-27). The increased volume entering this chamber causes it to enlarge. The right ventricle and main pulmonary artery, which are also involved in transporting this increased volume, subsequently enlarge (Fig. 4-27). The left atrium and left ventricle both remain normal in size. Patients who have defects of the septum secundum are seldom symptomatic in the neonatal period through early childhood.

A defect of the septum primum is quite different, since it represents a form of endocardial cushion defect. The defect is at the location of the ostium primum and is therefore located low, above the tricuspid valve, and is almost always associated with a cleft an-

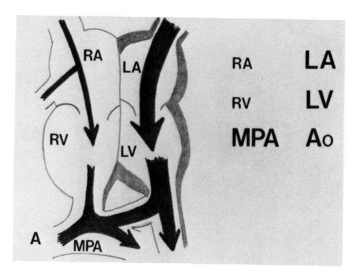

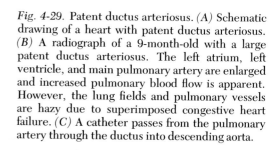

Fig. 4-29. Patent ductus arteriosus. *(A)* Schematic drawing of a heart with patent ductus arteriosus. *(B)* A radiograph of a 9-month-old with a large patent ductus arteriosus. The left atrium, left ventricle, and main pulmonary artery are enlarged and increased pulmonary blood flow is apparent. However, the lung fields and pulmonary vessels are hazy due to superimposed congestive heart failure. *(C)* A catheter passes from the pulmonary artery through the ductus into descending aorta.

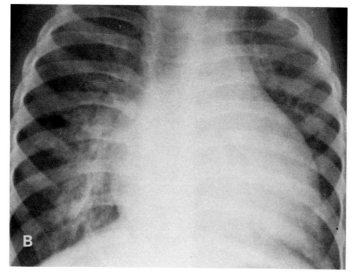

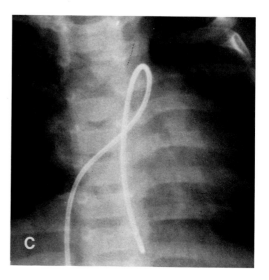

terior leaflet of the mitral valve. Therefore, mitral insufficiency may be present and may influence the degree of symptomatology and time of presentation. In the presence of mitral insufficiency, left atrial and left ventricular enlargement are present. However, the left atrium may not appear to be enlarged, since it is decompressed due to the atrial septal defect. When there is no significant mitral insufficiency, this defect resembles a defect of the septum secundum.

A ventricular septal defect is the most common congenital heart disease, comprising 20 to 25 per cent of all disorders. A large ventricular septal defect, in contrast to an atrial septal defect, quite often results in early congestive failure. In this anomaly the left atrium, left ventricle, and main pulmonary artery are enlarged in the presence

of a normal heart on the right side (Fig. 4-28). Although the shunt is directed from the left ventricle to the right ventricle, the right ventricle does not become dilated in an uncomplicated ventricular septal defect. The shunt occurs during ventricular systole at the time when the pulmonary valve is open and the right ventricle contracted. The blood passes directly into the main pulmonary artery. The left ventricle and left atrium alone accomodate the increased volume and therefore become dilated. The right ventricle eventually enlarges when a large shunt is present that results in increased pulmonary pressure, so called "dynamic pulmonary hypertension." The main differences between an atrial septal defect of the septum secundum and a ventricular septal defect are the relatively late onset and the right-sided

Table 4-2. **Radiographic Features of Acyanotic Cardiomegaly With Increased Pulmonary Blood Flow**

Lesion	Chamber and Vessel Enlargement
Artrial septal defect	Right atrium
Partial anomalous pulmonary venous drainage	Right ventricle Main pulmonary artery (Right side)
Ventricular septal defect	Left atrium Left ventricle Main pulmonary artery (Left side)
Patent ductus arteriosus	Left atrium Left ventricle Main pulmonary artery Aorta (Left side plus aorta)

involvement in the former compared to left-sided involvement in the latter.

Patent ductus arteriosus is the second most common congenital heart disease. Anatomically, the ductus is a structure that connects the pulmonary artery and the aorta just beyond the origin of the left subclavian. This structure is necessary during fetal life and usually closes shortly after birth. However, if the ductus persists, a shunt from the aorta to the pulmonary artery is created and the pulmonary artery increases in size. The increased return from the lungs is then accommodated by the left heart, resulting in left atrial, left ventricular, and aortic enlargement (Fig. 4-29). The right ventricle enlarges late, and only after alterations of the pulmonary circulation have occurred. A patent ductus arteriosus is therefore easily differentiated from an atrial septal defect, in which only the right-sided chambers are involved. However, distinguishing a patent ductus arteriosus from a ventricular septal defect may be more difficult, since the left side of the heart is affected in both. However, aortic dilatation is associated with a patent ductus arteriosus and not with a ventricular septal defect.

Partial anomalous pulmonary venous drainage occurs when the pulmonary veins draining the right lung communicate not with the left atrium, but with the systemic venous circulation (e.g., the right atrium, the superior vena cava). Its similarity to an atrial septal defect is striking, since in both the right-sided chambers and pulmonary vessels are involved. Moreover, anomalous pulmonary veins draining into the right atrium are associated with 9 per cent of all atrial septal defects.

Endocardial cushion defects consist of a number of disorders. The endocardial cushions contribute to the formation of the mitral and tricuspid valves, and parts of the atrial and ventricular septa. Consequently, defects in the development of these cushions lead to a range of abnormalities, from the partial form of a septum primum defect to complete atrioventricular communication. The complete form consists of an atrial septal defect, a ventricular septal defect, and one common atrioventricular valve orifice. Therefore, communication exists between all four cardiac chambers. In general the heart is quite large, and exhibits multiple chamber enlargement as well as marked pulmonary hyper-circulation (Fig. 4-30). In the incomplete form the anterior leaflet of the mitral valve is cleft, producing mitral insufficiency with corresponding enlargement of the left atrium and ventricle. In addition to the shunting at the atrial and ventricular levels, cushion defects can also be associated with a shunt directed from the left ventricle to the right atrium.

Discussion

The age of the patient and manner of presentation, in addition to the radiographic findings, are helpful features in differentiating the number of lesions responsible for acyanotic heart disease with shunt vascularity. The ductus arteriosus closes shortly after birth in the full term infant. It may persist in patients with congenital rubella syndrome and may be sporadic in some normal patients. Delayed closure occurs more frequently in premature infants and in infants suffering from hyaline membrane disease. Unfortunately, this further complicates the patient's underlying pulmonary problem. However, with present-day, sophisticated respiratory therapy it is possible to manage these patients without surgical closure, which is now employed infrequently.

Ventricular septal defects are rarely a problem in newborns, since high pulmonary vascular resistance prevents the usual left-to-right shunt. However, as the pulmonary vascular resistance falls, the left-to-right shunt

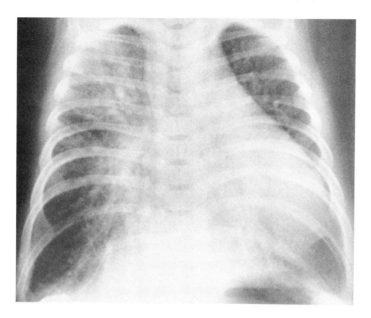

Fig. 4-30. Endocardial cushion defect. A 5-month-old with Down's syndrome. There is cardiomegaly associated with marked pulmonary hypervascularity. The lungs are hyperinflated and demonstrate localized emphysema, probably related to extrinsic compression of the bronchi.

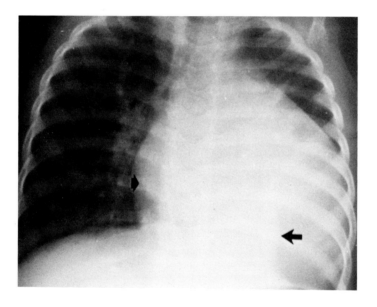

Fig. 4-31. Endocardial fibroelastosis. A 2-month-old with massive cardiomegaly consisting mainly of left ventricular and left atrial enlargement *(small arrow)*. Left lower lobe atelectasis is present behind the heart *(large arrow)*. However, the pulmonary vascularity is normal.

becomes manifest, and the chest radiograph then demonstrates cardiomegaly, mainly left-sided, with increased pulmonary arterial blood flow. When congestive heart failure becomes manifest, the vessels become hazy and indistinct. A long-standing large shunt, if untreated, may terminate in pulmonary arterial hypertension with secondary histologic changes that are associated with increased pulmonary resistance. The radiographic changes are then altered, and the left-to-right shunt diminishes, with subsequent reduction of the pulmonary blood flow and a decrease in heart size. The central arteries remain dilated and appear to be abruptly cut off or

pruned from the remaining peripheral branches. This pattern is typical of pulmonary hypertension and indicates a steady progression toward irreversible disease.

An atrial septal defect of the septum secundum is usually not symptomatic in infancy. This lesion is often an incidental finding detected during a preschool examination. When this disorder is familial, it is frequently associated with other abnormalities, such as the Holt-Oram syndrome and Noonan's syndrome. An atrial septal defect is rarely associated with development of pulmonary arterial hypertension.

Endocardial cushion defects of the complete form are found in approximately 50 per cent of cases of Down's syndrome and congenital heart disease. The mode of presentation is often similar to that of ventricular septal defect and is similarly related to the fall of pulmonary vascular resistence. Patients with severe valvular insufficiency may present earlier than those with an uncomplicated left-to-right shunt. Development of pulmonary arterial hypertension is frequent and occurs relatively early, even before the age of two.

ACYANOTIC CARDIOMEGALY WITH NORMAL PULMONARY BLOOD FLOW

Cardiomegaly associated with normal pulmonary blood flow excludes the presence of a left-to-right shunt. Other possible disorders that may affect cardiac structure should then be considered: cardiac muscle disease (primary or secondary), coronary artery disease, obstructive lesions, metabolic and rhythm disorders, and pericardial effusion. The radiographic appearance in some is nondistinctive. Therefore the correct diagnosis is most often determined by correlating the radiographic features with the clinical and laboratory findings.

Disease Entities

Endomyocardial disease
    Endocardial fibroelastosis
    Viral myocarditis
    Hypertrophic cardiomyopathy
    Glycogen storage disease
Disease of the coronary arteries
    Aberrant origin of the left coronary artery
        from the pulmonary artery
    Calcification of the coronary arteries
    Periarteritis nodosa
    Mucocutaneous lymph node disease
Obstructive congenital heart disease
    Critical aortic stenosis of infancy
    Severe coarctation of the aorta in infancy
Metabolic disorders
    Infants of diabetic mothers
    Severe anemia
    Atrioventricular fistula (cerebral and hepatic)
Pericardial effusion, pericarditis, and rhythm disorders
    Paroxysmal supraventricular tachycardia with cardiac failure

Differential Diagnosis

Most of the entities above present with cardiomegaly with or without clinical evidence of congestive heart failure. If generalized cardiomegaly is the only presenting feature, it may be difficult to differentiate one disease from the other. Consequently, it is helpful to know the age of the patient, the mode of the presentation, any positive physical findings, and the changes on the electrocardiogram.

Endomyocardial disease, whatever the cause, is usually associated with marked cardiomegaly that consists basically of an enlarged left ventricle and left atrium. A frequent finding is left lower lobe atelectasis. This is related to mechanical compression of the left main stem bronchus between the enlarged left atrium and the pulmonary artery (Fig. 4-31). In this group of diseases endocardial fibroelastosis and myocarditis are most frequently encountered. Endocardial fibroelastosis is characterized pathologically by the presence of a thick left ventricular myocardium and a glistening, thick, silvery, endocardial layer that involves primarily the left atrium and ventricle. Endocardial fibroelastic proliferation is predominant. Because of these changes, the ventricle contracts poorly with abnormal orientation of the papillary muscle, resulting in mitral insufficiency.

The peak incidence varies somewhat in each entity. Endocardial fibroelastosis is encountered between the ages of 1 to 6 months. Viral myocarditis occurs rarely as a fulminant congenital disease but presents more commonly between the ages of 6 months to 2 years. Despite the slight differences between the two, it is now believed that they may be the same process. There is increasing evidence that endomyocardial disease may represent the final stage of an intrauterine viral infection with the Coxsackie B virus.

Glycogen storage disease is recognized by its familial incidence and associated physical findings such as a large tongue, muscle hypotonia, and hypoglycemia. It is usually fatal, with death occuring within the 1st year of life.

Disease of the coronary arteries includes aberrant origin of the left coronary artery (Fig. 4-32). Changes associated with this disorder are indistinguishable clincally from endocardial fibroelastosis or myocarditis. The lesion may present at 2 to 6 months of age if

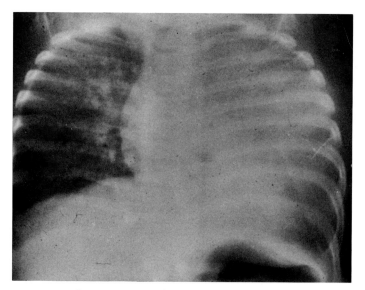

Fig. 4-32. Aberrant origin of the left coronary artery. The chest radiograph in this 3-month-old reveals massive cardiomegaly and some left lung collapse. The fundus of the stomach is indented by the massively enlarged left ventricle. The pulmonary arterial vessels are normal, although venous engorgement is evident by the haziness surrounding the right hilum.

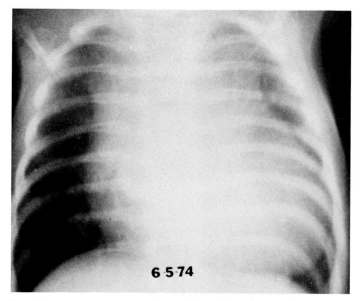

Fig. 4-33. Aortic stenosis. The cardiac silhouette is enlarged, exhibiting mainly left ventricular and left atrial enlargement. The great vessels are obscured by the overlying thymus, and the pulmonary vascularity is normal.

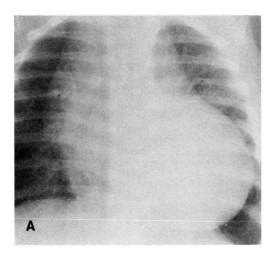

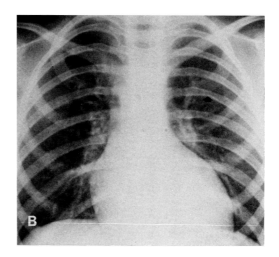

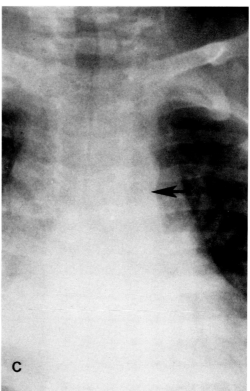

Fig. 4-34. Coarctation of the aorta. *(A)* The heart is markedly enlarged in this 5-week-old infant, with congestive changes apparent throughout the lung fields. *(B)* A chest film in a 5-year-old reveals distinct rib notching *(arrows)*. The heart is enlarged and there is some widening of the ascending aorta. *(C)* A detailed view of the aortic knob in a patient with coarctation demonstrates the dilated aorta proximal and distal to the stenosis, a "figure three" *(arrow)*.

there are inadequate collateral vessels between the left and right coronary arteries. As the pulmonary arterial resistance decreases, the pulmonary arterial pressure is not sufficient to perfuse the left coronary artery. As a consequence, myocardial ischemia and subsequent infarction result. The electrocardiogram is often helpful, displaying a pattern of anterolateral myocardial infarction.

Calcification of the coronary arteries is rare. Deposition of calcium occurs in the tunica media of the coronary arteries and in other arteries. Associated calcification of the arteries in the neck is diagnostic.

Periarteritis nodosa is also extremely rare, especially in patients under 6 years of age. It has been associated with aneurysmal dilatation of the coronary vessels, as well as calcification. It is usually accompanied by fever, leucocytosis, and hypertension. A recently described disorder, mucocutaneous lymph node disease, shows a similar cardiac presentation.

Obstructive congenital heart disease con-

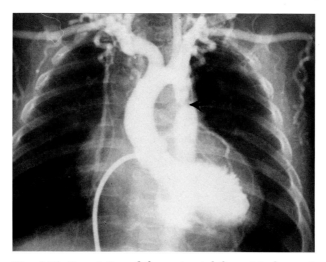
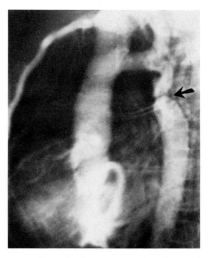

Fig. 4-35. Coarctation of the aorta. A left ventricular angiogram reveals a distinct coarctation *(arrow)* associated with post-stenotic dilatation of the descending aorta. Note the prominent internal mammary artery descending anteriorly and other collateral vessels.

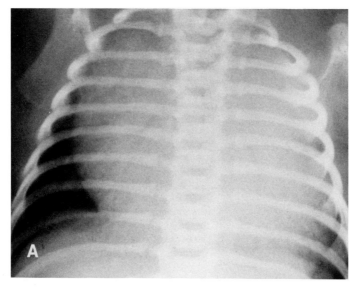

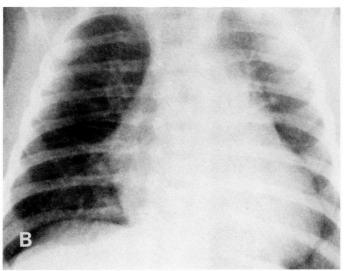

Fig. 4-36. Infant of a diabetic mother. *(A)* A large cardio-thymic silhouette is present with normal pulmonary blood flow. *(B)* Thirty-two days later the heart size has regressed. The pulmonary vessels are still normal.

174

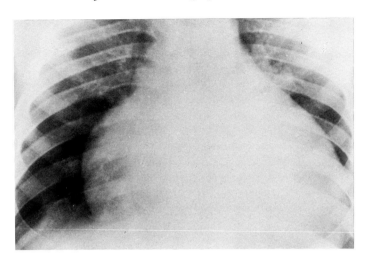

Fig. 4-37. Pericarditis. The heart is markedly enlarged in its transverse diameter. It is somewhat shapeless and resembles a "water bottle."

sists of critical aortic stenosis (Fig. 4-33) and severe coarctation of the aorta (Fig. 4-34A) when they occur in infancy. These two have been confused with the entities above, especially since endocardial fibroelastosis is often an associated finding in left ventricular obstructive disease. Uncomplicated coarctation of the aorta consists of a distinct narrowing of the aorta, usually at the level of the isthmus just beyond the origin of the left subclavian artery (Fig. 4-35). Severe coarctation may present in newborns with profound heart failure, a weak pulse, and no differential blood pressure between the upper and lower extremities. Similarly, the cardiac output can be so reduced in critical aortic stenosis with severe heart failure that neither a murmur nor a click is audible. In older patients with significant coarctation, the site of coarctation on the aortic knob is actually visible as a distinct notch or "figure three" (Fig. 4-34C). Rib notching (Fig. 4-34B) that results when large intercostal arteries serve as collateral vessels which bypass the coarctate segment is not usually seen in infancy.

Metabolic disorders may be associated with cardiomegaly. The infant of a diabetic mother will occasionally present with severe cardiomegaly (Fig. 4-36A) that is associated with macrosomatia. If such an infant is also hypoglycemic, congestive heart failure may be present. Most often, however, the cardiomegaly is asymptomatic and subsides within a few weeks.

Severe anemia or the presence of a large arteriovenous fistula either in the liver or the brain is associated with early, high-output congestive heart failure. Laboratory data and the presence of a cranial or hepatic bruit facilitates the diagnosis.

Pericardial effusion and pericarditis, although quite rare in infants, should always be considered in any rapidly enlarging heart without associated congestive failure. The silhouette expands in its transverse diameter and soon becomes globular, producing the so called "water bottle" heart (Fig. 4-37). At this stage, cardiac pulsations are no longer detected under fluoroscopy. The epicardial fat pad is occasionally seen through the fluid as a radiolucent, pulsating crescent. Isotope scanning of the heart, echocardiography, and angiography, performed to localize the wall of the right atrium within the surrounding fluid, are other modalities that can be utilized to substantiate the diagnosis. The most common cause of pericardial effusion in the pediatric age-group is rheumatic heart disease. In areas where rheumatic fever is on the decline other diseases, such as viral, bacterial, tubercular, and Histoplasma pericarditis, should be considered. Juvenile rheumatoid arthritis and lupus erythematosus are other known causes of pericarditis. Although it may be difficult to determine the cause of pericarditis by radiographic examination alone, associated lymph node enlargement and pneumonic infiltrations indicate a granulomatous or neoplastic etiology.

Paroxysmal supra-ventricular tachycardia with cardiac failure can have similar radiologic features. However, a diagnosis cannot be made on this basis. A physical examination and ECG are necessary.

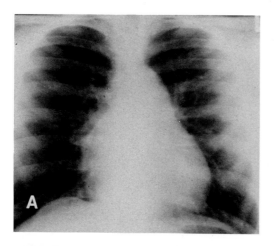

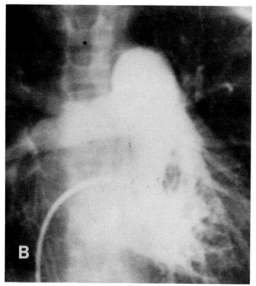

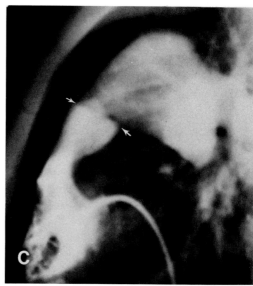

Fig. 4-38. Mild pulmonary stenosis. *(A)* Mild cardiac enlargement with a prominent pulmonary artery, a prominent right atrium, and a right ventricle are apparent. *(B, C)* Right ventriclular injection demonstrates only a mild stenosis of the pulmonary valve *(arrows)*. However, the pulmonary artery is hugely dilated in its cephalocaudad diameter.

ACYANOTIC CONGENITAL HEART DISEASE WITH NORMAL PULMONARY BLOOD FLOW (WITH OR WITHOUT CARDIOMEGALY)

The diseases discussed in this section are not accompanied by severe cardiac enlargement. In fact, the cardiac size in some is no indication of the severity of the lesion.

Disease Entities
Pulmonary valvular stenosis
Aortic stenosis and regurgitation
Mitral valvular stenosis and regurgitation

Differential Diagnosis

Pulmonary valvular stenosis is a common lesion ranking fourth among congenital heart diseases. It is often associated with other lesions. Only "pure" pulmonary stenosis, pulmonary stenosis with intact ventricular septum, is discussed here.

The lesion consists of thickening and fusion of the valve cusps. In the most severe form the valve is thickened, dome-shaped, and has only a pinpoint opening. The main pulmonary artery exhibits post-stenotic dilatation. The cause of this dilatation is not completely understood, and the degree of dilatation is not related to the severity of the stenosis. The true size of the pulmonary artery is not always apparent in the frontal view, since the main pulmonary artery is often dilated in a cephalocaudad dimension.

In order to overcome the valvular obstruction, the right ventricle becomes hypertrophied. The overall cardiac silhouette,

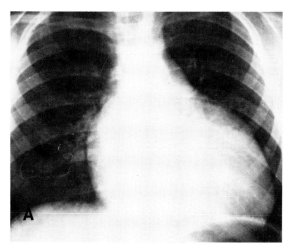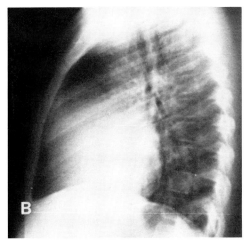

Fig. 4-39. Severe pulmonary stenosis. *(A)* This 4-year-old has severe cardiomegaly manifested mainly by a large right atrium and ventricle. *(B)* On the lateral projection the retrosternal space is obliterated.

however, may not appear enlarged and the pulmonary blood flow in an uncomplicated stenosis, regardless of the severity, is usually normal (Fig. 4-38). In the presence of critical stenosis right ventricular failure may develop, resulting in right ventricular dilatation and cardiomegaly (Fig. 4-39). A right-to-left shunt through a dilated foramen ovale subsequently develops, and radiographic evidence of decreased pulmonary blood flow and clinical cyanosis becomes apparent. The radiologic appearance of this lesion ranges from a normal-looking heart with an enlarged main pulmonary artery in mild cases, to cardiomegaly with decreased pulmonary blood flow and an enlarged pulmonary artery in severe cases.

Because of the enlarged pulmonary artery, an atrial septal defect and idiopathic dilatation of the main pulmonary artery should be considered in the differential diagnosis. The former exhibits enlargement of the right atrium and ventricle and an associated increased pulmonary blood flow. Idiopathic dilatation of the pulmonary artery cannot be differentiated from mild pulmonary stenosis on conventional chest radiographs.

Aortic valvular stenosis constitutes approximately 5 per cent of all congenital heart diseases. The cusps are thickened and the valve is frequently bicuspid. The stenotic valve forms a dome-shaped diaphragm, usually with an eccentric opening. Supravalvular and subvalvular stenosis are other forms of left ventricular outflow obstruction. Supravalvu-

lar stenosis can occur as an isolated lesion or as part of a familial disease associated with infantile hypercalcemia, elfin facies, and peripheral pulmonary stenosis. Idiopathic hypertrophic subaortic stenosis is the most common form of subaortic stenosis, the second most common being a discrete diaphragm. The etiology of idiopathic hypertrophic subaortic stenosis is known, but it is often familial. The principle hemodynamic disturbance is pressure overload of the left ventricle, which responds with concentric hypertrophy but not dilatation. The radiographic features of aortic valvular stenosis are, for the most parrt, non-distinctive. The heart is usually of normal size since it is rarely related to the severity of the disease. The left ventricle may be prominent and the aorta dilated (Fig. 4-40). Critical aortic stenosis of infancy is different and often presents with severe heart failure and evidence of poor systemic perfusion in the first few weeks of life. A radiograph shows generalized cardiomegaly with normal pulmonary arterial markings, and it often resembles the chest radiograph of cardiomyopathy patients (Fig. 4-33). The clinical presentation is helpful in the differential diagnosis.

Subvalvular and supravalvular stenosis should be suspected when left ventricular enlargement is present without post-stenotic aortic dilatation.

Isolated aortic insufficiency is an uncommon lesion. It is usually acquired as a result of rheumatic fever or, occasionally, a high ventricular septal defect. It is also associated

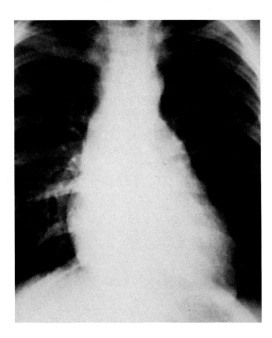

Fig. 4-40. Aortic stenosis. The ascending aorta is dilated and there is associated left ventricular enlargement. The overall cardiac size, however, is not remarkably enlarged.

with a dilated aorta. Aortic insufficiency usually presents with large left ventricle related to the volume overload, in contrast to aortic stenosis.

Isolated congenital mitral stenosis without associated lesions is rare in pediatrics. It usually is due to congenital parachute mitral valve or is a part of the hypoplastic left heart syndrome. Mitral stenosis associated with rheumatic heart disease is far more common, although its incidence is decreasing rapidly in this country. The incidence of rheumatic fever itself has been steadily declining, and improved streptococcal prophylaxis prevents recurrences and therefore the development of mitral stenosis. However, it still remains a distinct problem in the newly developing countries.

The radiographic appearance of mitral stenosis is similar regardless of its etiology. The chambers and vessels proximal to the obstructed valve are affected, and the left ventricle is usually spared. This fact helps differentiate mitral stenosis from mitral insufficiency (Fig. 4-4A). When significant stenosis is present, there is often evidence of pulmonary venous obstruction.

Mitral insufficiency is mostly acquired and related to rheumatic fever. Congenital mitral insufficiency is exceedingly rare. Mitral insufficiency, however, can be associated with sickle cell cardiomyopathy, viral endocarditis, and myocardial infarction related to an anomalous left coronary artery. Marfan's syndrome is often associated with prolapse of the mitral valve.

In the presence of significant mitral insufficiency, the cardiac silhouette shows an enlarged left atrium and ventricle. Patients with rheumatic mitral insufficiency often exhibit a large left atrial appendage. The main difference between mitral stenosis and mitral insufficiency is the left ventricular enlargement associated with the latter.

REFERENCES

1. Bloomfield, K. D.: The natural history of ventricular septal defect in patient surviving infancy. Circulation, *29:*914, 1964.
2. Dunbar, J. S.: Plain film diagnosis of congenital heart disease in the newborn. Curr. Probl. Radiol., *1:*29, 1971.
3. Collet, R. W., and Edwards, J. E.: Persistent truncus arteriosus. A classification according to anatomic types. Surg. Clin. North Am., *29:*1245, 1949.
4. Elliot, L. P., and Schiebler, G. L.: A roentgenologic electrocardiograph approach to cyanotic form of heart disease. Pediatr. Clin. North Am., *18:*1133, 1971.
5. Garman, J. E., Hensen, R. E., and Eyler, W. R.: Coarctation of the aorta in infancy. Detection of chest radiographs. Radiology, *85:*418, 1965.
6. Hastreiter, A. R., and Miller, R. A.: Management of primary endomyocardial disease. The Pediatr. Clin. North Am., *11:*401, 1964.
7. Kirkling, J. W., and Karp, R. B.: The tetralogy of Fallot. Philadelphia, Saunders, 1970.

8. Meszaros, W. T.: Lung changes in left heart failure. Circulation, *47*:859, 1973.

9. Nadas, A. S.: Pediatric Cardiology. ed. 3. Philadelphia, Saunders, 1972.

10. Rabinowitz, J. G., and Moseley, J. E.: Lateral lumbar spine in Down's syndrome. A new roentgen feature. Radiology, *83*:75, 1964.

11. Reid, M., et al.: Cardiomegaly associated with neonatal hypoglycemia. Acta. Paediatr. Scand., *60*:295, 1970.

12. Rowe, R. D., and Mehrizi, A.: The neonate with congenital heart disease. Philadelphia, Saunders, 1968.

13. Taybi, H. Roentgen evaluation of cardiomegaly in the newborn period and early infancy. Pediatr. Clin. North Am., *18*:1031, 1971.

14. Thibeault, D. W., Emmanouilides, G. C., Nelson, R. J., Lachman, R. S., Rosengart, R. M., and Oh, W.: Patent ductus arteriosus complicating the respiratory distress syndrome in preterm infants. J. Pediatr., *86*:120, 1975.

5
Robert L. Siegle, M.D.

Radiographic Patterns of Thoracic Diseases in the Newborn

AIR SPACE DISEASE

The radiographic pattern of air space disease occurs when air normally present within the alveoli is replaced by a substance of higher density (e.g., exudate, transudate, blood). The resulting appearance varies in severity from patchy minute areas of increased radiodensity to complete consolidation of one or both lung fields. In its most severe form the thorax looks like a homogenous, soft-tissue radiodensity and has been referred to as a "whiteout" (Fig. 5-1). An important radiographic feature indicative of air space disease is the air bronchogram, which results when air-containing bronchi are surrounded by non-aerated alveoli. A difference in density is created, and the bronchi become visible as linear, branching, air-containing tubules (Fig. 5-1B). An air bronchogram is the radiographic equivalent of bronchial breathing, and may be the only significant radiographic finding when minimal pulmonary disease is present. Occasionally, the air within the bronchi as well as the alveoli is replaced by a substance of higher density. Air space disease may then be recognized by its fluffy, confluent appearance if the infiltration is smaller than a lobe.

Differential Diagnosis

The most common air space disorder in newborns is hyaline membrane disease. This disease should be the initial consideration in

Disease Entities

Hyaline membrane disease (HMD; respiratory distress syndrome)
Transient tachypnea of the newborn (respiratory distress syndrome Type II)
Hemolytic streptococcal pneumonia
Oxygen toxicity
Meconium aspiration
Pulmonary hemorrhage
Pulmonary edema
Congenital lymphangiectasia
Total anomalous pulmonary venous return with obstruction
Pneumonia
Infant of diabetic mother
Transient symptomatic neonatal hypoglycemia
Chronic pulmonary insufficiency of prematurity (CPIP)

all premature newborns with respiratory distress, unless the radiographic development or the clinical presentation suggests otherwise. Hyaline membrane disease is usually present at the time of birth and progresses during the 1st hours. Alveolar atelectasis is the basic pathology. Radiographically the lung looks finely stippled or as if it contained ground glass (Fig. 5-2). Air bronchograms are almost universally present. In severe disease the lungs may be completely consolidated (Figs. 5-1, 5-2) but are never overexpanded.

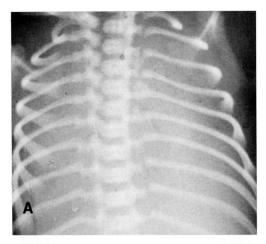

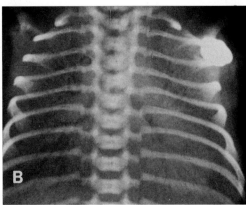

Fig. 5-1. Hyaline membrane disease. "Whiteout." (A) Both lungs are opacified by an alveolar process equal in density to that of the heart. As a result the entire thorax presents as a uniform radiodensity ("whiteout"). Air bronchograms on the left indicate the alveolar nature of the process. (B) Air bronchogram. This chest radiograph demonstrates the early phase of a "whiteout" in both lung fields. Note that the entire tracheobronchial tree is outlined with air.

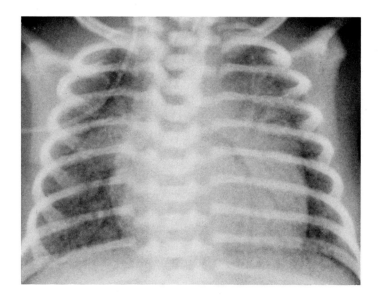

Fig. 5-2. Hyaline membrane disease. Both lungs manifest a stippled appearance. This is due to diffuse alveolar atelectasis. Air bronchograms are also quite apparent.

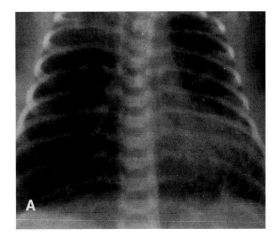

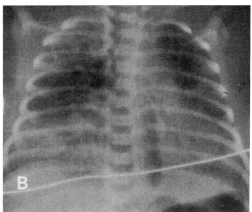

Fig. 5-3. Beta hemolytic streptococcal pneumonia. *(A)* The lungs demonstrate a diffuse stippled infiltration that grossly resembles hyaline membrane disease. However, the coarseness of the infiltration within the left lower lung field is more suggestive of pneumonia. *(B)* The patient's condition progressively worsened, and pneumomediastinum, interstitial emphysema, and further consolidation developed. Consolidation is more characteristic of pneumonia.

If the infant does not succumb to the disease in the 1st few days, gradual improvement occurs, and 1 to 2 weeks may be necessary for complete resolution in some patients. Clearing begins initially in the upper and peripheral lung fields.

Hyaline membrane disease must be differentiated from the severe form of transient tachypnea or wet lung of the newborn, and from beta hemolytic streptococcal pneumonia. Both are clinically and radiographically similar. In one series of patients with beta hemolytic steptococcal pneumonia, careful retrospective analysis of all radiographs failed to detect any distinguishing findings (Fig. 5-3). However, at autopsy pleural effusion was present in 50 per cent of the cases. The detection of fluid is distinctive and should be followed by antibiotic therapy; early antibiotic therapy has a positive influence on the survival of infants with beta hemolytic streptococcal pneumonia. Our experience indicates that the pulmonary pattern in beta hemolytic streptococcal pneumonia may be somewhat coarser than that of hyaline membrane disease, and asymmetrical areas of consolidation develop as the disease progresses (Fig. 5-3B).

In wet lung disease the alveoli are filled with unabsorbed alveolar fluid (Fig. 5-4). The milder forms demonstrate alveolar infiltrations predominantly within the central and lower lung fields. This disease is also associated with a degree of hyperaeration, in comparison to the deficiently aerated lungs of hyaline membrane disease, and a slightly depressed diaphragm. The alveolar fluid is drained by way of the lymphatic system and the disease therefore changes from an early alveolar to an interstitial process during resolution. Small amounts of pleural fluid are frequently present and are identified by thickening of the horizontal fissure. This is significant and occasionally is the only radiographic finding in mild cases (Fig. 5-5). Regardless of the degree to which the alveoli are affected, resolution occurs within 72 hours with only minimal supportive care (Fig. 5-4B).

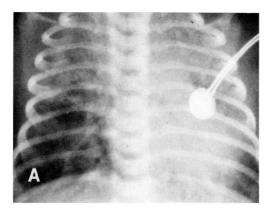
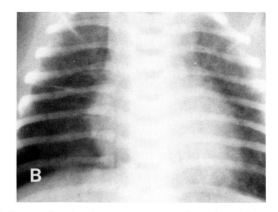

Fig. 5-4. Transient tachypnea in the newborn. *(A)* Severe alveolar disease is present throughout the lung fields. The pattern resembles pulmonary edema or advanced hyaline membrane disease. *(B)* The pulmonary infiltrations resolved within 48 hours. Minimal wetting of the horizontal fissure and some distended vessels on the left are still present.

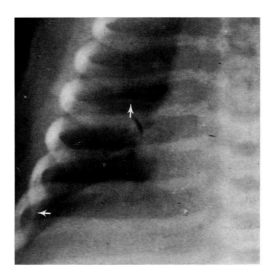

Fig. 5-5. Mild, transient tachypnea of the newborn. Pleural fluid is apparent in both the horizontal and oblique fissures *(arrows)*. Alveolar disease is barely noticeable.

Neonates with fetal distress may aspirate meconium. This substance obstructs the bronchi and produces a combination of pathologic findings that consist of patchy, nonuniform air space disease and peripheral air trapping. Radiographically, the lungs demonstrate hyperinflation and scattered areas of patchy pneumonia. The diaphragm is usually quite depressed (Fig. 5-6). Interstitial emphysema, pneumomediastinum, and pneumothorax are common complications.

Oxygen toxicity consists of a number of stages that have a specific appearance and time of onset. A period of time must elapse before this condition develops, and therefore it does not appear simultaneously with the diseases above. Oxygen toxicity presents late in the 1st week of life; it is almost always sequentially superimposed on moderate to severe hyaline membrane disease which has been treated with high concentrations of oxygen over a prolonged period. The initial manifestation is the recurrence of air space diseases that has resolved partially or completely. It takes the form of diffuse opacification of the lungs (Fig. 5-7). The process soon develops a diffuse reticular and cystic pattern, and the infant's demand for increasing concentrations of oxygen does not abate.

There may be no way to distinguish the pulmonary changes of bilateral pneumonia,

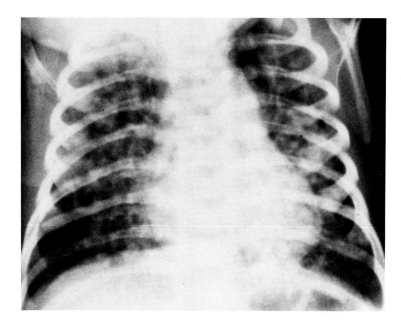

Fig. 5-6. Meconium aspiration. Both lung fields are hyperaerated and contain patchy infiltrations. The findings are coarser than those of hyaline membrane disease.

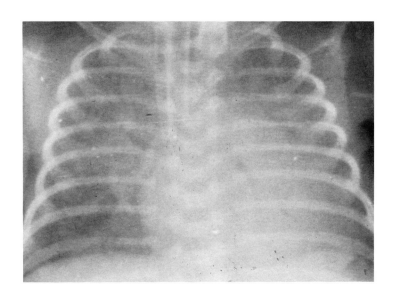

Fig. 5-7. Early oxygen toxicity. Both lung fields are opacified by a diffuse homogenous process. This stage is radiographically difficult to differentiate from any diffuse air space disease. The process developed in a newborn with hyaline membrane disease.

pulmonary edema, and pulmonary hemorrhage by radiographic means alone. Each may cause a complete "whiteout" of the lung fields in their most severe forms and may be patchy and less diffuse in moderate forms.

Lymphangiectasia and total anomalous pulmonary venous return with obstruction are rare disorders that have been confused both clinically and radiographically with hyaline membrane disease (Fig. 5-8). However, the pulmonary manifestations and the clinical features of respiratory distress are basically different and persist well beyond the anticipated duration of hyaline membrane disease.

Respiratory distress in lymphangiectasia is quite severe and often associated with marked cyanosis. The pulmonary changes are due to distended lymphatics that result in a coarsely nodular or reticular pattern. This is easily differentiated from the fine ground-glass pattern of hyaline membrane disease. The combination of alveolar and interstitial edema is the predominant radiographic feature of total anomalous venous return with obstruction (Fig. 5-8).

Infants of diabetic mothers also manifest moderate to severe bilaterally symmetrical alveolar infiltrates. The lesions are commonly

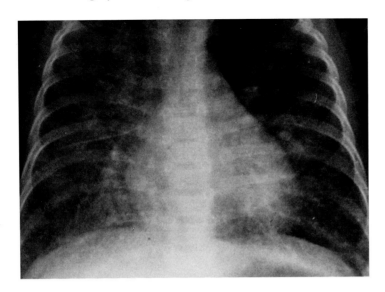

Fig. 5-8. Total anomalous pulmonary venous return. A chest radiograph in a newborn with respiratory distress consists mainly of diffuse and alveolar interstitial edema. Kerley's A and B lines are quite apparent, and the horizontal fissure is thickened with fluid.

homogenous but occasionally present in a diffuse, granular pattern. Mild cases show no pulmonary disease. In general, the pulmonary features are associated with gross cardiac enlargement and increased vascularity. This combination of findings is quite distinctive. Not surprisingly, similar changes are noted in infants with transient neonatal symptomatic hypoglycemia. The hypoglycemia which is common to both may be responsible for all of the pathologic features.

More recently it has been noted that some apparently healthy, premature infants, generally under 1500 gms., developed a delayed respiratory distress 4 to 7 days after birth. This has been termed chronic pulmonary insufficiency of prematurity. Unlike hyaline membrane disease it persists for 2 to 4 weeks. Although the pathophysiology suggests a loss of surfactant, the radiologic picture does not resemble that of hyaline membrane disease, bronchopulmonary dysplasia, or Wilson-Mikity syndrome. In fact, the changes are subtle and manifest a slow reduction in volume with atelectasis.

Discussion

The mechanism responsible for hyaline membrane disease has not been completely elucidated. Inadequate production of surfactant in the lungs of premature infants is still considered a major factor. This substance is responsible for lowering the surface tension within the alveolar walls. Decreased surface tension permits the alveoli to remain open, thus preventing alveolar collapse. The capacity of the lung to produce surfactant increases gradually, and the disease resolves within 3 to 14 days if the infant survives the initial critical phase. The incidence of complications, such as pneumomediastinum, pneumothorax, and oxygen toxicity, is high in this disease.

One must bear in mind that all premature infants are not secure once they survive the first days of life without developing hyaline membrane disease. This false sense of security can be destroyed by the development of chronic pulmonary insufficiency of prematurity, which is also related to reduced surfactant production.

In newborns the lung normally produces intra-alveolar fluid that is rapidly extruded or absorbed. Infants born in the breech presentation or by Cesarean section are deprived of the natural thoracic squeeze that occurs during delivery and will retain the fluid for longer periods of time. The delayed clearing of fetal fluid results in transient episodes of tachypnea. The fluid, however, is gradually absorbed by way of the lymphatic system, and the symptoms abate within 2 to 3 days.

The classic case of meconium aspiration consists of an anoxic, postmature baby who is passing meconium. However, a recent study by Gooding and Gregory has shown that a wide spectrum exists and that the severity of respiratory distress is related to the radiologic changes. Meconium is a tenacious substance and when aspirated results in

Table 5-1. **Differential Characteristics of Air Space Disease**

Disease	Onset	Distribution	Type	Hyperaeration	Progress
Hyaline membrane disease	At birth	Diffuse	Stippled to homogeneous	None	Resolves
Wet lung	At birth	Diffuse	Homogeneous	Minimal	To interstitial process
Hemolytic streptococcal pneumonia	At birth	Diffuse	Stippled to homogeneous	None	May consolidate
Meconium aspiration	At birth	Diffuse	Patchy and coarse	None	May consolidate
Oxygen toxicity	One week after oxygen therapy	Diffuse	homogeneous	Minimal	To reticular nodular pattern
Hemorrhage	Variable	Patchy to diffuse	Homogeneous	None	Resolves
Lymphangiectasis	At birth	Patchy to diffuse	Homogeneous	None	Persists
Total anomalous pulmonary venous return	At birth	Patchy to diffuse	Homogeneous	None	Persists
Chronic pulmonary insufficiency of prematurity	4-7 days after birth	Normal to patchy		Reduced	Resolves in 2-4 weeks or more

bronchial blockage and inflammation. The amount aspirated is therefore quite critical. A significantly high incidence of pneumomediastinum and pneumothorax complicates this entity. However, the lung parenchyma is mature and able to exchange gases so that the overall prognosis, even with complications, is relatively good in comparison to that of hyaline membrane disease.

Neonatal pulmonary hemorrhage is usually caused by septic shock and decreased platelets, hemorrhagic pneumonia, platelet inactivation during dextran therapy for necrotizing enterocolitis, and endotracheal tube manipulation causing tracheal bleeding.

Congenital pneumonia is especially critical, and premature rupture of the membranes and resulting amnionitis is a well known cause of severe intrauterine pneumonia. Respiratory distress associated with pneumonia, however, is commonly due to hemolytic streptococcal pneumonia.

Pulmonary edema in the newborn is the result of cardiovascular disease. It presents early when associated with either atrioventricular malformations or anomalies of the left side of the heart, such as valvular stenosis and the hypoplastic left heart syndrome. Fortunately, these diseases are rare. Far more common today is a persistent ductus arteriosus superimposed upon hyaline membrane disease, which perpetuates the high resistance accompanying the fetal circulation and thus prevents closure of the ductus. Therefore, the resulting cardiac failure does not appear in the immediate neonatal period. Its presence is suggested by the persistence of the ground glass appearance characteristic of hyaline membrane disease and by other features of cardiac failure which eventually become obvious (Fig. 5-9).

Congenital pulmonary lymphagiectasia is rare and is considered a non-cardiac form of pulmonary edema. Survival beyond the neonatal period is unusual. The lesion occurs by itself, in association with congenital heart disease, or as part of generalized lymphangiectasia. Pathologically, the lungs are wet and demonstrate a number of dilated, almost cystic lymphatic channels. Similar changes have been described in patients with total anomalous pulmonary venous drainage with obstruction. The pulmonary drainage is most often below the diaphragm. The obstruction may be due to severe stenosis of the draining vessel or to stenosis of the vessel with which it communicates, such as the portal vein or inferior vena cava. The liver itself behaves as a high resistance bed and produces the same obstructive changes when all communicating vessels are normal and patent.

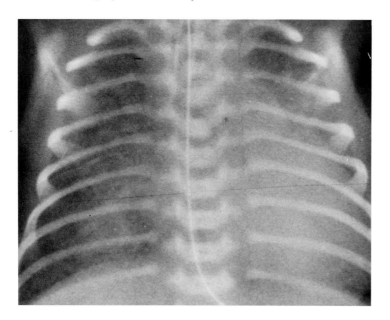

Fig. 5-9. Hyaline membrane disease with patent ductus arteriosus. This infant had hyaline membrane disease and developed pulmonary edema because of a persistent patent ductus arteriosus. Note the perihilar consolidation associated with hyperlucent peripheral lung fields and a wet horizontal fissure.

DISEASES WHICH RESULT IN NONUNIFORM PATTERNS

Most of the disorders discussed in this section reflect interstitial lung disease and consist of lung infiltrations that result in a number of nonhomogenous radiographic patterns. Basically the findings consist of a combination of linear and irregular, patchy infiltrations that may be too small to be better defined on the neonatal chest film.

Disease Entities

Transient tachypnea of the newborn (wet lung syndrome)
Fetal aspiration syndrome
Congenital pneumonia
Acquired pneumonia
Aspiration pneumonia
Oxygen toxicity (bronchopulmonary dysplasia, respirator lung)
Mikity-Wilson syndrome
Interstitial emphysema
Pulmonary lymphangiectasia
Total anomalous pulmonary venous return

Differential Diagnosis

Transient tachypnea of the newborn, also referred to as wet lung syndrome, is manifested at birth by tachypnea. The radiographic appearance varies according to the stage of development and the severity of the

disease. The initial, and most severe stage is manifested by the retention of considerable fluid in the alveoli, which produces an alveolar process (Fig. 5-4). The typical case involves an infant who does not appear severely ill and who responds well to oxygen. In moderate cases or in cases which are improving, the radiographic pattern consists of an interstitial process with distended lymphatics. Pleural fluid and often hyperaeration complete the picture (Fig. 5-4B). Mild cases may present with tachypnea and nominal radiographic findings.

Fetal aspiration syndrome is a result of intrauterine aspiration and produces a radiographic spectrum similar to the wet lung syndrome. When severe, it may be confused with pneumonia; when mild, it resembles transient tachypnea of the newborn (Fig. 5-10). The moderate to severe form demonstrates streaky or patchy radiodensities involving both lungs and is usually associated with air-trapping, indicated by flattened diaphragms and an increased anteroposterior diameter of the chest. In milder forms there may only be air-trapping and a minimal increase in interstitial markings. This entity should not be confused with aspiration pneumonia, since its radiographic appearance is quite different despite the similar terminology. Aspiration pneumonia presents in a patchy, coarse pattern (Fig. 5-6) and its distribution reflects the baby's position at the time of aspiration. This is obviously different

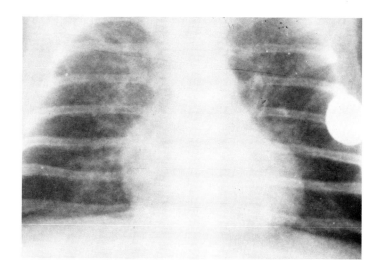

Fig. 5-10. Mild fetal aspiration. The patchy infiltrations throughout the lung fields strongly resemble the wet lung syndrome. However, there is no evidence of pleural thickening.

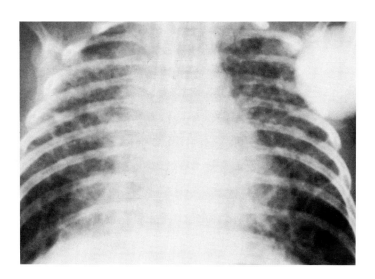

Fig. 5-11. Oxygen toxicity. Stage II. This somewhat advanced stage of oxygen toxicity is characterized by diffuse and coarse interstitial changes intermixed with cystic air collections throughout the lung fields.

from fetal aspiration syndrome in which the lungs are uniformly involved.

In congenital and acquired aspiration pneumonia, the pulmonary infiltration is diffuse and patchy to some degree in the initial stages. As the disease progresses this is superseded by coalescense of the infiltrations and lung consolidation with alveolar opacification. However, congenital viral pneumonias, such as those caused by herpes or rubella, present with a reticular nodular pattern.

Bronchopulmonary dysplasia, or oxygen toxicity as it develops beyond the initial stages of the disease, produces a coarse reticular appearance (Fig. 5-11). This pattern should not be confused with that of congenital or aspiration pneumonia. Oxygen toxicity usually follows treated hyaline membrane

disease after a certain interval of time, and it requires some weeks or months for it to resolve. However, the disease begins with a diffuse alveolar exudate (Fig. 5-7).

The Wilson-Mikity syndrome (pulmonary dysmaturity) is a disease which is closely related radiographically to oxygen toxicity. It presents with a characteristic pattern of diffuse interstitial and cystic changes. The term "bubbly lung" has become synonomous with the Wilson-Mikity syndrome. The main features that distinguish this syndrome from oxygen toxicity are a late onset e.g. (usually during the 3rd week of life), no previous incidence of hyaline membrane disease, and no history of oxygen administration.

Interstitial emphysema is a consequence of dissection of air into the lung interstitium. It arises as a complication of hyaline membrane

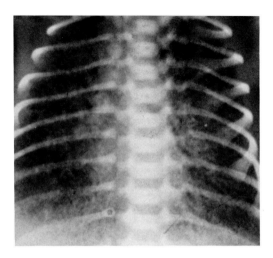

Fig. 5-12. Interstitial emphysema. Diffuse linear and circular radiolucencies are noted throughout the lung fields. This pattern is easily confused with air bronchograms but is generally more thick and coarse.

disease or any abnormality associated with increased intra-alveolar pressure with subsequent rupture of the alveolar walls. Interstitial emphysema can assume many forms. Basically, it presents with multiple radiolucencies that are surrounded by opacified lung. The radiolucencies have a wormy or tortuous configuration that radiates toward the hilum (Fig. 5-12). These findings at first glance suggest resolution of the underlying disease or a diffuse air bronchogram. The mottled and coarse pattern associated with interstitial emphysema is relatively distinctive. As opposed to the other diseases which result in nonuniform patterns, the interstitium in this entity is radiolucent within a background of underlying radiodense lung. Congenital lymphangiectasia and total anomalous pulmonary venous return with obstruction are classic examples of interstitial disease if alveolar edema is not superimposed. The distended lymphatics produce a fine reticular pattern throughout the lung fields that superficially resembles hyaline membrane disease (Fig. 5-8).

Discussion

The fetal aspiration syndrome is presumed to be the result of an intrauterine insult to the fetus with resulting fetal anoxia. Such an episode leads to fetal gasping attempts, aspiration of amniotic fluid, and passage of meconium into the amniotic fluid. Amniotic fluid in the lung causes a chemical pneumonitis. However, this becomes more severe if meconium is also present within the fluid.

Aspiration pneumonia often presents in the right upper lobe, since the infant usually lies in the supine position (Figs. 5-13). Prematurity is a common cause of aspiration because of incomplete muscular and neurologic development. It may also be secondary to vomiting as a result of gastrointestinal disease. Congenital diseases such as amyotonia congenita, familial dysautonomia, and esophageal atresia also result in neonatal aspiration.

Congenital and acquired pneumonias are either viral or bacterial in origin. The bacterial pneumonia that originates in utero following premature rupture of the membranes is probably the most severe. Most bacterial pneumonias elevate the levels of serum globulins. Such a laboratory finding is useful in elucidating difficult diagnostic problems. Sepsis leads to marked platelet deficiency and results in the additional problem of pulmonary hemorrhage.

Pulmonary oxygen toxicity has become a significant problem in newborn intensive care nurseries. Increased concentrations of ambient oxygen greater than 80 per cent delivered over a prolonged period (e.g., 150 hours) cause deleterious effects on the lung. Because of the inadequate gas exchange in hyaline membrane disease, only the lung parenchyma is exposed to these high levels of oxygen. The result is an initial alveolar exudate that appears radiographically like that of hyaline membrane disease. This is followed by proliferative inflammatory changes within the lung interstitium that result in the characteristic honeycomb pattern. Because of the cellular dysplasia seen in this syndrome,

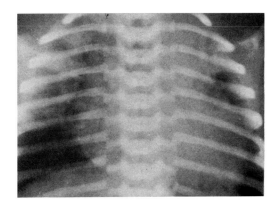

Fig. 5-13. Aspiration pneumonia with atelectasis of both upper lobes occurred following removal of an endotracheal tube. This resolved completely.

recent experimental studies performed on newborn mice indicate that the effect may be related to inhibition of DNA synthesis and cell replication.

A similar radiographic pattern is seen in the Mikity-Wilson syndrome, also known as bronchopulmonary dysmaturity. It is probable that this disease and oxygen toxicity constitute variations of the same process and that both diseases represent an abnormal response of immature lung tissue to variable concentrations of oxygen at different pressures. The effect of pressure alone may be significant, since many premature infants so afflicted are assisted with continuous positive airway pressure or positive end expiratory pressure.

In addition to the coarse reticular pattern characteristic of oxygen toxicity and the Mikity-Wilson syndrome, fleeting areas of atelectasis may appear for 1 to 2 days in one part of the lung and then reappear in another as a result of mucous plugs, which are caused by altered mucous secretion, cilial inactivation, and other unknown effects of oxygen and pressure. The effects of oxygen toxicity are variable. Some infants recover in a matter of weeks or months. Other infants maintain a smoldering pattern of mild to moderate chronic lung disease, and some die of progressive lung disease with superimposed cor pulmonale.

Unlike other diseases which result in nonuniform lung patterns, interstitial emphysema involves the presence of abnormally positioned air and not an infiltration or fluid of greater density. It most commonly arises as a complication of hyaline membrane disease or as a result of assisted ventilation in hyaline membrane disease. Any process causing sudden elevation in al-

veolar or bronchiolar pressure can also produce interstitial emphysema. The air initially accumulates within the lung interstitium and then dissects proximally through the interstitium and along the major vessels back to the mediastinum. Less commonly encountered complications of interstitial emphysema include pneumopericardium and pulmonary air embolus if the air dissects into the pulmonary veins.

Swischuck has recently classified the air bubbles observed in infants with hyaline membrane disease on the basis of size, appearance, location, and pathology. Type I are small, round, and uniform and are the result of terminal bronchial and alveolar distention. Consequently, they deflate upon expiration and are more prominent and prevalent in infants receiving some form of positive pressure ventilation. Air bubbles of Type II remain intact upon expiration and assume a wormy, sinuous course, toward the hilum. The entire pathoradiologic picture is therefore compatible with interstitial emphysema. Air bubbles of Type III are larger, round, poorly defined, thick-walled, and are associated with distention but not air-trapping, since the bubbles do not deflate upon expiration. Air bubbles of Type III are found with bronchopulmonary dysplasia.

DISEASES WHICH RESULT IN THE UNILATERALLY OPACIFIED CHEST

As the title indicates, this section refers to uniformly homogenous radiodense lesions occupying either an entire or part of the hemithorax. The changes may arise either within the lung or within the pleural space. The majority of lesions which cause radiodense opacification as a result of air

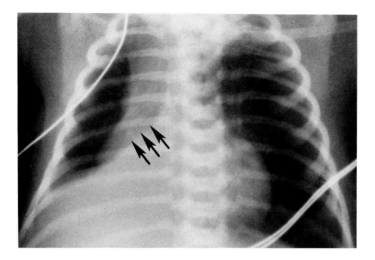

Fig. 5-14. Atelectasis. Mucous plug. The right lower and middle lobes are collapsed. Note the triangular radiodensity projecting behind the heart *(arrows)*. The mediastinum is pulled toward the right. Obstruction was caused by a mucous plug within the bronchus intermedius.

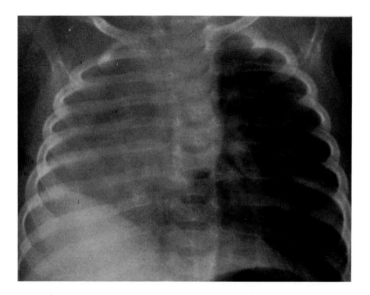

Fig. 5-15. Hypoplastic right lung. The right hemithorax is relatively radiopaque. All the mediastinal structures are displaced to this side and the right hemidiaphragm is elevated. These findings resemble atelectasis of the right lung, although the chronicity of the lesion suggests a congenital abnormality.

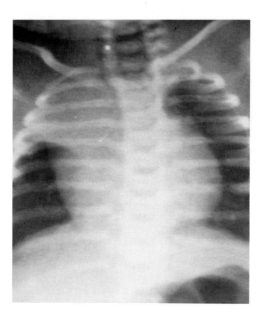

Fig. 5-16. Right upper lobe pneumonia in esophageal atresia. Homogeneous consolidation occupies the right upper lobe. Note the distended proximal esophageal pouch suggesting esophageal atresia and gas within the stomach indicating a fistulous communication between the trachea and lower esophagus.

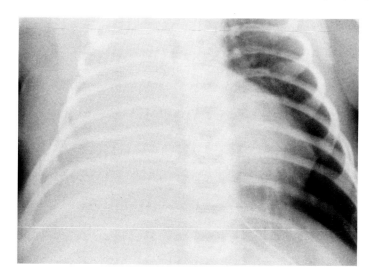

Fig.5-17. Pneumonia of the right lung. The entire right lung is homogenously radiodense with no detectable shift of the mediastinum.

space disease demonstrate air bronchograms and a distribution conforming to lung morphology (containment within a segment of lobe or lung). Other disease processes arising within the pulmonary parenchyma that are not caused by air space disease have a specific configuration. Occasionally they are diagnosed only by exclusion. Fluid within the pleural space, regardless of its nature, is always of uniform density and obliterates the cardiac and diaphragmatic borders.

Disease Entities

Atelectasis (segmental or lobar)
Absent or hypoplastic lung
Lung consolidation secondary to pneumonia or hemorrhage
Cystic adenomatoid malformation
Lobar emphysema
Diaphragmatic paralysis
Tumors
Chylothorax
Cardiomyopathy
Diaphragmatic herniation or eventration

Differential Diagnosis

The position of the mediastinum is an important feature in determining the cause of unilateral opacification in newborns. For example, a shift of the mediastinum toward the affected side indicates lung volume loss and suggests atelectasis due to an obstructed bronchus (Fig. 5-14). Depending upon the location of the obstruction, a segment, lobe,

or an entire lung may be affected. The collapsed segment or lobe frequently assumes a triangular configuration on the frontal projection, with the apex of the triangle originating at the hilum. Atelectasis of a lung may be more confusing, since an entire hemithorax becomes radiodense. The resulting alterations resemble congenital hypoplastic lung. The bronchial tree is patent, however, in the congenital hypoplastic lung (Fig. 5-15). In both of these diseases the uninvolved, normal lung is often hyperlucent as a result of compensatory hyperinflation.

A unilateral homogenous opacification associated with minimal or no mediastinal shift and lung volume loss is often caused by pneumonia. The presenting configuration depends upon the extent of the pneumonia. Most often the lesion affects segments of a lobe or an entire lobe. Right upper lobe pneumonia with or without atelectasis is sometimes the initial finding in newborns with esophageal atresia and should alert the physician to this possibility. The right upper lung field is opacified and assumes a triangular radiodensity (Fig. 5-16). This can be confused with an enlarged thymus. Right middle and lingular lobe pneumonias are recognized by location and the effect on the adjacent cardiac border, which is obliterated by the infiltration. This phenomenon is called the "silhouette" sign and indicates that the borders of two contiguous structures of equal radiodensity merge. Rarely is an entire lung affected (Fig. 5-17). Unilateral pulmonary hemorrhage produces a similar radiographic appearance. This condition is often iat-

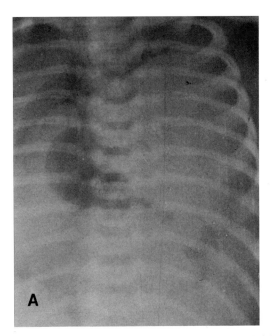
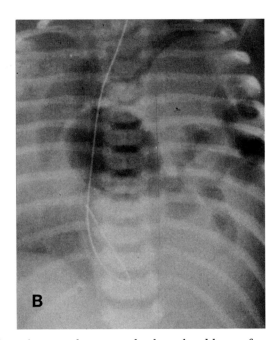

Fig. 5-18. Diaphragmatic herniation. *(A)* The left hemithorax is almost completely replaced by a soft-tissue mass. The mediastinum is displaced to the right. The round, central radiolucency is the "hole in the bassinet". *(B)* After the insertion of a naso-gastric tube air accumulates in the bowel within the left hemithorax.

rogenic, as a result of trauma produced by the tip of an endotracheal tube. When pleural effusion occupies an entire hemithorax, the affected hemithorax is homogeneously radiodense but is often associated with some mediastinal displacement to the contralateral side because of the increased thoracic volume.

Lesions that result in an increase in lung volume cause mediastinal displacement away from the opacified lung. This is commonly encountered in congenital diaphragmatic hernia or eventration of the diaphragm (Fig. 5-18). These lesions occur frequently on the left side and present as a radiopaque mass in the immediate postnatal period, when the abdominal viscera are not yet aerated (Fig. 5-18A). The abdomen itself looks non-aerated and scaphoid. The introduction of a few milliliters of air into the stomach by means of a feeding tube quickly elucidates the problem (Fig. 5-18B).

Paralysis of the diaphragm presents as a unilateral radiodense lesion within the lower thorax. It is also associated with a slight mediastinal shift to the opposite side (Fig. 5-19) and therefore resembles congenital diaphragmatic hernia and eventration. As in

eventration, a recognizable diaphragmatic curvature is always present. The diagnosis can be verified by fluoroscopy. Upon expiration the mediastinal structures, especially the heart, are in the center of the chest, and both leaves of the diaphragm are at equal levels. Upon inspiration, however, the heart falls precipitously to the side of the normally descending hemidiaphragm.

Cystic adenomatoid malformation consists of a mass that arises within the lung and can be large enough to occupy an entire hemithorax. The radiographic features depend upon the morphology of the malformation and the time of discovery. It is always radiodense when the lesion consists mainly of adenomatous tissue. Moreover, the cystic structures are frequently filled with fluid in the immediate neonatal period, and as a result the malformation may be uniformly radiopaque. Congenital lobar emphysema may also present at birth. It too is a mass-like lesion which may be fluid filled. Both lesions cause displacement of the residual normal lung and the mediastinum. However, lobar emphysema becomes progressively worse and atelectasis of the ipsilateral normal lung also results. The cystic nature of the lesion

Diseases Which Result in the Unilaterally Opacified Chest

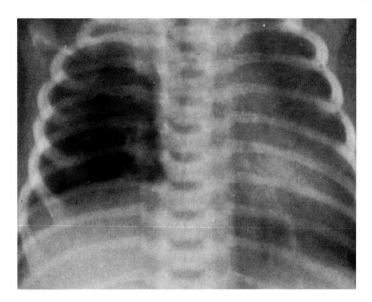

Fig. 5-19. Paralysis of the diaphragm. The right leaf of the diaphragm is slightly elevated and displaces the mediastinum slightly to the left. The soft-tissue radiodensity maintains its characteristic diaphragmatic curvature regardless of its height.

soon becomes apparent as the fluid is displaced or absorbed from the affected area.

In some cases of cardiomyopathy the heart becomes so large that it does not conform to any recognizable cardiac configuration and is mistaken for an abnormal mass. It causes mediastinal shift and respiratory embarrassment as well as compression atelectasis of the left lung. Abnormal electrocardiographic changes, however, identify the structure. Myocarditis, an aberrant left coronary artery, pericardial tumors, and even pericardial effusion have been known to cause similar, confusing radiographic presentations.

Hydrothorax or chylothorax always results in a radiodense hemithorax. The mediastinum may or may not be deviated to the contralateral side. The opacified hemithorax is homogeneously radiodense, and the underlying lung, although frequently normal, is difficult to visualize. An absolute diagnosis can be established only by thoracentesis. A small to moderate amount of accumulated fluid is easily recognized. The costophrenic sinus is the first area obliterated. Loss of the cardiac and diaphragmatic contours are also typical findings. Thickening of the fissures and a lateral meniscus are other features of pleural effusion. Larger amounts result in opacification of the affected hemithorax with mediastinal shift toward the normal side.

Congenital pneumonias, either bacterial or viral, usually present as streaky and patchy perihilar radiodensities, much the same as

fetal aspiration syndrome. In severe cases, the disease becomes confluent and lobar in distribution. The lesions may be unilateral but are more often bilateral. Secondary hemolysis and pulmonary hemorrhage may ensue, resulting in death. Radiographically, the lungs become consolidated, without mediastinal shift. With superimposed pulmonary hemorrhage, they appear even more radiodense. Pneumonia acquired during the perinatal period also shows a lobar distribution without mediastinal shift.

Discussion

Atelectasis may affect only a segment or an entire lung. Premature infants have only a limited ability to handle secretions, and mucous plugs resulting in atelectasis are common. Similar forms of atelectasis also complicate oxygen toxicity (respirator lung) in which the problem is essentially the same. The high level of oxygen and high pressures result in the formation of viscous secretions and simultaneously incapacitate or actually destroy cilial activity, allowing for mucous plug formation and atelectasis. The areas of atelectasis often demonstrate a characteristic ephemeral pattern, with involvement of a lobe one day, followed by clearing, and then involvement of another lobe or segment the next day (Fig. 5-20). In newborns, atelectasis with pneumonia of the right upper lobe is a common complication of esophageal atresia and

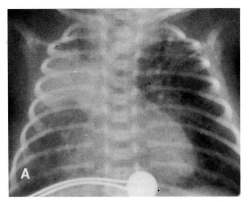 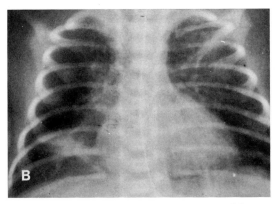

Fig. 5-20. Wandering atelectatic radiodensities. Mucous plugs. *(A)* Atelectasis of the right upper lobe is associated with bilaterally diffuse segmental changes. *(B)* The same patient the following day. All previous atelectatic changes have disappeared and another has formed within the right lower lobe.

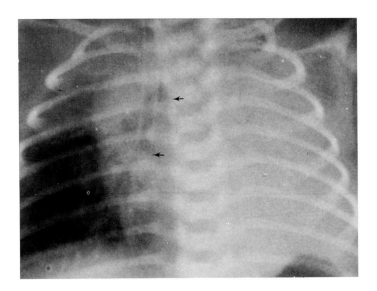

Fig. 5-21. Atelectasis. Malpositioned endotracheal tube. The left hemithorax is completely opacified. An endotracheal tube *(lower arrow)* is located within the right intermediate bronchus occluding the left main bronchus. (The upper arrow is at the level of the carina.)

tracheoesophageal fistula. It occurs following aspiration from the upper esophageal pouch and from gastric reflux occurring through the lower esophageal pouch into the right upper lobe when the lower esophageal pouch communicates with the trachea.

An unfortunate form of atelectasis develops when an endotracheal tube is wedged into a bronchus and occludes the remaining bronchi (Fig. 5-21). The anatomy of the tracheobronchial tree predisposes to easy access to the right bronchus. If the tube is wedged further into the bronchus intermedius, the right upper lobe as well as the entire left lung is obstructed.

The severity of lung hypoplasia is variable, ranging from a diminished number of

bronchial branches to complete agenesis. The degree of decreased aeration and loss of lung volume is therefore proportional to the severity of the defect. Total agenesis of a lung results in complete opacification of the affected side because of severe displacement of all the mediastinal components to that side. The left side is more commonly affected. It is usually asymptomatic unless associated with an anomalous pulmonary vein, as in the venolobar syndrome, or with other congenital cardiac defects, such as tetralogy of Fallot.

Pulmonary hypoplasia is often associated with malformations in other organ systems. When it is associated with renal agenesis, Potter facies is always present. Vertebral anomalies are commonly encountered in

Table 5-2. **Differential Characteristics of the Unilateral Opacified Chest**

Diseases	Mediastinal Shift			Air Bronchograms
	Shift to Radiodense Side	*Shift Away from Radiodense Side*	*No Shift*	
Atelectasis secondary to obstruction	+	−	−	±
Hypoplasia	+	−	−	−
Lobar pneumonia	−	−	+	+
Pulmonary hemorrhage	−	−	+	±
Hernia or eventration	−	+	−	−
Diaphragmatic paralysis	−	+	−	−
Cystic adenomatoid malformation or congenital lobar emphysema	−	+	−	−
Cardiomyopathy	−	+	−	± (depending on related atelectasis)
Hydrothorax or chylothorax	−	±	±	−

pulmonary hypoplasia. Congenital diaphragmatic herniation and eventration, when they occur early in fetal life, interfere with normal lung development and result in varying degrees of pulmonary hypoplasia.

Congenital lobar emphysema is most often the result of obstruction due to cartilaginous abnormalities, a ball-valve type of mucosal flap, or inflammatory disease. In the neonatal period the affected lobe may look like a solid mass, since the underlying obstruction impedes drainage of the already present intrapulmonary fluid. It is more commonly recognized, however, as a progressively enlarging hyperlucent structure. Congenital lobar emphysema results in increasing respiratory difficulty as it expands and shifts the mediastinum to the opposite side. A similar radiographic transition occurs with cystic adenomatoid malformation. Progressive compression of surrounding lung also results in a mediastinal shift away from the mass.

There should be no difficulty in establishing the diagnosis of diaphragmatic herniation when air filled bowel is identified in the chest. In newborns, however, when the gut

is airless, the intestines form a mass that displaces the mediastinal and pulmonary structures to the unaffected side. Occasionally the herniated loops become incarcerated and a closed loop obstruction develops. This is a rare situation, and the radiographic presentation consists of a persistent mass of radiodensity in a very sick infant. Although diaphragmatic hernias are more common on the left than the right, they occasionally occur on the right, with the liver or the right kidney within the thorax.

Diaphragmatic eventration is quite similar although the area of opacification is usually more limited. The overlying fibrous sheath limits the elevation of the abdominal contents, and consequently the entire hemithorax is frequently not opacified. Although eventration appears less extensive than herniation, surgical repair may be more difficult because of the absence of actual muscle mass.

Paralysis of the diaphragm is most commonly the result of trauma at birth and should be considered in a newborn with a fractured clavicle or Erb's palsy. Occasion-

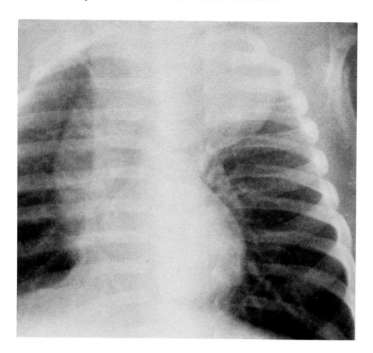

Fig. 5-22. Congenital neuroblastoma. This radiograph shows a posterior mediastinal mass that could be mistaken for pneumonia. However, the oval configuration and tapering margins indicate its extrapleural origin.

ally, it occurs as a complication of neonatal cardiac surgery. The injury is often not permanent, since the phrenic nerve has usually been traumatized but not avulsed. The primary mode of treatment is watchful waiting.

Chylothorax is an unusual accumulation of chyle that arises following an apparent lymphatic disruption of the thoracic duct. Although the actual mechanism is still not clear, trauma at birth is believed to be highly probable. True chyle does not develop until the infant has been fed, and prior to the first feeding the fluid resembles a transudate. As in diaphragmatic paralysis, initial treatment is watchful waiting, since the duct often closes spontaneously.

Bronchial and neurenteric cysts as well as mediastinal tumors are exceedingly rare in the newborn period (Fig. 5-22).

DISEASES ASSOCIATED WITH ABNORMAL AIR IN THE CHEST

This section includes a number of pathologic entities that cause noticeable abnormal accumulations of air in the chest and simultaneous distortion of adjacent structures in neonates. Radiographically, areas of increased radiolucency are produced and most often are recognized with little difficulty. The main problem is to identify the site as well as the cause of the air collection.

Disease Entities

Pneumomediastinum
Pneumothorax
Pneumopericardium
Pneumocardium
Cyst
Pneumatocele
Cystic adenomatoid malformation
Lobar emphysema
Hyperlucent lung secondary to obstruction
Bowel in chest
Esophageal atresia

Differential Diagnosis

A pneumomediastinum is produced when air collects within the potential space of the mediastinum. The findings vary from a collection of small linear or cystic bubbles (Fig. 5-23) to the well known "spinnaker sail" sign. In both presentations, the thymus is displaced laterally away from the mediastinum (Fig. 5-23). The "spinnaker sail" sign is the result of both superior and lateral displacement of the thymic lobes which produces a crescent-shaped soft-tissue configuration (Fig. 5-24). This sign should not be confused with the other nautical terms that denote a normal thymus (Fig. 5-25). The "sail" sign refers to the triangular configuration that the normal right lobe of the thymus assumes as it projects from the mediastinum. The "thymic

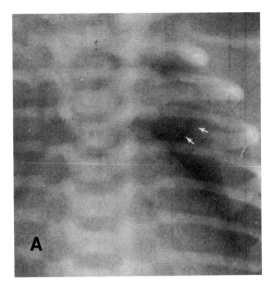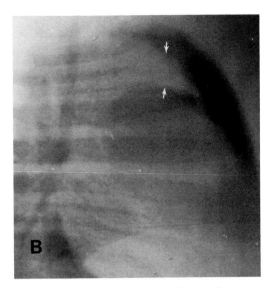

Fig. 5-23. Minimal pneumomediastinum. *(A)* A suggestive corona of air surrounds a soft-tissue radiodensity in the left upper lung field *(arrows)*. This is the only indication of mediastinal air in this projection. *(B)* The lateral radiograph, however, demonstrates a characteristic amount of air anterior and superior to the cardiac shadow. The thymus is displaced away from the cardiac structure and appears as a triangular soft-tissue radiodensity *(arrows)*.

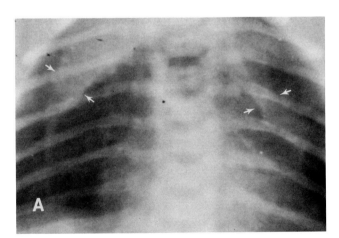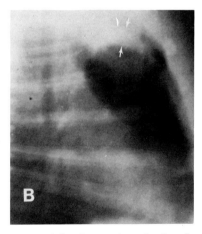

Fig. 5-24. Pneumomediastinum. The "spinnaker sail" sign. *(A)* The thymic lobes *(arrows)* are displaced both laterally and superiorly by a cystic collection of air within the mediastinum. The soft-tissue lobes assume a crescent configuration, hence the term "spinnaker sail." The borders of the lobes are outlined by mediastinal air and the lateral borders by the lungs. *(B)* Lateral projection again confirms the presence of a pneumomediastinum. The large collection of air is located anterior and superior to the cardiac shadow and the thymus is floating high within this air space *(arrows)*.

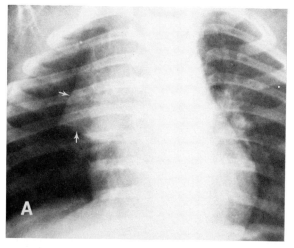
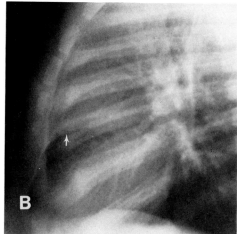
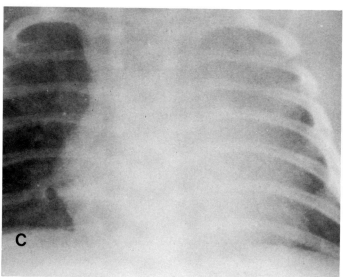

Fig. 5-25. Normal thymus. (*A, B*) The normal thymus in this patient presents as a triangular mass ("sail" sign). The base of the triangle projects along the horizontal fissure (*lower arrow*). The lateral margin (*upper arrow*) has a wavy appearance ("wave" sign). (*C*) The normal thymus can occasionally be quite large and simulate cardiomegaly. In this patient, the thymus is recognized by its soft radiodensity and wavy margin.

wave" is a term describing the lateral lobular contour of the thymus that is caused by the rib indentations.

A cross-table lateral projection with the infant in the supine position is very useful in evaluating free mediastinal air. Normally the anterior space above the heart is occupied by thymus and consists of soft-tissue radiodensity. When air accumulates in this area it becomes radiolucent and the thymus is displaced superiorly (Figs. 5-23B, 5-24B).

Air collecting within the pleural space is almost always associated with partial or complete collapse of the lung (Fig. 5-26). The lung is displaced away from the chest wall, and the border of the lung is sharply delineated by a surrounding radiolucent zone. One must take care not to confuse superimposed skin folds that present as thin, linear lines, extending down the length of the chest, as the margin of the lung. Pneumothorax is often overlooked and difficult to evaluate on the frontal projection if underlying hyaline membrane disease is present. The lung in this disease is fluid filled, noncompliant, and inherently stiff. As a result it refrains from collapsing and maintains its usual configuration (Figs. 5-26, 5-27). A cross-table lateral view performed in the supine position, however, confirms the actual amount of air located anteriorly and shows the lung pancaked dorsally (Fig. 5-26B). This view is also valuable in distinguishing medial pneumothorax from pneumomediastinum. Both lesions may resemble each other in the supine position. The lung tends to fall laterally away from the mediastinum and the air within the pleural cavity rises to occupy this

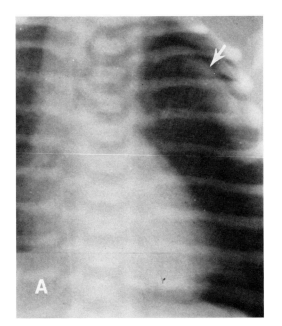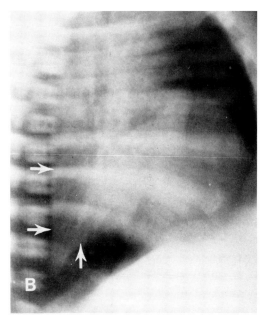

Fig. 5-26. Pneumothorax. *(A)* The left hemithorax appears more radiolucent than the right. However, only a margin of the upper lobe is outlined by the surrounding free air *(arrow)*. *(B)* On the lateral film a large pneumothorax is defined. The posterior and inferior borders of the lungs are sharply demarcated *(arrows)*.

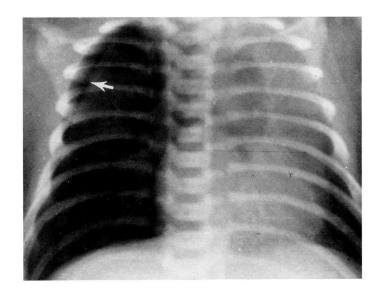

Fig. 5-27. Pneumothorax. The right hemithorax is markedly hyperlucent. The mediastinum is displaced to the left and is accompanied by free air herniating across the midline. The right lung is partially collapsed *(arrow)*.

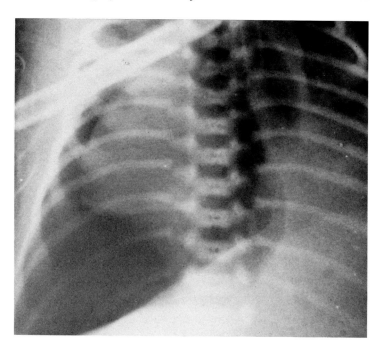

Fig. 5-28. Tension pneumothorax. A huge amount of air is loculated within the right hemithorax completely collapsing the right lung. Note the depression of the right diaphragm and the displacement of the mediastinum despite the presence of a thoracotomy tube.

region. If the mechanism causing the pneumothorax persists, and air continues to enter without adequate means of escape, a ball-valve mechanism is established that results in a tension pneumothorax. The result is severe depression of the ipsilateral diaphragm, and a mediastinal shift away from the affected side (Fig. 5-28). In fact, the opposite lung may be compressed.

A pneumopericardium may also be difficult to distinguish from pneumomediastinum. However, in the supine position air within the pericardium projects along the inferior cardiac border (Fig. 5-29A). This configuration is not possible with air located within the mediastinum, since the heart by means of its surrounding pericardium is attached inferiorly to the diaphragm and occupies the center of the mediastinum. In the erect position, intrapericardial air remains within the anatomic limits of the pericardium, and in the lateral projection does not rise to displace the thymus away from the heart to any obvious extent (Fig. 5-29B).

Air within the heart itself is an even graver complication. It is exceptionally rare and not compatible with life. In this entity, the radiolucencies are located within one or more cardiac chambers, and the internal and not the external margin of the heart is outlined. Air is almost always present within the major vessels and looks like linear, radiolucent streaks arising from the heart (Fig. 5-30).

Esophageal atresia can be mistaken for mediastinal air, since the proximally distended esophagus produces a prominent oval air collection in the superior mediastinum. This is best recognized in the lateral projection (Fig. 5-31). Regurgitation in newborns is often the first clinical symptom, and installation of a few drops of contrast material into the esophagus adequately defines the level of the atresia (Fig. 5-31C). However, this procedure is not necessary and may result in the aspiration of the contrast agent. Insertion of a tube alone to detect esophageal atresia is inconclusive.

Cystic accumulations of air in the lung include a number of lesions that range from congenital malformations to pulmonary cysts and pneumatoceles. Pneumatoceles and simple lung cysts have the same radiographic appearance and present as relatively thin-walled, rounded, air radiolucencies of variable size within the lung parenchyma. Not all cysts are radiolucent in newborns. Some may present as fluid filled masses if no bronchial communication exists. Pneumatoceles occur following infection or other pulmonary disease and are unusual in newborns (Fig. 5-32). They have been seen in infants with hyaline membrane disease as a result of loculated interstitial emphysema.

Adenomatoid malformation is a rare intrapulmonary multicystic lesion. This mass consists of small cysts lined with pseudo-

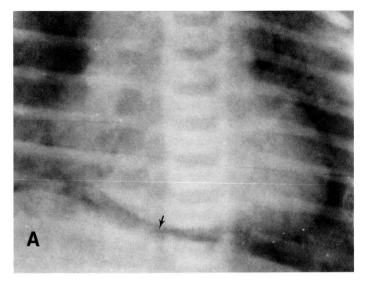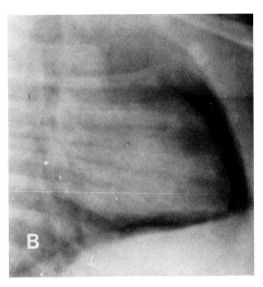

Fig. 5-29. (A) A halo of air outlines the cardiac silhouette. The inferior border *(arrow)* is clearly demarcated by the air. Diffuse pulmonary disease and interstitial emphysema are also apparent. *(B)* In the lateral projection, the air surrounds the heart inferiorly and anteriorly. The superior anterior mediastinum is still occupied by soft tissue.

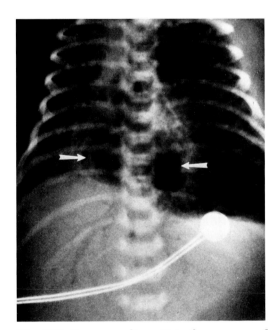

Fig. 5-30. Pneumocardium. Note the presence of air within the chambers of the heart *(arrows)* and the radiolucent, linear streaks of air within the hepatic veins, aorta, and great vessels. Diffuse interstitial emphysema is present within the lungs.

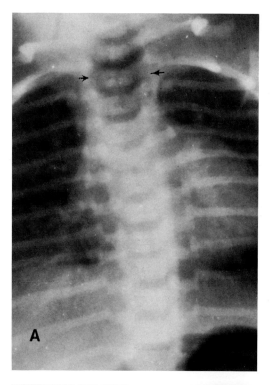

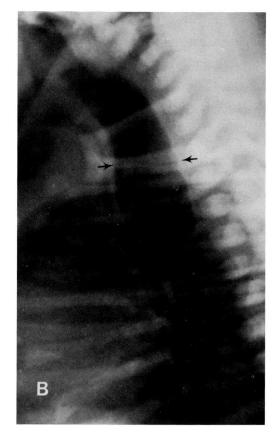

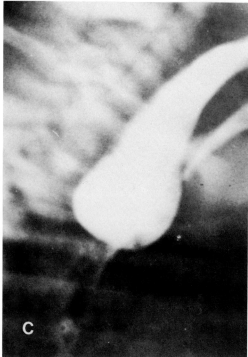

Fig. 5-31. Esophageal atresia with tracheoesophageal fistula. *(A)* A large oblong collection of air is present in the superior mediastinum *(arrows).* Note the presence of air within the stomach that indicates tracheoesophageal communication. *(B)* On the lateral projection the air collection *(arrows)* is located posterior to an anteriorly displaced trachea. *(C)* Installation of radiopaque material into the upper pouch confirms the diagnosis. In this instance the amount of contrast material administered was excessive and aspiration occurred.

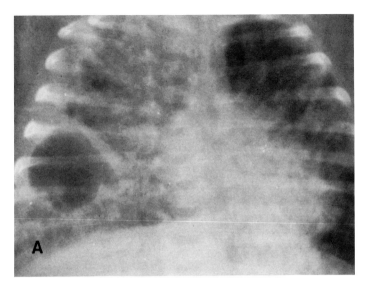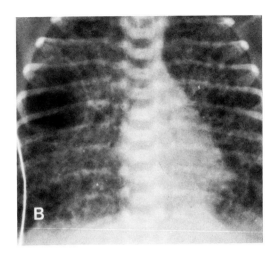

Fig. 5-32. Pneumatoceles. *(A)* A large air cyst within the right mid-lung is associated with diffuse pneumonia. The surrounding infection differentiates this pneumatocele from a congenital cyst. *(B)* Note the pneumatocele in the right upper lobe in a patient with severe hyaline membrane disease and bilateral pneumothorax.

stratified, columnar epithelium containing abundant mucin production. Some lesions are formed largely of dense soft tissue, although in most lesions cyst formation is prominent and morphologically resembles a honeycomb. The radiographic pattern is also a mixture of radiodense and radiolucent structures that vary according to the amount and ultimate size of the cysts. The malformed lobe is greatly increased in size and weight and compresses the remaining lung, causing severe respiratory distress. Moreover, the heart, mediastinum, and the involved lung may all be displaced to the opposite side. All of these changes encroach upon the great vessels and interfere with the venous return to the heart. As a result there is a high incidence of anasarca associated with this lesion. In infants, where the malformation consists of both dense and cystic tissue elements, the radiographic pattern can be mistaken for herniated bowel in the thorax.

Bowel herniation usually has a distinct appearance. Bowel loops, when partly fluid filled or air filled, have a striking radiographic appearance. Should the herniated bowel be entirely fluid filled in the immediate newborn period, its appearance resembles a tumor or lung consolidation (Fig. 5-18A). Instillation of or the normal swallowing of air into the stomach demonstrates the abnormal location of the bowel (Fig. 5-18B). The ipsilateral lung is usually hypoplastic and the mediastinum is displaced to the contralateral side. Sometimes the diaphragm is obscured by air filled bowel located immediately above and below, while at other times it may be quite clearly seen in its customary location.

Congenital lobar emphysema is characterized by an expanding hyperlucent area in the lung (Fig. 5-33). This abnormality is usually associated with deficiencies in the bronchial cartilage and results in air-trapping within the affected lung, lobe, or segment. The left upper and right middle lobes are most commonly involved. This lesion may resemble other cystic malformations. However, the progressively expanding feature associated with collapse of the remaining normal lung on the affected side is characteristic. Similar development may follow acquired bronchial disease. In these instances, however, the lower lobes are just as likely to be involved.

Discussion

Hyaline membrane disease is a common cause of abnormalities associated with air in the chest. The increased intra-alveolar pressure that arises as part of the disease process or as a result of therapy may rupture the alveolar walls allowing for dissection of air into

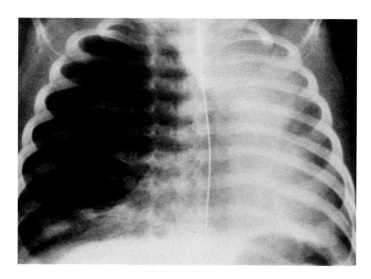

Fig. 5-33. Lobar emphysema. Note the expanding large cystic collection in the right upper lung field that displaces the mediastinum and the adjacent lung.

the lung interstitium. Interstitial emphysema is the first manifestation of this complication and appears as diffuse, linear or stippled radiolucencies throughout the lung. Unfortunately this is not always easily recognized. Further dissection of air occurs in a centripetal pattern along the course of the bronchi and major vessels and culminates in pneumomediastinum and/or pneumothorax. These are frequently the initial manifestations of alveolar rupture, since interstitial air is sometimes not apparent.

Dissection of air into the pericardium is a less frequent complication. Clinically, the heart sounds decrease or even disappear. If a tension pneumopericardium develops, tamponade may result. Even more disastrous, but quite rare, is the dissection of air into the heart. The pathogenesis is basically similar, although the air does not remain confined to the interstitium but ruptures into the pulmonary veins.

It is vital to recognize the presence of interstitial emphysema and the complications above, particularly if positive pressure assisted ventilation is being utilized. Its use must be reduced to an absolute minimum to prevent further dissection into the tissues.

Pneumothorax and pneumomediastinum are frequent complications of meconium aspiration and result from the air-trapping and increased respiratory effort characteristic of this syndrome. With meconium aspiration the lungs are mature, and the outcome is more favorable than when pneumothorax and pneumomediastinum complicate hyaline membrane disease.

Esophageal atresia occurs in a number of forms, and a specific diagnosis can often be made from a single examination of the chest. Five types have been described: Type A, atresia without tracheoesophageal fistula (Fig. 5-34); Type B, atresia with upper pouch fistula; Type C, atresia with lower pouch fistula (the most common, with an incidence of 84 per cent); Type D, atresia with upper and lower pouch fistula; and Type E, tracheoesophageal fistula without atresia, the classic "H" Type (Fig. 5-35). The radiologic diagnosis of Type C is established by noting the presence of air within the stomach and remaining gastrointestinal tract associated with esophageal atresia (Fig. 5-31). This feature is also seen with the rare Type D. When no air can be detected within the gastrointestinal tract, Type A is suggested. Type B results in continual aspiration. The "H" Type fistula is rather infrequent but is nevertheless commonly discussed as a cause of repeated aspiration pneumonia.

Survival of patients with esophageal atresia is determined by the weight of the patient and the associated congenital defects. Cardiovascular anomalies are the most significant. However, many anomalies are possible, such as an imperforate anus, malrotation, and duodenal atresia in the gastrointestinal tract, vertebral and rib anomalies in the skeletal system, and a ventricular septal defect and patent ductus arteriosus in the cardiovascular system.

Pneumatoceles are usually the sequelae of bacterial pneumonia, particularly staphylococcal pneumonia, which is rare in the

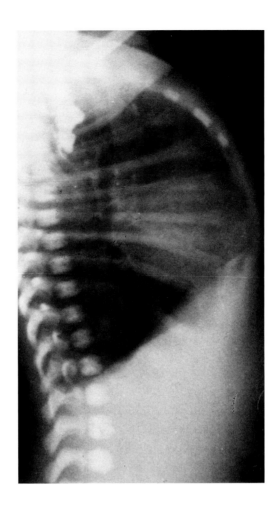

Fig. 5-34. Esophageal atresia without tracheo-esophageal fistula. Note the radiopaque material retained within the atretic proximal esophageal pouch in the upper thorax and no air within the stomach.

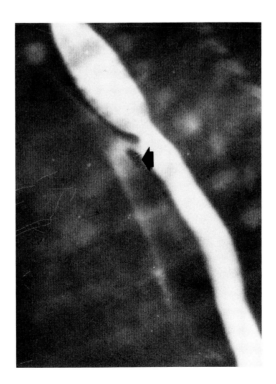

Fig. 5-35. "H" type fistula. The entire esophagus is outlined with barium. A small fistulous communication originates in the upper third of the esophagus and extends superiorly to reach the trachea (arrow).

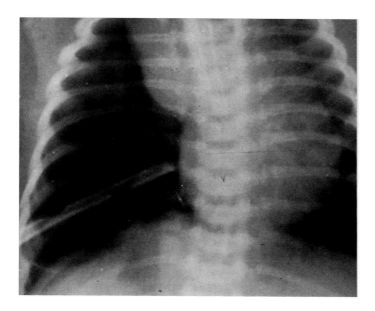

Fig. 5-36. Pneumothorax after diaphragmatic repair. A huge collection of air persists within the right hemithorax. The right lung is still collapsed superiorly and the mediastinum is still located on the left.

1st few days of life. *Escherichia coli* and Pseudomonas infections are more common in this period. Most pneumatoceles arising in this way resolve spontaneously and may require a long period of time, during which the patient is asymptomatic. If a history of previous pneumonia is questionable, there may be no way to distinguish a true lung cyst from a pneumatocele.

A portion of the bowel may appear to be in the chest because of a diaphragmatic eventration, or it may actually be present in the chest because of herniation through a defect in the diaphragm. Herniation occurs more frequently through posterior diaphragmatic defects, such as the foramen of Bochdalek, than through anterior defects, such as Morgagni's Foramen. Bowel in the thoracic cavity from whatever cause may result in serious respiratory sequelae even after surgical repair. The lung on the affected side is often hypoplastic because of pressure from the invading bowel during its development. Postoperatively the hemithorax on the involved side remains hyperlucent, since the hypoplastic lung fails to expand adequately and fill this space (Fig. 5-36). Complete expansion of the lung on the affected side may never occur in some patients. Follow-up studies of surgically treated patients have shown radiographic evidence of distention and marked reduction in perfusion of the lower lobes on the herniated side, possibly due to a persistently increased vascular resistance.

RESPIRATORY DISTRESS WITH NORMAL HEART AND LUNGS

Respiratory difficulties in neonates may seem mysterious when the heart and lungs appear to be clinically and radiographically normal. Other possibilities must then be considered.

Disease Entities

Esophageal atresia
Vascular anomalies
Choanal atresia
Idopathic apnea
Neurological abnormality

Differential Diagnosis

Clearly, the chest radiograph plays a small but nevertheless important role in distinguishing the entities above. Although the lungs are clear, other features may be present to suggest a specific diagnosis. For example, in esophageal atresia the dilated proximal esophageal segment can be detected as a superior mediastinal radiolucent structure (see p. 202). This may be present with or without right upper lobe pneumonia.

Anomalies of the great vessels are often asymptomatic but can result in stridor and wheezing. The clinical findings depend upon the nature of the lesion and the amount of extrinsic pressure exerted upon the trachea. An anomalous innominate or left common ca-

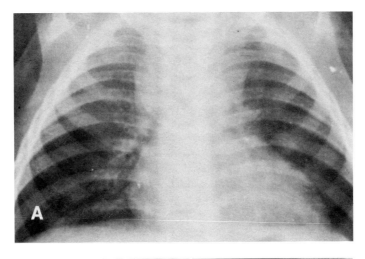

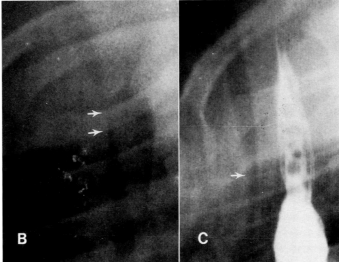

Fig. 5-37. Aberrant right innominate artery. *(A)* Normal chest radiographic in an infant with stridor. *(B)* Note the soft-tissue mass indenting the upper trachea anteriorly *(arrows)* on the lateral projection. *(C)* Again the anterior indentation upon the trachea is visualized on the barium swallow.

rotid artery that arises more distally than usual is a common occurence. Both of these vessels must cross in front of the trachea to reach the parts of the body which they supply. In infants with a narrow thoracic inlet the trachea is compressed. The problem is identified when the lateral chest examination and specifically the upper thoracic region demonstrates an anterior impression upon the trachea at the level of the thoracic inlet (Fig. 5-37). This finding is characteristic, and arteriographic confirmation is not necessary.

The detection of a right aortic arch on the chest radiograph frequently indicates the existence of a vascular ring (see Figs. 4-19, 4-20). A right aortic arch is recognized on the frontal projection as a prominent mass in the right mediastinum. The convex aortic knob is absent, and the trachea is deviated to the left. The esophagram is an important diagnostic study, since it not only identifies the arch but also clarifies the position of the descending aorta. A posterior defect of the esophagus is the result of the descending aorta passing posteriorly to the left. If the descending aorta passes to the right, it produces an anterolateral impression upon the esophagus. A right-sided descending aorta produces a linear paravertebral line on the right. There is no customary line on the left. A right-sided aortic arch alone is often associated with a ligamentum arteriosum, or an anomalous left subclavian artery which completes the ring around the trachea as in truncus arteriosus Type II. The subclavian artery may arise from an aortic diverticulum, the diverticulum of Kummerall. This produces an indentation on the barium filled esoph-

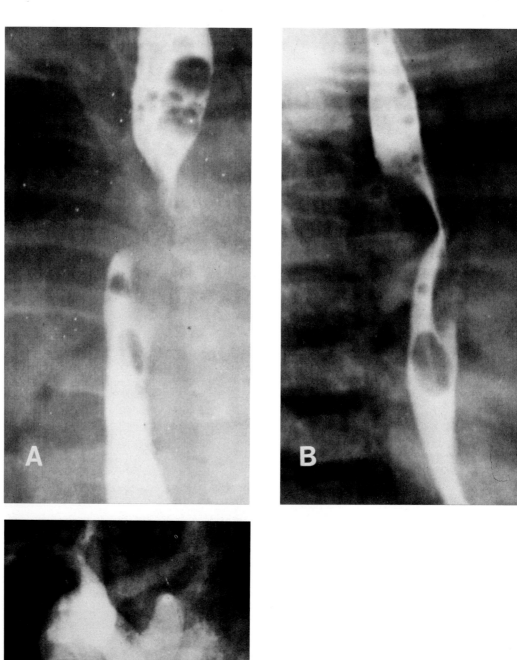

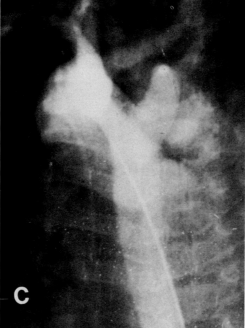

Fig. 5-38. Double aortic arch. *(A)* Barium esophagram in an infant with respiratory difficulty reveals bilateral indentations upon the esophagus in the frontal projection. *(B)* A large posterior indentation is also identified on the lateral projection. *(C)* The aortogram demonstrates two aortic arches. The right is larger and more superiorly positioned.

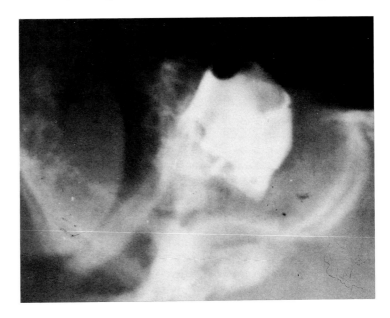

Fig. 5-39. Choanal atresia. Contrast material was instilled into both nostrils with the infant in a brow up position. The contrast material remains in the nose.

agram that looks like a double aortic arch. A right aortic arch is also a common finding in some cases of cyanotic heart disease (e.g., tetralogy of Fallot, truncus arteriosus). However, in truncus arteriosus Type I, the great vessels arise as a mirror image of the left arch and cause no tracheal compression. A double aortic arch should be considered when a large right and a small left aortic arch are identified. The barium swallow is diagnostic and manifests a bilateral indentation of the esophagus in the frontal projection (Fig. 5-38A). The right arch is the most dominant and superior of the two types in 75 per cent of cases (Fig. 5-38C).

A pulmonary sling results when the left pulmonary artery arises from the right pulmonary artery and not as an individual branch from the main pulmonary artery. The right pulmonary artery ascends anteriorly and to the right of the esophagus. The left pulmonary artery encircles the right bronchus and passes through the mediastinum between the trachea and the esophagus. The lateral projection is vital and demonstrates the vessel as a mass situated between the trachea and esophagus, just above the level of the carina. The right lung is often hyperlucent because of the pressure created by the aberrant vessel during the development of the right bronchus.

Choanal atresia may result in immediate and prolonged respiratory distress, since infants are basically nose breathers. Mouth breathing is learned. Some infants with choanal atresia adapt quickly, and respiratory embarrassment diminishes. Nevertheless, during feeding, even the adaptable ones can develop cyanosis, apnea, and may aspirate. To confirm the disorder radiographically, several drops of a radiopaque material are introduced into each nostril in the supine position (Fig. 5-39). If the contrast material remains in the anterior nasal passage, choanal atresia is present. Other atresias or stenoses of the upper respiratory tract are rare, such as tracheal stenosis and laryngeal web.

Apnea is a neonatal problem of major proportions. There is a much higher incidence in premature infants, and its etiology usually remains unexplained. In some instances a specific cause is recognized. Neurological deficit, as with cerebral hemorrhage, must be considered. Sepsis may also result in apnea, just as it results in other central nervous system abnormalities, such as loss of temperature control. With all of these the chest film is frequently normal.

Respiratory difficulty with stridor and apnea is sometimes associated with upper airway obstruction, such as that due to enlarged tonsils and adenoids. In fact, any lesion causing narrowing of the upper airway (e.g., laryngomalacia, Crouzon's disease, Pierre Robin syndrome) can result in right-sided cardiac failure and cor pulmonale. This phenomon has become increasingly more significant in the past few years.

Table 5-3. **Radiographic Characteristics of Vascular Rings**

	Location		
Vascular Anomalies	*Thorax*	*Esophagus*	*Defect on Esophogram*
Aberrant innominate artery	Inlet	Anterior to trachea and esophagus	None
Aberrant right subclavian artery	Upper 3rd	Posterior	Linear upwards from left to right
Aberrant left subclavian artery	Upper 3rd	Posterior	Linear upwards from right to left (right aortic arch)
Double aortic arch	Upper 3rd	Posterior and lateral	Round and oval lateral indentations
Pulmonary sling	Middle 3rd	Between esophagus and trachea	Round and oval anterior indentation

WHERE IS THE TUBE?

Catheters and tubes are becoming more necessary as part of the life support systems for sick neonates. It is important, therefore, to identify the position of any given tube and to decide if the position is ideal. Consequently, some basic anatomy must be considered along with the purpose and direction of insertion of the tube.

Tube Types

Peripheral venous catheter
Umbilical vein catheter
Umbilical artery catheter
Naso-gastric and naso-jejunal tube
Chest tube
Endotracheal tube

Discussion

Peripheral venous catheters can be threaded through veins of the upper extremity, just as in adults. If positioned centrally, they can be used for hyperalimentation or to measure central venous pressure. Ideally, the catheter should end in the superior vena cava near the level of the right atrium. The most common error in placement of peripheral venous catheters is either inadequate advancement of the catheter, with the tip remaining in the arm, or improper advancement, with the catheter terminating in an undesirable vessel (Fig. 5-40).

For example, if the end of the tube crosses the midline horizontally, the catheter is located in the contralateral subclavian vein (Fig. 5-40A). Should the end of the catheter be directed superiorly into the neck, it has probably reached a jugular vein (Fig. 5-40B). Although such faulty placements may suffice for normal intravenous administration, there is inadequate venous flow for hyperalimentation. A catheter placed in an upper extremity may occasionally terminate caudad to the heart as it passes through the right atrium into the inferior vena cava. Poor insertion may occasionally perforate the vessel, and the catheter tip may enter the pleural space or the lung. As a result, pleural effusion due to feeding or a pneumothorax may develop (Fig. 5-40C).

There is also a significant risk of abnormal catheter placement in the chest when the catheter has been passed cephalad by way of the umbilicus. Ideally, an umbilical vein catheter should end either in the thoracic segment of the inferior vena cava or in the right atrium (Fig. 5-41). Obviously, if it is pushed too far, it may cross the foramen ovale and enter the left atrium, or rarely it may cross the tricuspid valve to end in the right ventricle or pulmonary outflow tract (Fig. 5-42).

Currently, an umbilical artery catheter is the most acceptable modality. However, improper catheter placement adjacent to or within major abdominal vessels results in the severe complication of vascular thrombosis with bowel necrosis. The catheter tip should therefore be located some distance from the origin of these vessels. The descending thoracic of the lower abdominal aorta are acceptable sites (Fig. 5-43).

Any vascular catheter that has been placed beyond its ideal location can be accurately re-

(Text continued on p. 216.)

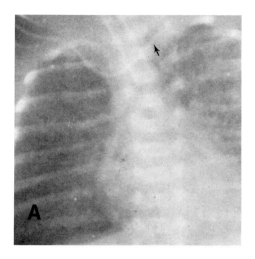

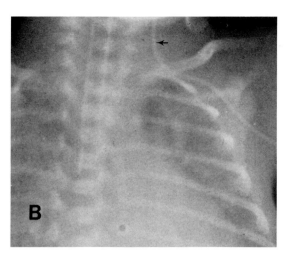

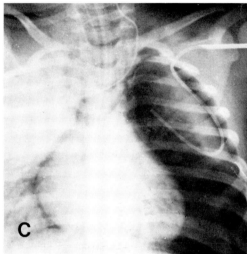

Fig. 5-40. Abnormal peripheral vein catheter placements in the upper arm. (A) This catheter extended from the subclavian vein on the right to the subclavian vein on the left (arrow). (B) This upper vein catheter was passed cephalad into the jugular vein (arrow). (C) This catheter was passed through the vessel into the lung causing a pneumothorax on the left and a pneumomediastinum.

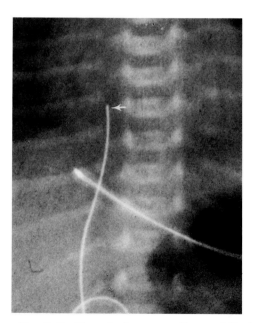

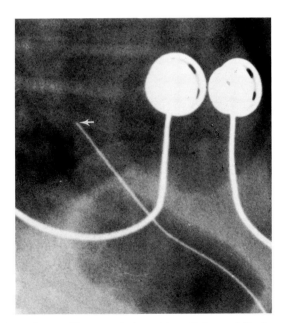

Fig. 5-41. Normal placement of an umbilical vein catheter. The terminal position of the umbilical vein catheter is at the level of the right atrium (arrow). Note the normal upward and posterior direction of the catheter as it passes through the liver to reach the inferior vena cava and the right atrium.

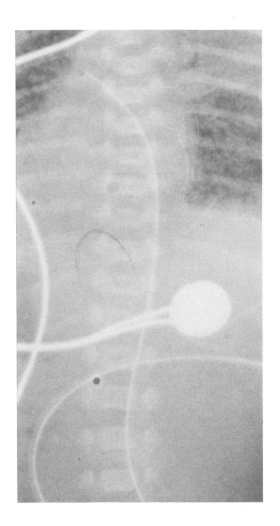

Fig. 5-42. Abnormal placement of an umbilical vein catheter. This venous catheter was passed through the foramen ovale into the left atrium.

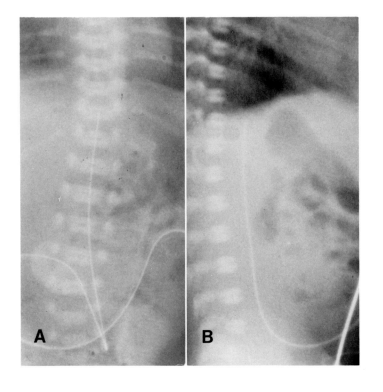

Fig. 5-43. Normal arterial catheter. (A) The initial path of an arterial catheter is through the umbilical artery downward into the hypogastric artery. It then turns cephalad to terminate above the major abdominal vessels. (B) On the lateral projection the posterior location of the catheter within the aorta is well outlined.

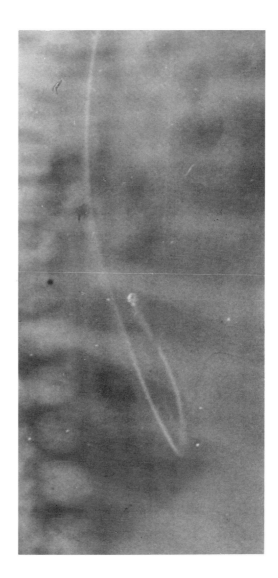

Fig. 5-44. Naso-gastric tube within the esophagus. This lateral projection demonstrates the naso-gastric tube coiled within the esophagus.

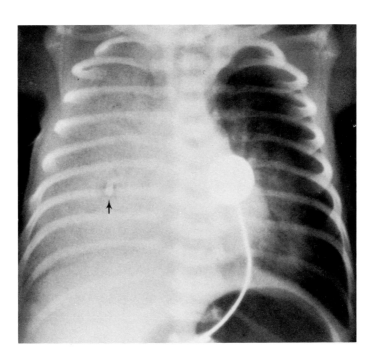

Fig. 5-45. Naso-gastric tube malpositioned within the right lower bronchus. Note the tip of a nasogastric tube within the right lower lobe *(arrow).* The entire lung is opacified following the introduction of fluid into the lung by means of this tube.

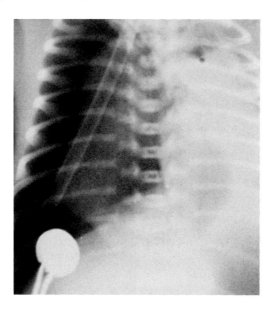

Fig. 5-46. Abnormal intubation. The endotracheal tube was passed somewhat agressively through the lungs causing a massive tension pneumothorax.

tracted to the desired location. However, a catheter that is positioned short of its goal should not be treated in a similar manner. The catheter segment resting on the patient's skin is no longer sterile, and the entire catheter must be replaced by a fresh, sterile one.

Naso-gastric and naso-jejunal tubes are also important lifelines in neonatal care. The end of these tubes should be clearly identified below the diaphragm in the intended viscus. Radiographs for placement are essential. Clearly, if the tube is coiled in a distended cervical esophagus, esophageal atresia should be strongly considered. However, it is not uncommon for an alimentation tube directed toward the stomach to coil back into the esophagus (Fig. 5-44). In addition, it is not impossible to intubate the tracheobronchial tree with a feeding tube. This can be quite detrimental to the lung (Fig. 5-45).

Endotracheal tubing is often minimally radiopague, which makes the determination of position somewhat difficult. Ideally the tube should be centrally positioned and terminate above the carina within the trachea. If the tube is positioned too high it may easily slip back above the epiglottis. If the tube passes below the carina, it will slip into a main broncus, especially the right bronchus, with resulting airway obstruction, blocking the contralateral lung (Fig. 5-21). If the tube becomes wedged in the bronchus intermedius, the right upper lobe may also be obstructed.

Occasionally the endotracheal tube may be pushed even further than the mainstem bronchus by an inexperienced hand. The result is potentially disastrous if the catheter perforates the lung and causes a pneumothorax (Fig. 5-46).

Chest tubes are probably the largest foreign bodies encountered in the chest. They are essential in the treatment of a pneumothorax, a relatively common but severe complication of hyaline membrane disease and fetal aspiration syndrome. The placement of more than one tube in a hemithorax is not uncommon. In some situations air is seen beneath the lung. It is conceivable that this air is, in fact, extrapleural, since it persists despite the placement of the chest tubes superiorly. In such a situation it is appropriate to place another chest tube between the diaphragm and the lung.

REFERENCES

Air Space Disease

1. Avery, M. D.: The Lung and its disorders in the newborn infant. *In* Schaffer, A. J. (ed.): Major Problems in Pediatrics. Philadelphia, Saunders, 1968.
2. Gooding, C. A., and Gregory, G. A.: Roentgenographic analysis of meconium aspiration of the newborn. Radiology, *100:*131, 1971.
3. Hemming, V. G., McCloskey, D. W., and Hill, H. R.: Pneumonia in the neonate associated with Group B streptococcal septicemia. Am. J. Dis. Child., *130:*1231, 1976.
4. Kraus, A. N., Klain, D. B., and Auld, P. A.:

Chronic pulmonary insufficiency of prematurity (CPIP). Pediatrics, *55:*55, 1975.

5. Northway, W. H., Jr., and Rosan, R. C.: Radiographic features of pulmonary oxygen toxicity in the newborn: bronchopulmonary dysplasia. Radiology, *91:*49, 1968.

Diseases Which Result in Nonuniform Patterns

6. Northway, W. H., Pereau, L., Petriceles, R., Bensel, K. G.: Oxygen toxicity in the newborn lung: reversal of inhibition of DNA synthesis in the mouse. Pediatrics. *57:*41, 1976.

7. Northway, W. H., Rosan, R. C., and Porter, D. Y.: Pulmonary disease following respirator therapy of hyaline membrane disease (bronchopulmonary dysplasia) N. Engl. J. Med., *276:*357, 1967.

8. Swischuck, L.: Bubbles in hyaline membrane disease. Radiology, *122:*417, 1977.

9. Thibeault, D. W., Lachman, R. S., et al.: Pulmonary interstitial emphysema, pneumomediastinum and pneumothorax. Am. J. Dis. Child., *126:*611, 1973.

Diseases Associated With Abnormal Air in the Chest

10. German, J. C., Mahour, G., H., and Woolley, M. D.: Esophageal atresia and associated anomalies. J. Pediatr. Surg., *11:*299, 1976.

11. Gross, R. E.: The surgery of infancy and childhood. Philadelphia, Saunders, 1953.

12. Moskowitz, P. S., and Griscom, N. T.: The medial pneumothorax. Radiology, *120:*143, 1976.

13. Wohl, M. E. B., Griscom, N. T., et al.: The Lung following repair of congenital diaphragmatic hernia. J. Pediatr., *90:*405, 1977.

6 | Robert L. Siegle, M.D.
Jack G. Rabinowitz, M.D., F.A.C.R.

Radiographic Patterns
of Thoracic Disease
in the Infant and Child

THE PARTIALLY OR TOTALLY OPACIFIED LUNG

An area of uniformly increased radiodensity that partially or completely opacifies a hemithorax may originate within the lung, extend into the lung from other tissues, or represent pleural fluid. The basic radiographic features of each in infants and children are the same as in adults, although the incidence of the underlying disease varies with the age-group.

Disease Entities

Alveolar pneumonia
Tumor mass
Pulmonary hemorrhage
Pseudotumor
Pulmonary edema
Pleural effusion
Atelectasis

Differential Diagnosis

Alveolar pneumonias are easily recognized if the overall opacification is relatively homogeneous and conforms to an anatomic segmental or lobar distribution (Figs. 6-1, 6-2). Air bronchograms are usually apparent when the radiographic detail is adequate. In its early stages of development, the distribution of an alveolar pneumonia may be lobular or acinar, and as a result its appearance consists only of multiple, patchy infiltrations. The presence of air bronchograms within the infiltrations and a fluffy, soft margin surrounding each lesion are of great importance in determining the alveolar nature.

Fortunately, tumor masses are rare in children. Primary neoplasms usually arise from structures contiguous with the lungs, such as the thymus, lymph nodes, or neurogenic tissue, but a single metastasis may occur in the lungs. In general, a neoplastic mass is solid, with irregular borders if it arises within the parenchyma, rounded if it is metastatic, and oval with an incomplete margin if it arises outside the lung (Fig. 6-3).

Some forms of pneumonia may assume a spherical configuration during their development. Such an appearance has been called pseudotumor pneumonia because of its striking resemblance to an abnormal mass (Fig. 6-4). It is seen almost exclusively in children and at this stage appears to defy anatomic boundaries within the lung. Close observation, however, reveals features characteristic of an alveolar process (e.g., air

(Text continued on p. 222.)

219

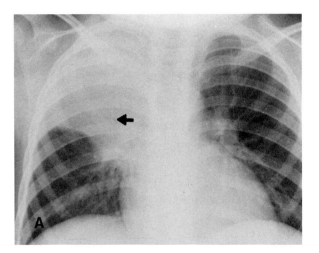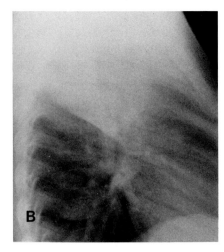

Fig. 6-1. Pneumococcal pneumonia of the right upper lobe. *(A)* A homogeneous radiodensity occupies the entire right upper lobe. Note the air bronchogram *(arrow).* *(B)* The lateral film reveals minimal elevation of the anterior segment and mildly enlarged hilar nodes.

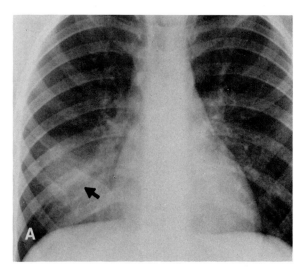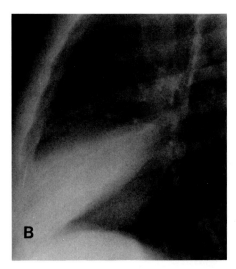

Fig. 6-2. Pneumonia of the right middle lobe. *(A)* A relatively homogeneous infiltration with an air bronchogram *(arrow)* occupies the right middle lobe. The superior margin is demarcated by the horizontal fissure and the cardiac border is obscured. *(B)* In the lateral projection the lobe assumes a triangular configuration with some volume loss. The horizontal fissure is slightly depressed. The lesion is quite radiodense on the lateral film because of the superimposed cardiac silhouette.

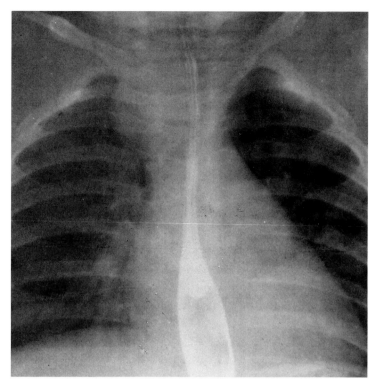

Fig. 6-3. Bronchogenic cyst. A well-defined oval mass is noted within the upper mediastinum. The proximal trachea and esophagus are displaced to the left, and only the border of the mass surrounded by lung is seen. This is not a common location for a bronchogenic cyst.

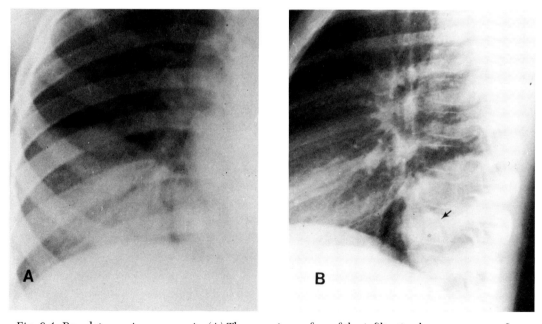

Fig. 6-4. Pseudotumor in pneumonia. (A) The superior surface of the infiltration has a concave configuration. (B) On the lateral film the infiltration resembles a pleural-based tumor. Air bronchograms indicate the pneumonic nature of the lesion (arrow).

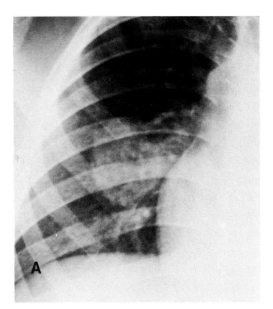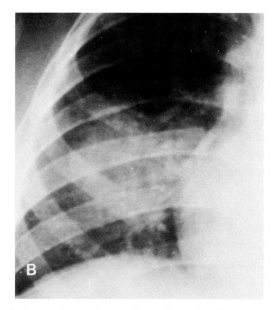

Fig. 6-5. Pseudotumor in pneumonia. *(A)* The initial chest radiograph reveals a spherical infiltration within the right lower lobe that strikingly resembles a tumor mass. *(B)* Within 24 hours, however, the infiltration spread into other portions of the lobe confirming its alveolar location.

bronchograms and ill-defined, fluffy borders). This presentation is only a transient stage in the pneumonic process, and reexamination 1 to 2 days later demonstrates the more characteristic segmental or lobar distribution of the lesion (Fig. 6-5).

An extensive pleural effusion may occasionally be confused with a lung consolidation when it produces a homogeneous opacification of most or all of a hemithorax and completely obliterates the underlying lung (Fig. 6-6). The absence of air bronchograms, or the conformity to any segmental or lobar anatomy, suggests the presence of pleural fluid. Further confusion may arise when the radiograph is exposed with the patient in a supine position. The pleural fluid becomes layered posteriorly, adding uniform density to the entire hemithorax. Every effort should then be made to obtain erect and/or lateral decubitus studies to confirm the presence of an effusion.

For pleural fluid to become loculate in a fissure and produce a mass-like configuration, pre-existing pleural adhesions must be present. Therefore, such an occurrence is unusual in children but not in adults. The collection assumes an oval configuration with tapering margins, best observed on the lateral projection.

Pulmonary edema is usually the cause of bilateral and symmetrical opacification of the lungs. The radiodensity is fluffy and coalescent and demonstrates features of underlying alveolar disease. The peripheral lung fluids are spared, and as a result a radiolucent halo is produced around the central core of the lung.

Extensive pulmonary hemorrhage is uncommon in the pediatric age-group. It is seen more often in neonates (see Chapter 5). Severe pulmonary injury manifested by a hematoma represents a localized pulmonary hemorrhage. This is the result of blunt or penetrating chest trauma and results in the serosanguineous filling of air spaces in the region of the trauma. The radiographic appearance differs from most forms of pneumonia, since pulmonary hemorrhage is not usually manifested by a segmental distribution. However, it presents as alveolar disease, with air bronchograms and ill-defined margins, and most often assumes an oval configuration (Fig. 6-7). A hematoma requires more time (usually weeks) to resolve than do most acute pneumonias. During the period of resolution, the lesion decreases in size and becomes more oval in configuration. Liquification of the hematoma results in the formation of a cavity (Fig. 6-7). The radiographic find-

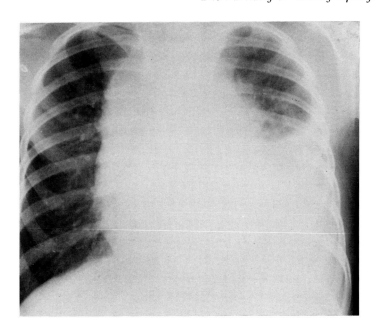

Fig. 6-6. Leukemic infiltration of the thymus with pleural effusion. A large pleural effusion obliterates most of the left hemithorax. The anterior mediastinum is widened because of leukemic infiltration.

ings of pulmonary contusion without hemorrhage basically indicate the presence of a transudate, and resolution is a matter of a few days.

Atelectasis resembles a consolidated lung but with volume loss. When atelectasis of a lobe occurs, the fissures not only define a smaller than normal area for that lobe but deviate toward the mediastinum (Fig. 6-8). As a result, they often assume a triangular configuration. Secondary thoracic changes also occur to compensate for the loss of volume (e.g., elevation of the diaphragm and mediastinal shift to the atelectatic side). If the volume loss is great, compensatory hyperaeration of the neighboring lung occurs, and a relatively hyperlucent lung results. The features of shift and hyperlucency are especially prominent in the presence of an entire lung collapse.

Discussion

Most bacterial pneumonias appear radiographically similar in many respects, although there are some basic differences. Lobar consolidation is frequently a result of pneumococcal pneumonia and occurs commonly in the late winter or early spring (Fig. 6-1). Pneumococci gain entrance into the lungs by way of the respiratory passages. A rapid outpouring of edematous fluid from the alveoli occurs, which not only helps support bacterial growth but further aids in

the spread of organisms to adjacent alveoli. This explains how and why the underlying lobe undergoes such rapid consolidation. With present-day antimicrobial therapy, the pathologic stages of red and white hepatization, which were considered characteristic of pneumococcal pneumonia, are no longer witnessed.

Hemophilus pneumonia is also frequently lobar (Fig. 6-9). As such, it may be difficult to differentiate from disease caused by pneumococcus. However, Hemophilus pneumonia has an insidious onset, in comparison to the sudden onset characteristic of a pneumococcal pneumonia. Bronchopneumonia and disseminated disease may also occur, as in most forms of pneumonia. The disease is almost always associated with pleural effusion and is usually preceded by some form of nasopharyngeal disease. Epiglottitis, otitis media, and meningitis may also occur.

A patchy or lobar homogeneous consolidation accompanied by a pleural exudate is, in all likelihood, the result of a Staphylococcus infection. This type of pneumonia may occur at any age but is most likely to occur during the 1st year of life. Infection of the right lung is more probable than the left, and pneumatoceles or abscesses develop early. Pneumatoceles tend to persist and even increase in size despite an overall regression of the pneumonic process. Other bacterial pneu-

(Text continued on p. 227.)

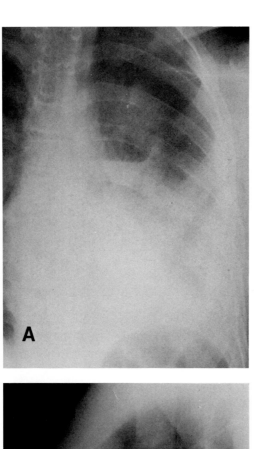

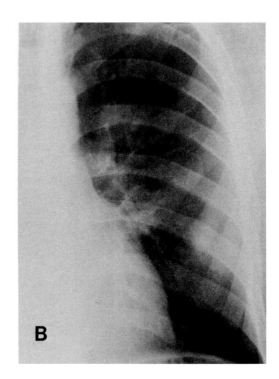

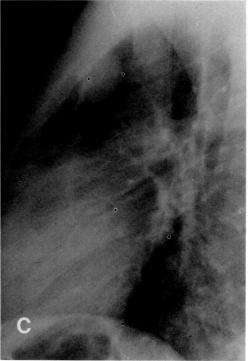

Fig. 6-7. Pulmonary hematoma. *(A)* The initial film taken a few days following blunt trauma to the chest reveals an area of infiltration, with cavitation in the left perihilar region, a diffuse pneumonic infiltration within the left lower lobe, and some pleural effusion. Subcutaneous emphysema is also apparent. *(B, C)* A few weeks later, most of the hematoma has resolved. The lesion in the left perihilar region now appears spherical and on the lateral projection is surrounded by a halo of air. The round mass represents a fibrin ball.

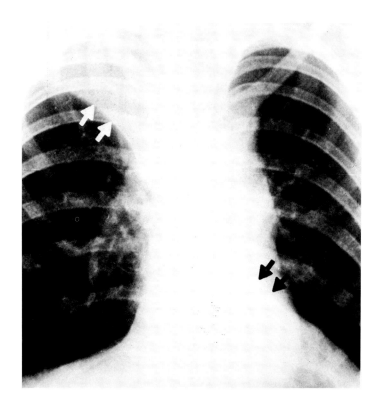

Fig. 6-8. Atelectasis of the right upper lobe and left lower lobe. A patient with an acute attack of asthma. Both the right upper and left lower lobes are collapsed. Note that there is deviation of the fissures toward the mediastinum *(arrows).* The collapsed lobes are homogeneously radiodense and triangular in configuration. The left lower lobe is seen through the cardiac structure.

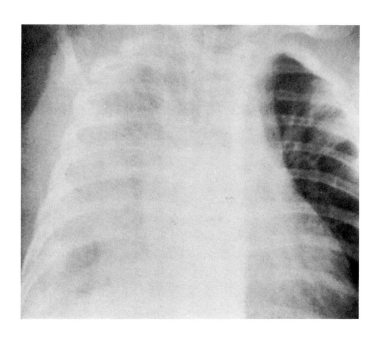

Fig. 6-9. Hemophilus pneumonia. A diffuse lobar pneumonia within the right lung field is associated with a large pleural reaction. Hemophilus was cultured from the pleural fluid.

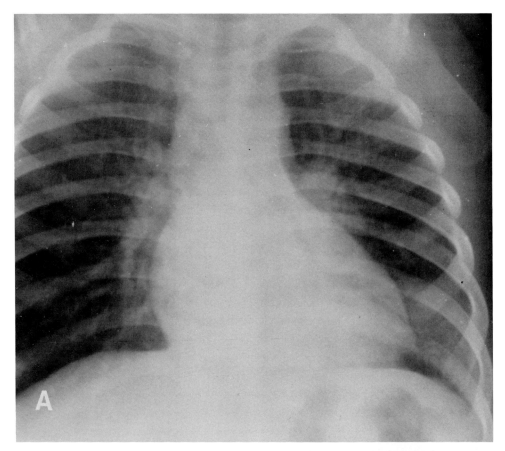

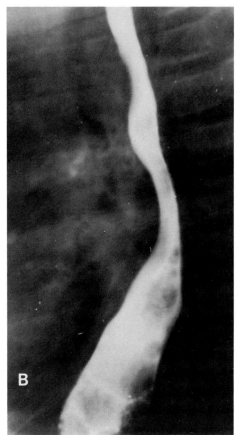

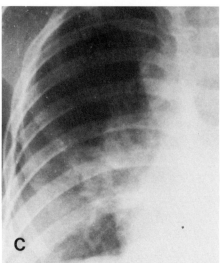

Fig. 6-10. Pneumonia with involvement of the lymph nodes. *(A)* Primary tuberculosis. Pulmonary infiltration is present within the left lower lung field, associated with well-defined left hilar nodes. *(B)* The size of the nodes are well demonstrated by the impression formed upon the anterior margin of the esophagus. *(C)* Rocky mountain spotted fever. Note the nonspecific alveolar consolidation in the right lower lobe and the enlarged right paratracheal lymph node.

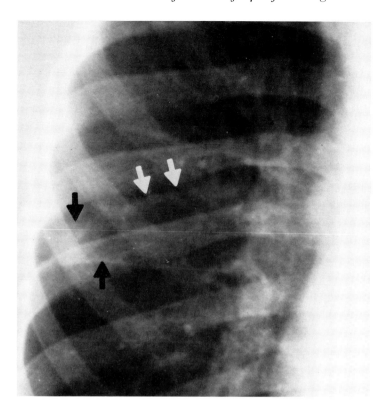

Fig. 6-11. Primary tuberculosis (Ghon complex). A small parenchymal focus is noted in the right lateral lung field adjacent to the horizontal fissure *(upper black arrow)*. A distended lymph channel extends from the lesion toward the hilum *(white arrows)*. The hilar nodes are slightly enlarged. The horizontal fissure adjacent to the infiltration is thickened by a small exudate *(lower black arrow)*.

monias that cause empyema or pneumatocele formation are the result of infection with Streptococcus, Klebsiella, and Hemophilus.

Mycoplasma pneumoniae shows an unusual pattern of infection. It demonstrates an increasing incidence of reinfection in young children, with progressive severity as the child becomes older. This phenomenon is paradoxical and indicates an increasing sensitivity to the organism with repeated infections. Because the *Mycoplasma pneumoniae* attaches superficially to the bronchial mucosa and probably never penetrates the lung parenchyma, more than one infection may be required to stimulate a symptomatic response. This may explain why two distinct clinical and radiographic syndromes have been described: one in which nonspecific symptoms are associated with a reticulonodular pattern, and another in which the symptoms suggestive of bacterial pneumonia are associated with segmental and lobar consolidation. The latter may be accompanied by a pleural reaction.

Most bacterial pneumonias have some degree of associated hilar lymph node involvement. The size and degree of the affected lymph nodes are related to the infecting or-

ganism, since some are more likely to affect the regional lymph nodes (Fig. 6-10). Tuberculosis is always a major consideration when pulmonary consolidation is associated with obvious hilar adenopathy (Fig. 6-10A, B). The primary infection is frequently within the lower lung fields. The size of the original focus is usually small and limited to an acinus or lobule. Occasionally, a segment or a lobe may be involved, often the result of atelectasis caused by bronchial occlusion or endobronchial disease. The infection may be limited to regional draining lymph nodes but can spread to adjacent lymph nodes and to both sides of the mediastinum. The combination of the parenchymal focus and the enlarged lymph nodes has been termed the primary or Ghon complex. The degree of consolidation is variable and may not even be apparent when the disease is found. The only manifestation may be unexplained unilateral hilar adenopathy. A mild pleural reaction and lymphangitis comprise the rest of the tuberculous Ghon complex (Fig. 6-11). It is unusual to see all features simultaneously.

In certain parts of the country, this complex of radiographic findings is the result of other infections, such as histoplasmosis in the

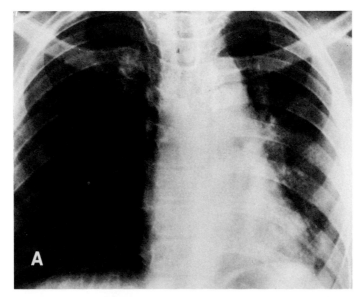

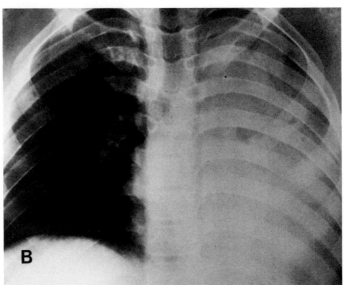

Fig. 6-12. Histoplasmosis. Endobronchial disease. *(A)* Early left lower lobe collapse and an enlarged left hilum are noted. *(B)* Five days later the entire left lung is collapsed and early tissue necrosis is apparent. The esophagus was indented by mediastinal lymph nodes, and bronchoscopy revealed Histoplasma granulomas.

Mississippi Valley and coccidiodomycosis in California and Arizona. Histoplasmosis differs slightly from tuberculosis in its parenchymal distribution. Although single focal lesions occur, multiple, patchy lesions that vary in size from a few centimeters to an entire segment are more frequently seen in this disease and are characteristic of overwhelming infection. Calcification occurs more rapidly and extensively in histoplasmosis. It is not unusual, therefore, to see multiple focal areas of parenchymal calcification. The presence of calcified nodes is an indicator of previous histoplasmosis. In contrast to tuberculosis, a pleural reaction in histoplasmosis is distinctly unusual.

Histoplasmosis is an acquired infection that has a worldwide distribution, with the greatest incidence being in the Ohio, Mississippi, and Missouri valleys. Colder areas appear to be free of Histoplasma spores and infection. The source of infection is bird or bat droppings. Once the spores reach the alveoli, they change to the yeast form and stimulate an infiltration associated with a regional lymph node reaction similar to tuberculosis.

Atelectasis is the result of an obstructing lesion. An effort to determine the nature of the obstruction is therefore mandatory. The detection of associated adenopathy is important, since enlarged nodes can obstruct a bronchus either by compression or by the ac-

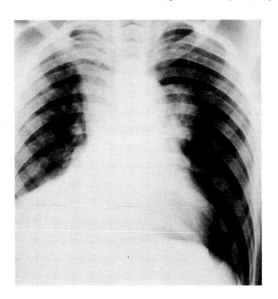

Fig. 6-13. Mediastinal histoplasmosis with atelectasis of the right middle and lower lobes. Huge nodes are present on both sides of the mediastinum. Complete atelectasis of right middle and lower lobes are present because of compression and endobronchial histoplasmosis in the right intermediate bronchus.

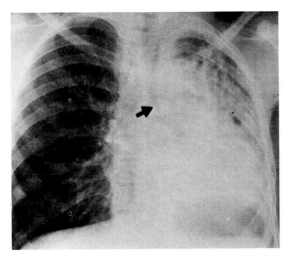
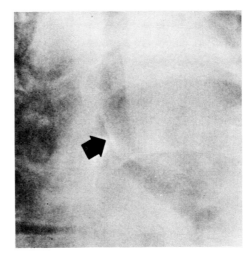

Fig. 6-14. Obstructive pneumonia with abscess. The left lung is completely collapsed and demonstrates multiple cavities. Volume loss is manifested by an overt mediastinal shift, unilateral elevation of the diaphragm, and overcrowding of the thoracic cage. A metallic object *(arrow)* which proved to be the snap of a metal can is present within the left main bronchus.

tual invasion of the bronchus, producing endobronchial disease. Both phenomena are commonly encountered in tuberculosis and histoplasomsis (Figs. 6-12, 6-13). Atelectasis of the right middle lobe (the right middle lobe syndrome) is not common because of the anatomy of the right bronchus. It originates from the bronchus intermedius at almost a right angle and is therefore prone to extensive compression. Sarcoidosis and lymphosarcoma rarely cause bronchial obstruction, despite the relatively large size of the nodes associated with these diseases. An un-

fortunate and potentially dangerous cause of atelectasis in the pediatric age-group is foreign body aspiration (Fig. 6-14). Foreign bodies are either radiopaque or radiolucent. Since they are poorly visualized, if at all, they are implicitly more dangerous. Foreign body aspiration should be suspected whenever atelectasis occurs suddenly, and no obvious radiographic cause can be detected. One of the most common and potentially destructive foreign bodies is the peanut. When a peanut remains long enough in a bronchus, it decomposes, releasing enzymes that have a lo-

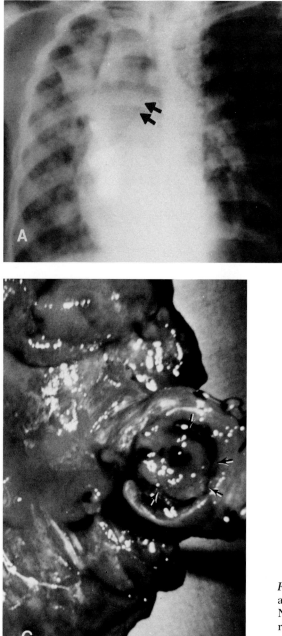

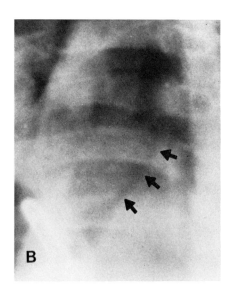

Fig. 6-15. Carcinoid tumor. *(A)* Atelectasis with abscess formation is present in the right lung. Note the extent of the mediastinal shift. *(B)* The right main bronchus is narrowed by a soft-tissue mass that is best seen on the detailed view. *(C)* A surgical specimen reveals the fleshy, intrabronchial, carcinoid tumor *(arrows)*.

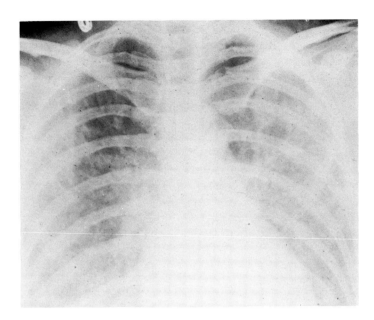

Fig. 6-16. Chickenpox pneumonia in the adult. A fine reticular nodular infiltration diffusely involves both lung fields, producing an overall haziness.

cally destructive effect on lung parenchyma. A foreign body may not cause atelectasis initially but may produce air-trapping by means of a ball-valve phenomenon. Prolonged retention of any foreign body can result in progressive pulmonary consolidation and eventual bronchiectasis (Fig. 6-14). The peak incidence of foreign body aspiration is between 1 and 2 years of age, and the right bronchial tree is involved in 50 to 70 per cent of the cases.

Extensive cardiomegaly, such as cardiomyopathy and aberrant origin of the left coronary artery, may cause collapse of the left lower lobe by direct pressure. Obstruction by primary neoplasm is quite rare. The most common neoplasm in this age-group is the carcinoid tumor (Fig. 6-15). Bronchogenic carcinoma is almost never encountered.

A pulmonary hematoma arises following a blow to the chest wall which is of sufficient force to compress the pulmonary parenchyma and cause disruption of and hemorrhage into the alveoli. Such an occurrence is rare under the age of 14 years because of the resiliency of the thorax in a child.

THE DIRTY LUNG

In some thoracic diseases, the chest radiograph demonstrates a myriad of pathologic features that consist of a combination of alveolar, interstitial, cystic, and bronchiectatic changes. As a result, assorted radiodensities of varying dimensions and shapes are encountered, and the term dirty lung has been applied to this overall, nonspecific radiographic appearance. It is futile to attempt to differentiate alveolar from interstitial disease, since all too often both the interstitium and the air spaces are simultaneously involved. Although the majority of the lesions associated with this type of presentation are usually chronic, some diseases of acute origin are manifested by a similar type of pattern.

Disease Entities
Infectious pneumonia
Aspiration
Cystic fibrosis
Tracheoesophageal fistula
Immunodeficiency disease
Chronic granulomatous disease of childhood
Alpha$_1$-antitrypsin Deficiency
Granulomatous diseases
Histiocytosis
Collagen diseases
Desquamative interstitial disease
Bronchiectasis

Differential Diagnosis

An acute disease consisting predominantly of a diffuse, streaky interstitial process that may or may not be associated with some degree of nodularity most likely represents a

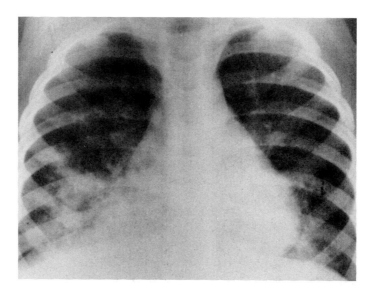

Fig. 6-17. Pneumonia due to hydrocarbon aspiration. Bilateral patchy pneumonic infiltrations are noted within both lower lung fields. Some coalescence has occurred on the right. Air bronchograms are well-defined.

viral pneumonitis. This form of pneumonia is nonspecific but not difficult to recognize (Fig. 6-16). It has been seen in measles, chicken pox, and rubella, as well as in patients in the early stages of mycoplasma pneumonia. The presence of an alveolar consolidation associated with measles is almost always due to superimposed pneumonia.

The recent onset of a largely irregular nodular pattern with some degree of coalescence is probably more indicative of bronchopneumonia or extensive aspiration pneumonia. In children most infectious pneumonias, regardless of the origin, initially are more often acinar in location than lobar and as a result may be confused with interstitial disease. Bronchopneumonia is relatively uniform in distribution, with much of the radiodensity presenting in a perihilar configuration and with some extension to various peripheral or basilar portions of the lungs. Children often demonstrate tachypnea and/or air-trapping associated with pneumonia. As a result, depressed diaphragms and relative hyperlucency of the lungs are often present.

Aspiration pneumonia usually involves the dependent portions of the lungs, relative to the patient's position at the time of aspiration. The changes result from a combination of the effects of the aspirated material, chemical irritation, and developing pneumonia. The findings, therefore, are usually in the basilar lung fields and consist of patchy, ill-defined radiodensities intermixed with streaky infiltrations that radiate toward the

hilum (Fig. 6-17). Hydrocarbon ingestion, particularly furniture polish, is a common problem in childhood. The manifestations disappear rapidly unless complicated by cavity or superimposed bacterial pneumonia.

Early perihilar development with extension into the peripheral lung fields is the main finding in *Pneumocystis carinii* pneumonia (Fig. 6-57). Essentially this disease is encountered in patients with underlying neoplastic disease.

Most other diseases manifested by a dirty lung are characterized clinically by recurrent and chronic episodes that lead to progressively worse pulmonary findings. The end stage consists of fibrosis and bronchiectasis, associated with linear or cystic air pockets with thin or thick walls, and recurrent areas of pneumonia.

Barium swallow examination should always be performed in patients with a dirty lung to exclude lesions that may cause aspiration. An H-type tracheoesophageal fistula is often considered but not often diagnosed. It is, nevertheless, a cause of recurrent lung infection in children and can be cured. The fistula is difficult to demonstrate under ordinary circumstances, since it is located high in the esophagus and is directed superiorly from the esophagus to the trachea (see Fig. 5-35). The child should be studied in a position which is as prone as possible to allow the contrast material to flow anteriorly into the trachea and to afford visualization of the small connection between the esophagus and trachea.

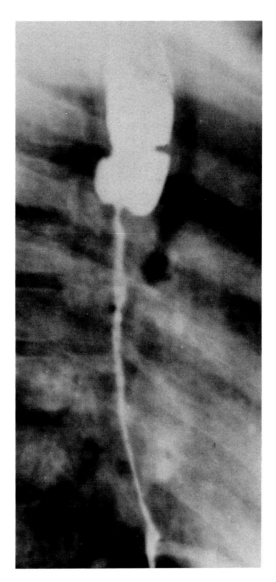

Fig. 6-18. Esophageal stricture due to ingestion of lye. A severe stricture is located at the junction of the proximal and central third of the esophagus. The margins are smooth, and the distal portion of the esophagus is narrowed and somewhat irregular.

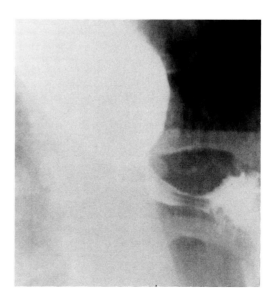

Fig. 6-19. Achalasia. The entire esophagus is dilated. The narrowed segment is located just below the diaphragm and demonstrates a smooth and intact mucosa.

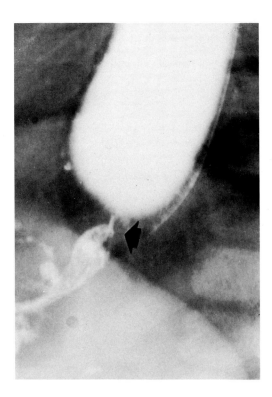

Fig. 6-20. Esophageal stenosis with pulmonary and bronchial remnants. The esophagus is markedly dilated. At the level of the diaphragm a short but smooth stenotic segment is visualized *(arrow)*. A serial section of this segment revealed pulmonary tissue and bronchial cartilage. (The clefts characteristic of this lesion are not apparent.)

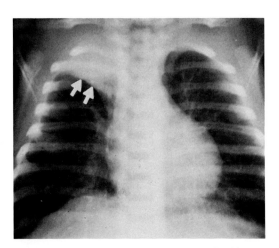
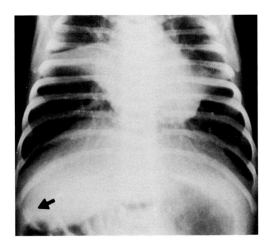

Fig. 6-21. Cystic fibrosis. This 2-month-old patient presented with recurrent episodes of airway obstruction and atelectasis. This was initially observed in the right upper lobe *(white arrows)* and then shortly after in the right middle lobe. Calcifications are present on the liver surface, indicating previous meconium peritonitis *(black arrow)*.

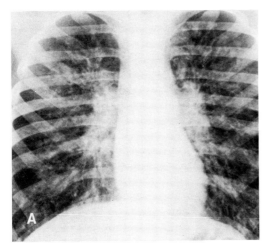

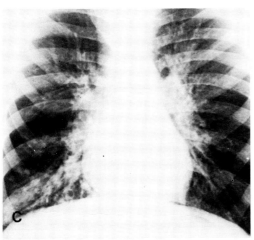

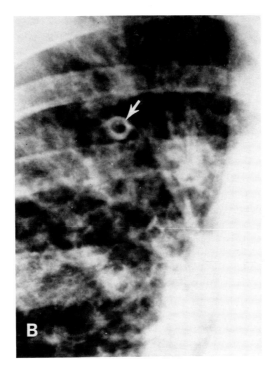

Fig. 6-22. Cystic fibrosis. *(A)* Diffuse interstitial changes as well as alveolar infiltrations are present throughout the lung fields. Multiple, small cystic lesions are also noted. *(B)* A detailed view of the right upper lung field better shows these changes. The walls of the cystic structures vary in thickness. A single, thick-walled cavity is present ("blob bronchiectasis"; *arrow*). *(C)* Another patient with similar findings but with evidence of air-trapping in the lower lung fields.

Selective introduction of the contrast material at various levels by way of an endotracheal tube offers the best possibility of success.

Recurrent aspiration due to a dysfunction of the swallowing mechanism can also be elucidated during the barium swallow. Contrast material passes into the trachea continually as the patient swallows.

Esophageal obstruction is an obvious cause of aspiration pneumonia due to overflow from the dilated obstructed esophagus. Food is retained in the esophagus and is aspirated when the individual is in a supine position. Esophageal obstruction may be due to stricture, peptic esophagitis, achalasia, and, rarely, neoplasm. The esophagus proximal to the stenotic area is usually dilated. Except in the case of a neoplasm, the esophagus tapers smoothly at the narrowed area. There is no mucosal destruction or overhanging margin. A stricture can occur anywhere within the

esophagus (Fig. 6-18). However, the distal end of the esophagus is affected in peptic esophagitis. In achalasia, a smooth, nondistensible segment of the esophagus is observed at or below the diaphragm (Fig. 6-19). Moreover, diffuse abnormal and irregular contractions can occur throughout the esophagus. In patients with achalasia, an injection of urocholine (Mecholyl) elicits strong contractions of the esophagus within a few minutes. This response is diagnostic. Patients with achalasia most often present with complaints related to the esophagus, such as pain upon swallowing or fullness.

Congenital strictures have been found in the distal esophagus, associated with tracheobronchial remnants (Fig. 6-20). Radiographically, multiple clefts are present which resemble diverticula and lead from the stenotic area to intramural cystic spaces that are lined by ciliated, pseudo-stratified, columnar epithelium.

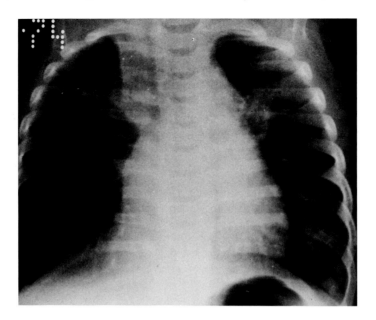

Fig. 6-23. Chronic lung disease secondary to oxygen toxicity and persistent patent ductus arteriosus. Markedly hyperlucent lungs are present in the lung fields due to air-trapping. Infiltrations and cystic changes are also apparent despite the overexposed quality of the radiograph.

There are a significant number of diseases caused by immunodeficiency states, either qualitative or quantitative, that result in recurrent lung infections. The diagnosis can be suggested by the radiologist but is most often confirmed by immunoelectrophoresis. Certain radiographic findings are present that are relatively characteristic. Most frequently, the thymus has not developed or is exceedingly small, and the epipharynx is hyperlucent because there is no adenoid tissue, which is normally prominent in children. A relatively similar disease is chronic granulomatous disease of childhood. This is the result of defective phagocytosis and results in recurrent pneumonia. Quite often diffuse pulmonary changes are recognized by spherical, encapsulating infiltrations. Enlarged hilar and paratracheal nodes are also prominent.

In a young child recurrent episodes of tachypnea with evidence of air-trapping and atelectasis should immediately suggest obstructive airway disease, particularly cystic fibrosis. The early phases of cystic fibrosis consist of hyperlucent lungs, a depressed diaphragm, bulging intercostal spaces, and areas of streaky infiltrations that probably represent bronchial plugging. Segmental or lobar atelectasis completes the radiographic findings (Fig. 6-21). Repeated pneumonias eventually supervene, and chronic changes consisting of a reticular nodular pattern, "honeycombing," patchy atelectasis or consolidation, and air-trapping with mucous plugs develop within the lung fields (Fig. 6-22). Large areas of cystic change, as well as multiple peribronchiolar abscesses, are typical. The peribronchiolar abscesses eventually communicate with the adjacent bronchus, producing a thick-walled but relatively small abscess cavity. This has been called "blob bronchiectasis" by some physicians (Fig. 6-22C). As the pulmonary involvement becomes greater, severe emphysema and cor pulmonale eventually develop. Extrapulmonary abnormalities are always present in cystic fibrosis (e.g., pansinusitis, malabsorption). Abnormally high levels of electrolytes in the sweat confirms the diagnosis. Unfortunately, some newborns who survive initial episodes of hyaline membrane disease and/or oxygen toxicity develop a pulmonary pattern resembling chronic lung disease. Radiographically, this consists of a diffuse, coarse reticular pattern often interspersed with small atelectatic segments and air way obstruction (Fig. 6-23). In many patients a patent ductus arteriosus causes further complications and increases the overall parenchymal markings, with shunt vascularity.

A child presenting with any form of chronic lung disease should be tested for abnormal alpha $_1$-antitrypsin levels. Deficient levels are associated with an obstructive pulmonary syndrome that consists of bronchitis, asthma, or emphysema.

Certain collagen diseases, such as scleroderma, present with diffuse fibrosis.

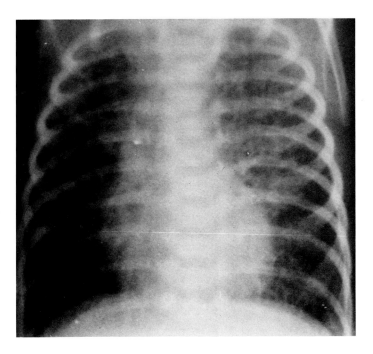

Fig. 6-24. Gaucher's disease. In a young infant a diffuse reticular nodular infiltration is shown in both lung fields producing a "honeycomb" appearance.

However this is distinctly rare in the pediatric age-group.

Chronically diseased lungs with thickened reticular nodular infiltrations associated with "honeycombing" have been seen in children with Gaucher's disease (Fig. 6-24), Niemann-Pick disease, and histiocytosis (Fig. 6-25). In the latter, the infiltrations may produce fibrosis with resulting cystic changes. An associated pneumothorax is not uncommon in eosinophilic granuloma.

Desquamative interstitial disease and lymphocytic interstitial disease are unusual interstitial lesions that are rarely seen in children, although the clinical and pathologic features are the same as those described in adults. The usual presentation is a nonproductive cough, weight loss, anorexia, and easy fatigability. Both lesions manifest a radiographic pattern that extends from the hilum to the basilar portions of the lung. It consists mainly of a wedge-shaped, hazy, "ground glass" infiltration that radiates along both cardiac borders to both lung bases, sparing the costophrenic angles. Lymphadenopathy has been reported, but it may represent lymphoid hyperplasia. Without therapy the lesions persist and progress, resulting in cor pulmonale.

Chronic upper airway disease such as pansinusitis results in chronic recurrent pneumonia. The result may eventually be bronchiectasis and fibrosis. Radiographically, a mixture of alveolar consolidation and thickened, dilated bronchi are associated with cystic lung disease. Kartagener's syndrome, consisting of situs inversus, pansinusitis, and bronchiectasis, is considered a chronic upper airway disease, despite its familial nature.

Congenital bronchiectasis due to deficiency of bronchial cartilage, the Williams-Campbell syndrome, can occur within a lobe or throughout the lung fields. The characteristic clinical features are persistent cough, wheezing, and emphysema after a mild respiratory infection. It is still uncertain whether the lesion is congenital or acquired.

Discussion

Acute aspiration pneumonia is a very common home catastrophe. It is rarely seen until 1 year of age, when, unfortunately, inquisitiveness and mobility mature together. The most commonly aspirated agents are cleaning fluids, especially furniture polish. In most homes cleaning fluids are readily accessible, and the aromatic nature makes them quite attractive. It is likely that the very low surface tension of such agents allows some of it to slide under the epiglottis and into the trachea during swallowing. Vomiting with aspiration accounts for only a small part of the pulmonary changes. If chemical aspiration is

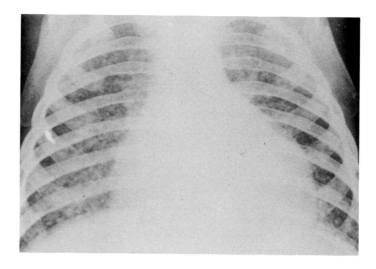

Fig. 6-25. Letterer-Siwe disease. A reticular nodular pattern exists in both lung fields. The cardiac silhouette is also enlarged, indicating pericardial infiltration.

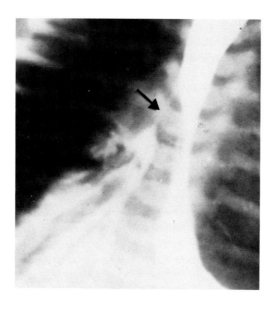

Fig. 6-26. Bronchoesophageal fistula. This patient presented with right lower lobe pneumonia and bronchiectasis. The right lower lobe bronchus originates from the esophagus *(arrow)*.

suspected, the child should be observed for 24 hours, since it may take this long for the radiographic appearance of chemical pneumonitis to develop.

Of all tracheoesophageal anomalies, the H-type fistula is the one that remains undetected longest. The fistula is usually small and is not associated with obstruction of either the esophagus or trachea. This results in repeated episodes of pneumonia due to small aspirations. The H-type fistula is only one of several esophageal or pharyngeal abnormalities that cause recurrent aspiration. A pharyngeal diverticulum and disfigurement of the epiglottis may produce recurrent aspiration. Disfigurement may be the result of trauma from insertion of an endotracheal tube or cicatrization from previous epiglot-

titis. A rare esophagobronchial communication has also been noted (Fig. 6-26).

Abnormalities in deglutition are often seen in the Riley-Day syndrome (familial dysautonomia), as well as in muscular dystrophy and cerebral palsy. Familial dysautonomia is the result of dysfunction in the central nervous system. It occurs predominantly in children of Jewish extraction. The pulmonary effects of the disease produce the worst of the many clinical manifestations, which include excessive perspiration, defective lacrimation, emotional instability, motor incoordination, and even indifference to pain. Two thirds of patients have severe pulmonary changes that eventually lead to death.

Aspiration is also relatively common in seizure disorders and chalasia. Chalasia is com-

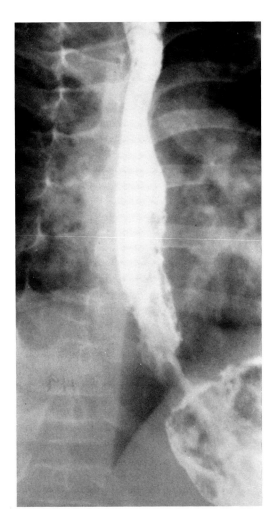

Fig. 6-27. Moniliasis of the esophagus. The esophagus shows irregular superficial ulcerations involving the central and distal third.

mon in neonates and is due to an immature esophageal sphincter mechanism.

There are a number of immunodeficiency states that relate to cellular and humoral immunologic mechanisms. Combined immunodeficiency disease is probably related to stem cell abnormality and results in both a cellular and humoral deficiency state. For the most part, the pulmonary findings are widespread, with recurring alveolar infiltrates, as well as interstitial disease. There is no thymus in the mediastinum, and occasionally monilial esophagitis (Fig. 6-27) and malabsorption are present. The pulmonary disease is the most severe problem and is most responsible for the morbidity in immunodeficient patients. One must bear in mind that superimposed infection with *Pneumocystis carinii* or viral pneumonias are not uncommon. Abnormalities of cellular immunity alone have been noted in DiGeorge's syndrome, a disease related to

maldevelopment of the third and fourth pharyngeal pouches, with no thymus and parathyroids. Other anomalies of the mandible, aortic arch, and ear are related to this embryologic abnormality. Because there are no parathyroids, tetany is exhibited early in life. However, recurrent infections, especially with viruses, fungi, and acid-fast bacteria, are typical. The diagnosis can be confirmed by the absence of delayed sensitivity and the presence of normal immunoglobulins.

Humoral immunodeficiency (Bruton's disease) is characterized by a lack of immunoglobulins in affected patients. Cellular immunity, however, is intact. Histologically, the lymph nodes reveal a paucity of plasma cells and germinal centers. Following an initial normal period of 6 to 9 months, patients begin to show signs of repeated and chronic severe infections that are associated with atelectasis, bronchiectasis, and emphysema.

Table. 6-1. **Characteristics of Infectious Pneumonia**

Infecting Organism	Parenchymal Predominance	Lymph-adenopathy	Empyema or Pleural Reaction	Pneumatocoele or Abscess
Pneumococcus	Lobar	Small	Rare	
Hemophilus	Lobar		Common	
Staphylococcus	Patchy to lobar		Common	Common
Klebsiella	Lobar		Infrequent	Common
Mycoplasma	Variable		Occasional	
Virus	Patchy	Minimal	Occasional	
Mycobacterium	Patchy to lobar	Predominant	Infrequent	Unusual in primary tuberculosis
Histoplasma	Patchy	Predominant		Can occur

The infections are usually pyogenic. All patients are susceptible to recurrent infections and develop an ongoing pattern of combined interstitial and alveolar disease intermixed with scarring from previous inflammation. Radiographically, there is no way to distinguish thymic aplasia or hypoplasia from a shrunken thymus caused by stress. Before the age of 6 moths, it may be difficult to establish the diagnosis radiographically, since lymphoid tissue such as the adenoids may still be normal but not evident radiographically.

The ataxia-telangiectasia syndrome, also known as the Louis-Bar syndrome, is associated with immunoglobulin deficiency and reflects a disturbance in T cell function and decreased IgA. Sino-pulmonary disease begins in late childhood and leads to severe bronchiectasis. The syndrome is an autosomal recessive disease in which thymic abnormalities are noted at postmortem. Ataxia and progressive teleangiectasia become obvious in early childhood.

The Wiskott-Aldrich syndrome, also associated with immunoglobuoin deficiency, is an X-linked recessive disorder manifested by eczema, thrombocytopenia, and a wide spectrum of infection that begins late in the 1st year. The abnormality in affected patients may be related to selective inability to respond to polysaccharide antigens.

Cystic fibrosis is a disease that is manifested by widely varying degrees of severity and is due to a generalized dysfunction of exocrine glands. The mucous secretions are abnormal physicochemically, forming concretions which obstruct ducts of glandular and organ systems. Every organ seems to be involved, and chronic pulmonary disease is present in almost all patients. The bacterial flora cultured from the nasopharynx, sputum, and lungs consists primarily of *Staphylococcus aureus* and *Pseudomonas aeruginosa*. Cystic fibrosis is the most common lethal hereditary disease among Caucasians and is less common among Blacks.

Radiographically, the last stage of respirator lung or oxygen toxicity may closely resemble the pulmonary manifestations of cystic fibrosis. Chronic obstructive lung disease and cor pulmonale are common to all three. In oxygen toxicity, the changes characteristic of the last stage become evident at a much younger age than do changes associated with cystic fibrosis. In addition there is normally a history of prematurity and hyaline membrane disease.

Recently, improved diagnostic criteria have allowed the distinction of distinct entities from the large group of nonspecific diffuse lung disease. Desquamative interstitial pneumonia is such a disease and consists of nodular and stiff lungs. Microscopically, there is a proliferation of cells lining the aleveoli and accumulation of cells that are probably alveolar macrophages. Many contain PAS-positive, golden-brown pigment granules. Interstitial infiltration is also present but minimal.

When a patient continues to have recurrent infection and extensive lung involvement radiographically, and when diagnostic tests have been inconclusive, by exclusion of diagnosis of idiopathic chronic lung disease remains. In our own institution, more than 50 per cent of the children evaluated for such problems fall into this category. The treatment is symptomatic. Many outgrow the disease, whereas others continue to progress with fibrosis and end-stage pulmonary disease, the Hamman-Rich syndrome.

NODULAR THORACIC MASSES

The spectrum of nodular masses encountered in the chest of infants and children is extensive, as in adults, although the actual number of possible diseases is lower. Most lesions manifest certain features that suggest a specific diagnosis. The location, the configuration, and the consistency (e.g., calcium or bone) are important, as well as the nature of the surrounding margin.

Disease Entities

Small pulmonary lesions
  Miliary tuberculosis
  Sarcoidosis
  Chicken pox pneumonia
  Extrinsic allergic alveolitis
  Granuloma
Large pulmonary lesions
  Pseudotumor
  Collagen disease
  Bronchopulmonary sequestration
  Primary malignancy
  Metastasis
Anterior mediastinal lesions
  Lesions of the thymus
  Hygroma
  Desmoid
  Hodgkin's disease
  Pericardial cyst
Middle mediastinal lesions
  Lymphadenopathy
  Bronchogenic cyst
  Duplication
  Posterior mediastinal lesions
  Neuroblastoma
  Neuroganglioma
  Neurofibroma
  Extramedullary hematopoiesis

Differential Diagnosis

Nodular masses may arise either in the lung, the mediastinum, the pleura, or the chest wall. Obviously, it is not difficult to recognize the location of a mass within the lung. However, lesions lying close to the mediastinum or pleura may require several projections. Mediastinal and pleural masses have a distinct and recognizable configuration. The entire circumference of these lesions is almost never completely delineated, since only a portion of the mass is surrounded by lung (Fig. 6-3). The configuration of the lesion is frequently oval, in comparison to the customary round and well circumscribed intrapulmonary mass. As a result, the vertical axis is usually longer than the transverse axis, although this feature is not always obvious.

The mediastinum is basically divided into three compartments, anterior, middle, and posterior. Many of the lesions which affect the mediastinum tend to occur in one compartment. A superior mediastinum also exists, although it is of little practical importance. The anterior mediastinum is bounded anteriorly by the sternum and posteriorly by the pericardium, aorta, and great vessels. In the pediatric age-group, the thymus is the most common site of anterior mediastinal lesions. Although the thymus is not normally well-defined in infants and children occasionally it becomes hyperplastic and looks like a tumor (Fig. 6-28). Primary thymic tumors are rare in children, and the majority of thymic masses are cysts. Some tumors which are not thymic in origin may present as thymic masses (e.g., histiocytosis, lymphoma, leukemia). Other lesions which occur in the anterior mediastinum include teratomas, anterior mediastinal nodes, hemangiomas, and cystic hygromas. A hygroma can be quite large and may extend from the soft tissues of the neck beneath the sternum into the anterior mediastinum (Fig. 6-29). This presentation closely resembles the enlarged substernal thyroid of the adult. Teratoid lesions are well circumscribed, although on the lateral projection they are flattened against the sternum. They seldom demonstrate a sulcus sign, a well circumscribed biconvex border along the anterior, superior, and inferior surface. In addition, calcium or bony structures are often evident in these masses, facilitating a preoperative diagnosis (Fig. 6-30). Twenty per cent of teratomas are malignant; males exhibit a higher incidence of malignancy than females. Hodgkin's disease, particularly the nodular, sclerosing form, is the most commonly encountered lymphoma in the anterior mediastinum and is most often seen in young adults. The lesion is often ill-defined on the lateral film. Pericardial cysts are benign and communicate with the pericardium in 10 per cent of the cases. They occur predominantly in the right cardiophrenic angle and rarely produce a sulcus sign in the lateral projection. Lymphoid hyperplasia is proba-

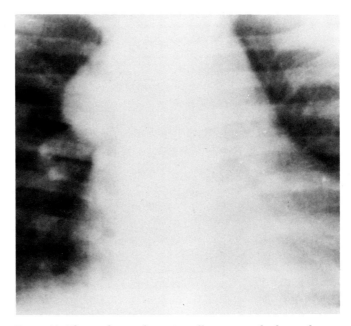

Fig. 6-28. Thymic hyperplasia. A well circumscribed round mass is superimposed over the right paratracheal region. This was located in the anterior mediastinum and histologically consisted of hyperplastic thymic tissue.

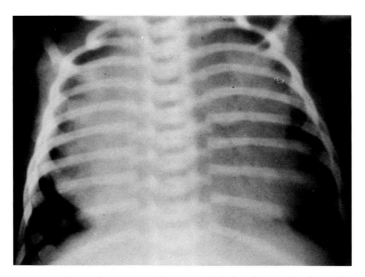

Fig. 6-29. Cystic hygroma. A huge, well-defined mass displaces the entire mediastinum to the left. A large hygroma was removed.

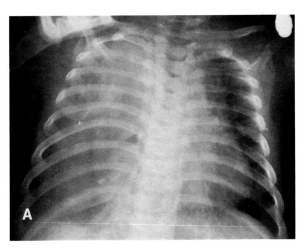

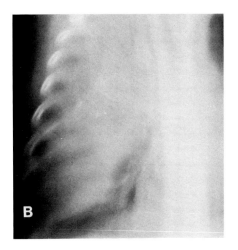

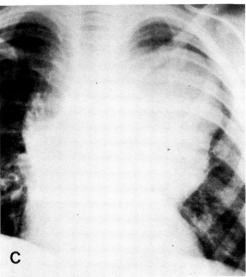

Fig. 6-30. Benign cystic teratoma. *(A, B)* A huge mass containing calcifications arises from the right side of the mediastinum and obscures most of the right hemithorax. The mass appears soft, since little displacement of the mediastinum is noted despite the overall size of the mass. *(C)* Another huge teratoma with a lobular contour.

bly a postinflammatory response and is indistinguishable from lymphoma. Rarely, neurogenic tumors, cardiac tumors, and bronchogenic cysts present anteriorly. In cases where some confusion arises because of an enlarged thymus, several days of administration of systemic steroids will involute the thymus but will not affect most other anterior mediastinal lesions.

The posterior mediastinum lies behind the posterior border of the heart and the anterior aspect of the vertebral bodies. It contains the descending aorta, esophagus, thoracic duct, azygous and hemiazygous veins, and sympathetic chains. However, posterior mediastinal masses consist mainly of tumors of neural origin, ranging from malignant neuroblastomas to mature ganglioneuromas or neurofibromas. Posterior mediastinal le-

sions frequently bulge into the adjacent lung, making it difficult to distinguish one tumor from another radiographically, since all produce bone distortion and rib erosion and widen the adjacent foramen. The presence of rib erosion and intraspinal extension is more common in neuroblastoma, and an elongated mass occupying a large vertebral area is more characteristic of a ganglioneuroma than of the oval and spherical neuroblastoma (Fig. 6-31). Consequently, the mass is greater in ganglioneuroma. Both lesions may demonstrate calcium deposits, and biopsy is often necessary for absolute diagnosis.

Posterior mediastinal masses may arise from the vertebral bodies, as with a metastasis, Pott's disease, and discitis. The vertebral bodies show distinct changes in such diseases (see Chapter 8).

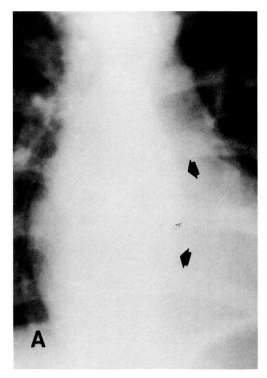

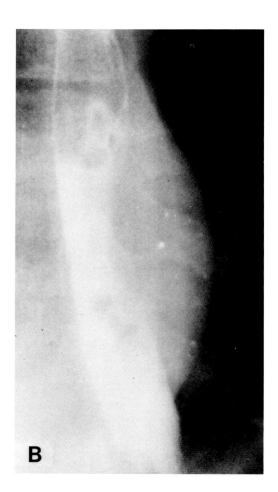

Fig. 6-31. Ganglioneuroma. (A) A spindel-shaped mass is noted in the left paravertebral area (arrows). (B) The extrapleural component of this mass is well visualized on the esophagram. The elongated spindle-shaped configuration is characteristic for this tumor.

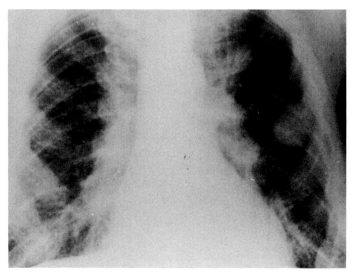

Fig. 6-32. Extramedullary hematopoiesis. Cooley's anemia. Multiple, bilateral, paravertebral, nodular masses are noted. Other soft-tissue masses arise from the ribs which are widened and demonstrate thin cortices and thickened trabeculae.

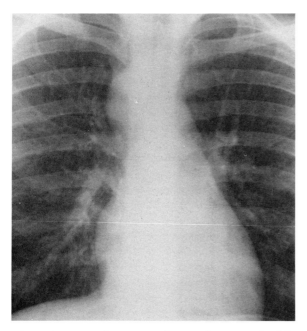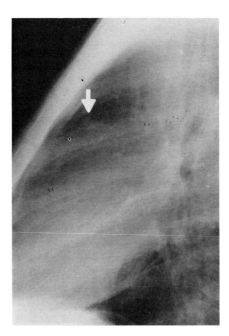

Fig. 6-33. Histoplasmosis. A large right paratracheal lymph node is visualized. A small single primary focus is noted within the anterior segment *(arrow)*.

Extramedullary hematopoeisis is an unusual entity associated with severe anemias, such as thallasemia. It presents on the chest film as a pseudotumorous mass or masses that lie adjacent to and originate from the vertebral column associated with bone changes of thallesemia, or other findings of anemia, and no evidence of bone destruction (Fig. 6-32).

The middle mediastinum contains the heart, pericardium, ascending and transverse arch of the aorta, superior and inferior vena cavae, trachea, bronchi, and the pulmonary arteries and veins. Nodular masses in the middle mediastinum most commonly represent enlarged lymph nodes which result from a number of diseases. Slightly enlarged nodes may be difficult to distinguish from hilar vessels in the frontal projection. The lateral radiograph is useful in this regard. Normal hilar structures ordinarily blend into the parenchyma in this projection, whereas the presence of sharply defined radiodensities are definitely abnormal and suggest lymphadenopathy. Infection and neoplasm are mainly responsible for nodal enlargement, although infection probably has the higher incidence. Most pulmonary infections are accompanied by some degree of adenopathy, and in some lesions this is a major feature of the disease. Primary tuber-

culosis and histoplasmosis are excellent examples. In fact, nodal enlargement may be the most important element in both, since the initial parenchymal focus is not always apparent and may have resolved by the time the disease is discovered. Caseation is far more extensive in the lymph nodes than in the parenchyma and accounts for the number and size of the nodes involved, as well as the prolonged duration of the disease. This feature is more pronounced in histoplasmosis and is frequently bilateral. Lymphnode enlargement without obvious parenchymal involvement is called mediastinal granuloma (Fig. 6-33).

Sarcoidosis frequently affects the lymph nodes but is uncommon in children, usually being diagnosed at a later age. The classical presentation consists of enlarged bilateral hilar nodes, alone or associated with an enlarged right paratracheal node. These nodes are quite large and circumscribed and present a "potato node" appearance. The patients are usually asymptomatic, and as a result the disease is frequently undiagnosed.

Neoplastic disease, especially leukemia or lymphoma, encompasses another group of diseases that may present with enlarged medistinal lymph nodes (Fig. 6-34). Neoplastic disease should be strongly considered

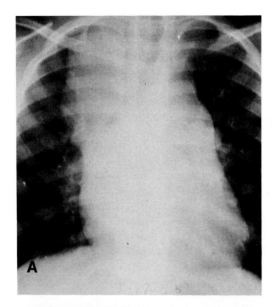

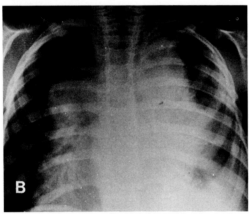

Fig. 6-34. Mediastinal neoplasms. *(A)* Letterer-Siwe disease. The entire middle mediastinum is filled with enlarged nodes. A huge mass is present in the right paratracheal region displacing the trachea to the left. Nodes on the left side and in the infracarinal area compress the main bronchus. Destructive bone lesions were also present in this child. *(B)* Acute lymphosarcoma. Huge nodes assuming a grossly lobular configuration occupy the greater part of the mediastinum. Pleural involvement is also noted on the left.

when additional features, such as systemic symptoms, bone changes, and generalized lymphadenopathy, are present. Chronic granulomatous disease of childhood also presents with large, non-regressive lymph nodes.

A bronchogenic cyst is commonly located in the middle mediastinum. It is usually an incidental but obvious finding in older children and in adults. In infants and young children, however, the mass is not easily visible on plain film and is responsible for causing severe respiratory distress because of airway obstruction. Hyperaeaation or atelectasis is the initial presentation. A barium swallow should always be performed in these situations to exclude the presence of a mediastinal mass, since occult bronchogenic cysts cause some displacement of the esophagus. In older children, this lesion is

recognized by a single, well circumscribed, round mass that is typically located at the level of the carina (Fig. 6-35).

A barium swallow also aids in detecting and diagnosing esophageal duplication. The abnormal mass not only causes indentation of the esophagus but is inherently fixed to it. The lesion can be cystic or tubular, and two-thirds of them are right-sided. They are often associated with more than one duplication (e.g., unrelated tubular jejunal lesions).

When analyzing pulmonary parenchymal nodular lesions, it is convenient to categorize them by size, configuration, and amount. A single, well circumscribed, small nodule in an asymptomatic juvenile lung is in all likelihood a granuloma, most frequently a tuberculoma or a result of histoplasmosis. A Histoplasma granuloma can be distinguished from a tuberculous granuloma only when it

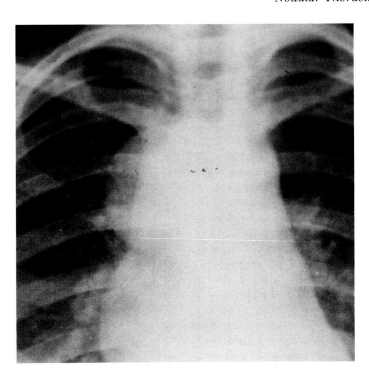

Fig. 6-35. Bronchogenic cyst. Note the well circumscribed spherical mass located at the level of the right carina.

presents with more than one lesion. Visibly enlarged hilar nodes, as well as calcifications, are present in both. Histoplasma granulomas occasionally increase in size over a period of time and have been mistaken for neoplasms. The circumferential growth is related to a continual apposition of fibrotic tissue around the periphery of the lesion.

Many pulmonary lesions produce multiple, uniformly distributed, nodular radiodensities of a few millimeters in size. The result is a fine granular or tiny nodular appearance throughout both lung fields. Tuberculosis should always be the prime consideration because of its high incidence and mortality (see p. 252).

Multiple, round radiodensities that vary in size from a few millimeters to perhaps centimeters in diameter may represent infection or metastatic disease. A serious infection with Histoplasma commonly presents with this pattern. The lesions are diffuse, of almost uniform size, and symmetrical, except in areas of coalescence (Fig. 6-36A). The inflammatory nature of the process is easily recognized by the soft, fluffy border of each lesion. As healing supervenes, the lesions become smaller and the margins sharper (Fig. 6-36B). Calcium is subsequently deposited in each lesion, a typical finding.

Wilm's tumor and a number of bone and soft-tissue sarcomas are the most common lesions which may disseminate to involve the lungs. Metastatic disease is usually radiographically distinguisable from miliary disease in which all lesions do not arise simultaneously. Metastatic lesions are rarely miliary and are often larger and variable in size. The configuration of each lesion usually consists of a sharply demarcated, spherical mass (Fig. 6-37).

A single, large, round mass found in the lung of an infant or child is rarely a primary pulmonary neoplasm. More often, the mass is a pneumonic pseudotumor, and a reexamination after a few hours will clearly demonstrate a more recognizable lesion with segmental or lobar distribution (Fig. 6-4, 6-5). A pseudotumor is not uncommon in pneumococcal pneumonia. The term encapsulating is used to describe types of pneumonia which produce infiltrations that are consistently spherical in appearance. Chronic granulomatous disease of childhood and pneumonia in measles are two such entities. Should a rounded mass present along a fissure it is probably a form of pseudotumor caused by effusion. An interesting pseudotumor is produced by the reparative process of an inflammatory lesion. It presents as a

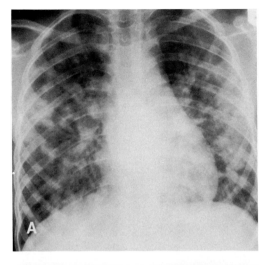
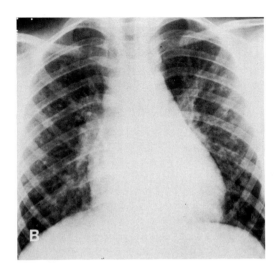
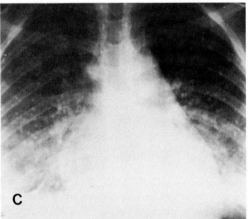

Fig. 6-36. Diffuse histoplasmosis. *(A)* Overwhelming infection reveals a soft nodular infiltration throughout both lung fields. In the periphery the lesion appears more homogeneous because of conglomeration and no coalescence. *(B)* Approximately 6 months later the lesions are smaller and more sharply circumscribed. *(C)* In another patient diffuse symmetrical calcifications are shown due to multiple chronic histoplasma granulomas. (Cardiomegaly and pleural effusion are due to superimposed acute glomerulonephritis.)

distinct, well circumscribed mass that may be discovered following an acute pneumonic process or on a routine chest radiograph. Over 50 per cent of the patients are asymptomatic at the time of discovery; cough and hemoptysis are occasionally encountered in the others. With such a combination of findings, this form of pseudotumor is often mistaken for a neoplasm, unless previous radiographs that demonstrate the development of the lesion are available. The size of an inflammatory pseudotumor is variable, and in some instances it measures several centimeters in diameter. It is often uniform in radiodensity but can have a necrotic center and occasionally massive calcific deposits. Calcification is an excellent radiographic indicator of benign disease; a calcified pseudotumor simulates a hamartoma. Hilar adenopathy has occasionally been observed but pleural effusion or metastasis is never present.

Other well-defined pulmonary lesions include arteriovenous malformations and pulmonary sequestration. Arteriovenous malformations may be single or multiple (Fig. 6-38) but are always supplied by large vessels that radiate back toward the hilum. The vascular nature can be further substantiated under direct fluoroscopic observation by noting the alteration in size of the lesion during various phases of respiration. Angiography, nevertheless, best demonstrates the lesion. Multiple pulmonary arteriovenous malformations should suggest the Weber-Rendu-Osler syndrome. Similar vascular malformations may be present throughout other parts of the body.

Pulmonary sequestration is quite variable in appearance and configuration. It may be round, triangular, or may even demonstrate no recognizable form. Its location, posterior in the lower lobe adjacent to the vertebral column, is characteristic. The radiographic

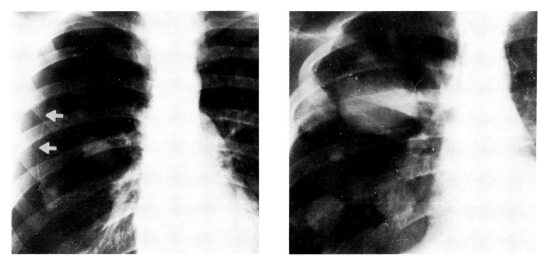

Fig. 6-37. Metastatic sarcoma with pneumothorax. (A) Multiple, large, well-defined nodules are visualized, associated with a pneumothorax on the right *(arrows)*. (B) Six months later, the lesions have increased in size and amount and demonstrate pleural involvement.

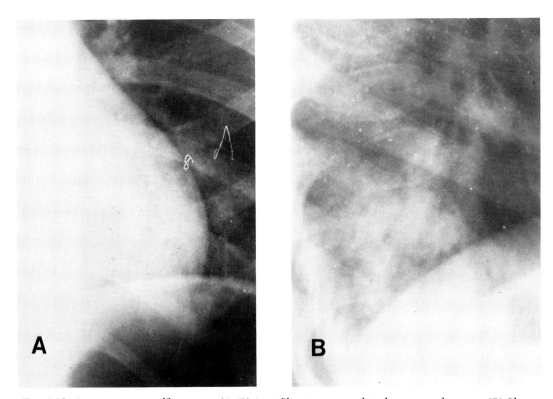

Fig. 6-38. Arteriovenous malformation. (A, B) An infiltration is noted in the retrocardiac area. (B) Close observation on the lateral film suggests the multiple nodular defects characteristic of an arteriovenous malformation.

presentation depends mostly upon its pathologic structure; when completely cystic pulmonary sequestration may be almost impossible to observe unless it is rendered radiopaque by infection (Fig. 6-50). Sequestrations do not communicate with a bronchus and are most often supplied by a systemic artery arising from the aorta below the diaphragm.

Mucous impaction and mucocele are rare causes of pulmonary nodular lesions. Both are similar since they represent a gradual accumulation of mucous within a bronchus. However, a mucocele arises only in an occluded bronchus caused by congenital atresia or by an inflammatory or neoplastic stricture. Mucoid impaction is almost exclusively confined to patients with asthma, chronic bronchitis, and cystic fibrosis. Radiographically, a mucocele is manifested by a well rounded, spherical mass, surrounded by an area of emphysema. A mucoid impaction may also look rounded, but, unlike a mucocele, it demonstrates an oblong branching pattern that radiates from the hilum.

Malignant primary lesions are indeed rare in infants and children; carcinoid tumors are probably the most common and are recognized by a well circumscribed mass that commonly obstructs the bronchus, producing atelectasis. Benign tumors are occasionally found in the pediatric age-group.

Discussion

A neurogenic tumor is the most common cause of a mediastinal mass in children under the age of 4 years. Beyond this age, lymphomas predominate. Neurogenic tumors are found mainly in the posterior mediastinum, and neuroblastoma is probably the most frequent tumor encountered. In general, 10 to 15 per cent of these tumors arise in the thorax, and the higher the lesion is in the thorax, the better is the prognosis. In patients with a neuroblastoma, the survival rate is higher if it is discovered before 1 year of age. At any time, a neuroblastoma may be transformed spontaneously into a more benign form, such as a ganglioneuroblastoma or a mature ganglioneuroma. Calcification within a neural tumor is not distinctive; both benign and malignant lesions contain deposits of calcium. This may not be apparent on plain films but is often seen on body sections or computerized tomography.

A paravertebral mass resulting from an infectious process can be confusing. Quite frequently no organism can be identified, and the diagnosis of discitis is made based on the presence of inflammatory tissue on biopsy. The treatment is quite variable; the patient may receive no therapy, may be advised to rest, or may be given broad spectrum antibiotics. Most paramediastinal masses caused by infection are still the result of tuberculosis. The tubercule bacillus is difficult to culture, and a positive tuberculin patch test should almost be sufficient to establish the diagnosis. If this low grade infection remains untreated, the lesions progress slowly producing extensive kyphotic changes.

Esophageal duplications comprise 15 per cent of all alimentary tract duplications. Most are found in children but 25 to 30 per cent are discovered later in life. The wall of the duplication often contains gastric intestinal mucosa and smooth muscle. If gastric mucosa is present, it can cause severe symptoms, such as pain and bleeding.

Nodal disease occurring in tuberculosis and in histoplasmosis is quite extensive, since the major portion of the infecting organisms drain into these structures. As a result, the infection is more severe and persists for a longer period of time. Sometimes lymphadenopathy is the only radiographic finding, and differentiation from neoplasm may be difficult, since progressive enlargement of the lymph nodes can occur in histoplasmosis. At one time, the term mediastinal granuloma was used to designate caseous or fibrocaseous mediastinal nodes in which no causative agent could be isolated. Now with more refined techniques, histoplasmosis has been shown to be the most frequent cause. Mediastinal histoplasmosis can present with fever, weakness, cough, and even dysphagia. The lymph nodes compress neighboring mediastinal structures and can produce atelectasis, pericarditis, and superior vena cava syndrome. In some cases, the nodes fail to regress but progress to a chronic stage, in which the continual deposition of fibrous tissue is the main pathologic finding. Fibrosis involves and compresses some or all of the mediastinal tissues. Superior vena cava syndrome, esophageal stricture, stenosis of the

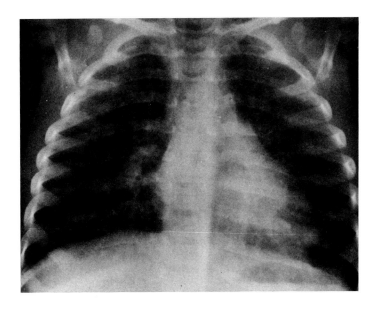

Fig. 6-39. Miliary tuberculosis. An early but distinct miliary dissemination is apparent in both lung fields. No obvious primary lesion is noted in this patient, except for a suggested infiltration in the left retrocardiac area.

tracheobronchial tree, and occlusion of the pulmonary arteries and veins all follow. Fibrous mediastinitis is probably the result of a hypersensitivity response of the patient to an unidentified antigen that oozes from the periphery of the nodes into the surrounding tissues. This phenomenon also accounts for the apparent growth of the Histoplasma granuloma.

Post-inflammatory pseudotumors have been given a variety of names that include xanthoma, xanthofibroma, sclerosing hemangioma, histiocytoma xanthogranuloma, and plasma cell tumor. These are all variations of the same entity, which begins as an acute pneumonic process that incompletely resolves and forms a granulomatous process. The predominance of one cell type may represent a particular phase of development. Histiocytes, foam cells, lymphocytes, and giant cells have all been found and account for the number of pathologic descriptions.

Bronchopulmonary sequestration is a congenital anomaly within the thorax that is not connected with the normal bronchial tree and is supplied by a systemic vessel arising from the lower thoracic aorta or upper abdominal aorta. It is basically a unilocular or multilocular cyst that, if uninfected, may remain completely undetected. Two forms of sequestration are noted, intrapulmonary and extrapulmonary. The lesions, except for location and venous drainage, are remarkably similar. By definition, the intrapulmonary le-

sion is contained within the lung and drains into the pulmonary veins. Extrapulmonary lesions are distinct, are enclosed in a pleural envelope, and drain by way of the azygous system.

A mucocele with hyperinflation is rare and is due to bronchial atresia. It seems to affect the left upper lobe most frequently. The pathogenesis of focal air trapping with bronchial atresia remains unknown, but it is probably best explained by an air drift through the pores of Kohn. The atretic bronchus must, therefore, be segmental and not lobar to allow for transsegmental collateral drift.

DISEASES WHICH RESULT IN A MICRONODULAR PATTERN

A diffuse micronodular pattern is manifested radiographically by pinpoint shadows distributed throughout the lung fields. The lesions measure approximately 1 mm. in diameter (Fig. 6-39) but under certain circumstances may attain the size of 2 to 3 mms. in diameter. At this time, they appear more confluent and produce a "snowstorm" appearance (Fig. 6-40). This pattern has occasionally been confused with that of pulmonary edema because of the overall haziness within the lung fields. However, close observation demonstrates a diffuse nodularity that is obviously not as homogeneous as the radiodensity produced by alveolar fluid.

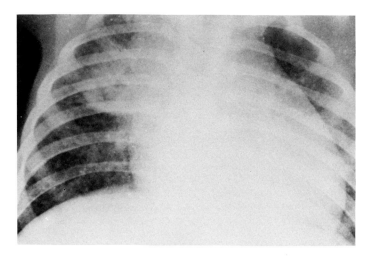

Fig. 6-40. Primary tuberculosis with miliary spread. A large pneumonic focus is present within the right upper lobe. An obvious miliary dissemination is also present throughout the lung fields. The lesions are larger and more confluent than the previous case.

Disease Entities

Miliary disease
Allergic hypersensitivity pneumonia
Sarcoidosis
Diffuse bronchopneumonia
Metastatic disease
Pulmonary alveolar microlithiasis

Differential Diagnosis

Miliary tuberculosis, because of its high morbidity and mortality, should be the initial consideration when one is confronted with a diffuse micronodular pattern in a sick child. This radiographic feature reflects hematogenous spread of the disease and, unfortunately, requires an interval of approximately 6 weeks from the actual time of dissemination to the time the lesions become radiographically evident. In the early phases detection may be difficult, since the nodules tend to merge with the vascular markings (Fig. 6-39). However, as the disease progresses, the lesions enlarge and become more obvious. Tuberculosis should be strongly suspected if residual evidence of a primary focus is recognized (Fig. 6-40).

Other infectious diseases of either fungal or bacterial origin also undergo hematogenous dissemination, but are not common in the pediatric age-group.

Extrinsic allergic alveolitis is a term which describes the response of the lung to specific antigens contained in organic dust. The size of the dust particle is decidedly important, since it must be small enough to penetrate deep into the most distal portions of the lung parenchyma. Clinically, extrinsic allergic alveolitis is manifested and heralded by the onset of dyspnea accompanied by radiographic manifestations of a diffuse micronodular pattern. The lung fields appear granular, and demonstrate a diffusely scattered mottling throughout the lungs that tends to spare the upper and lower lung fields. Individual nodules range from 1 mm. or less to several millimeters in diameter (Fig. 6-41). They may be discrete but are usually ill-defined. The diameter of the lesions in the lower lung fields may be larger (Fig. 6-42). Associated enlarged lymph nodes have been described, with variable degrees of incidence. The presence of enlarged nodes, however, is unusual.

Sarcoidosis is also associated with diffuse micronodular changes throughout the lung field. Sarcoidosis, in general, is quite unusual in the pediatric age-group. The radiographic manifestations of the disease at the time of diagnosis are, surprisingly, already limited to the pulmonary effects that consist of mottling, nodular infiltrations, and miliary nodules. The hilar nodes are frequently in the process of regressing and at this stage the hilum demonstrates evidence of increased radiodensity or size and, in addition, a hazy border. Clinically, there should be no difficulty in distinquishing the disease from extrinsic allergic alveolitis, since the overall clinical picture is much more dramatic in extrinsic allergic alveolitis. The majority of patients with sarcoidosis are relatively asymptomatic and, as a result, are not detected during the initial stage of the disease.

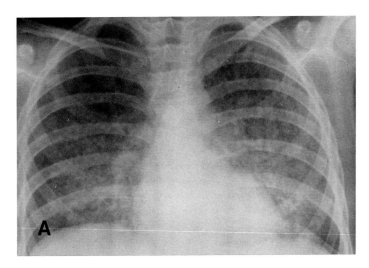

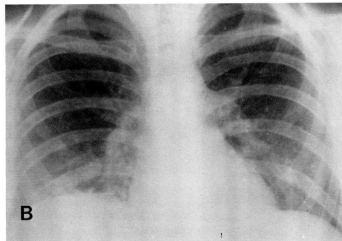

Fig. 6-41. Extrinsic allergic alveolitis (farmer's lung). *(A, B)* A diffuse micronodular pattern is present producing an overall haziness in both lung fields in a young male with severe dypsnea. After a few days in the hospital the entire process regressed without therapy.

Bronchopneumonia often presents in a diffuse nodular pattern and occasionally may involve both lung fields. A variety of etiological agents may be responsible. The lesions produced can be uniform in size but more often show evidence of areas of coalescence of variable size and configuration.

Viral pneumonia produces a variety of pulmonary manifestations that range from interstitial infiltration to gross consolidation. In many, interstitial infiltration is produced. Viral pneumonias complicating measles and chicken pox are known to produce this appearance. Chicken pox may resolve with diffuse calcification.

Metastatic disease may occasionally present with a micronodular pattern. Close observation of the lesions demonstrates well-defined and sharp surrounding margins. Knowing the source of the metastasis is helpful.

The radiographic manifestations of alveolar microlithiasis are diagnostic, despite a rare occurrence in infants and children. The fundamental feature is a fine, sand-like micronodulation that involves both lungs diffusely (Fig. 6-43). Each nodule is usually well-defined and measures less than 1 mm. in diameter. Because of the total effect, the overall radiodensity of the lower lung fields is greater than that of the upper fields. Complications, such as pneumothorax and calcification of the pericardium, have been noted.

Discussion

Most extrinsic allergic alveolar diseases occur as a result of occupational or environmental exposure, and the amount of identifiable antigens is becoming increasingly larger. Farmer's lung is the earliest named and probably most thoroughly understood condition which causes allergic alveolitis.

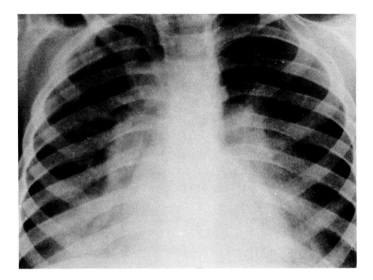

Fig. 6-42. Extrinsic allergic alveolitis (chicken breeder's disease). Coalescence of the fine micronodular infiltration has occurred and appears almost homogeneous. Close observation, however, reveals the exact nature of the lesion. The lungs cleared shortly after entering the hospital. (The patient lived adjacent to a chicken market and responded positively when challenged.)

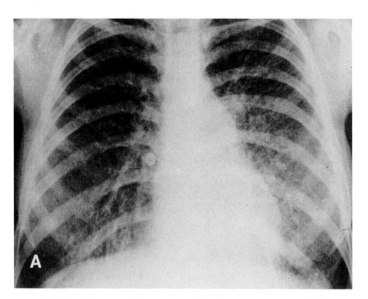

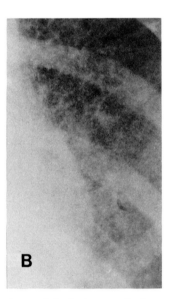

Fig. 6-43. Pulmonary alveolar microlithiasis. *(A)* Note the diffuse dense micronodular lesions producing a sand-like appearance throughout the lung fields. *(B)* A detailed view of the lung field demonstrates the intra-alveolar calculi.

The antigen responsible is a thermophilic actinomycetes. The clinical picture depends on the degree of exposure to antigens (present in moldy hay) and the sensitivity of the subject. Recent studies indicate that many farmers have the clinical syndrome without all of the immunologic and radiological manifestations commonly described in the literature. The classical, acute onset occurs in perhaps no more than one third of all cases. The most common presentation is insidious, characterized by gradual progression of dyspnea, cough, weight loss, fever, and chills. Allergic aleveolitis also occurs in mushroom worker's disease, bagassosis, chicken breeder's disease, and maple bark disease. The knowledge of definite exposure to these antigens is helpful in establishing the diagnosis. Much more specific is the demonstration of precipitating antibodies. Regardless of the marked variation in antigens, the target organ, the lung, is the same and its response, both pathologically and radiographically, is similar in all diseases.

Pulmonary alveolar microlithiasis is a disease of unknown etiology that is characterized by the presence of tiny calculi (calispherocytes) within the pulmonary alveoli. Some degree of familial incidence has been recorded and as such seems to be restricted only to siblings. Other pathogenic mechanisms, environmental and metabolic, have been proposed but not proven. In the early stages of the disease, the alveolar walls remain normal. However, interstitial fibrosis associated with giant cell formation eventually occurs, and blebs and bullae may form. Cor pulmunale is the final result.

ABNORMAL AREAS OF RADIOLUCENCY IN THE THORAX

Abnormal radiolucent collections in the thorax are encountered less commonly in children than in neonates or adults. Many of the basic causes are the same. A lesion associated with air in the lungs is reflected as an area of diffuse or localized hyperlucency that may or may not be surrounded by a zone of increased radiodensity. Any radiolucent structure appearing in the soft tissues of the thorax is abnormal.

Disease Entities

Thoracic lesions
  Pneumothorax
  Pneumomediastinum
  Pneumopericardium
  Hiatal hernia
  Colonic interposition
  Duplication
Pulmonary lesions
  Local
    Pneumatocele
    Cavitation
    Pulmonary sequestration
    Congenital cyst
  Diffuse
    Emphysema
    Unilateral hyperlucent lung
    Absence of the pectoralis muscle
    Hypoplastic lung
    Lobar emphysema

Differential Diagnosis

A unilateral hyperlucent hemithorax may be caused by a number of entities, such as a pneumothorax (Fig. 6-44, 6-51). The radiographic manifestations of a pneumothorax

depend upon the amount of free air, the position of the patient, and the phase of respiration at the time of exposure. A small pneumothorax is not easily recognized on routine chest radiographs but is best demonstrated if the film is exposed during an expiratory phase or in a decubitus position. During expiration, the overall pulmonary volume is decreased, and the lung markings are crowded together. In the decubitus position, the lung falls and the air rises. Both processes help to exaggerate the difference in density between the lung and the surrounding pleural air. As a result, a radiolucent halo (pneumothorax) is seen, sharply outlining the visceral pleura (Fig. 6-44). Extreme caution must be exercised when evaluating a chest radiograph taken in the supine position for a pneumothorax. In this position the lung falls posteriorly and the pleural air rises anteriorly. As a result, it is often difficult to discern the boundary of the collapsed lung. The only radiographic suggestion of free pleural air is a slight increase in radiolucency on one side of the chest. A unilateral hyperlucent lung may also be found in the hyperlucent lung syndrome and in lesions resulting from air-trapping, as in foreign body aspiration and lobar emphysema (see p. 197). A hyperlucent lung is differentiated from a pneumothorax by the absence of a demonstrable visceral pleural edge.

The unilateral hyperlucent lung syndrome, or the Swyer-James syndrome, is an acquired disease characterized by a hyperlucent lung with normal or more frequently, decreased pulmonary volume that is associated with a corresponding shift of the mediastinum toward the hyperlucent lung (Fig. 6-45). The lung changes little in volume during respiration. Bronchography reveals dilated and clubbed bronchi, with no filling of the bronchial tree or alveoli beyond the obstructed bronchi. The ipsilateral pulmonary artery is small and its branches are narrow and diminished in caliber. Additional lesions which produce unilateral hyperlucency of the hemithorax are relatively uncommon: (1) Unilateral absence of the pectoralis muscle is readily noted by physical examination; (2) a hypoplastic lung is small in size and is more often radiodense than radiolucent because of poor ventilation, and the bronchial tree is unusually small in caliber but normal in appearance; (3) lobar emphysema or com-

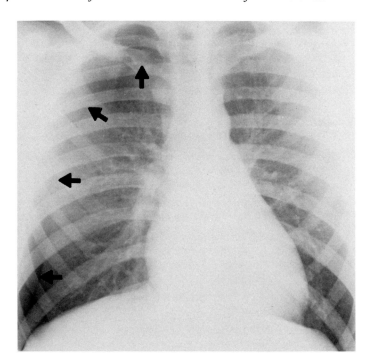

Fig. 6-44. Pneumothorax. A fairly prominent pneumothorax is visualized on the right *(arrows).* The lung is partially collapsed. A slight increase in radiolucency within the periphery of the right lung field is present.

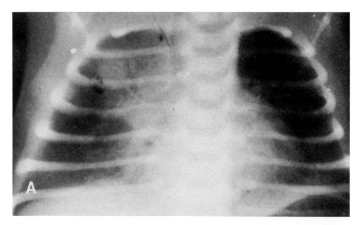

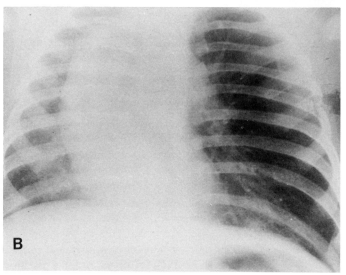

Fig. 6-45. Swyer-James syndrome. *(A)* Both the trachea and mediastinum are shifted slightly to the right. The right lung is somewhat radiodense because of a superimposed pneumonia. *(B)* Upon inspiration the mediastinum moves toward the side of the involved lung.

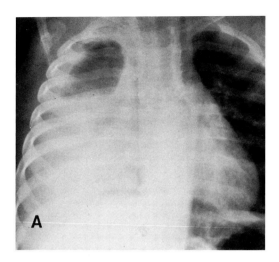

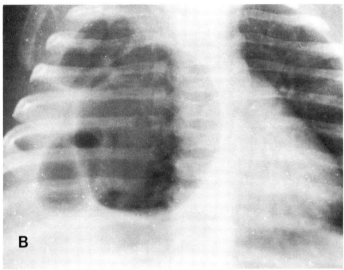

Fig. 6-46. Staphylococcal pneumonia with pneumatocele. *(A)* Extensive pneumonia with a developing, thin-walled pneumatocele within the right upper lobe. A large empyema is also present. *(B)* Multiple large pneumatoceles are shown in a patient with staphylococcal pneumonia. Note the thin wall surrounding each lesion.

pensatory emphysema produces an overall increase in size and radiolucency in the corresponding hemithorax.

Localized accumulations of air such as pneumatoceles, congenital cysts, and abscesses, also occur within the lung. Pneumatoceles are thin-walled collections of intrapulmonary air that arise as a result of air-trapping. They frequently occur in the course of a suppurative pneumonia and have been known to occur in 61 per cent of cases of staphylococcocal pneumonia. They vary in size from 0.5 cms. in diameter to large cysts that may expand and coalesce to produce ten-

sion cysts in some cases. Pneumatoceles usually appear within 1 week after the onset of the illness and disappear in an average of 6 weeks (Fig. 6-46).

Pneumatoceles are also known to occur following trauma and hydrocarbon aspiration. An average time of 9 days is required for a pneumatocele to develop following hydrocarbon aspiration. The pneumatocele gradually enlarges and may be irregular in shape (Fig. 6-47). Compartmentalization is common. The pathogenesis is related to air-trapping secondary to parenchymal disruption.

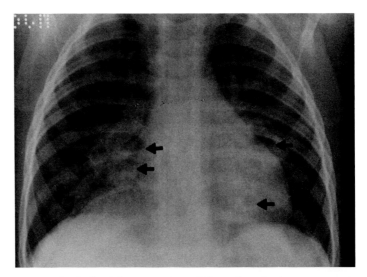

Fig. 6-47. Hydrocarbon ingestion. Bilateral aspiration pneumonia with multiple cavities *(arrows)* containing air fluid levels is shown. The patient aspirated furniture polish 2 weeks previously.

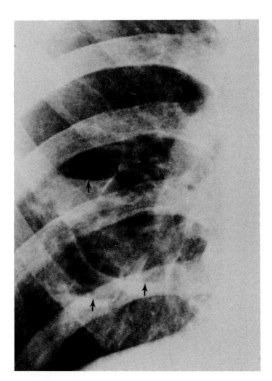

Fig. 6-48. Infected congenital cysts. Multiple congenital cysts containing minimal fluid are present within the right lung field *(arrows)*. The cysts subsequently became completely filled.

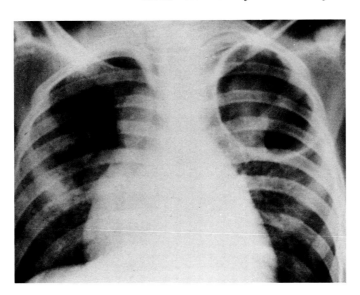

Fig. 6-49. Lung abscess. A patient with rheumatic heart disease on steroid therapy demonstrates a large, thick-walled abscess in the left upper lung field.

It is important to distinguish congenital cysts of the lung from the air cysts that occur during staphylococcal pneumonia. Such air cysts may persist for long periods of time, although it is unusual to find a cyst 1 year after the initial infection. The congenital cyst not only persists but maintains a constant size, whereas the size of the pneumatocele fluctuates. Congenital cysts frequently remain unrecognized until infection supervenes (Fig. 6-48). Histologically, the true congenital cyst is lined by bronchial epithelium.

Pneumatoceles must also be distinguished from actual cavitary lesions. Cavitation is the result of parenchymal necrosis, and the surrounding wall is initially thick and irregular. However, this becomes smoother and decreases in thickness as the cavity resolves or progresses into a more chronic stage (Fig. 6-49).

Congenital bronchiolar cysts that communicate with the main bronchus have been described elsewhere. These lesions in many respects demonstrate features similar to sequestration. However, pulmonary sequestration is manifested by a mass of nonfunctional lung tissue, often cystic in nature, that does not communicate with the tracheobronchial tree and is characteristically located in the lower medial posterior lung fields, with or without fluid (Fig. 6-50).

Loculated mediastinal air collections may occur within a dilated esophagus or within esophageal lesions, or may be due to free air penetrating the mediastinal tissues.

Gastrogenic cysts are gastric-lined, congenital foregut cysts. These are uncommon mediastinal cysts that manifest a cystic, oval appearance, and they are often associated with spinal anomalies. Radiopertechnetate imaging is a safe and accurate means of diagnosing these cysts, since the nucleitide is concentrated in the parietal cells. By contrast, duplications or cysts arising from the esophagus rarely communicate with the lumen of the parent structure and present primarily as soft-tissue masses within the mediastinum and not as cystic structures. (Fig. 6-51).

Empyema is a purulent process that occurs within the pleural space. It may originate as a primary pleural process but more often arises subsequent to adjacent infection (e.g., pneumonia, subphrenic abscess). The accumulation of air in the pleural fluid assumes the form of multiple, loculated air fluid collections. This indicates the presence of a bronchopleural fistula, unless the air has been introduced artificially.

Air within the mediastinum is usually not difficult to recognize. The typically loculated, cystic collection of air encountered in newborns is only rarely observed beyond the neonatal period. In older children as in adults, the radiographic appearance mainly consists of linear, strip-like collections of air that dissect the normal solid mediastinal structures (Fig. 6-52). Small amounts are difficult to observe because of the adjacent lung tissue. If the air collects below the peri-

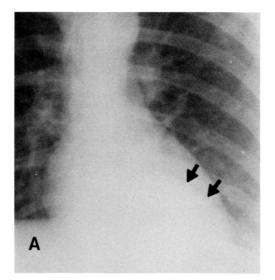
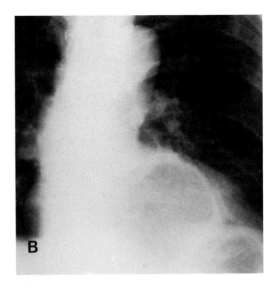
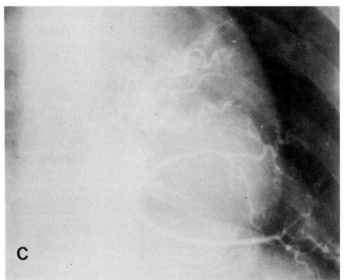

Fig. 6-50. Intrapulmonary sequestrations in adults. *(A)* Sequestration in this patient assumes a triangular configuration in the retrocardiac area. *(B)* In this patient the sequestation appears as a large, cystic, thick-walled structure. *(C)* An aortogram reveals multiple vessels arising from the thoracic aorta to supply the lesion.

cardium, the diaphragm is well outlined. Occasionally, mediastinal air surrounds the cardiac structure and simulates a pneumopericardium. Air within the pericardium remains localized, and the outer margin of the heart is usually sharply outlined. The pericardium itself is a thin, fine structure. However, when involved with a purulent exudate it becomes thick and irregular (Fig. 6-53). Mediastinal air dissects freely into the cervical and supraclavicular spaces, occasionally the first clinical manifestation of a pneumomediastinum.

A hiatal hernia can present as abnormal loculi of air or a large single air fluid level restricted to the retrocardiac area. This radiographic feature is common in adults but may also occur in the pediatric age-group.

An enlarged, dilated esophagus may represent achalasia, stricture, or other esophageal disorders. The esophagus descends along the right paravertebral region and is occasionally mistaken for an enlarged heart. The presence of an air fluid level indicates the structure involved and the nature of the lesion (Fig. 6-54). An air fluid level is best manifested after the patient drinks some water.

A colon interposed between the proximal esophagus and the stomach in order to bypass

(Text continued on p. 264.)

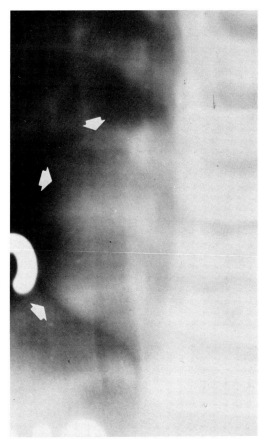

Fig. 6-51. Duplication. An oval-shaped mass is present within the posterior mediastinum *(arrows).* The lateral margins of the vertebral bodies are slightly deformed. Histologic examination revealed a duplication lined with gastric mucosa.

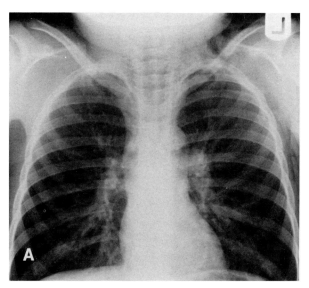
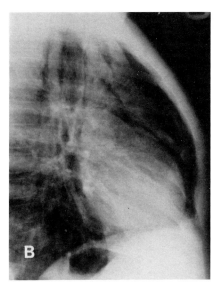

Fig. 6-52. Pneumothorax and pneumomediastinum in asthma. *(A)* In a young teenager with an acute asthmatic attack and severe chest pain, subcutaneous emphysema is noted in the soft tissues of the left thorax and cervical regions. A pneumomediastinum is not evident on the frontal film. *(B)* In the lateral projection extensive air dissects the entire mediastinum and displaces the thymus away from the cardiac silhouette.

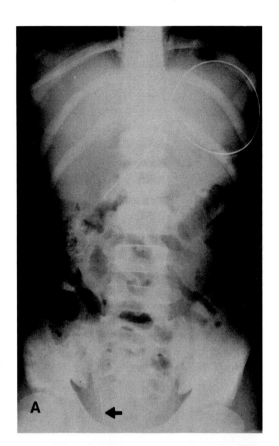

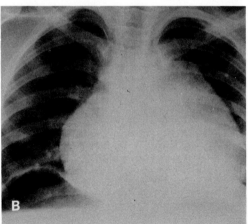

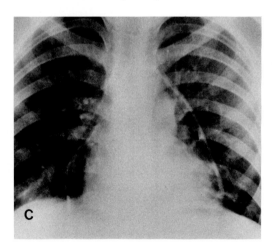

Fig. 6-53. Acute purulent pericarditis. (A) An abdominal film reveals a pin lying free within the abdomen in the right lower quadrent. Note free air overlying the liver shadow. (B) A few days later a subphrenic abscess developed, producing a huge air fluid collection below the right diaphragm. The cardiac silhouette at this time has enlarged and demonstrates evidence of pericarditis. (C) Following pericardiocentesis, the pericardium is thick and irregular and already shows evidence of adhesions (arrow).

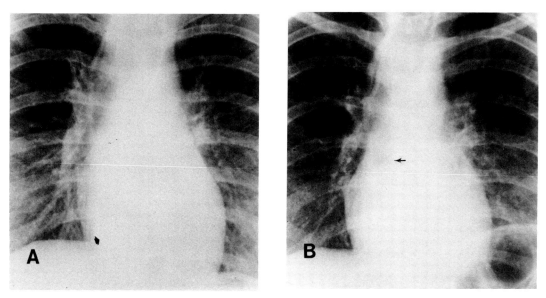

Fig. 6-54. Achalasia. (A) A large paravertebral elliptical radiodensity is noted through the cardiac structure (arrow). (B) An air fluid level is observed during different examination (arrow).

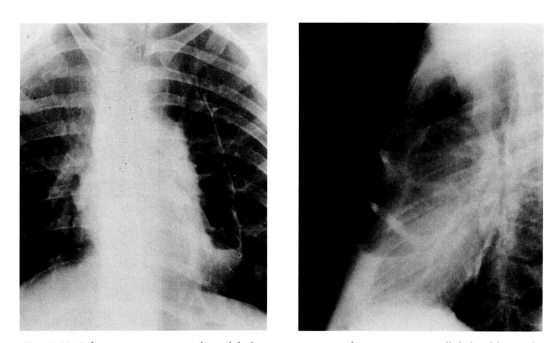

Fig. 6-55. Colonic interposition. A large lobular cystic structure demonstrating a well-defined haustral pattern is located anteriorly on the chest wall.

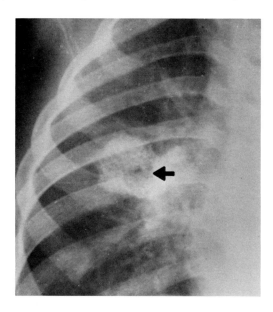

Fig. 6-56. Primary tuberculosis with pseudo-cavity. A large, calcifying, primary focus is noted within the right mid-lung field, associated with calcified lymph nodes. The center of the lesion appears radiolucent because of the accumulation of high lipid containing caseating material *(arrow).*

esophageal strictures often looks like a cystic structure containing air. This can descend on either side of the midline. Careful scrutiny reveals that the overall cystic configuration is comprised of haustral markings (Fig. 6-55).

Discussion

Asthma is a common cause of pneumothorax and pneumomediastinum in young adolescents (Fig. 6-44). The pathogenesis is similar to neonatal respiratory distress syndrome, except that in asthma bronchospasm is the basic cause of increased alveolar pressure. Pneumothorax should always be suspected in an individual who continues to demonstrate shortness of breath following an acute episode. A pneumothorax associated with asthma is usually small, self-limited, and relatively asymptomatic. An important but uncommon cause of pneumothorax is foreign body aspiration, which should be suspected in any case of unexplained pneumomediastinum and pneumothorax. Airway obstruction caused by foreign body aspiration results in severe respiratory difficulty, with peripheral air trapping and rupture of the alveolar membranes. Other causes of spontaneous pneumomediastinum include lower respiratory tract infection associated with cough, pertussis, influenza, bronchopneumonia, and isolated Valsalva's maneuver. Pneumothorax may also be the result of blunt or penetrating injury to the thorax. However, with blunt trauma rib frac-

tures must be present. This is uncommon in childhood due to the overall elasticity of the rib cage.

It is likely that spontaneous pneumothorax may be a common manifestation of pulmonary involvement in histiocytosis. This seems to occur in one of four patients with eosinophilic granuloma. A few physicians maintain that some cases of spontaneous pneumothorax may represent formes frustes of this disease. Formation of cysts and blebs in histiocytosis readily explains the development of pneumothorax. Although not common, malignant neoplasms, and particularly peripheral metastatic sarcomas, are associated with spontaneous pneumothorax. The actual mechanism is unknown, but some physicians believed it is caused by acutal rupture of necrotic tumor into a bronchus and into the pleural space.

Swyer and James reported the first case of unilateral hyperlucent lung in a 6-year-old boy with recurrent lower respiratory tract infection. The underlying pathogenesis is now believed to be bronchiolitis obliterans. Most commonly this follows an adenovirus infection, although hydrocarbon ingestion, radiation therapy, measles, and pertussis have also been implicated.

The development of an abscess and a pneumatocele in staphylococcal pneumonia are quite similar in many respects. Staphylococcus causes destructive parenchymal changes as it spreads distally into the

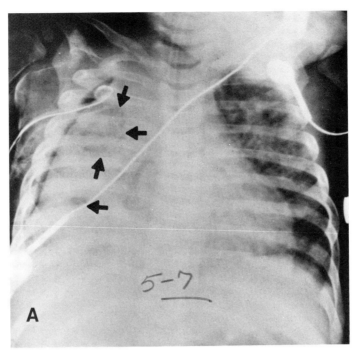

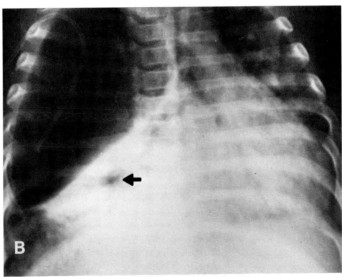

Fig. 6-57. Primary progressive tuberculosis. *(A)* The initial chest film shows disease in both lung fields. Caseous pneumonia with obvious cavity formation *(arrows)* and a small pneumothorax is noted on the right. A bronchogenic spread is apparent on the left. *(B)* Progression of the pneumothorax due to bronchopleural fistula is quite evident 2 days later. The cavity is now well-defined *(arrow).*

smallest bronchi and into the interstitial tissues. In addition, the exudative process leads to obstruction of small bronchioles resulting in local consolidation. A pneumatocele may arise when small areas of necrosis occurring in the peribronchial interstitial tissue perforate the bronchial wall, permitting air to enter; these continue to inflate by way of a check-valve action caused by the edematous bronchial mucosa or by luminal secretions. Or, pneumatoceles may arise by air-trapping due to bronchial obstruction caused by inflammation and edema. An abscess, by con-

trast, is basically a large area of necrosis produced from multiple, coalescent microabscesses. Not all necrotizing pneumonias occurring in children are caused by Staphylococcus; Streptococcus, acid-fast bacilli, and a number of fungi are also responsible for tissue breakdown.

Tuberculosis in infants and children most frequently occurs in the form of a primary infection. Caseation plays an important role in the underlying pathologic process, but cavitation demonstrable by radiograph is indeed rare. A pseudo-cavity occasionally arises

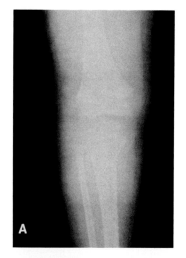
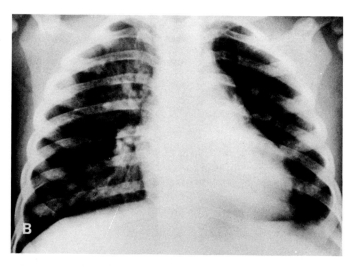
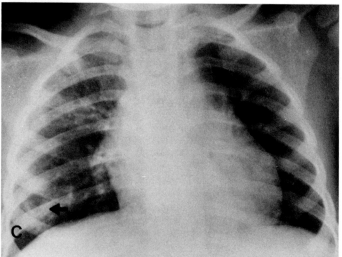

Fig. 6-58. Septic emboli caused by Streptococcus. *(A)* This patient presented with diffuse cellulitis in the right leg. Note the severe soft-tissue swelling. *(B)* A few days later chest pain developed and multiple nodular radiodensities appeared in both lungs. On the right early cavitation is demonstrated. *(C)* Following antibiotic therapy most of the lesions disappeared. A large cavity persists within the right lower lobe *(arrow).*

when excessive amounts of caseating material accumulate in the center of a primary focus. The material which has a high lipid content is then surrounded by a zone of dense tissue (Fig. 6-56). Actual cavity formation occurs in children whose defense mechanisms are overwhelmed by the disease. This has been called primary progressive tuberculosis (Fig. 6-57). The cavities vary in size and appearance but are mainly thick-walled, with irregular inner surfaces. Commonly, they begin in the upper lung field and spread to other areas of the lung. The entire process represents a rapid evolution of primary tuberculosis to a reactivation phase without passing through an inactive latent period.

Many fungal lesions simulate tuberculous lesions and are distinguished only by the identification of the causative organism or by

positive skin or serologic reactions. Histoplasmosis, caused by *Histoplasma capsulatum,* is such a fungus. It often begins as a single focus, but multiple foci are more characteristic. Occasionally, the development of smooth, thin-walled or moderately thick-walled cavities occurs as a manifestation of the primary infection. This presentation strongly resembles that of septic emboli or underlying vasculitis. However, the patients look relatively normal, despite the severe radiologic appearance.

The development of most other fungal infections simulates tuberculosis in both a primary acute phase, as well as a chronic phase. Blastomycosis, coccidiomycosis, and actinomycosis are rarely manifested in the pediatric age-group. Nocardiosis, however, is presently assuming a prominent role in immunodeficient patients. Nocardia are aerobic, unencapsulated, nonmotile, gram-positive, and partially acid-fast organisms that produce pulmonary findings of bronchopneumonia and cavitation, not unlike other mycotic infections.

Pneumatocele formation following hydrocarbon ingestion is a not an uncommon problem and occurs in approximately 10 per cent of children who accidentally ingest furniture polish, nail polish remover, benzene and other hydrocarbons. The findings are also the result of tissue breakdown and edema, which creates a ball-valve phenomenon. The cysts require a few days to weeks to resolve, depending upon the type of hydrocarbon ingested.

An unusual cause of cavitation is the resolving hematoma. This occurs with consolidation approximately 2 weeks following the initial episode of trauma. Initially a crescent of air surrounds the retracting hematoma, a radiographic presentation that resembles a fungus ball and an echinococcus cyst.

Septic emboli are infrequent causes of cavitation (Fig. 6-54). These arise from distant foci of infection and are transported by way of the blood stream to the lungs. The lower lobes, therefore, are most frequently involved, and the initial lesions consist of patchy pneumonic consolidations that quickly undergo necrosis (Fig. 6-58).

As in adults, metastatic malignancy in children may produce cavitation when tumor growth exceeds its vascular supply. The central core of tissues is then deficient in vascularity, resulting in ischemia, subsequent necrosis, and breakdown. The appearance of a cavitating malignant mass resembles a combination of pyogenic pneumonia and granulomatous disease. The mass is normally well-defined, without extensive surrounding consolidation, and the walls are thicker and more nodular than are those usually seen in granulomatous disease. Should multiple metastatic masses cavitate simultaneously, there is a strong likelihood that the patient is undergoing chemotherapy. This is especially common in extra-nodal lymphoma.

Although the actual demonstration of a hiatal hernia is uncommon in the pediatric age-group, increasing evidence suggests the frequency of hiatal hernia and gastroesophageal reflux is much higher than previously suspected. Identification of gastric mucosal folds, as well as the hernia itself, is best accomplished with multiple spot films on prone oblique and supine positions, with thick barium (Fig. 6-59). Hiatal hernias and reflux should be suspected in all infants who spit or vomit frequently and are irritable, and who manifest poor appetite and recurring aspiration pneumonia. Reflux esophagitis with esophageal stricture is an unfortuante complication which occurs if the lesion remains unrecognized for prolonged periods of time.

Some infants and children with hiatal hernia undergo bizarre, athetoid motions in an effort to reduce the hernia and thus the reflux. Until physicians realized that hiatal hernias and esophagitis were responsible for these movements, such infants were thought to be victims of degenerating neural disease.

DIFFUSE PERIHILAR INFILTRATIONS

Radiographically, diffuse perihilar infiltrations originate from the central hilar area and spread toward the peripheral lung fields. As a result, the lung fields become hazy and radiopaque. In some lesions, the peripheral lung fields are clear and radiolucent, producing a halo around the radiodense, central region. In others, the entire lung fields may be completely infiltrated. When the peripheral regions are radiolucent, the appearance of the radiopaque lungs has been likened to a butterfly or a bat wing. In general, the majority of the lesions producing this appearance are located within the alveoli.

Disease Entities
Pulmonary edema
Diffuse exudative pneumonia
Opportunistic infection (*Pneumocystis carinii* pneumonia)
Pulmonary alveolar proteinosis
Pulmonary hemorrhage
Aspiration pneumonia
Extrinsic allergic alveolitis
Veno-occlusive disease

Differential Diagnosis

In infants and children, pulmonary edema is by far the best example and probably the most common cause of diffuse perihilar infiltrations. Usually, the lungs are unblemished

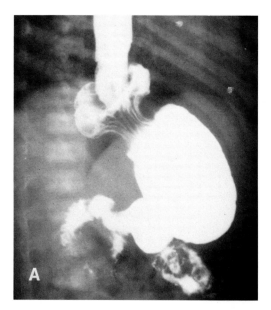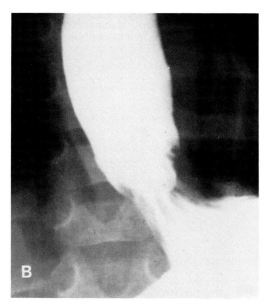

Fig. 6-59. Hiatal hernia. *(A)* A large sliding hiatal hernia is present. The gastric fundus with its many mucosal folds is seen "mushrooming" into the thorax. *(B)* A more subtle manifestation. The hiatal ring is patulous and multiple gastric folds are present.

in this age-group. As a result, fluid accumulation is not impeded by the presence of underlying disease within the lung (e.g., fibrosis or cysts) and disseminates uniformly and symmetrically throughout. The accumulation of fluid may not be easily recognized early, since it may be located within the insterstitium (Fig. 6-60) and can be confused with interstitial disease. The presence of distended upper lobe veins and Kerley's B lines are important radiographic findings, indicating edema. As the venous pressure continues to rise, alveolar filling begins, resulting in the classical "butterfly" pattern, with the perihilar and central lung regions involved and the peripheral lungs clear. The infiltrate, in addition, demonstrates all the radiographic manifestations of alveolar disease, with air bronchograms and ill-defined borders (Fig. 6-60).

Although pulmonary edema is often symmertrical and bilateral, it can sometimes present in a segmental, lobar, or unilateral distribution (Fig. 6-60). This presentation is usually transient and depends upon the stage of development of the edema, the position of the patient, and preexisting disease. Unilateral disease is occasionally seen after rapid re-expansion of the lung following pneumothorax.

An overwhelming infectious process may produce a diffuse exudate throughout the entire lungs that simulates edema. In this presentation, the infecting organisms are poorly contained and spread centrifugally throughout the bronchial passages. The initial changes, therefore, are more or less perihilar in distribution, although the entire lung fields are quickly involved. The absence of cardiac enlargement, congested veins, and lymphatics in a patient who appears septic, should suggest a diffuse exudative process. It is absolutely necessary to isolate the specific organism in order to determine the proper therapy.

Pneumocystis carinii pneumonia is an unusual infection caused by a protozoa. The radiographic presentation is somewhat characteristic, despite its remarkable similarity to that of pulmonary edema and diffuse exudative pneumonia. The pulmonary infiltrate begins in a specific perihilar distribution and slowly disseminates throughout the lung fields, with areas of coalescence (Fig. 6-61). The peripheral lung fields are spared initially, since the disease spreads centrifugally through the bronchial passages. Early in the course of the disease, a diffuse acinar pattern is produced that may resemble intersitial disease. As coalescense occurs, the alveolar nature of the disease becomes

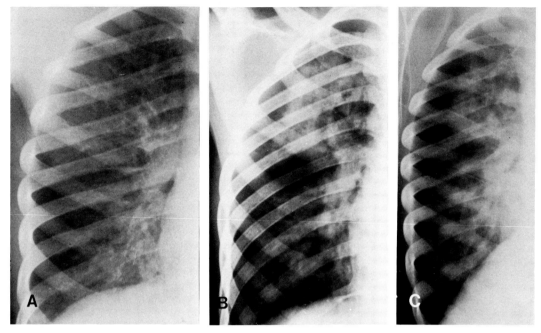

Fig. 6-60. Degrees of pulmonary edema. *(A)* Fluid is present within the interstitium. A diffuse reticular pattern throughout the upper and lower lung fields is apparent, with thickening of the horizontal fissure and Kerley's B lines. *(B)* Fluid accumulates within the upper lung field. *(C)* The classical picture of pulmonary edema is present with ill-defined margins and air bronchograms. The surrounding lung field is remarkably clear.

evident. In fact, when the entire lung fields are affected, the disease may completely resemble pulmonary edema. A specific diagnosis almost always depends upon identification of the organism, and lung biopsy is an important diagnostic modality in this respect.

A similar presentation occasionally occurs with pulmonary hemorrhage. Recurrent episodes are characteristic for idiopathic pulmonary hemosiderosis and Goodpasture's syndrome (Fig. 6-62). The radiographic findings are identical. In the early stages, the pattern is one of diffuse, mottled areas of radiopacity scattered evenly throughout the lungs. Distribution is widespread but is prominent in the perihilar area simulating pulmonary edema (Fig. 6-62D, E, F). The pulmonary infiltration resolves in a few days and becomes a reticular pattern as the intra-alveolar contents are transported by macrophages to the intersititial space and lymphatics. With repeated episodes, subsequent deposition of hemosiderin occurs, with intersititial fibrosis. Cor pulmonale eventually develops due to intersititial fibrosis.

Aspiration of gastric contents produces a chemical pneumonitis that can irritate the interalveolar septa, causing a diffuse transudation into the lungs. This stage is difficult to distinguish from ordinary edema if the antecedent is unobserved.

Many physicians compare the classical presentation of alveolar proteinosis to that of pulmonary edema. However, alveolar proteinosis, in contrast to most lesions with this presentation, is insidious and progressive in its development. Moreover, the disease has a strong propensity to begin in the lower lobes and progressively involves the entire lungs.

The important radiographic manifestations of pulmonary veno-occlusive disease consist of findings which indicate post-capillary hypertension, such as Kerley's B lines, pulmonary edema, and pleural fluid, and findings which indicate pulmonary arterial hypertension, such as dilated central pulmonary arteries. Large pulmonary venous engorgement is usually not seen, which allows differentiation from mitral stenosis and other disorders of the major pulmonary veins. Although there

(Text continued on p. 272.)

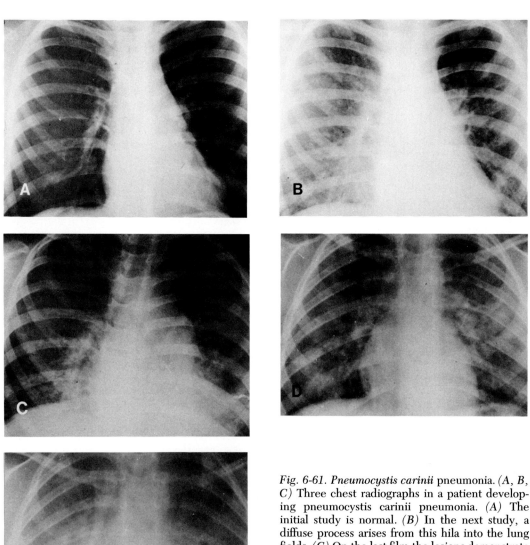

Fig. 6-61. *Pneumocystis carinii* pneumonia. (*A, B, C*) Three chest radiographs in a patient developing pneumocystis carinii pneumonia. (*A*) The initial study is normal. (*B*) In the next study, a diffuse process arises from this hila into the lung fields. (*C*) On the last film the lesions demonstrate further consolidation, and the alveolar character becomes obvious. (*D*) In another patient with diffuse changes throughout the lung fields, the initial film is somewhat patchy. (*E*) In a few days, despite the alveolar and interstitial location, the process is diffusely homogeneous.

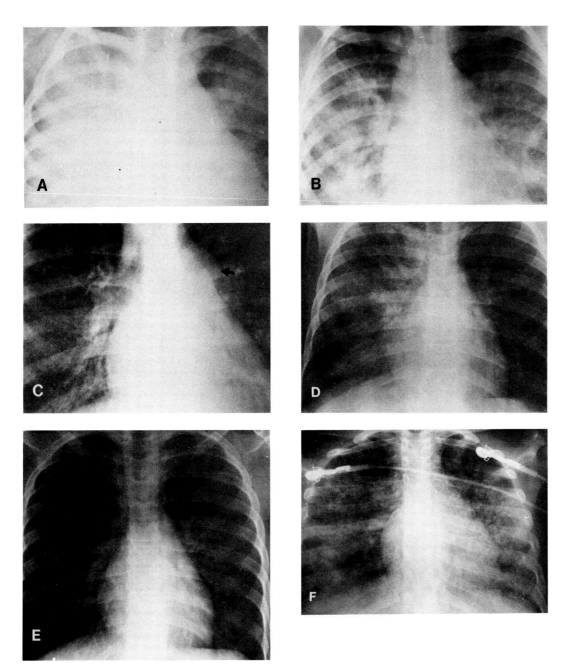

Fig. 6-62. Pulmonary hemorrhage. *(A, B, C)* Progression of idiopathic pulmonary hemosiderosis. *(A)* The initial study was performed at 2.5 years of age. Massive hemorrhage is seen throughout the lung fields, resembling pulmonary edema. *(B)* The patient returned to the hospital 5 years later with another episode of diffuse hemorrhage that appeared more patchy on the right. *(C)* At 14 years of age the chest radiograph demonstrates diffuse interstitial fibrosis associated with pulmonary hypertension. Note the size of the pulmonary artery *(arrows). (D, E, F)* Goodpasture's syndrome. *(D)* This is the initial film of an 8-year-old female with pulmonary hemorrhage, iron deficiency anemia, and renal disease. Patchy perihilar infiltration is noted on the right. *(E)* The patient's chest quickly returned to normal. *(F)* Eight days later, massive pulmonary hemorrhage recurred. Note the diffuse air bronchogram.

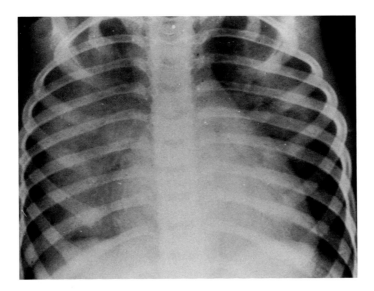

Fig. 6-63. Pulmonary edema and acute rheumatic fever with pericarditis. Pulmonary edema is present and is more extensive on the right than on the left. The peripheral lung fields are remarkably clear. Gross cardiac enlargement is obvious.

is moderate to severe elevation of the pulmonary artery pressure, the pulmonary wedge pressure is usually normal or slightly elevated because of venous runoff by way of collateral vessels.

Although extrinsic allergic alveolitis can be confused with edema because of its diffuse distribution, the main radiographic features are not homogenous but consist of a granular or nodular mottling of the lung fields.

Discussion

Pulmonary edema is likely to involve the central part of the lung or an individual lobe probably because of the underlying anatomy and physiology of the lung. A lobe can be structurally divided into a medulla and cortex. There is reason to believe that the outer cortex is involved in the ventilatory mechanics to a greater extent than is the central medulla; therefore, the outer cortex undergoes the greatest volume changes because of its ready distensibility. Lymphatic drainage, in general, depends upon the movement of adjacent structures and is thus greatly stimulated in the well ventilated parts, such as the cortex. This action is also aided in part by the compressing motions of the thoracic cage. The internal lymphatics lying deep within the parenchyma drain centrally toward the hilum and in pulmonary edema are unaided and incapable of emptying the boggy, swollen central lung fields.

The superficial, rapid respiratory motion of the lungs exerts no influence upon the central lymphatics.

Pulmonary edema is caused by a number of entities:

Cardiac Enlargement
1. Congenital heart disease
2. Rheumatic heart disease (acute or chronic)
3. Acute glomerulonephritis
4. Myocarditis
5. Cardiomyopathy

No Cardiac Enlargement
1. Neurogenic enlargement
   a. Head trauma
   b. Subarachnoid hemorrhage
2. Near drowning
3. Smoke inhalation
4. Aspiration
5. Allergic reaction (blood transfusion)
6. Drug abuse
7. Snake bite
8. Iatrogenic pulmonary edema

The causes of pulmonary edema can be divided into two categories based on the presence or absence of cardiac enlargement. In the group with cardiac enlargement, the size and configuration of the heart, as well as other associated radiographic findings, often indicates specific disease. However, the radiographic features in pulmonary edema

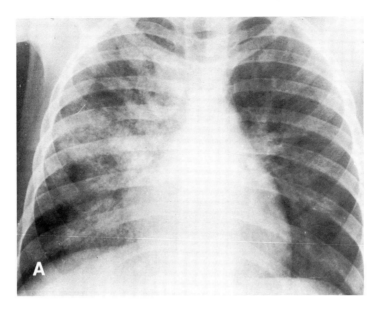

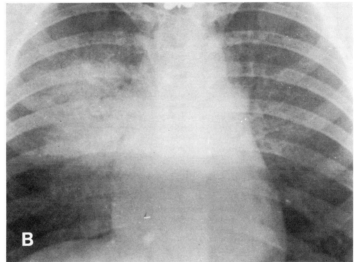

Fig. 6-64. Pulmonary edema. *(A)* Head trauma. Fairly well-defined perihilar edema is noted on the right. Early interstitial changes are also noted on the left. The patient had recent head injury. *(B)* Near drowning. Diffuse bilateral edema is noted. Note the predominant perihilar distribution on the right. Projected above the upper thoracic vertebra is a butterfly pendant.

without cardiac enlargement are nonspecific, and only close correlation with a precipitating event distinguishes the causative entities.

In general, rheumatic and congenital heart disease demonstrate specific characteristics (see Chapter 4). In most myocardiopathies the heart is grossly large. The left atrium is frequently dilated because of the restrictive motion of the left ventricle. Acute pulmonary edema associated with recent cardiac enlargement is often the result of acute rheumatic fever (Fig. 6-63), viral myocarditis, or glomerulonephritis.

A wide spectrum of abnormalities is re-

sponsible for producing pulmonary edema without cardiac enlargement, such as increased intracranial pressure due to recent brain injury (Fig. 6-64), convulsions, tumor, or hemorrhage. The pathophysiology is not completely understood, although bradycardia and peripheral vasoconstriction followed by lowered cardiac output and elevated venous and arterial pressures are believed to be responsible. Exposure to fire with smoke inhalation results in pulmonary edema. The onset of edema may not be instantaneous, and a victim of smoke or superheated air inhalation should be observed for at least 24 hours following exposure. Near drowning as a cause of pulmonary edema is becoming an increasing problem. In the state of Florida, drowning ranks third as the most common cause of death in children. Near drowning is defined as survival following asphyxia or aspiration due to submission in a fluid medium. Fluid aspiration is not required, in 10 to 20 per cent of the cases laryngospasm alone results in asphyxia. Although fresh and salt water aspiration behave physiologically somewhat differently, the final pathologic result in most cases is pulmonary edema. Hypertonic salt water draws water into the alveoli, producing immediate pulmonary edema. Fresh water, however, is hypotonic and water flows from the alveoli into the blood stream, causing hemodilution. In addition, the fresh water washes out the existing surfactant. This results in alveolar collapse, atelectasis, intrapulmonary shunting, and pulmonary edema (Fig. 6-64B). Pulmonary edema is more significant pathologically than hemodilution, which is only transient. If proper therapy is instituted the resulting pulmonary edema resolves in 3 to 5 days. Persistent pulmonary infiltrations beyond this time indicates superimposed infection. The introduction of excessive intravenous fluids results in iatrogenic pulmonary edema due to circulatory overload. Severe allergic responses to medication, contrast agents, and insect bites result in pulmonary edema in addition to urticaria, bronchospasm, and shock.

It is difficult to suggest what kind of mechanism is responsible for the development of unilateral pulmonary edema. However, rapid re-expansion of a lung causes a sudden increase in the negative intrapleural pressure, to which the lung responds with a rapid increase in pulmonary capillary pressure and blood flow, resulting in fluid transudation across the capillary and alveolar membranes. An associated anoxic effect upon the capillary membrane increases the probability of fluid accumulation.

Idiopathic pulmonary hemosiderosis and Goodpasture's syndrome have identical thoracic manifestations. Goodpasture's syndrome however, is also manifested by renal disease. The incidence of the two diseases differs, since hemosiderosis occurs mostly in young children, below the age of 10. Goodpasture's syndrome, by contrast, is a disease of young adults, over the age of 16. Iron deficiency anemia, hemoptysis, and specific radiographic changes usually indicate a diagnosis of idiopathic pulmonary hemosiderosis. Both diseases probably reflect an autoimmune process, affecting the alveolar capillary membrane. In Goodpasture's syndrome, however, hemoptysis usually precedes the clinical manifestations of renal disease by months.

Diffuse exudative pneumonia can be of either bacterial, fungal, or viral origin. There is often no radiographic means of distinguishing the three. The diagnosis is suggested by known exposure to a specific organism or by isolation of the organism. A diagnosis should be made as quickly as possible so proper antimicrobial therapy can be given before the patient is overwhelmed by infection.

Pneumocystis carinii pneumonia was originally recognized in Eastern European nurseries following World War II. It has been reported almost exclusively as an opportunistic infection in patients with congenital or acquired immunologic defects. It is now being encountered with increasing frequency as a common cause of diffuse progressive pneumonia in patients with underlying malignant disease. Percutaneous lung biopsy has markedly increased the number of early diagnoses.

Pulmonary alveolar proteinosis is a rare disease of unknown eitiology characterized by the deposition within the air spaces of a somewhat granular material, high in protein and lipid content, that is PAS-positive. It is believed that the material is derived from or is secreted by the Type II pneumocyte.

The pathologic hallmark of pulmonary veno-occlusive disease is narrowing and obliteration of the lumina of small pulmonary veins and venules by minimal fibrous tissue proliferation. Although the occlusions are thrombotic in origin, the basic cause still remains a mystery.

REVERSE PULMONARY EDEMA

Reverse pulmonary edema has a radiographic appearance which is the photographic negative, or the reversal, of the usual shadows noted in pulmonary edema. The infiltrative process is located peripherally within the lung fields. The central lung fields are relatively normal and radiolucent.

Disease Entities
Chronic eosinophilic pneumonia
Sarcoidosis
Löffler's pneumonia
Collagen disease
Parasitic infestation

Differential Diagnosis

The radiographic presentation is remarkably similar in all of the diseases above, despite the different clinical presentations. Chronic eosinophilic pneumonia, which represents the prototype of diseases which produce reverse pulmonary edema, has not yet been encountered in children. The characteristic radiographic feature, however, is a "ground glass" infiltration that arises in the peripheral lung fields. The lesion consists of multiple radiopaque areas with ill-defined margins that do not conform to any segment or lobe but border the periphery of the lungs, apposed to the pleura. More often the lesions involve the upper or lower lateral lung and occasionally occur first in one lung and then the other. The lesions vary in size but may fill an entire lung field if untreated. Laminography will show a clear central zone. If the lesions regress and then recur, they usually involve the same part of the lung. In general, an elevated level of eosinophils is present, and the clinical and radiographic response to steroid therapy is dramatic.

Pulmonary sarcoidosis presents in a number of patterns, one of which is a soft, fluffy infiltration that involves the outer peripheral borders of the lung. In contrast to chronic eosinophilic pneumonia however, it is likely to affect the outer central third of the lung. It is relatively homogeneous in appearance, manifests air bronchograms, and has therefore been described as alveolar sarcoidosis. This description is somewhat ambiguous, since sarcoidosis is basically a process restricted to the interstitium. However, a number of findings may account for this presentation. Histologic sections through nodular infiltrates often demonstrate massive conglomerations of large granulomas compressing and squeezing alveoli, thus producing a pseudoalveolar pattern. We have also noted actual filling of the alveoli with cells that resemble histiocytes. Lastly, cholesterol pneumonia due to bronchial obstruction has been described as another contributing factor.

Certain collagen disorders present with peripheral infiltrations. In all probability the underlying pathology is related to a vasculitis and therefore resembles the pattern of a hemorrhagic infarction.

A changing peripheral pattern may be encountered in Löffler's pneumonia, in which infiltrations disappear and then reappear in other portions of the lung fields. In addition, during their life cycle certain parasites migrate through the lung fields before reaching the intestine. Some individuals respond with an allergic reaction during this migration. The common parasites responsible are Ascaris, Strongyloides, and Schistosoma.

RADIODENSE, THICKENED PLEURAL SPACE

The healthly, normal pleurae are almost too fine and thin to be radiographically visible, although interlobar fissures are occasionally demonstrable when viewed end on. The azygous fissure extends as a vertical line from the apex toward the hilum. This fissure varies in thickness because two layers of complete pleurae are present on both sides of the anomalous cleft in the lung that is produced by the azygous vein. The caudal end of the oblique fissure is occasionally visualized when it projects somewhat ectopically forward so that part of it is exposed in an axial projection. This occurs in association with cardiomegaly or deficient aeration of the lung.

Disease Entities
Pleural effusion
Pleural fibrosis
Neoplasm

Differential Diagnosis

Pleural fluid is usually manifested by a thickened, lateral pleural stripe or by blunting of the costophrenic space. Pleural fluid may assume many configurations. In general, it begins in the subpulmonary region and may remain there for a period of time, where it generally assumes the contour of the diaphragm (Figs. 6-65, 6-66). It looks like a relatively high and flat curve, and on the left the fundus of the stomach is located lower than anticipated. If the film is exposed with the patient in a supine position, pleural fluid is

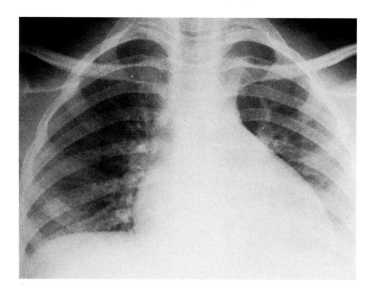

Fig. 6-65. Acute glomerulonephritis. Note the classic triad: Diffuse congestive changes are associated with cardiac enlargement and bilateral infrapulmonary pleural effusions.

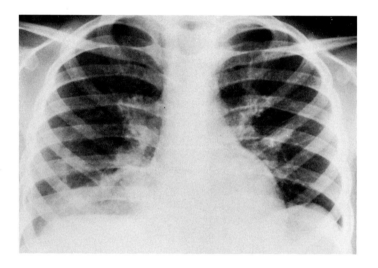

Fig. 6-66. Nephrotic syndrome. Bilateral subpulmonary effusions are present. Some fluid extends along the lateral chest wall and in the oblique fissure. The right diaphragm appears flat, and the apex of the curve is displaced laterally. The heart is of normal caliber.

positioned along the dorsal surface of the thorax, producing an overall increase in radiodensity within the hemithorax. A large accumulation of fluid is easy to recognize, since it obscures the underlying lung and diaphragm (Fig. 6-6). If the fluid fills an entire hemithorax, that side is completely obscured by a homogeneous radiodensity. The underlying lung is obviously compressed, and the diaphragm is flattened. Eventual inversion of the diaphragm with associated paradoxical respiratory motion of the diaphragm ensues, causing severe respiratory difficulty.

Radiographic examination of the chest in different positions, such as a lateral decubitus position, usually alleviates some of the problems that may arise when trying to distinguish free pleural fluid from a mass or loculate fluid. Free fluid generally separates into layers under the influence of gravity. Loculate fluid resembles a pleural-based tumor. Both present as a round or oval mass that projects away from the pleural surface. A pleural tumor in this age-group, however, is quite rare.

Discussion

A number of types of fluid collect within the pleura, depending upon the nature of the underlying disease process. For example, hydrothorax occurs readily in hypoproteinemia states, such as nephrosis and protein enteropathy. Hydrothorax is commonly

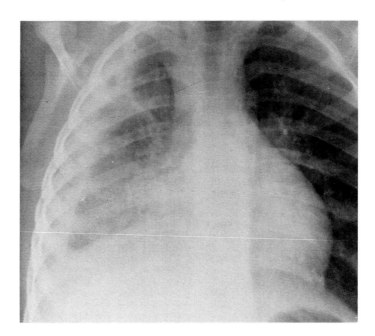

Fig. 6-67. Pneumococcal pneumonia with empyema. A pneumococcal pneumonia of the right lower and middle lobes associated with a large empyema is present in the right hemithorax.

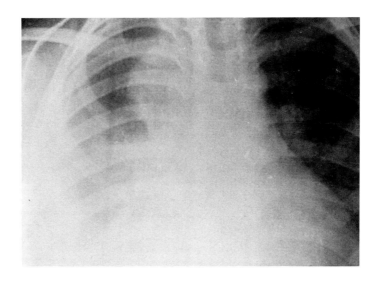

Fig. 6-68. Primary tuberculosis with large pleural effusion. A huge lymph node is located in the right paratrachael area associated with a large pleural effusion. A poorly visible pneumonic infiltration is present in the right lower lobe.

bilateral and without symptoms and, although a common finding in adults with congestive heart failure, it is not often seen in the pediatric age-group, surprisingly.

Inflammation of the pleura is the result of bacterial infection and a number of viral diseases. Pleural involvement in rheumatic fever is not unusual and occasional association with collagen disease has also been observed.

Small to moderate accumulation of pleural fluid is encountered in any form of pneumonia. Consequently, the presence of an ipsilateral, widened pleural stripe adja-

cent to an area of pneumonia is not unusual. Prior to the introduction of antibiotic therapy, this was seen in 10 per cent of all pneumococcal pneumonias (Fig. 6-67). Staphylococcal pneumonia, however, is notoriously associated with the highest incidence of pleural reactions. The fluid accumulation is often an empyema. In the early stages of the disease, the effusion may appear sterile on gross inspection. However, eventually it becomes thick and greenish due to the presence of cells and fibrin. Hemophilus and Klebsiella pneumonias, although far less frequent, are commonly associated with em-

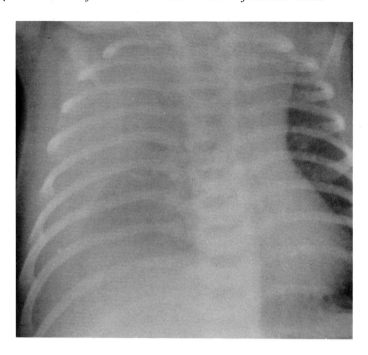

Fig. 6-69. Chylothorax. A large fluid collection is shown within the right hemithorax; lymph was revealed upon thoracentesis.

pyema. In one series of 10 patients with *Hemophilus influenzae* pneumonia, pleural effusion or thickening was noted on admission in all 10 patients (Fig. 6-9). The effusion is always located on the side of the pneumonia and persists for some time following resolution of the parenchymal infiltration. The usual features of primary tuberculosis, consisting of a primary parenchymal focus plus regional nodal enlargement, are frequently accompanied by a pleural effusion of variable size. As opposed to other bacterial infections, the patient is usually asymptomatic and the effusion is only of short duration. In the young adult, tuberculous effusions can be quite massive (Fig. 6-68) and may be the only manifestation of the disease, since the underlying parenchymal focus may be too small to be visible or may be completely obscured by the effusion.

Pleural effusion is an important manifestation of acute glomerulonephritis. It occurs in approximately 75 per cent of afflicted patients. The effusion is frequently infrapulmonary and is consequently often unobserved (Fig. 6-65). The fluid collects in such a location because of its high protein content, which decreases its mobility. Other characteristic radiographic findings noted in acute glomerulonephritis are cardiomegaly and congestive changes (Fig. 6-65). The presence

of this classic triad on the chest radiograph is almost pathognomonic. Pulmonary edema and pneumonia complete the spectrum but are less common. In general, the findings are caused by water rentention and overload and disappear rapidly following diuresis.

The nephrotic syndrome is also associated with bilateral pleural effusions. However, the heart size is small because of the diminished intravascular volume (Fig. 6-66).

Pleural effusions may also be the result of metastatic disease. This is relatively uncommon in children, although any tumor has the potential of affecting the pleura and provoking a reaction. Of diseases which affect the pleura, acute leukemia is the most important.

A hemothorax may result following trauma to the chest if at the time of injury a fractured rib perforates an intercostal vessel. We have witnessed an unusual accumulation of pleural fluid a few days following blunt trauma to the chest; there was no apparent rib injury and the consistency of the fluid was that of a transudate. The fluid accumulation was probably related to pleural contusion, since it regressed rapidly.

An interesting and rare form of pleural effusion is chylothorax (Fig. 6-69). Distinction from other forms of pleural effusion can be made only by examining the fluid. However, in newborns this fluid may be clear initially.

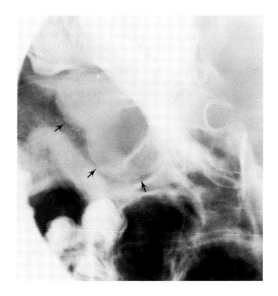

Fig. 6-70. Adenoid hyperplasia. Large lobular adenoids are noted within the epipharynx *(arrows).*

Fat globulins are responsible for producing the opalescent fluid and become established only after milk feeding. In newborns, the etiology is unclear. Lymphedema may also be present.

In older children, chylothorax is usually the result of trauma with rupture of the duct, although pressure exerted by a tumor or enlarged lymph nodes can cause leakage of chyle.

UPPER RESPIRATORY TRACT OBSTRUCTION

Upper respiratory tract obstruction is a significant problem in infants and children. There are a number of diseases, which can be acute or chronic, and some may be life-threatening. The radiologic examination plays an important role in locating and diagnosing these lesions. However, certain basic facts should considered before approaching the major problems. The lateral film of the neck and pharynx is the most important examination in evaluating obstructions in the upper respiratory tract.

The physician should be aware that adenoid tissue is not well developed in the first 6 to 8 weeks of life but becomes quite prominent in older children. Also, the retropharyngeal soft tissues vary in thickness during normal respiration. Considerable anterior buckling of the trachea occurs during the expiratory phase and may, at times, result in the false impression of a re-

tropharyngeal mass. Examination of the neck should therefore be made in both inspiratory and respiratory phases, with the neck held absolutely straight during the examination.

Disease Entities
Lesions of the nasopharynx
   Adenoid hyperplasia
   Tumors
Lesions of the oropharynx
   Enlarged tongue (Pierre Robin syndrome)
   Tonsillar abscess
   Hygroma
   Goiter
   Cysts
Lesions of the hypopharynx and larynx
   Foreign body
   Web
   Stenosis
   Epiglotitis
   Tracheobronchitis
   Tumor

Differential Diagnosis

On the lateral radiograph masses in the epipharynx are large, composed of soft tissue, and occupy most of the normal air column. Although the size and location may be determined on the radiographic examination, the exact nature of the lesion often requires tissue diagnosis. Adenoid tissue alone can become quite hyperplastic and simulate a neoplasm (Fig. 6-70). For the most part, it

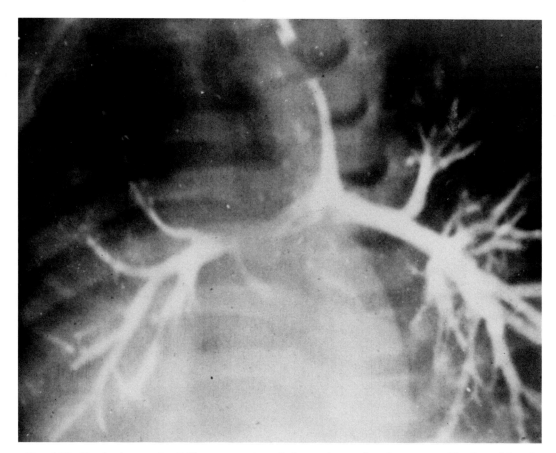

Fig. 6-71. Tracheal stenosis. Diffuse narrowing of the entire trachea is present. The bronchi and their branches appear normal.

remains localized in the area of its origin and maintains its original configuration to some degree. Tumors in this area are uncommon in children and give rise to symptoms of respiratory obstruction, nasal discharge, and epistaxis. Recurrent or persistant sinusitis is another clinical manifestation. The most common tumor encountered may be the nasal polyp, which is not a true lesion of the nasopharynx but originates in the paranasal sinus and prolapses posteriorly. Papillomas are structurally similar to the polyp but differ histologically. The tumor is found commonly at the base of the uvula and has a propensity to recur following removal. Nasopharyngeal angiofibroma is a highly vascular tumor that occurs in the nasopharynx, particularly in males between the ages of 10 and 20 years. Epistaxis is a common clinical finding. The tumor is relatively benign and does not metastasize. It does, however, have a strong capacity to grow, infiltrate, and destroy neighboring bone and soft tissues. The main

radiographic features consist of a large, highly invasive tumor that grows into the neighboring nasal cavity and paranasal sinuses. An "antral" sign, which depicts bowing of the posterior walls of the maxillary bone of the involved side, has been described and is considered pathognomonic of nasopharyngeal angiofibroma. Other tumors, such as rhabdomyosarcoma and lymphoepithelioma, are also encountered in this area. Carcinomas of this region are rare and are most likely related to lymphoepithelioma.

A large tongue is an important finding in the Pierre Robin syndrome. This is associated with a hypoplastic mandible and posterior prolapse and retrodisplacement of the tongue itself, which impinges upon the posterior wall of the pharynx and is responsible for respiratory obstruction. Other abnormalities associated with a large tongue are Down's syndrome, Cretinism, and the Beckwith-Wiedemann syndrome.

Diseases arising in the retropharyneal area

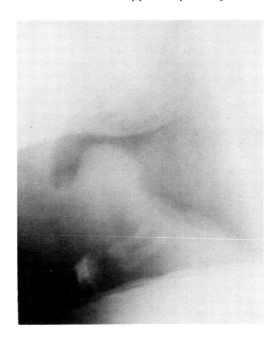

Fig. 6-72. Epiglottitis. The entire epiglottis and aryepiglottic folds are markedly swollen.

are easily diagnosed by the presence of a large, soft-tissue mass causing anterior displacement of the trachea. In the 1st years of life this arises secondary to infection from penetrating injury. Some of these masses are relatively asymptomatic and appear later as a paraesophageal diverticulum. Diagnosis of a retropharnyngeal abscess must be established early and treated in order to prevent further growth of this lesion into the esophagus, mediastinum, or the surrounding tissues. Retropharyngeal goiter and cystic hygroma are usually fairly well-defined and present in the neonatal period for the most part. They are not often seen in older children. Both are benign lesions and produce little symptomatology aside from the results of size and location.

Foreign bodies in the hypopharynx and larynx usually deposit in the region of the cricopharyngeal muscle, cause difficulty in swallowing, and are associated with drooling. However, if sufficient edema occurs the airway is narrowed and respiratory difficulties ensue. Similar airway narrowing occurs following inflammatory disease, particularly severe burns of the pharynx following ingestion of caustic substances. This can cause fibrosis and destruction of the cartilage and bony structures. Developmental abnormalities of the larynx, such as congential web, glottic stenosis, and cartilage dysplasia, result in respiratory difficulties. Generally, these are found in newborns. Congenital or acquired

tracheal stenosis may also result in airway obstruction (Fig. 6-71).

Inflammatory lesions are the most common laryngeal abnormalities which cause respiratory distress. The two principal considerations are epiglottitis and croup (laryngotracheobronchitis). Both are often acute and marked by air hunger associated with substernal inspiratory retractions, tachypnea, and tachycardia. The epiglottis is swollen and displaced posteriorly. Most often the diagnosis can be established by direct inspection. However, radiographic examination of the neck is useful in those cases where the diagnosis is in doubt. The epiglottis appears enlarged and swollen. The aryepiglottic folds are also quite thickened (Fig. 6-72). Diffuse edema caused by an allergic reaction, angioneurotic edema, produces a similar radiographic appearance. However, the findings differ in croup, where the subglottic portion of the trachea is thin and narrow. This usually extends below the glottis, with the glottis and epiglottis remaining normal (Fig. 6-73). Traumatic lesions of the larynx may result in respiratory obstruction. Foreign bodies and tumors in this area are quite unusual and rare (Fig. 6-74, 6-75).

Discussion

Recent attention has been drawn to upper respiratory tract obstruction caused by hypertrophic tonsils and adenoids. In some children this abnormality has resulted in

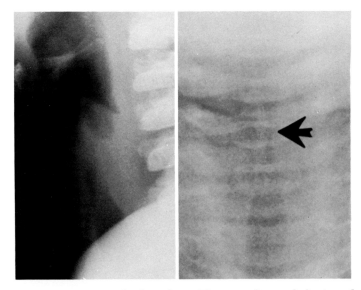

Fig. 6-73. Acute tracheobronchitis. The immediate subglottic and upper tracheal region is distinctly narrowed *(arrow).* Although the patient's symptoms are identical to those of epiglottis, the radiographic findings reveal that the inflammatory process is below the region of the glottis, and the epiglottis is normal.

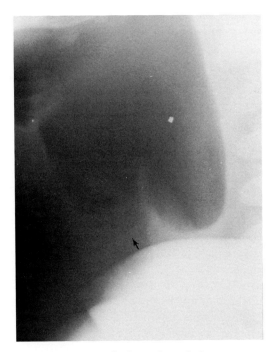

Fig. 6-74. Foreign body in the subglottic region. The epipharynx is markedly distended due to obstruction of the upper airway. A barely discernible foreign body is noted in the subglottic region *(arrow).*

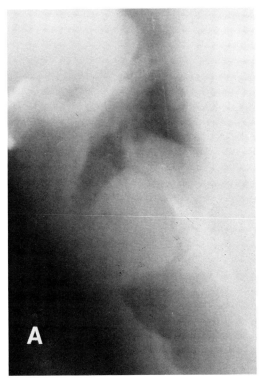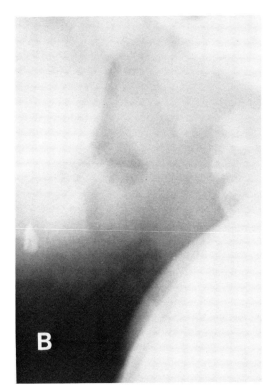

Fig. 6-75. Masses in the larynx. *(A)* Subglottic papilloma. A large, well-defined soft-tissue mass occupies and obstructs the glottis. *(B)* Subglottic hamartoma. A mass is present within the subglottic area. This lesion simulates a hemangioma.

pulmonary hypertension and congestive heart failure. In general, obstruction of the airway results in hypoxia and hypercapnia. Pulmonary hypertension is thought to be the find result of chronic hypoxia or carbon dioxide retention. Acute obstruction may present with pulmonary edema.

A papilloma is a true neoplasm composed of masses of stratified squamous tissue in papillary formation and therefore differs from a nasopharyngeal polyp. Polyps are more frequently inflammatory in origin and recur if the primary abnormality is not controlled.

REFERENCES

The Partially or Totally Opacified Lung

1. Fernald, G. W., Collier, A. M., and Clyde, W. A., Jr.: Respiratory infection due to *Mycoplasma pneumoniae* in infants and children. Pediatrics, 55:327, 1975.
2. Putman, C. E., Curtis, A., Simeone, J. E., and Jensen, P.: Mycoplasma pneumonia. Am. J. Roentgenol. Radium Ther. Nucl. Med., 124:417, 1975.
3. Reed, M. H.: Radiology of airway foreign bodies in children. J. Can. Assoc. Radiol., 28:111, 1977.
4. Specht, E. E.: Pulmonary hematoma. Am. J. Dis. Child., 111:559, 1966.
5. Vinik, M., Altman, D. H., and Parks, R. E. Experience with *Hemophilus influenzae* pneumonia. Radiology, 86:701, 1966.

The Dirty Lung

6. Anderson, L. S., Schaekelford, G. D., Mancilla-Jimenez, R., and McAlister, W. H.: Cartilaginous esophageal ring: cause of esophageal stenosis in infants and children. Radiology, 108:665, 1973.
7. Kirkpatrick, J. A., Capitanio, M. A., and Pereira, R. M.: Immunologic abnormalities: roentgen observation. Radiol. Clin. North. Am., 10:245, 1972.
8. Liebow, A. A., Sher, A., and Billingsly, J. G.: Disquamative interstitial pneumonia. Am. J. Med., 39:369, 1965.
9. Mitchell, R. E., and Bury, R. G.: Congenital bronchiectasis due to deficiency of bronchial cartilage (William-Campbell syndrome). J. Pediatr., 87:230, 1975.
10. Schneider, R. M., Durius, D. B., and Brown, H. Z.: Disquamative interstitial pneumonia in a 4-year-old child. N. Engl. J. Med., 277:1056, 1967.

Nodular Thoracic Masses

11. Bar-Ziv, J., and Nogrady, M. D.: Mediastinal neuroblastoma and ganglioneuroma: differentiation between primary and seconary involvement on the chest roentgenogram. Am. J. Roentgenol. Radium Ther. Nucl. Med., *125:* 380, 1975.
12. Bower, R. J., and Kiesewetter, W. B.,: Mediastinal masses in infants and children. Arch. Surg., *112:*1003, 1977.
13. Eraklis, A. J., Griscom, N. T., and McGovern, J. B.: Bronchogenic cysts of the mediastinum in infancy. N. Engl. J. Med., *281:*1150, 1969.
14. Kinkabwala, M. H., Becker, J. A., and Rabinowitz, J. G.: Osle-Weber-Render syndrome with multiple angiographic findings. Br. J. Radiol., *45:*534, 1972.
15. Pearl, M., and Wooley, M. W.: Pulmonary xanthomatous post-inflammatory pseudotumors in children. J. Pediatr. Surg., *8:*255, 1973.
16. Siltzbach, L. E., and Greenberg, G. M.: Childhood sarcoidosis—a study of 18 patients. N. Engl. J. Med., *279:*1239, 1968.
17. Talner, L. B., Gnelich, J. T., Liebow, A. A., and Greenspan, R. H.: The syndrome of bronchial mucocoele and regional hyperinflation of the lung. Am. J. Roentgenol. Radium Ther. Nucl. Med., *110:*675, 1970.
18. Wieder, S., and Rabinowitz, J. G.: Radiographic findings of fibrosing mediastinitis. Radiology, *125:*305, 1977.

Diseases Which Result in a Micronodular Pattern

19. Fraser, R. G., and Pare, J. A. P.: Extrinsic allergic alveolitis Semin. Roentgenol., *10:*31, 1975.
20. Siltzbach, L. E., and Greenberg, G. N.: Childhood sarcoidosis—a study of eighteen patients. N. Engl. J. Med., *279:*1239, 1968.
21. Rabinowitz, J. G., Ullrich, S., and Soriano, N. G.: Usual unusual manifestations of sarcoidosis and the hilar haze. Am. J. Roentgenol. Radium Ther. Nucl. Med., *120:*821, 1974.

Abnormal Areas of Radiolucency in the Thorax

22. Darling, D. B., Fisher, J. H., and Gellis, S.: Hiatal hernea and gastroesphogeal reflux in infants and children: Analysis of the incidence in North American children Pediatrics, *54:*450, 1974.
23. Dines, D. E.: Diagnostic significance of pneumatocoele of the lung. J.A.M.A., *204:* 1169, 1968.
24. Dines, D. E., et al.: Malignant pulmonary neoplasmas predisposing to spontaneous pneumothorax. Mayo Clin. Proc., *48:*541, 1973.
25. Harris, V. J., and Brown, R.: Pneumatoceles as a complication of chemical pneumonia after hydrocarbon ingestion. Am. J. Roentgenol. Radium Ther. Nucl. Med., *125:*531, 1975.
26. Kogett, M., Swischuk, L., and Goldblum, R.: Swyer-James syndrome in children. Am. J. Dis. Child., *125:*614, 1973.
27. Roland, A. S., Merdinger, W. F., and Froeb, H. F.: Recurrent spontaneous pneumothorax. A clue to diagnosis of histiocytosis. N. Engl. J. Med., *270:*73, 1964.
28. Swyer, R., and James, G.: A Case of unilateral pulmonary emphysema. Thorax, *8:*133, 1953.

Diffuse Perihilar Infiltrations

29. Fandel, I., and Bancalari, E.: Near drowning in children: clinical aspects. Pediatrics, *58:*573, 1976.
30. Felman, A. H.: Neurogenic pulmonary edema—observation in 6 patients. Am. J. Roentgenol. Radium Ther. Nucl. Med., *112:*393, 1971.
31. Fleischner, F. G.: The butterfly pattern of acute pulmonary edema. Am. J. Cardiol., *20:*39, 1967.
32. Forrest, J. V.: Radiographic findings in *Pneumocystis carinii* pneumonia. Radiology, *103:*539, 1972.
33. Harle, T. S., Kountoupis, J. T., Boone, M. L. M., and Fred, H. L.: Pulmonary edema without cardiomegaly Am. J. Roentgenol. Radium Ther. Nucl. Med., *103:*555, 1968.
34. Schackelford, G. D., Sacks, E. J., Mullens, J. D., and McAlister, W. H.: Pulmonary veno-occlusive disease: case report and review of literature. Am. J. Roentgenol. Radium Ther. Nucl. Med., *128:*643, 1977.
35. Steckel, R. J.: Unilateral pulmonary edema after pneumothorax. N. Engl. J. Med., *289:*621, 1973.

Upper Respiratory Tract Obstruction

36. Capitanio, M. A., and Kirkpatrick, J. A.: Upper respiratory tract obstruction in infants and children. Radiol. Clin. North Am., *6:*265, 1968.

7 | Barry Gerald, M.D.

Systematic Radiographic Evaluation of the Abnormal Skull

Diagnostically, radiographs of the skull in infants and children are far more important than in adults, since they are often associated with bone changes in disease that affects the skull or brain. Moreover, the multiple congenital defects that may appear in childhood are often associated with abnormalities that are detectable on skull radiographs. The malleability of the skull in children allows for easier and earlier recognition of increased intracranial pressure, although determination of the underlying process may require more extensive investigation. Infections of the central nervous system are often associated with intracranial calcifications and increased intracranial pressure. The use of radiographic examinations in trauma to the skull is very well known and probably excessive.

In children skull radiographs are more difficult to interpret than in adults because of the continual change in size, contour, and degree of ossification that occurs from year to year due to growth of the brain and body. Therefore, physicians must be familiar with the normal appearance of the skull at several stages of development in order to interpret any abnormality.

Computerized tomography is becoming a vital modality in evaluating diseases of the brain in all age-groups.

SINGLE RADIOLUCENT DEFECTS OF THE SKULL

When a radiolucent defect of the skull is recognized the physician must decide if it represents a normal structure, an anomaly, or a pathologic process. Important considerations are the location of the defect, whether there is soft-tissue involvement, the table or tables of bones of the skull involved, and whether the borders of the defect are sharp, ill-defined, or sclerotic.

Disease Entities

Anomalous apertures
   Emissary veins
   Parietal foramina
Meningoencephalocele
Dermal sinus
Epidermoid tumor (cholesteatoma)
Fracture of the skull
Leptomeningeal cyst ("growing" fracture)
Eosinophilic granuloma
Hemangioma
Osteomyelitis
Neurofibromatosis
Operative defects
Abnormal intracranial masses

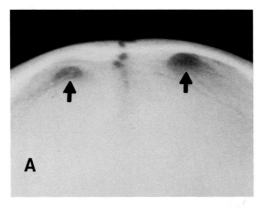
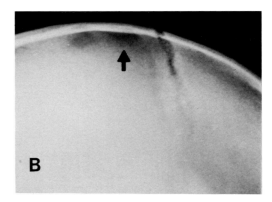
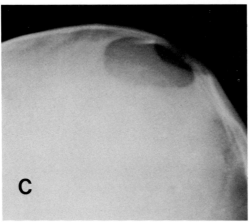

Fig. 7-1. Parietal foramen. *(A)* Frontal and *(B)* lateral projections demonstrate symmetrical, radiolucent defects with sharp borders in both parietal regions *(arrows). (C)* Similar, but larger, defects are shown in the posterior parietal region.

Differential Diagnosis

Anomalous apertures in general have sharp and often sclerotic borders. Transosseous emmissary veins are usually seen in the mid-portion of the occipital bone and in the posterior parietal regions. These structures have no pathologic significance but may enlarge with chronically increased intracranial pressure. Parietal foramina (Fig. 7-1) are seen in the superior and posterior portions of the parietal bones. Usually these apertures are paired and symmetrical. However, they can be asymmetrical in size and occasionally even fuse, forming a single foramen. Closely related but rarely observed are the anteriorly located frontal foramina (Fig. 7-20).

Meningoencephaloceles are severe malformations located in the midline of the skull and most frequently in the frontal or occipital regions (Fig. 7-2). The bony defects produced are radiolucent, with sharp borders that are occasionally beveled. A soft-tissue mass is prominent. In the 1st 3 months of life, a lucunar skull, or lückenshädel, is often present with this malformation.

A dermal sinus also occurs in the midline of the skull and presents as a radiolucent defect with sharp, slightly sclerotic borders (Fig. 7-3). Overlying soft-tissue changes, such as a nevus or lipoma, may be present. These lesions may have an intracranial component which requires extensive radiologic procedures for documentation.

Epidermoid tumors (Fig. 7-4) develop from a congenital inclusion of epithelial cells within the calvarium. Although referred to as cholesteatomas, these lesions are distinctly different from the inflammatory mastoid process which involves the petrous bone and results in extensive bone destruction. Radiographically, an epidermoid tumor has sharp, well circumscribed, sclerotic borders, which may be lobulated. These lesions are not likely to occur in the midline, in contrast to the dermal sinus.

Linear, non-depressed fractures (Fig. 7-5) are the most common radiolucent, pathologic defects seen in the skull. The possibility of incorrectly identifying a fracture is a continuing source of worry to many physicians. However, it is doubtful that identification of a

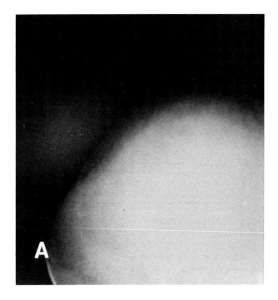

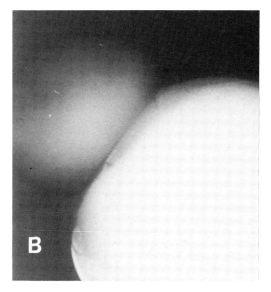

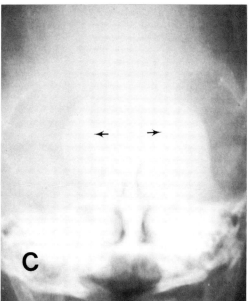

Fig. 7-2. Encephalocele. *(A)* A large midline bony defect is present in the posterior parietal region. *(B)* The same film, but of a different radiodensity, better manifests the soft-tissue mass. *(C)* A bony defect in the fronto-ethmoid area associated with a soft-tissue mass indicates a frontal encephalocele. Note the increased distance between the medial walls of the orbit (orbital hypertelorism).

linear fracture on a radiograph is of great importance; a careful neurologic examination is more informative.

A fracture is manifested by a thin, radiolucent line with sharp borders. This line is basically straight, but acute deviations and branching may occur. Fractures usually occur at the site of trauma. Contrecoup fractures are rare, although contrecoup brain damage is frequent. Therefore, a radiolucent line located beneath a hematoma is more significant than one which is not located at the site of trauma. A fracture must be differentiated from a suture and from vascular markings. A suture is in a predictable location and

in older children has serrated, sawtooth edges. The metopic suture (running vertically in the mid-portion of the frontal bone) and the mendosal suture (in the occipital bone) are two common accessory sutures.

Vascular grooves have ill-defined borders and an undulating course (Fig. 7-6). The groove for the middle meningeal artery and vein near the coronal suture is the most frequently seen. Short, straight, vertical lines may be seen in the squamosal portion of the temporal bone. These are grooves along the outer table of bones of the skull, formed by branches of the superficial temporal artery.

(Text continued on p. 290.)

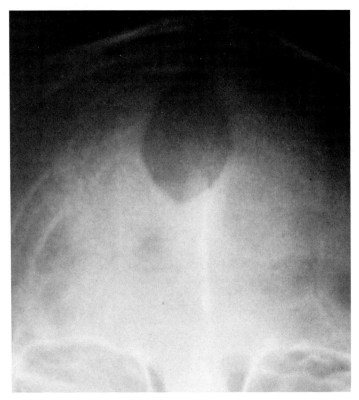

Fig. 7-3. Dermal sinus. A midline bony defect is shown with sharp, slightly sclerotic borders.

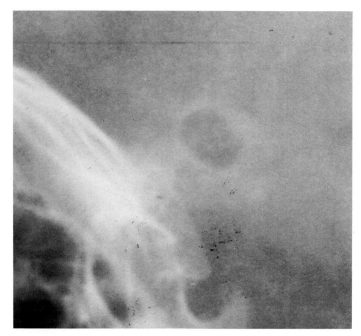

Fig. 7-4. Epidermoid tumor. Note the oval-shaped, bony defect with a sharp, sclerotic border.

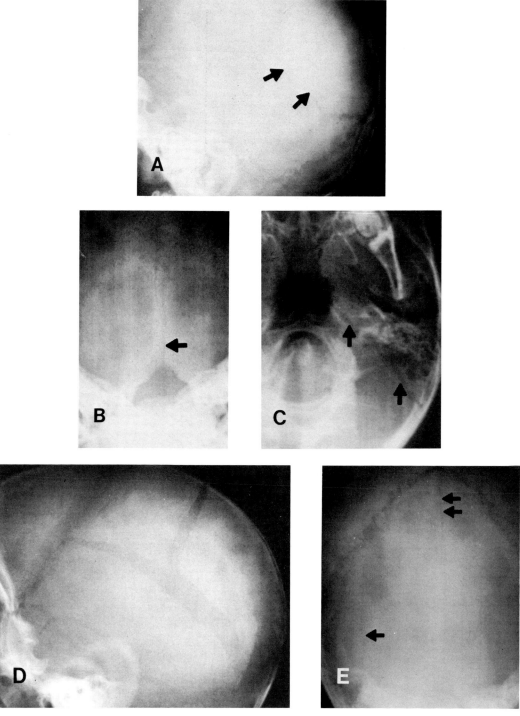

Fig. 7-5. Linear skull fractures. *(A)* A parietal linear fracture is shown *(arrows)* with sharp borders and abrupt changes in course. *(B)* An occipital fracture extending into the foramen magnum *(arrow)*. A fracture in this location is difficult to differentiate from the midoccipital synchondrosis. Correlation of the site of trauma with the radiographic abnormality is essential. *(C)* A basal skull fracture. The fracture *(arrows)* extends from the occipital bone through the medial portion of the left petrous pyramid. It is unusual to see a fracture of the skull base this well. *(D)* A wide fracture line extending from the coronal to the lamboid suture. A vertical limb extends to the sagittal suture. *(E)* A fracture *(single arrow)* in the right occipital area. The vertical line extending from the lambda *(double arrow)* is an anomalous suture but can easily be confused with a fracture.

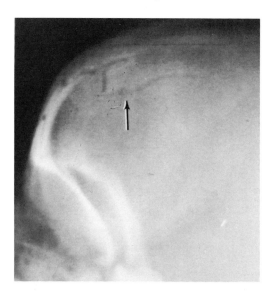

Fig. 7-6. Venous grooves in the frontal bone. These venous grooves look like a fracture but have an undulating course with ill-defined margins *(arrow)*.

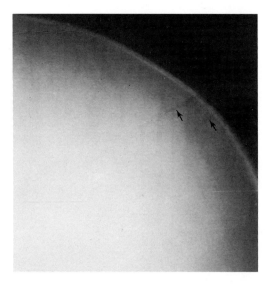

Fig. 7-7. Parietal fissures. These normal radiolucent defects *(arrows)* resemble fractures but represent strips of unossified membrane.

In newborns, short, radiolucent lines may be seen extending from the sagittal suture into the parietal bones (Fig. 7-7). These are normal strips of unossified membrane.

A depressed fracture has a more unfavorable prognosis than a linear fracture. Usually the trauma is severe, and clinical findings of brain damage are often present. Radiographically the depressed, overlapping bone fragments present as an area of increased radiodensity. This area may be surrounded on one side by a radiolucent halo where there is no bone, or it may demonstrate actual fracture lines radiating from the depressed area (Fig. 7-8). It may be necessary to obtain radiographs with oblique views, taken with the beam tangential to the fracture, to be certain that a depressed fragment is present (Fig. 7-8C).

In infants the skull may be depressed inward as a result of trauma; this is called a "ping-pong" fracture. A definite fracture line may not be seen. Again, tangential views may be required to show the lesion well.

It is most difficult to estimate the age of a fracture radiographically. Healing is accompanied by blurring of the sharp margins of the fracture, but progressive change is quite slow. The average time for a fracture to heal in a child is estimated at 1 year.

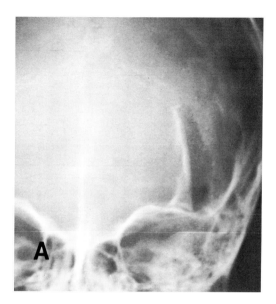

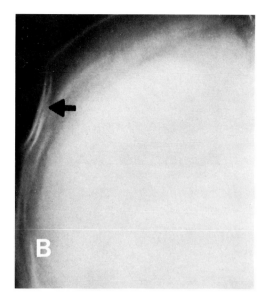

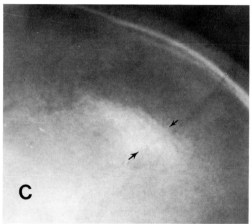

Fig. 7-8. Depressed fractures. *(A)* A depressed frontal fracture as shown by increased bone density surrounded by a zone of radiolucency. *(B)* On the lateral view, only an area of increased bone density is seen in the mid-parietal region *(arrows)*. *(C)* This is a tangential view of a depressed fracture *(arrow)* in the parietal bone.

A leptomeningeal cyst is a complication of a fracture seen particularly in children. It originates when the dura beneath the fracture is torn, and the arachnoid membrane herniates through the dura and into the bony defect. The pulsations of the brain and the enlarging arachnoid collection then cause progressive enlargement of the fracture line. Some physicians believe that a cyst need not always be present in a "growing" skull fracture, but that the pulsations of the brain through a dural defect cause expansion of the fracture.

The bony defect in a leptomeningeal cyst may have a scalloped appearance with sharp, non-sclerotic borders (Fig. 7-9). The border may look beveled, since the inner table of bones of the skull is more eroded than the outer table. Clinically this complication is often associated with underlying brain damage.

Radiographically, eosinophilic granuloma, the mildest form of the hystiocytosis diseases, is manifested by a single lytic lesion in the skull with a sharp, non-sclerotic border (Fig. 7-10). The edges of the lesion are often beveled. Occasionally, a small central fragment of bone may be present within the lytic defect. This is the button sequestrum and represents the mechanism by which the lesion heals from within. This finding is characteristic, although it has been infrequently described in inflammatory and neoplastic disease. The overlying soft tissues are normal. In patients with a clinical history of episodes of otitis, the external auditory canal may be

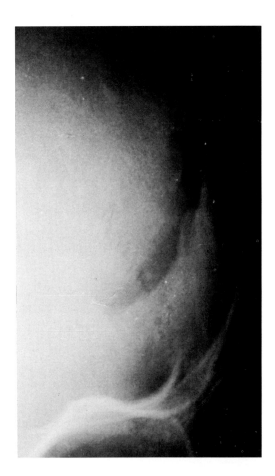

Fig. 7-9. Leptomenigeal cyst. Note the long, relatively wide radiolucent defect with well-defined borders in the left frontal region. This patient had a history of prior trauma to the left frontal region, and the cyst was surgically repaired.

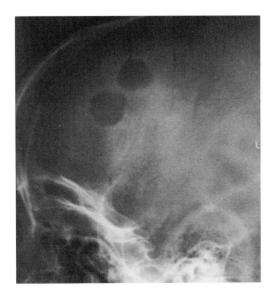

Fig. 7-10. Histiocytosis. Two large lytic defects are present in the frontal bone, and a small one is present in the parietal region. The borders are sharp but not sclerotic. The ill-defined radiolucencies in the central and lower portions of the parietal area are normal convolutional markings.

Table 7-1. **Single Radiolucent Oval Defects**

Type of Lesion	Characteristics
Lesions without sclerotic margins	
Meningoencephaloceles	Midline; associated with mass formation
Leptomeningeal cyst	Previous fracture line recognizable
Eosinophilic granuloma	Sharp, beveled edge
Infection	Ill-defined border
Burr hole	Sharp margins
Intracranial lesions	Ill-defined, beveled inner table of bones of the skull
Lesions with sclerotic margins	
Anomalous apertures	Sharp, sclerotic margins
Dermal sinus	Midline; slightly sclerotic margin
Epidermoid tumor	Sharp, sclerotic margin
Hemangioma	"Honeycombed" appearance; lobular, slightly sclerotic margin

affected by granuloma formation. Interstitial lung disease with a predisposition to spontaneous pneumothorax also occurs. The other forms of histiocytosis are discussed on pages 383, 388.

Infections of the skull are rare and are often associated with direct trauma or arise secondary to infection elsewhere in the body. The findings for any specific infection are not distinctive and the early radiographic presentation typically consists of a mottled, irregular area of lysis (Fig. 7-11). This soon consolidates, becoming a larger lesion with ill-defined margins. The demarcation of the margins depends greatly upon the nature of the lesion. In acute infections this is more irregular and ill-defined. Adjacent soft tissues are often involved and swelling, heat, and pain in the scalp may be the patient's initial complaint.

A hemangioma is a benign tumor that originates in the middle table of bones of the skull and expands the outer table. The inner table may be normal. The vascular diploic space is widened and looks like a honeycomb. Radiating spicules of bone are often seen. The borders of the lesion may be sclerotic (Fig. 7-12).

A rare manifestation of neurofibromatosis is the absence of bone along the margins of a suture. These areas are soft upon palpation. Radiographically, the lytic defect lies along a suture and has fairly well demarcated, nonsclerotic borders. The lesions are not related to adjacent neurofibroma but rather represent a widespread defect of mesenchyma.

A surgical defect in the skull may embarrass the unwary physician who makes an exotic diagnosis, only to find the child had a burr hole introduced early in life. Obviously surgical defects may be different sizes and may involve all three tables of bones of the skull. The margins are sharp but non-sclerotic (Fig. 7-33B).

A rare cause of a single, lytic defect is erosion of the skull due to a slowly expanding intracranial mass, such as a tumor or cyst (Fig. 7-13). These lesions have poorly defined, non-sclerotic borders. The clinical findings usually provide the key to the diagnosis.

MULTIPLE RADIOLUCENT DEFECTS OF THE SKULL

The recognition of multiple radiolucent defects is usually not difficult. In general, the associated diseases have a more unfavorable prognosis than those which produce a single radiolucent defect. In contrast to single defects, congenital anomalies and modification of normal cranial imperfections are usually not responsible.

Disease Entities

Craniolacunia, lückenschädel
Convolutional markings
Wormian bones
Histiocytosis
Metastatic tumor
Osteomyelitis
Hyperparathyroidism

Differential Diagnosis

Craniolacunia is due to multiple defects in that portion of the skull that ossifies from membranous tissue. It is not an isolated defect but is part of a syndrome that includes encephalocele and meningocele. The bony

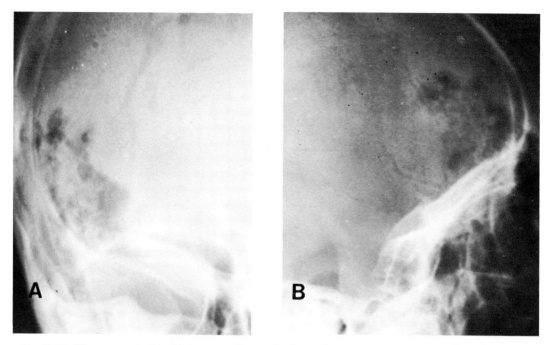

Fig. 7-11. Blastomycosis. *(A, B)* An area of irregular bone destruction is present in the right frontal region. The margins are poorly defined. Soft-tissue swelling was present as well as pulmonary infiltrate and areas of destruction in long bones. Widespread involvement such as this is common in blastomycosis.

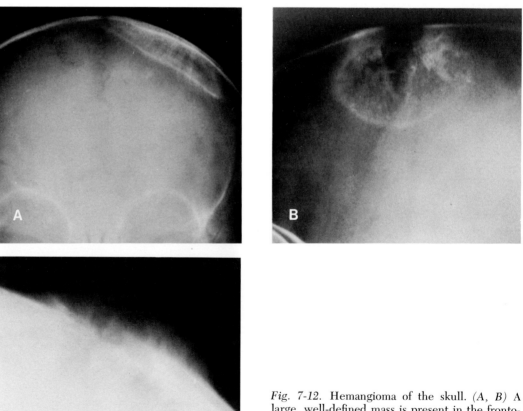

Fig. 7-12. Hemangioma of the skull. *(A, B)* A large, well-defined mass is present in the fronto-parietal region. It demonstrates a sharp sclerotic margin. *(C)* The characteristic spiculations of the tumor are well outlined on the tangential view.

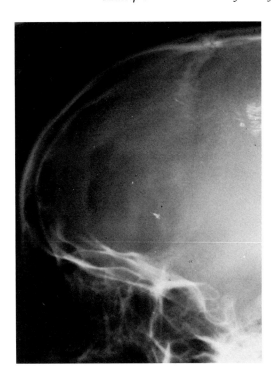

Fig. 7-13. Subarachnoid cyst. A lytic defect is present in the frontal bone. The margins are smooth and non-sclerotic. The bone destruction involved the inner and middle tables of bones of the skull (not readily apparent here). A subarachnoid cyst was demonstrated with angiography and pneumoencephalography and confirmed at surgery.

defects resolve spontaneously by 3 to 6 months of age and are not related to increased intracranial pressure. The increased intracranial pressure is a source of frequent confusion, since craniolacunia is rarely seen without the presence of an encephalocele or myelomeningocele, lesions often associated with hydrocephalus. However, craniolacunia does not develop because of increased intracranial pressure, its presence does not imply that increased pressure will develop, and, in fact, it does not have any prognostic significance other than its association with the encephalocele or myelomeningocele.

Craniolacunia is manifested by radiolucent defects scattered over the cranial vault, alternating with strips of normal bone that are directed in no predictable pattern (Fig. 7-14). The defects vary in size but are bilateral. They are most common in the parietal bone and the upper portion of the occipital bone. The intervening strips of normal bone at times appear more radiodense than the bone of a normal infant's skull, but this is not a steadfast rule.

Convolutional or digital markings refer to the normal molding of the inner table of bones of the skull. Presumably, the molding is due to pressure from the pulsating brain. There is some doubt about this, but no better

theory has been proposed. These defects can be seen as early as 6 months of age but are most marked at 4 to 6 years. They look like radiolucent areas with ill-defined margins (Fig. 7-31B). Their diameter does not usually exceed the diameter of a medium-sized finger. They are most prominent in the temporal areas but may involve the entire calvarium. Convolution markings should not be confused with crainiolacunia. The two occur in different age-groups, and have different appearances and entirely different implications. The extent of the markings varies from child to child. They may be markedly prominent with chronic increased intracranial pressure (Fig. 7-32), but because of the variation in extent, a diagnosis of increased pressure should never be based only on increased digital markings. Patients with a small brain, micrencephaly, usually have no convolutional markings.

Wormian bones are due to defective mineralization of the bone adjacent to sutures. Radiolucent lines extend from the sutures for a variable distance into adjacent bone (Fig. 7-15). The sutures themselves are often widened. An increased number of wormian bones are seen in cleidocranial dysostosis, osteogenesis imperfecta, hypothyroidism, and pyknodysostosis.

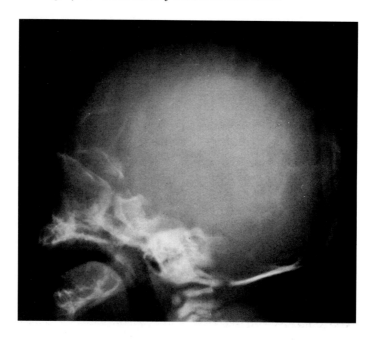

Fig. 7-14. Craniolacunia. Multiple radiolucent defects with somewhat sclerotic borders are present over the entire vault. A thoracolumbar myelomeningocele was present.

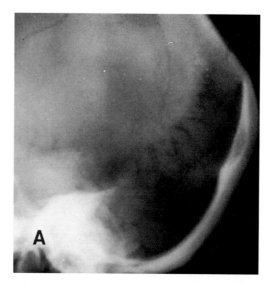

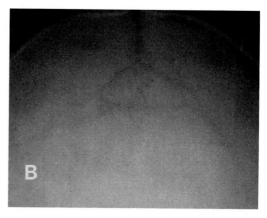

Fig. 7-15. Wormian bones. (*A, B*) Two patients are shown with wormian bones present in the lamboid suture. Note the excessive number of sutures containing the bones within.

The more malignant forms of histiocytosis, Hand-Schüller-Christian disease and Letterer-Siwe disease, have the same radiographic characteristics as eosinophilic granuloma but affect multiple areas of the skull (Fig. 7-10). These lesions are purely lytic with sharp, non-sclerotic borders. Soft-tissue changes are not seen radiographically. There often are other sites of bony involvement as well as visceral disease.

In most instances, metastases which affect the skull originate from neuroblastoma, Ewing's sarcoma, and leukemia. In each multiple lytic defects are present, of varying size and with irregular, non-sclerotic borders. The base of the skull as well as the vault may be affected (Fig. 7-16). The sutures may be widened due to increased intracranial pressure, due to direct invasion of the bone by a tumor or by a diffuse infiltration of the dura (as in leukemia), and due to the presence of a larger, bulky, extradural mass (as in neuroblastoma).

Osteomyelitis affecting multiple areas of

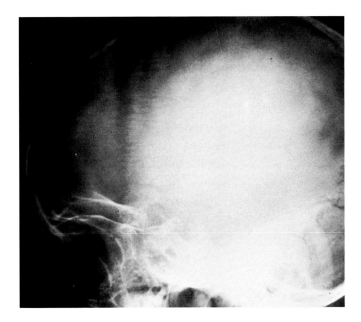

Fig. 7-16. Metastatic neuroblastoma. There is destruction of the anterior clinoids, planum sphenoidale, and orbital regions. The coronal sutures are wide, indicating increased intracranial pressure secondary to intracranial extension of the tumor.

the skull is rare and usually secondary to a focus elsewhere (Figs. 7-11, 7-12). The common infections are blastomycosis, coccidioidomycosis, actinomycosis, and tuberculosis. Radiographically, these lesions cannot be differentiated from the more malignant form of the histiocytosis, leukemia, and metastatic tumors. The borders of the lesions are irregular and non-sclerotic. Soft-tissue involvement may be prominent.

Hyperparathyroidism in children is usually secondary to renal disease rather than to a parathyroid adenoma. Mottled demineralization of the skull is seen radiographically. When there is minimal demineralization, the changes can be subtle and may be difficult to detect radiographically. Dural calcification is likely to occur in the secondary forms of hyperparathyroidism.

SCLEROTIC AREAS OF THE SKULL

There are several normal and pathologic processes which may be manifested by zones of increased radiodensity in the bony calvarium. However, the diseases are fewer and less common compared to lytic defects of the skull. Sclerotic lesions of the skull must be differentiated from calcific areas occurring in the brain or meninges. Usually, this problem is easily resolved by radiographs taken from a number of views, but occasionally stereoscopic views and tomography may be needed.

Disease Entities

Normal areas of sclerosis
Cephalohematoma
Fibrous dysplasia
Tuberous sclerosis
Rickets
Anemias
Osteoma

Differential Diagnosis

In infants the occipital bone and, to a lesser degree, the frontal bone look more radiodense than other bones of the calvarium. However, if the margins of the sutures are radiodense, fusion of the suture is present. This finding is of importance in the diagnosis of premature synostosis (Figs. 7-31, 7-32).

A cephalohematoma (Fig. 7-17) follows subperiosteal bleeding in an infant who experiences trauma at birth. The periosteum is fixed at the sutures, and as a result the swelling does not cross the suture line, in contrast to subcutaneous and subaponeurotic collections of fluid. It terminates at the midline when it occurs in the parietal regions but is centrally located when it involves the occipital and frontal areas. When it occurs in the frontal region, a cephalohematoma might be mistaken for an encephalocele. Fractures are occasionally seen beneath the cephalohematomas. Most often they resolve or undergo calcification, which occurs as early as 2 weeks

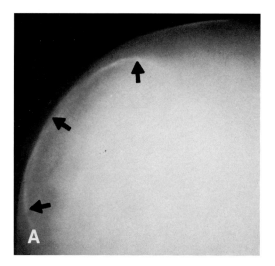
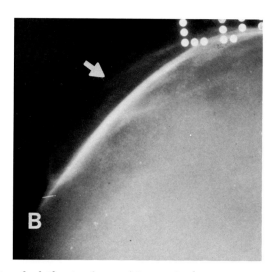

Fig. 7-17. Calcified cephalohematoma. *(A)* A thin rim of calcification *(arrows)* is seen in the posterior parietal region. *(B)* A tangential projection reveals the calcification outlining an oval soft-tissue mass. The calcification is best defined peripherally, along the margin of attachment.

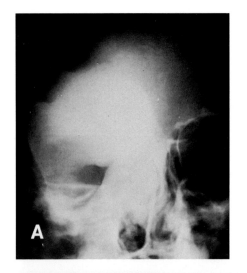
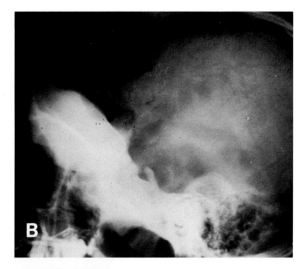
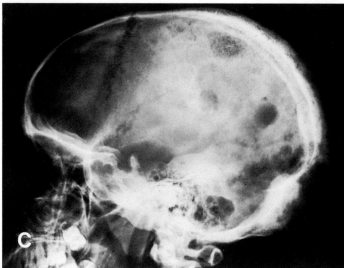

Fig. 7-18. Fibrous dysplasia. *(A, B)* The bone of the right orbital roof and the sphenoid ridge have a markedly increased density. The abnormal bone is sharply demarcated from the normal base in the lateral projection. Cystic lytic changes are also apparent superiorly within the frontal bone. *(C)* Another patient with polyostotic fibrous dysplasia. In this skull the lytic component predominates. Some areas are sharply bordered and beveled. Marked thickening along with cystic changes of the occipital bone are also present.

after birth. Initially, calcification occurs along the peripheral margins but eventually extends over the entire hematoma. Radiographically, the thickening of the outer table of the bones of the skull may remain after clinical regression of the mass. Rarely, a mass which is clinically apparent may persist into adult life, with hyperostosis being evident radiographically.

Fibrous dysplasia varies from a single lesion to an entire syndrome which occurs in females, with involvement of multiple bones, hyperpigmentation of the skin, and precocious puberty. In the skull the lesions are different and usually sclerotic due to thickened bone (Fig. 7-18). Normal trabecular markings are absent. The base of the skull, facial bones, mandible, and skull vault may be involved. The process encroaches upon adjacent foramina and paranasal sinuses. Cranial nerve deficits are quite rare.

Tuberous sclerosis is manifested by hyperostotic defects in the skull which are radiodense, with ill-defined borders, and which measure rarely more than 5 to 10 mms. in diameter. The disease is also characterized by adenoma sebaceum and mental retardation. Hamartomas affect multiple organs. Other radiographic findings include renal angiomyolipomas, interstitial pulmonary disease, cystic defects in the bones of the hands and feet, and sclerotic areas in the bony calvarium, spine, and pelvis. In the cerebral tissue these are manifested by intracranial calcifications.

Rickets involving the skull is now rarely seen. In this disease the outer table of the bones of the skull is thickened due to an accumulation of poorly mineralized bone. This eventually becomes dense with healing of the rachitic process, and radiographically the outer table is thickened and sclerotic. The process usually involves the frontal and parietal bones. The inner table is unaffected.

A number of forms of hemolytic anemia often affect the skull. The most severe changes occur in patients with familial erythroblastic anemia. In patients with severe iron deficiency anemia the skull may be affected, but rarely markedly. Radiographically, the diploic space is thickened, and in severe cases vertical bony striations extend through the middle and outer tables of the bones of the skull (Fig. 7-19). In severe cases of thalassemia, the bones of the face are involved, with obliteration of the sinuses.

An osteoma is the most common benign tumor affecting the skull and facial bones. It may project extracranially from the outer table of bones or originate from the inner table and extend intracranially. An osteoma is made up of dense, sclerotic bone with sharp, well circumscribed borders.

Several forms of bony dysplasia are associated with sclerosis of portions of the skull (see Chapter 10). The most marked changes occur in patients with osteopetrosis. The bones of the skull and face are thickened and radiopaque, most noticeably at the base of the skull (Fig. 7-20). Wormian bones are frequent, dentition is delayed, and the pituitary fossa looks small. The skull may be large due to hydrocephalus, but the cause is not known.

INTRACRANIAL CALCIFICATION

The correct interpretation of intracranial calcification is a valuable clue to the diagnosis of many intracranial and systemic diseases. The list of disease entities is long but several are associated with specific types of calcification and are easily recognizable.

Disease Entities

Physiologic calcification
    Calcification in the pineal gland
    Calcification of the choroid plexus
    Calcification of the habenular commissure
    Dural calcification
Artifacts
Familial, congenital, and metabolic diseases
    Tuberous sclerosis
    Sturge-Weber syndrome
    Hypoparathyroidism and pseudohypoparathyroidism
    Idiopathic familial cerebrovascular calcinosis (Fahr's disease)
    Idiopathic calcification of the basal ganglion
Inflammatory disease
    Cytomegalic inclusion disease
    Toxoplasmosis
    Abscess
Arteriovenous malformation
Intracerebral hematoma
Subdural hematoma
Neoplasm
    Craniopharyngioma
    Astrocytoma
    Oligodendroglioma
    Pinealoma

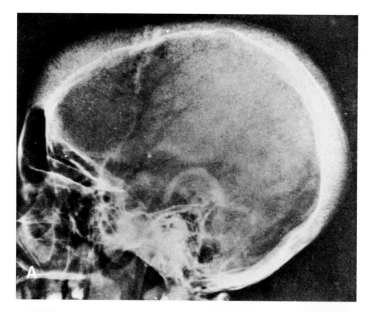

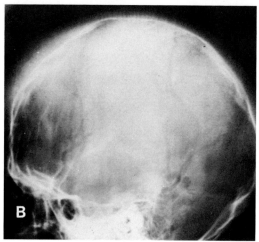

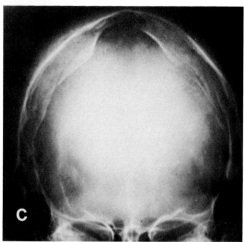

Fig. 7-19. Hemolytic anemias. (A) Sickle cell disease. The diploic space is thickened. Note the vertical, radiolucent strips contained in the diploë ("hair-on-end" appearance). This may be present in any severe hemolytic anemia but is relatively uncommon in sickle cell disease. (B) Spherocytosis. The diploic space is most notably thickened in the frontoparietal area. (C) The skull is somewhat elongated in the vertical dimension. Variations in shape, such as this, are fairly frequent in severe hemolytic anemia.

Differential Diagnosis

The most common site of intracranial physiologic calcification is the pineal gland. Calcification in this structure is rare prior to adolescence. The calcification is best seen in the lateral projection lying approximately 3 cms. above and posterior to the posterior clinoids. The midline position of the calcified gland in the anteroposterior projection is well known. The calcification may be nodular, amorphous, or lamellar. If the area of calcification exceeds 10 mms. in diameter or occurs in a child younger than 12 years, the possibility of pinealoma should be considered.

Calcification of the choroid plexuses of the lateral ventricles is more frequent than pineal calcification in young children. The calcifica-

tion is lateral and inferior to the pineal gland and is often bilateral and unequal in size. Choroid plexus calcification is of little, if any, help in determining whether there is an intracranial mass.

Calcification of the habenular commisure, just above and anterior to the pineal gland, has a characteristic crescentic shape, open posteriorly. It is rare in children and usually associated with calcification of the pineal gland.

Dural calcification in the falx and in the petroclinoid ligaments is not unusual in children. Both areas of calcification are easily recognized by their location. The calcification of the falx is seen most frequently anteriorly as a vertically oriented area of radiodensity with sharp borders on the anteroposterior projection. The petroclinoid ligaments are

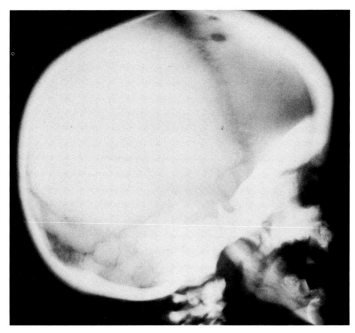

Fig. 7-20. Osteopetrosis. A lateral projection reveals markedly increased density and thickness of the base of the skull, the vault, and the face. The sella appears small and wormian bones are present posteriorly. Hydrocephalus may be present since the skull looks large, but this was not confirmed. Anterior frontal foramina are also apparent.

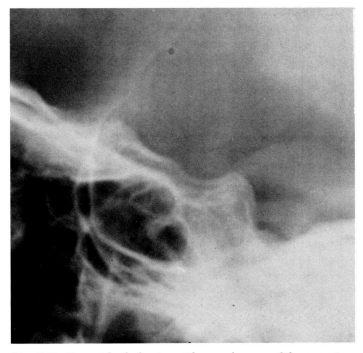

Fig. 7-21. Tentorial calcifications. The attachments of the tentorium to the anterior and posterior clinoid processes are calcified, preventing visualization of the sella. This extensive degree of dural calcification is unusual.

301

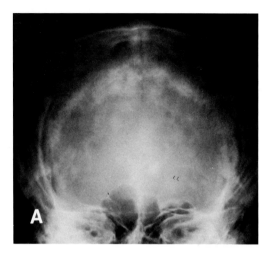

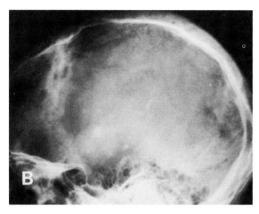

Fig. 7-22. Tuberous sclerosis. *(A, B)* Note the multiple areas of intracranial calcification.

the attachments of the tentorium to the petrous pyramids, the clinoid processes, and the dorsum sellae. The calcification is usually seen behind the posterior clinoid process but may extend between the anterior and posterior clinoid processes (Fig. 7-21).

Artifacts are a common source of embarrassment to the unwary physician. Jewelry, pins, needles, and other metallic objects have a greater radiodensity than calcium, and with a little experience these become a less frequent source of confusion. Pantopaque from prior myelography or ventriculography also has a metallic radiodensity. Dirt, rocks, grease, rubber bands, and braids have a lower radiodensity and as artifacts create more problems. A careful examination of the head, sometimes with thorough washing, and repeat radiographs will resolve the dilemma.

Adenoma sebaceum, epilepsy, and mental retardation are characteristic of tuberous sclerosis. Hamartomas occur in the brain as well as in many other sites. These masses consist of glial tissue and ganglion cells that calcify in approximately half of the affected patients. The calcifications lie in the subcortical, subependymal, or basal ganglion regions, are often paraventricular, and are usually multiple (Fig. 7-22). They vary in size and have no specific configuration. These intracranial calcifications should not be confused with the sclerotic lesions present in the bony calvarium that occur in association with tuberous sclerosis.

Another disorder frequently accompanied by mental retardation, epilepsy, and intra-

cranial calcification is the Sturge-Weber syndrome. Afflicted patients often have a cutaneous hemangioma distributed along the trigeminal nerve on the same side as the intracranial calcification. The calcification is usually in the parieto-occipital region and has a sinusoidal course with parallel linear calcifications, the "railroad track" appearance (Fig. 7-23). The calcification lies in the cerebral cortex under a meningeal angioma. Rarely, the meningeal angioma may also be calcified.

Calcification of the basal ganglia may occur in a variety of conditions but is most frequent in hypoparathyroidism and pseudohypoparathyroidism. The basal ganglia lie above the sphenoid ridge and sella turcica deep within the brain, approaching the midline (Fig. 7-24). The calcifications may assume a variety of forms, from small, punctate areas to large masses, and are almost always bilateral.

Irregular punctate areas of intracranial calcification, associated with severe growth disorder, progressive mental retardation, and a familial occurrence, indicate the presence of Fahr's disease. Microscopic deposits of iron and calcium occur in the subcortical centrum, basal ganglia, and cerebellar dentate nucleus and its adjacent white matter. The areas of ferrocalcinosis are widespread, irregular, punctate, and occasionally dustlike on the radiograph.

The two most common infections associated with intracranial calcifications are due to the cytomegalovirus and the parasite

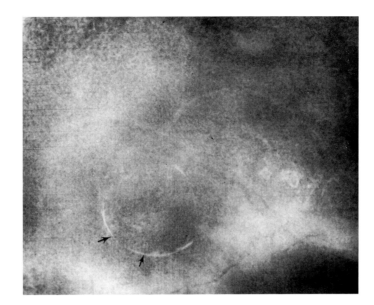

Fig. 7-26. Arteriovenous malformation. Note the many calcifications in the form of incomplete rings. The arc-shaped calcification with the greatest radius *(arrows)* is the vein of Galen.

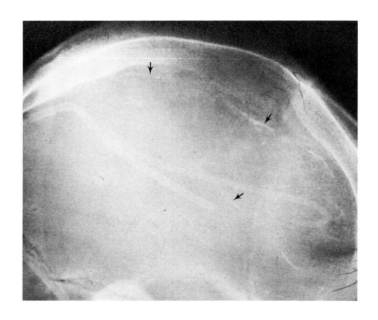

Fig. 7-27. Calcification in chronic subdural hematoma. A thin rim of calcification *(arrows)* covers a large area in the frontal region. The skull vault is thickened secondary to decreased brain growth. A ventricular shunt is present in the parietal area.

fants and young children. The clinical findings may include hydrocephalus, a loud cranial bruit, or congestive heart failure. The vein of Galen becomes markedly distended, and the condition is therefore called "aneurysm of the vein of Galen." The enlarged, thickened vein of Galen may become calcified (Fig. 7-26). The calcification is thin and crescentic, with the diameter of the arc exceeding 2.5 cms. It is located at the level of the pineal gland. The diagnosis is quite evident when these features are present.

Intracerebral bleeding is an uncommon cause of intracranial calcification. In children,

it is usually seen following trauma at birth. The calcification is non-distinctive.

Subdural hematomas may calcify, particularly if not evacuated surgically. The calcification outlines the margins of the hematoma and is usually linear. Changes in the contour of the skull due to restriction of brain growth may be associated with the calcification (Fig. 7-27).

A variety of intracranial neoplasms calcify (Fig. 7-28). The most common in children is craniopharyngioma. This tumor occurs in the suprasellar region and calcification is seen in approximately 75 per cent of the lesions. The

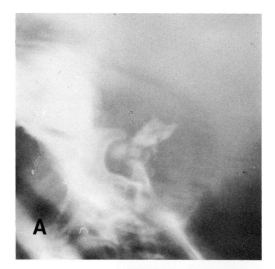
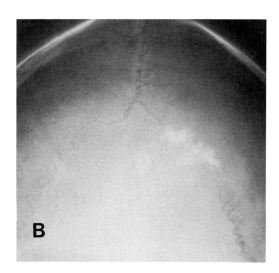
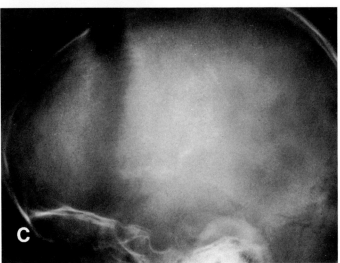

Fig. 7-28. Calcification within intracranial tumors. *(A)* Radiodense, suprasellar and intrasellar calcification is shown due to a craniopharyngioma. Intrasellar calcification is unusual with this tumor. *(B)* Two closely adjacent zones of moderately radiodense calcifications are seen to the left of the midline. These were present in an oligodendroglioma. *(C)* The sutures are widened indicating increased intracranial pressure. Amorphous calcifications covering a large circular area in the fronto-parietal area are present within an astrocytoma.

calcifications may be curvilinear, outlining the wall of the mass, or nodular, occuring within the tumor mass (Fig. 7-28A). A combination of both may also occur. It is important to bear in mind that suprasellar calcifications in children are almost always due to craniopharyngioma.

Supratentorial gliomas are not common in children but do occur and may calcify. Astrocytoma and oligodendroglioma are the two most frequent gliomas associated with calcification. Approximately 10 per cent of astrocytomas contain calcium that is demonstrable radiographically, as compared to 60 to 70 per cent of oligodendrogliomas. However, an

astrocytoma is far more common and, therefore, is a more frequent cause of calcification. The calcification may present as linear, nodular, or conglomerate masses. The type of calcification, however, is dependent upon which glioma is present (Figs. 7-28B, 7-28C).

ABNORMAL CONTOUR OF THE SKULL

The final contour of the skull is determined by the size and configuration of the intracranial contents, by the ability of the sutures to expand and, to lesser degrees, by extrinsic

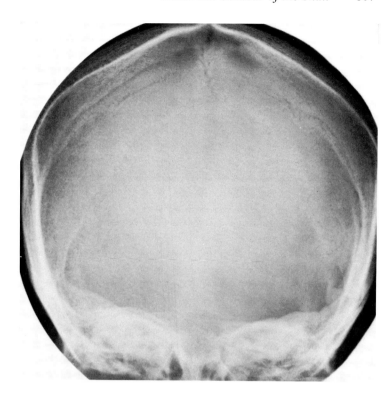

Fig. 7-29. Minimal atrophy of the right cerebral hemisphere. The diploic space on the right is thickened and the right petrous pyramid is elevated. There is minimal flattening of the skull in the right parietal area.

pressures which may shape the skull and by abnormal bone formation. An abnormality in any of these may result in a malformed calvarium.

Disease Entities
Abnormality of intracranial contents
    Unilateral cerebral atrophy (Davidoff-Dyke-Masson syndrome)
    Intracerebral cyst
    Subarachnoid cyst
    Subdural hematoma
Premature closure of suture
Extrinsic pressure
    Molding secondary to delivery
    Postural flattening
Abnormal bone formation
    Achondroplasia

Differential Diagnosis

In a patient with unilateral cerebral atrophy, the ipsilateral hemi-calvarium is smaller than the opposite side (Fig. 7-29). The tables of the bones of the skull are thicker. Occasionally there may be elevation of the ipsilateral petrous pyramid. This has been termed the Davidoff-Dyke-Masson syndrome.

Intracerebral and subarachnoid cysts may function as space-occupying masses and expand the adjacent bony calvarium (Fig. 7-30). The bony vault bulges outward and the inner table of the bones of the skull is thinned. Cysts of either type are most likely to occur in the temporal lobe.

A particular form of cyst, the Dandy-Walker syndrome, is due to congenital occlusion of the fourth ventricular outlets, the foramina of Magendi and Luschka. The fourth ventricle becomes markedly distended leading to bulging of the occipital bone and elevation of the lateral sinuses and the torcular Herophili. Dilatation of the lateral ventricles is usually present and is manifested radiographically by enlargement of the supratentorial portion of the calvarium.

Chronic subdural hematomas may cause expansion of the adjacent calvarium or may only erode the inner table (Fig 7-27). If calcification is present as well, the diagnosis of subdural hematoma is usually correct.

A suture allows expansion of the calvarium at right angles to the long axis of the suture. If the suture closes early, to accomodate the growing brain the calvarium expands to an abnormal degree in the direction of the axis of the fused suture. Therefore, premature closure of the sagittal suture prevents expan-

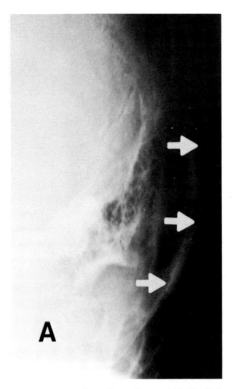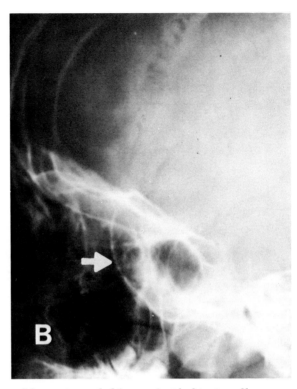

Fig. 7-30. Subarachnoid cyst. *(A)* The left temporal fossa is expanded *(arrows)* with thinning of bone on the frontal projection. *(B)* The frontal bone is thinned on the lateral view, and the middle cranial fossa, as shown by the thinned sphenoid wing *(arrow)*, is expanded. A subarachnoid cyst was identified with further studies.

sion in the coronal plane and leads to an elongated, narrow skull (Fig. 7-31A, 7-31B). Closure of both coronal sutures produces a short, wide skull. Unilateral coronal synostosis (Fig. 7-31C) produces elevation of the lateral portion of the ipsilateral orbital rim (the "harlequin" appearance), flattening of the forehead, prominence of the eye, and tilting of the nasal septum and cristi galli toward the affected side. Closure of two or more sutures leads to bizarre skull shapes, depending upon which suture closes first (Fig. 7-32). Generally, premature closure of a suture produces sclerosis of the bony margins, but the shape of the skull is a better index of premature closure than the appearance of the suture.

Premature synostosis of a single suture is a cosmetic defect, does not restrict brain growth, and is not a cause of mental retardation. If multiple sutures are involved, the restricted calvarial growth may be associated with brain damage.

The fetal skull is molded during vaginal de-

livery to conform to the bony and soft-tissue structures through which it must pass. Usually the parietal bones overlap the frontal and occipital bones. One parietal bone may override the other at the sagittal suture. Most changes disappear within 48 hours, but minor changes may persist for several days. If fetal molding persists, one should consider the possibility of micrencephaly.

If an infant is in one position for extended lengths of time, postural flattening may develop. This is characterized by flattening of the dependent portion of the bony calvarium and secondary deformities of the remaining portions. By taking a careful history, postural flattening can be differentiated from premature synostosis; in addition, the deformity does not correspond to the bony axis of a suture. In children with postural flattening, mental retardation may be the cause of the abnormal lack of movement.

Abnormalities of the calvarium are associated with a number of syndromes. Those abnormalities which accompany achondro-

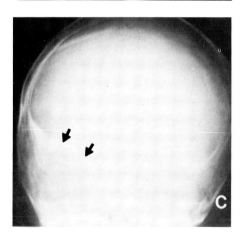

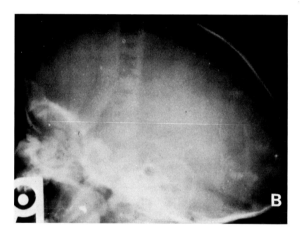

Fig. 7-31. Premature closure of suture. *(A, B)* Sagittal synostosis. The skull is long and narrow (scaphocephalic), and the sagittal suture is sclerotic. The digital or convolutional markings in the parietal region are quite apparent but normal. *(C)* Unilateral coronal synostosis. The right orbit is elongated with elevation of its superolateral border. The coronal suture is sclerotic.

plasia are worthy of mention. The bones at the base of the skull develop from cartilage and are therefore shortened in achondroplasia. Since the vault of the skull is formed from membranous bone, it is not affected directly. Slight ventricular enlargement is usually present. The result is a slightly enlarged calvarium, frontal bossing, flattening of the midface, and relatively large jaws. The foramen magnum may be small.

ABNORMAL INTRACRANIAL VOLUME

The calvarial size is dependent upon the size of the intracranial contents and is unrelated to the many factors that determine the size of the remaining portions of the body. Therefore, if the skull is large or small, physicians should be primarily concerned with determining whether an abnormality of the intracranial contents is responsible.

The cranial sutures are areas of unossified membranous tissue that allow for expansion of the calvarium. They are not analagous to the epiphyseal centers of long bones. As long as the intracranial contents are expanding, the normal suture remains open. When brain growth ceases, the cranial sutures will then close.

Probably the most accurate way to determine an abnormal cranial volume is to measure the skull directly and compare the measurements to standards for age and body size. Frequent measurements may be needed to detect minor abnormalities in growth of the calvarium. Standard radiographic measurements are available, but the simplest method is to compare the size of the skull to the size of the face. At birth, the volume of skull is approximately 4 times that of the face. This ratio decreases to approximately 3 to 1 by age 2 and to 1.5 to 1 by adulthood.

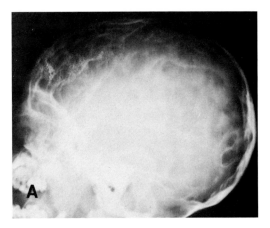

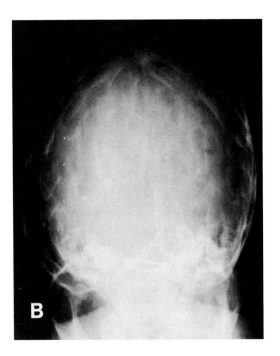

Fig. 7-32. Premature closure of multiple sutures. (A, B) The skull is elongated vertically (turricephaly), and the sutures are sclerotic. Digital or convolutional markings are prominent, a manifestation of increased intracranial pressure. (Radiodensities in the frontal region are artifacts.)

Disease Entities

Increased intracranial volume
    Hydrocephalus
    Macrencephaly
    Hydranencephaly
    Pituitary dwarfism
Decreased intracranial volume
    Micrencephaly
    Generalized premature craniostenosis
Increased intracranial pressure

Differential Diagnosis

Hydrocephalus simply refers to enlargement of the ventricular system and has a multitude of causes. The most common presentation consists of an infant with a large head and is cuased by congenital obstruction of the ventricular system. Usually, the intracranial pressure is not increased because the skull is able to expand to accomodate the increased volume. A specific diagnosis requires sophisticated neuroradiologic studies such as computerized tomography, encephalography, and angiography. Radiographically, the skull is large compared to the face (Fig. 7-33A). The bones of the calvarium may be poorly defined. Ordinarily, the sutures are not widened because the enlargement of the intracranial structures is slowly progressive, allowing bony apposition to proceed in an or-

derly fashion along the sutural margins. If expansion is rapid, bony apposition may not proceed at a comparable rate and the sutures become widened.

Macrencephaly is rare and is due to a large and malformed brain. Affected patients are usually mentally deficient. Radiographically this condition cannot be distinguished from milder forms of hydrocephalus. Soto's syndrome is associated with macrencephaly and increased bony maturity.

An unusual cause of macrocrania is neurofibromatosis. The mechanism in this disorder is unknown. Hydranencephaly may be an extreme form of hydrocephalus, or it may be due to primary failure of the brain to form. In either case, the calvarial size may be normal at birth but increases rapidly and may reach enormous proportions.

In pituitary dwarfism, the skull is not enlarged but somatic growth is retarded. Therefore, the normal skull appears to be enlarged compared to the somewhat small face. An incorrect diagnosis can be avoided by recognition of the overall small size of the patient.

A small skull is almost always due to a small brain, micrencephaly, and is accompanied by mental retardation. The contour of the skull is normal despite the small size (Fig. 7-34). Cranial sutures close early, but this is a result of micrencephaly and not the cause. The paranasal sinuses are usually quite large. Dig-

Fig. 7-33. Hydrocephalus. (A) The skull is large as compared to the face in this 1-year-old child. The sutures are normal, as expected, because of the chronic slow increase in intracranial volume. A ventricular shunting procedure was performed. (B) Two years after shunting the skull remains large, but the sutures appear to be closed and the tables of the bones of the skull are thick, indicating "arrested hydrocephalus." (C) Two years later, at age 5, symptoms of increased intracranial pressure were present. The sutures now appear to have reopened and the dorsum sella is eroded. Further studies indicated increased pressure due to a nonfunctioning ventricular shunt.

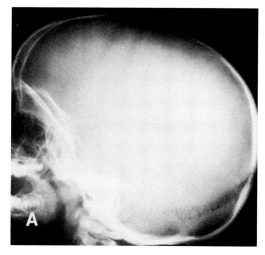

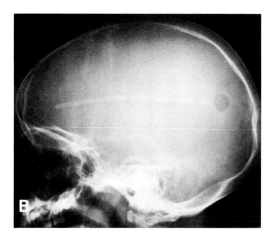

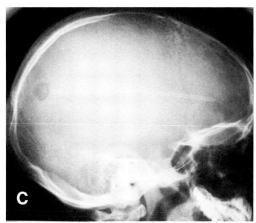

ital or convolutional markings are absent or decreased. In theory, a small skull of normal contour may be due to premature closure of all of the cranial sutures, but this is quite rare. When multiple sutures fuse prematurely, the fusion rarely occurs simultaneously at each suture. Therefore, the skull develops an abnormal contour as the calvarium tries to expand in unusual directions to accomodate the growing brain. Clinically, findings of increased intracranial pressure are present. A marked increase in number and early appearance of digital markings are present radiographically, as well as sclerosis of the margins of the suture.

An acute increase in intracranial pressure in a child has different manifestations depending upon whether the sutures are open or closed. If the sutures have not fused, they become wider due to the expansion of the intracranial contents (Figs. 7-16, 7-28C, 7-35). This manifestation is common until about 12 years of age. When the sutures are fused, the increased intracranial pressure is manifested by erosion of the dorsum sella and the posterior clinoids (Fig. 7-33C).

A few words of caution are necessary regarding the apppearance of digital or convolutional markings and the radiographic interpretation of increased intracranial pressure. An increased number of digital markings may be associated with raised intracranial pressure (Fig. 7-30). However, digital markings are so variable from patient to patient that an increased number, observed as an isolated radiographic finding, should not be interpreted as a manifestation of increased intracranial pressure.

Acute widening of the cranial sutures is not always the result of a rapid rise of intracranial pressure; it has been associated with deprivation dwarfism, perhaps due to rapid brain growth after the restoration of adequate nutrition.

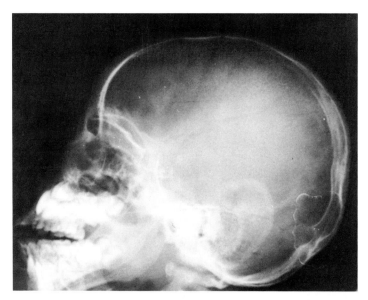

Fig. 7-34. Micrencephaly. The skull is small compared to the face in this 5-year-old child. The diploic space is thickened, the sutures are narrow, and the frontal sinus and mastoid areas are pneumatic. These features resemble those of the adult skull and are consistent with retarded growth of the skull due to a small brain.

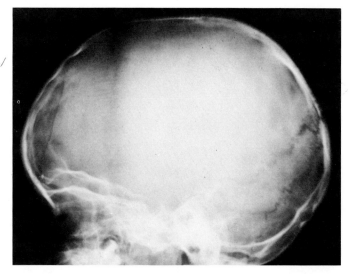

Fig. 7-35. Acute increase in intracranial pressure. The size of the skull is normal but the sutures are wide. As would be expected, the sella is normal.

INCREASED THICKNESS OF THE SKULL

Increased thickness of the bony calvarium is most often due to an increase in size of the middle table of bones of the skull or the diploic space. The diploic space begins to form in the 1st year of life and gradually increases in size as brain growth diminishes. Its maximum size is reached late in the 2nd decade of life. The middle table is formed of thin, bony trabeculae and vascular spaces, which serve as a site of hematopoiesis and reduce the weight of the calvarium. The vascular component may also aid in absorbing shock during external trauma.

An increased width of the diploic space may be due to an early cessation of brain growth or to increased hematopoiesis. Neoplasms and infections may involve the area and destroy surrounding bone, but the diploic space will not become larger.

Differential Diagnosis

Micrencephaly
Localized cerebral atrophy
"Arrested hydrocephalus"
Hemolytic anemia
    Thalassemia
    Sickle cell disease and other anemias

Differential Diagnosis

Micrencephaly, a small brain, leads to a small bony calvarium. The diploic space is formed early and is widened due to early cessation of brain growth (Fig. 7-34). The other radiographic features of micrencephaly have been discussed (see p. 310).

Localized cerebral atrophy produces an abnormal contour of the skull (Fig. 7-29). The diploic space on the ipsilateral side is thickened, again due to early cessation of brain growth.

Progressive hydrocephalus leads to a large bony calvarium and a decreased diploic space. However, if a ventricular shunt is performed and abnormal expansion ceases, ("arrested hydrocephalus") the cranial sutures close and the inner table of bones of the skull becomes thicker and the diploic space becomes larger (Fig. 7-33). A history of hydrocephalus and the presence of a ventricular shunt facilitate the correct diagnosis.

Hemolytic anemias produce hyperplasia of marrow in a number of sites, including the diploic space (Fig. 7-19). Thalassemia is associated with the most marked radiographic changes. The diploic space is widened with striking radial striations, the "hair-on-end" appearance. The diploic spaces of the facial bones, particularly the maxilla, are affected, leading to partial or complete obliteration of the paranasal sinuses.

Radial striations and thickening of the diploic space may be seen in sickle cell disease, but this is uncommon (Fig. 7-19). The facial bones are not involved. The milder forms of sickle cell disease, such as the sickle cell trait, rarely result in radiographic changes in the skull.

The other forms of hemolytic anemia, such as spherocytosis (Fig. 7-19) and iron deficiency anemia may be associated with radiographic changes similar to but less marked than those of sickle cell disease. The changes consist predominantly of minimal widening of the diploic space. Rarely, vertical striation is present.

REFERENCES

1. Afshani, E., Osman, M., and Girdancy, B. R.: Widening of the cranial sutures in children with deprivation dwarfism. Radiology, *109:*141, 1973.
2. Babbitt, D. P., Tang, T., Dobbs, J., and Berk, R.: Idiopathic familial archrovascular ferrocalcinosis (Fahr's disease) and review of differential diagnosis of intracranial calcification in children. Am. J. Roentgenol. Radium Ther. Nucl. Med., *105:*352, 1969.
3. Caffey, J.: Pediatric X-ray diagnosis. Chicago, Year Book Medical Publishers, 1972.
4. Carter, T. L., Gabeielson, T. O., and Abell, M. R.: Mechanism of split cranial sutures in metastatic neuroblastoma. Radiology, *91:*467, 1968.
5. Lagos, J. C., Holman, C. B., and Gomez, M. R.: Tuberous sclerosis, Neuroroentgenologic observations. Am. J. Roentgenol. Radium Ther. Nucl. Med., *104:*171, 1968.
6. Moseley, J. E., Rabinowitz, J. G., and Dziadiv, R.: Hyperostosis cranii ex vacuo. Radiology, *87:*1105, 1966.
7. Newton, T. H., and Potts, D. G.: Radiology of the skull and brain. *In* The Skull. St. Louis, C. V. Mosby, 1971.
8. Roberts, F., and Schopfner, C. E.: Plain skull roentgenograms in children with head trauma. Am. J. Roentgenol. Radium Ther. Nucl. Med., *114:*230, 1972.
9. Sholkoff, S. D., and Mainzer, F.: Button sequestrum revisited. Radiology, *100:*649, 1971.

8 | Barry Gerald, M.D.

Systematic Radiographic Evaluation of the Abnormal Spine

Lesions confined to the spine are relatively uncommon in the pediatric patient. Congenital malformations account for the majority of these abnormalities, with trauma, infection, and tumors being less common than in other parts of the body.

The normal radiographic appearance of the spine must be known before abnormalities can be recognized. This is complicated by the differences in appearance in different age-groups. Physicians should be aware of the ever-present possibility that an apparent abnormality may only be a manifestation of growth.

MALFORMATIONS OF THE VERTEBRAL COLUMN

To understand malformations of the vertebral column, a summary of the development of the vertebrae is necessary. The vertebral column forms around the notochord, lying on the ventral aspect of the neural tube. Each vertebral body forms initially from two lateral chondrification centers and then from anterior and posterior ossification centers which quickly fuse to form a single center, demonstrable radiographically in the 3rd fetal month. At birth, the vertebral bodies are somewhat rectangular in the thoracic region but more oval in the lumbar region. Small radiolucent defects are present in the midportions due to persistent vascular chan-

nels. A radiolucent line of unossified cartilage separates the vertebral body from the neural arch (Fig. 8-1).

As the child grows, the vertebral body assumes a more rectangular configuration. A step-like recess forms along the superior and inferior surfaces of the anterior portion of the vertebral body at approximately 7 to 8 years of age. This is the site of the ring apophysis which encircles the superior and inferior borders of the vertebral body but does not contribute to its vertical height. The apophyses begin to calcify at 8 to 9 years of age and fuse with the vertebral body between the ages of 12 and 15 years.

The neural arch includes the pedicles, laminae, superior and inferior articular facets, and the spinous and transverse processes. Growth occurs from two primary centers and is recognizable in the 3rd fetal month. Ossification begins initially at the first cervical vertebra and proceeds caudad. The centers gradually enlarge, fusing posteriorly to form the spinous process in the 2nd year of life. The neural arch fuses with the vertebral body between the 3rd and 6th year. The transverse processes form from secondary centers: the age at which they appear and the degree of fusion to the vertebral body are both highly variable.

The intervertebral disc is made up of an external annulus fibrosus, which is fused to the adjacent vertebral body, and a central nucle-

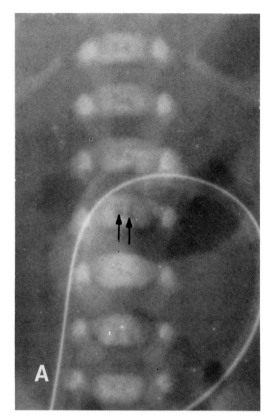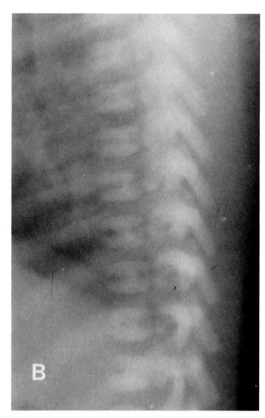

Fig. 8-1. Normal spine of newborn. *(A)* Note the lack of bony fusion of the vertebral body to the neural arch. Small, paired, oval radiolucencies, seen on the anteroposterior projection *(arrows)* over the mid-portions of the vertebral bodies, are openings for vessels supplying the vertebral bodies. The clefts in the mid-portions of the vertebral body, seen anteriorly on the anteroposterior projection and posteriorly on the lateral view *(B)*, are due to vascular channels.

us pulposus, a remnant of the notochord. The disc is quite large at birth and in some instances may approximate the size of the vertebral body. Its relative size progressively decreases, until it is one-third the height of the vertebral body in adults.

The first and second cervical vertebrae form in a different manner. The ring-like C1 arises from two lateral ossification centers and an anterior center. There are five centers for C2, an anterior and two lateral centers, plus two lateral centers for the base of the odontoid.

Abnormal formation and fusion of these ossification centers and persistence of the notochord are usually responsible for malformations of the vertebral column. Severe malformations are often lethal. Only those encountered relatively frequently are discussed here.

Disease Entities

Malformations of the vertebral body
   Coronal cleft
   Butterfly vertebrae
   Hemivertebrae
   Block vertebrae
   Diastematomyelia
   Anomalies associated with spinal malformations
Malformations of the neural arch
   Spina bifida occulta
   Meningocele
Alanto-axial anomalies
Sacral Agenesis

Differential Diagnosis

A coronal cleft in the vertebral body (Fig. 8-2A) occurs when the anterior and posterior ossification centers persist. The defect is

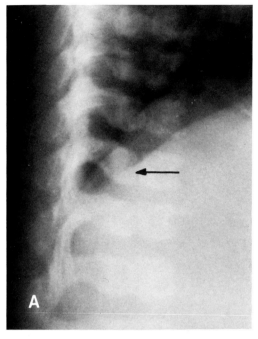

Fig. 8-2. Vertebral anomalies. (A) Coronal cleft vertebrae. A vertical radiolucent line (arrow) divides each vertebral body into two portions. (B) Hemivertebrae. The malformed vertebral bodies are seen at the levels of L2 on the right and T10 on the left (arrows) with scoliosis between the two. The vertebral bodies between the hemivertebrae are displaced obliquely because of inappropriate fusion of segments. (C) Dorsal hemivertebra and lumbar hypoplasia. A malformed and posteriorly placed vertebral body is present at the level of T12. Only two other lumbar vertebrae were present.

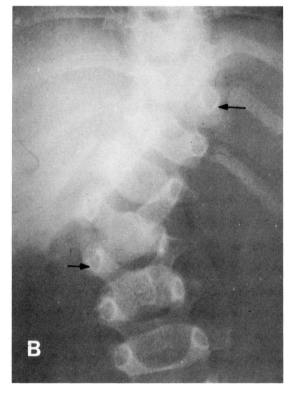

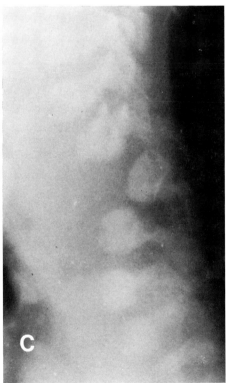

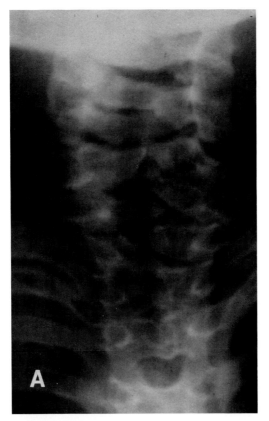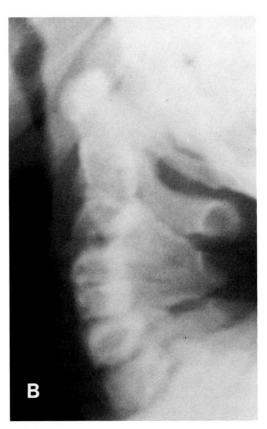

Fig. 8-3. Klippel-Feil deformity. *(A)* Multiple hemivertebrae are present in the lower cervical spine. Fused bodies are noted superiorly. *(B)* The lateral view better demonstrates the fusion of some vertebral bodies. The neck is short and the intervertebral disc spaces appear narrow.

manifested by a vertical, radiolucent line in the mid-portion of the vertebral body. It is most often seen in premature infants and involves the lower thoracic and lumbar regions. The anomaly is of no clinical significance and closes with normal growth. The possibility of associated anomalies, however, should be kept in mind. Interestingly, a coronal cleft is found more often in males than females, in a ratio of 9 to 1. This phenomenon has been used to predict the sex of an unborn infant.

Butterfly vertebrae result from persistence of notochordal tissue which prevents fusion of the lateral halves of the vertebral bodies. The halves are wedge-shaped medially, with a radiolucent defect dividing them. The width of the vertebrae is increased when seen in the anteroposterior projection. The neural arch and intervertebral disc may be malformed as well.

A hemivertebra occurs when the lateral half of the vertebral body is not formed due to the failure of a chondrification center to develop. The result is a triangular wedge of bone with the apex pointed medially (Fig. 8-2B). The vertebrae above and below the defect show compensatory deformation. This anomaly often involves several vertebral bodies and fusion defects are also found in the intervening vertebral bodies. It may be associated with other anomalies (e.g., hypoplasia of the lung, neurenteric cyst). Dorsal or ventral hemivertebrae result when one of the anterior or posterior ossification centers fails to develop. Dorsal vertebrae, which are due to underdevelopment of the anterior ossification center, are not common. They result in a gibbus deformity (Fig. 8-2C).

Formation of a block vertebra is due to abnormal segmentation of the segmental scleromere. There may be no intervertebral disc space, or the space persists as a thin, radiolucent line. The height of the affected vertebral bodies is usually normal, although some wedging or asymmetry may occur. The anomaly is most common in the lumbar region but occurs elsewhere.

The Klippel-Feil syndrome (Fig. 8-3) is

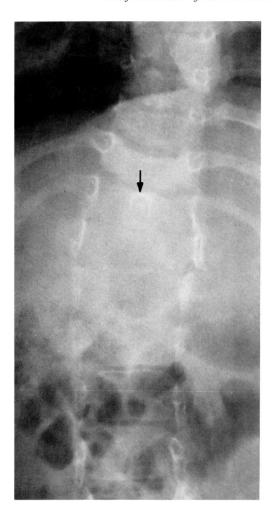

Fig. 8-4. Diastematomyelia. The distance between the pedicles in the lower thoracic and lumbar areas is increased. An oval bony density *(arrow)* superimposed over the middle of the vertebral body is seen at T12. This is the spur which bisects the cord.

due to fusion and deformity of several cervical vertebral bodies with a corresponding loss of height. The neural arches are also fused and malformed. The upper ribs may also be affected and are frequently fused or absent. The clinical features include a short neck, a low hairline, hyperextension of the head, and torticollis. Syndactylism, club foot, and kyphoscoliosis may also be present.

Diastematomyelia is a rare congenital anomaly in which the spinal cord is divided into two portions over a short segment. It may occur at any site but is most common in the lower thoracic or upper lumbar portions of the spinal cord. Tethering of the spinal cord is usually associated with diastematomyelia and may be the major cause of the clinical symptoms. The physical findings vary from minor defects in gait to incontinence and paraplegia. Deformities of the feet may also be present. Midline cutaneous defects,

such as a lipoma, nevus, or abnormal clumps of hair are not uncommon. The most frequent radiographic finding is the presence of multiple anomalies of the vertebral body, such as hemivertebrae and block vertebrae (Fig. 8-4). Neural arch anomalies, widening of the interpediculate distance, and kyphoscoliosis may also be present. A spur that varies in size, length, and consistency projects into the spinal canal from the posterior portion of the vertebral body. It can be identified on the conventional radiograph if it contains mineral such as calcium. Otherwise, myelography is required to demonstrate the defect.

Other organs may be affected when spinal anomalies are encountered. Neurenteric cysts, duplications of portions of the gastrointestinal tract, and agenesis or malformation of the kidneys are among those frequently found.

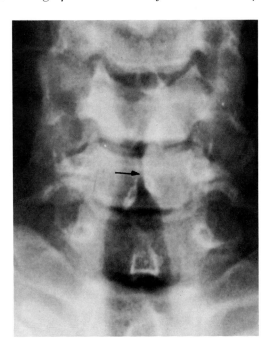

Fig. 8-5. Spina bifida occulta. A vertical radiolucent line *(arrow)* divides the spinous process of C6.

The most common anomaly of the neural arch is a cleft of the spinous process, often called spina bifida occulta (Fig. 8-5). The usual sites are at L5 and S1, but the cleft may occur at any level. These lesions are asymptomatic but when associated with other vertebral and cutaneous anomalies have a more serious prognosis. The separation is depicted radiographically as a vertical, radiolucent line in the spinous process.

A meningocele is a severe malformation in which the meninges protrude, sac-like, through the vertebral column. In a myelomeningocele the spinal cord also protrudes. These defects almost always occur posteriorly and are clinically obvious. The most frequent site is the lumbosacral region, but they may occur in the cervical or thoracic regions. Radiographically, the laminae are spread apart in a fusiform fashion, with the greatest widening at the mid-portion of the meningocele (Fig. 8-6). The neural arches are absent or malformed, and the pedicles are usually thinned. Anomalies of the vertebral bodies are not uncommon. The occurrence of craniolacunia or lacunar skull with these defects has been discussed (see Chapter 7).

Malformations involving the base of the skull and the first and second cervical vertebrae (Fig. 8-7) may produce confusing clinical symptoms, varying from neck pain, weakness, and tingling of the upper extremities to quadriplegia, a rare occurrence. The first cervical vertebra may be totally or partially fused to the occiput; the odontoid process may be hypoplastic or absent; and subluxation with anterior displacement of the skull and C1 as related to the odontoid process may be present. The last condition is of major concern due to the possibility of minor trauma, leading to damage of the spinal cord. It is not difficult to recognize such an anomaly on radiographic examinations. However, more sophisticated studies, such as tomography, are usually required to completely delineate the malformation.

Agenesis of the sacrum and coccyx may be partial or complete (Fig. 8-8). If complete agenesis occurs, the pelvis is narrowed with approximation of the iliac bones. Partial agenesis is most frequent, and usually it is easily recognized radiographically by absence of bony structures and associated malposition of the ipsilateral hemipelvis. Segmental defects also occur with clefts, hemivertebrae, and fusion of segments. Recognition of these anomalies is important because of frequent association with rectal and genitourinary malformations.

Flattening and beaking of the vertebral bodies and narrowing of the interpediculate spaces constitute a major part of the varying forms of bone dysplasia (see Chap. 10).

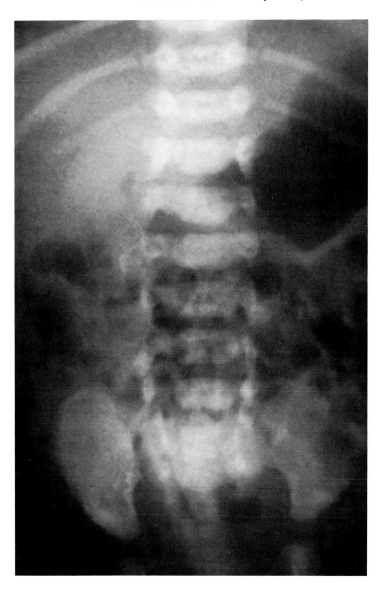

Fig. 8-6. Lumbar meningocele. The interpediculate distance is increased throughout the entire lumbar and sacral areas. The pedicles are also thinned.

ABNORMAL CURVATURE OF THE SPINE

Scoliosis, lateral curvature of the spine, and kyphosis, in which the curve is directed posteriorly, may occur separately or as a combined defect, kyphoscoliosis. When these are recognized early and appropriate treatment is begun, disabling deformities may be prevented. Radiographic examinations are required to establish the degree of the deformity, to evaluate its progression and the effect of treatment, and, perhaps most importantly, to aid in detecting the cause of the abnormal curvature. Scoliosis is more common than kyphosis and is therefore discussed primarily.

Before a radiographic diagnosis of scoliosis is established, the physician must be certain the patient is standing as erect as possible during the examination. The spine of a child too young to stand erect often has lateral and posterior curvatures which are normal. Radiographs in the supine, sitting, and erect positions are often required to establish the degree of scoliosis and the site of primary and secondary curves.

For the most part, diseases which cause abnormal curvature of the spine may be divided into three broad groups: those which directly affect the vertebral column, such as a malformation, bone dysplasia, and infection; those which affect the muscular system directly, such as muscular dystrophy, or indi-

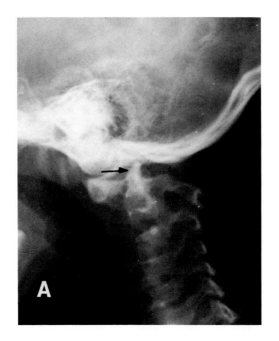

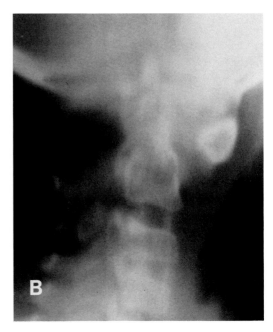

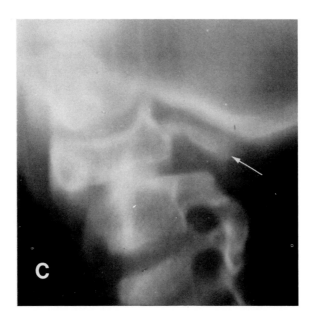

Fig. 8-7. Atlanto-occipital malformation. *(A)* A routine, oblique study of the spine demonstrates the tip of the odontoid *(arrow)* to extend into the inferior portion of the foramen magnum. *(B)* On lateral tomography the odonotid is somewhat posteriorly positioned as compared to the anterior portion of C1. *(C)* Oblique tomography shows that the lateral portions of C1 are incomplete and that the posterior portion *(white arrow)* is closely applied to the occiput and possibly fused to the skull.

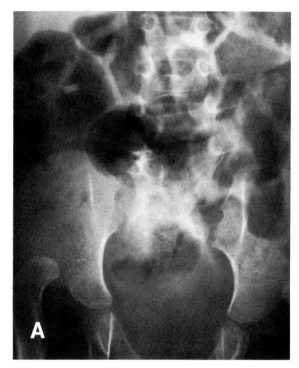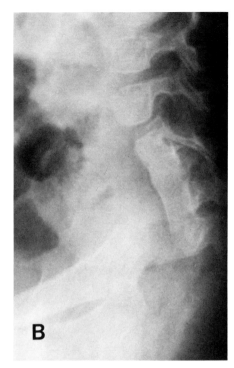

Fig. 8-8. Partial sacral agenesis. *(A, B)* The lower sacral segments and the coccyx are absent. Bilateral hip dislocation, a frequently associated anomaly, is also present in this patient.

rectly through the innervation of muscles, such as cerebral palsy; and idiopathic diseases, probably the most common cause of scoliosis.

Disease Entities

Idiopathic scoliosis
Neuromuscular disorders
Primary vertebral disorders
   Neurofibromatosis
   Infection
   Cardiopulmonary diseases
   Radiation therapy
   Congenital syndromes
   Malformations
   Tumors

Differential Diagnosis

Idiopathic scoliosis is by far the most common cause of abnormal curvature of the spine and is usually mild. It may occur as a rapidly progressive form in children 2 to 3 years of age or as a more slowly progressive form in the adolescent years. In general, the earlier the onset of scoliosis, the more likely the deformity will be severe. The degree of curva-

ture generally increases until growth of the vertebral column ceases and is then static. Radiographically, the spine is curved laterally with compensatory contralateral curves of the vertebral column above and below (Fig. 8-9). Scoliosis of the lumbar spine is only assoicated with a compensatory contralateral curve above the lumbar region, since the sacrum is a fixed structure. Rotation of the vertebrae occur with scoliosis and is manifested by displacement of the components of the neural arch in relation to the vertebral bodies. Articular facets may become locked because of rotation. Other than scoliosis and rotation of vertebrae, the radiographs are normal.

Neuromuscular disorders, such as poliomyelitis, meningoceles, cerebral palsy, and the different forms of muscular dystrophy, are often assoicated with severe scoliosis. In such cases the etiology of the deformity is obvious. Upon radiographic examination, in addition to scoliosis, decreased bone density secondary to lack of weight bearing is apparent.

In patients with familial dysautonomia, scoliosis is not uncommon. Recurrent aspira-

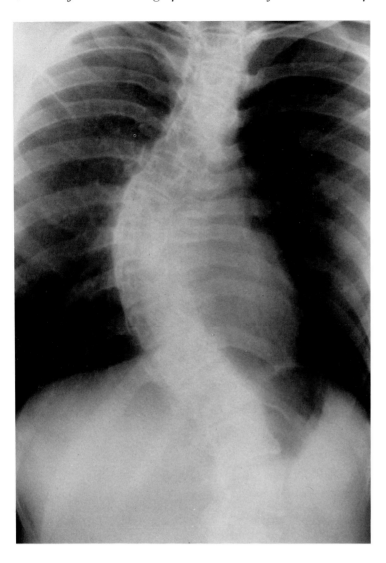

Fig. 8-9. Idiopathic scoliosis. The spine has an "S" shape. The vertebral bodies are normal but rotated, another feature of scoliosis.

tion pneumonias and other changes suggest the diagnosis.

A relatively high incidence of idiopathic scoliosis has also been recorded in patients with congenital heart disease, for reasons not well understood.

Some of the most severe forms of kyphoscoliosis are seen in patients with neurofibromatosis involving extensive segments of the vertebral column (Fig. 8-10). Most often the deformity is not related to the presence of neurofibroma. Scalloping of the posterior margins of the vertebral body and widening of intervertebral foramina are present. The presence of adjacent deformed ribs that appear narrowed and twisted (twisted ribbon deformity) is diagnostic.

Tuberculosis of the vertebral column may, in late stages, produce localized, abnormal curvatures of the spine. The abnormal curvature is due to destruction of vertebral bodies and the corresponding intervertebral disc spaces. The adjacent soft tissues are affected as well. The result is segmental collapse of a portion of the spine leading to a sharply angled, posterior curvature, a gibbus deformity. Radiographically, the destruction of the vertebral body and disc space as well as the abnormal curvature is evident. Calcification in the affected soft-tissue structures, a psoas abscess, is often present. Other forms of infections of the vertebral column are less likely to produce abnormal curvatures of the spine.

The most common pulmonary disease in children with kyphosis is cystic fibrosis. The progressive emphysema increases the anteroposterior dimension of the chest, arches

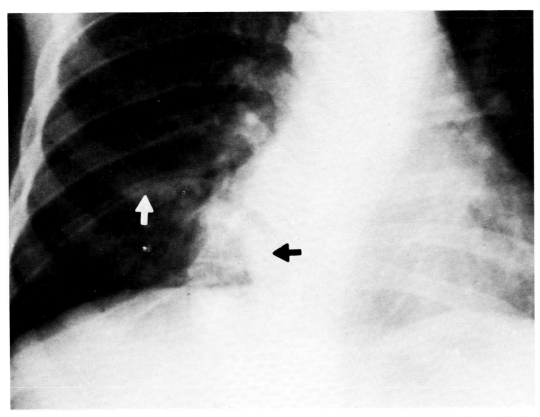

Fig. 8-10. Neurofibromatosis. Characteristic scoliosis associated with a deformed vertebral body *(black arrow)* is present. Note the associated twisted ribbon deformity of the right rib *(white arrow).*

the sternum anteriorly and the thoracic spine posteriorly, and flattens the diaphragm. The clinical and radiographic manifestations of cystic fibrosis are usually so marked that little attention is paid to the secondary deformity of the spine and chest.

The ultimate size of any bone is decreased if radiation therapy is given while growth potential remains. If a portion of a vertebral body is irradiated, the result may be decreased growth of that part of the body, with normal growth of the nonirradiated portion. The final result is wedging and scoliosis, with the concavity of the curve directed toward the irradiated side. Wilm's tumor is often treated with irradiation, and scoliosis is therefore a frequent complication. Now this is less common because the mechanism is understood. The radiographic findings only show nonspecific hypoplasia of a segment of the vertebral column. A history of prior irradiation is required for a specific diagnosis.

A number of forms of bone dysplasia and congenital malformations and syndromes are associated with scoliosis (Fig. 8-2C; see Chapter 10). Similarly, scoliosis may accompany an intramedullary tumor such as an astrocytoma (Fig. 8-25).

SCLEROTIC LESIONS OF THE VERTEBRAL BODY

In the pediatric age-group, sclerotic lesions of the vertebral body are rare. The list of diseases is short, and the clinical and radiographic characteristics of each are fairly characteristic.

Disease Entities

Neonatal central sclerosis
Renal disease
Hodgkin's disease
Tuberous sclerosis
Osteopetrosis

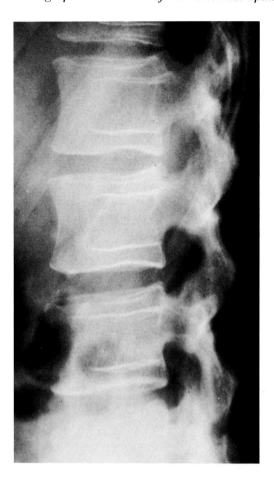

Fig. 8-11. Osteopetrosis. Adult with endo bone. Note the exact radiodense outline of a vertebral body enveloped within the adult bone. Similar bony changes were present throughout the body. (Contributed by Dr. David Wolstein.)

Differential Diagnosis

Sclerotic areas in the central portion of the vertebral body are frequently seen in neonates and most often in premature infants. These areas may follow the contour of the vertebral body and are most common in the thoracolumbar area. As the infant grows, these slowly disappear and are rarely seen after 1 year of age. The etiology is obscure, but such sclerotic areas are considered to be a variant of the normal state.

Hyperparathyroidism secondary to renal disease occurs in the form of renal osteodystrophy in the pediatric age-group. The basic process consists of bone resorption, producing decreased bone density radiographically. However, in the spine there are sclerotic zones at the superior and inferior portions of the vertebral bodies. These zones are more prominent than the decreased radiodensity of the remaining portions of the vertebral body. This mixture of sclerosis and radiolucency has been called "the rugger-jersey" deformity.

A single sclerotic vertebral body may be due to a number of disorders in adults. Although rare in pediatrics, it may still be seen in patients with Hodgkin's disease. This "unaggressive" neoplasm usually destroys bone in a pattern identical to bone destruction in leukemia, but occasionally a sclerotic reaction is produced. The normal trabecular pattern of bone is absent. The lesion is frequently accompanied by adjacent lymph node disease that causes erosion of the anterior margin of the body. Characteristically, the neural arch is not affected.

Sclerotic areas with irregular margins may occur in the vertebral column of patients with tuberous sclerosis. The vertebral body and the neural arch may be involved. These lesions are presumed to be caused by hamartomas with adjacent bone sclerosis. Clinical findings such as seizures, mental retardation, and adenoma sebaceum usually pinpoint the diagnosis.

Osteopetrosis is a congenital defect of bone formation. The bone produced is densely

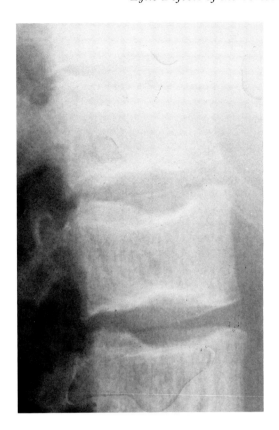

Fig. 8-12. Sickle cell disease. The vertical trabeculae are thickened. This appearance is exaggerated by the decrease in overall bone density. The defects in the superior and inferior margins of the bodies are characteristic of this disease.

sclerotic, but is more fragile than normal bone. The vertebral column is usually involved. The vertebral body and neural arch are densely sclerotic, with loss of the normal trabecular pattern of bone. Fractures are not uncommon. Radiolucent zones in the center of the vertebral body may be present, and on occasion have a contour resembling the vertebral body in miniature (Fig. 8-11).

LYTIC DEFECTS OF THE VERTEBRAL BODY

After recognizing a lytic lesion of the vertebral body, several radiographic criteria became important in arriving at a final diagnosis. For example, a different group of diseases must be considered if an entire vertebral body is uniformly involved and if more than one vertebral body is affected. The appearance of the borders of the lesion, whether sclerotic or ill-defined, is important. The presence or absence of bone expansion is often a clue to the final diagnosis, as is that portion of the vertebral body involved. Looking for associated lesions of the intervertebral disc space and neural arch is also important.

Disease Entities

Hemolytic anemia
  Thalasemia
  Sickle cell disease
Herniation of nucleus pulposus (Schmorl's node)
Neurofibromatosis
Metastatic neoplasm
Infection

Differential Diagnosis

Of all the anemias, thalasemia is associated with the most marked radiographic changes in bone. In the vertebral column, there is a diffuse decrease in bone density due to marrow hyperplasia. The remaining bony trabeculae appear prominent, producing a striated appearance. The cortical margins are thin and may bulge. Similar findings are present in the neural arch.

The radiographic changes in sickle cell disease (Fig. 8-12) are partially due to bone marrow hyperplasia but are also caused by vascular thrombosis, bone infarction and, rarely, osteomyelitis. Vertical bony trabeculae are prominent, but the overall effect is decreased

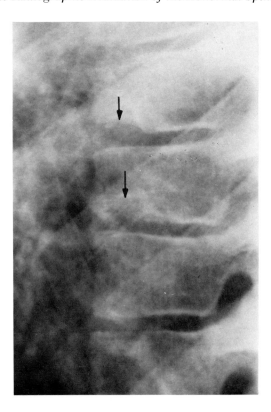

Fig. 8-13. Scheuermann's disease. This 16-year-old boy had recurrent episodes of back pain for approximately 1 year. Defects *(arrows)* are present in the anteroinferior margins of several thoracic and lumbar vertebral bodies. The margins are irregular but sclerotic.

bone density. In adults, bone repair may lead to increased density, but this is rare in childhood. Thrombosis or stasis due to sickling leads to minor degrees of infarction and growth retardation of the central portion of the vertebral body. The resultant deformity of the vertebral body assumes an appearance resembling a flat H, since the peripheral portion of the superior and inferior borders of the vertebral body continue to grow normally (Fig. 8-12).

Herniation of the nucleus pulposus through the surrounding annulus fibrosus may occur in any direction. The etiology, as proposed by Schmorl, is a congenital weakness of the annulus which, with repeated mild trauma, allows escape of the nucleus. It is most common in adolescent males. Defects in the vertebral body may be produced by the misplaced nucleus. These defects are manifested radiographically by smooth, lytic areas with sclerotic borders, usually in the central, anterior, or posterior portions of the superior or inferior borders of the vertebral body (Fig. 8-13). If the fragment extrudes anteriorly, it may also separate the ring apophysis from the vertebral body. The result is a small defect of the anteroinferior or anterosuperior border of the vertebral body,

with a small piece of bone separated from the vertebral body, the so called "lumbus vertebra." These defects are most often incidental, seen in adolescents and young adults. Occasionally pain may be associated, and, in extreme examples, loss of vertebral body height and kyphosis are present. This process is called Scheuermann's disease.

Neurofibromatosis, or von Recklinghausen's disease, produces variable manifestations. It may be associated with severe scoliosis. Scalloped defects are often present in the posterior margins of the vertebral bodies (Fig. 8-14). These defects have sharp, sclerotic borders and may involve several vertebral bodies. A neurogenic tumor is not usually present at the site of the bony abnormality. The etiology is obscure but presumed to be a defect of bone formation. Intraspinal tumors may occur.

Destruction of vertebral bodies due to a metastatic tumor is not as common in children as in adults. The two most common causes are neuroblastoma and leukemia. Soft-tissue sarcomas, such as rhabdomyosarcoma and fibrosarcoma, are less frequent. The different forms of reticuloendotheliosis are often radiographically indistinguishable from metastatic tumors. The changes are

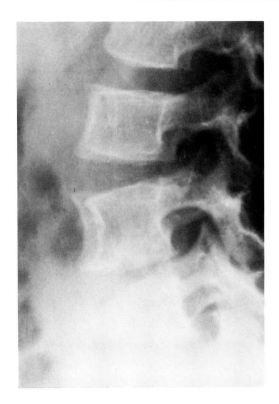

Fig. 8-14. Neurofibromatosis. The posterior borders of the vertebral bodies are convex anteriorly. The anterior margins appear to be duplicated by a thin margin of bone. These and other changes in bone caused by neurofibromatosis are difficult to explain but are thought to be due to be a defect in the mesoderm.

those of irregular bone destruction with cortical disruption. Wedging or complete collapse may be present. Several vertebral bodies are involved as well as the neural arches. The intervertebral disc space is not affected.

In infants and children, osteomyelitis involving the vertebral column (Fig. 8-15) is much less common than involvement of the long bones. A variety of organisms are encountered, ranging from Staphylococcus and Streptococcus to *Mycobacterium tuberculosis,* Brucella, and Blastomyces. The process usually begins in the subchondral bone. The bone is destroyed and the cortex penetrated with involvement of the intervertebral disc. Collapse of the vertebral body may occur as well as marked narrowing of the intervertebral disc space. Soft-tissue involvement is frequent, leading to paraspinal masses. Later, fusion of the bodies, bony bridging, sclerosis, and calcification in the paraspinal mass may be seen.

Osteomyelitis may be difficult to distinguish from metastatic disease. However, a metastatic tumor often affects several vertebral bodies, does not affect the intervertebral disc space, and need not be associated with a paraspinal mass.

A hemangioma is the most common primary tumor of the vertebral column and is usually confined to the vertebral body. The tumor rarely involves more than one vertebra and is most often found in the lower thoracic and upper lumbar areas. A hemangioma is usually incidental and of no clinical importance. Radiographically it is manifested by a generalized decrease in vertebral density, associated with vertical, relatively radiodense striations.

DECREASED VERTEBRAL BODY HEIGHT

A decrease in the height of a vertebral body is not common in the pediatric age-group, and therefore the possible causes are few. Usually, a specific diagnosis can be made with relative ease.

Disease Entities
Eosinophilic granuloma
Metastatic tumor
Trauma
Congenital defects

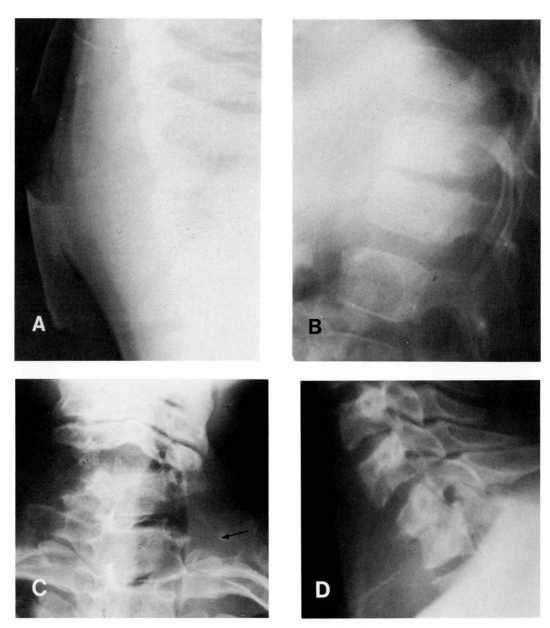

Fig. 8-15. Osteomyelitis. *(A)* A soft-tissue mass is associated with a destroyed spinous process. *(B)* The intervertebral disc space is narrowed, particularly anteriorly. The adjacent bony margins appear dense. *(C, D)* The disc space between C7 and T1 is narrowed and the lateral masses of C7 and T1 on the left are destroyed. (The presence of tuberculosis was proven in each of these cases, but the radiographic changes are indistinguishable from other forms of osteomyelitis.)

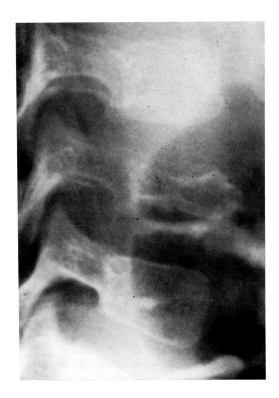

Fig. 8-16. Eosinophilic granuloma. There is decreased density and loss of height of a vertebral body. The body is collapsed and flat (vertebra plana).

Differential Diagnosis

Eosinophilic granuloma may involve any portion of the skeleton, including the spine (Fig. 8-16). Flattening of the entire vertebral body (vertebra plana) with preservation of the disc space and neural arch is so distinctive that its presence warrants a presumptive diagnosis of eosinophilic granuloma. A paraspinal soft-tissue mass is rarely present. Partial, rather than complete, collapse of the body also occurs. This may be difficult to differentiate from a single metastatic lesion. The disease is most common in the 2nd decade of life may occur in several age-groups. The course of the disease is unique, since the body is restored to a normal state within 12 to 18 months.

A metastatic tumor of the vertebral column produces bone destruction and collapse without affecting the intervertebral disc space. The bone destruction is more irregular than bone destruction in eosinophilic granuloma and often involves several vertebrae and the neural arch. Neuroblastoma, leukemia, and reticulum cell sarcoma are the most likely malignant tumors. The different forms of reticuloendotheliosis may involve the spine and are manifested by lytic defects involving multiple sites.

Compression fractures of the vertebral body produce a decrease in height (Fig. 8-17). Fractures of the vertebral column are unusual in young children but much more common in juveniles. The fracture most often involves the anterior portion of the vertebral body with anterior wedging. Several vertebrae in the same region may be involved. There is usually a history of trauma, since a major force is required to produce a fracture of the vertebral body. Other causes include convulsions and tetanus.

Several forms of congenital bone dysplasia produce decreased height of a few or all of the vertebral bodies. This is frequently seen in many of the storage diseases (e.g., mucopolysaccharidosis, lipidosis, gangliosidosis). Small deformed bodies, most often encountered at the level of T12 and L1, are characteristic (Fig. 8-18). Alteration of the anterior margin of the vertebral body due to an excessive accumulation of unossified cartilage is probably the main cause of the seemingly small vertebral body. However, the height of the remaining portion of the vertebral body is normal. The possibility that disc herniation produces this deformity has also been suggested.

A generalized decrease in size of all of the vertebral bodies is encountered in achondro-

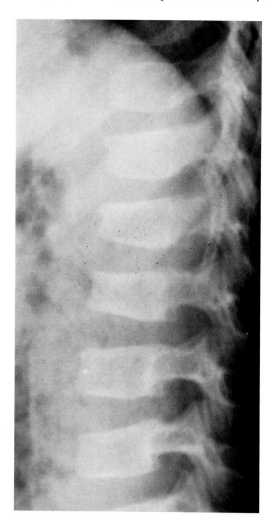

Fig. 8-17. Multiple compression fractures. There is loss of height anteriorly at the level of T12 through L2, with a wedge of bone along the anterosuperior borders. The fractures in this child were due to tetanus.

plasia and similar diseases, such as thanatophoric dwarfism, metatrophic dwarfism, and achondrogenesis. The decrease in size is related to decreased ossification and excessive cartilage. The more abnormal is ossification, the smaller are the vertebral bodies.

Morquio's syndrome is recognized by the presence of universal platyspondylisis.

INCREASED VERTEBRAL BODY HEIGHT

The configuration of a vertebral body changes with growth. In newborns the vertebral bodies are more or less cuboid in the thorax and round in the lumbar area. However, the horizontal diameter of the body is always greater than the vertical diameter.

Thus a vertebra looks like a rectangle lying on its larger side. Gooding and Neuhauser demonstrated the effects of gravitational pressure and stress upon the growth and development of the vertebral body. Growth in the vertical direction occurs along the cartilaginous layers that surround the superior and inferior surfaces of the vertebral body. Decreased or no pressure on these surfaces results in longitudinal overgrowth of the body, and, by contrast, excessive stress or pressure upon the body may result in an actual decrease in vertical growth. The presence of a tall vertebra in an older child, therefore, is the result of an inability to maintain an upright position and thereby allow for the normal effect of gravitational pressure on the growth plates. The cause of tall vertebrae in newborns is not understood.

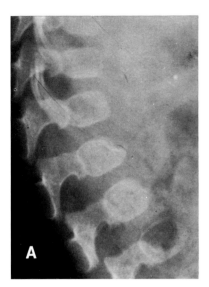
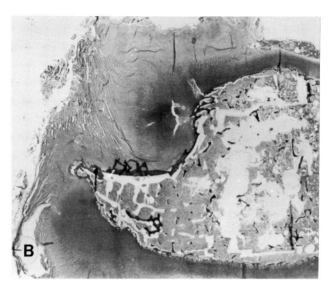

Fig. 8-18. Gangliosidosis. *(A)* Note the apparent small body at the level of L1 with its characteristic inferior notch. This appearance is typical of many of the storage disorders. *(B)* A cross section through the abnormal vertebra reveals an excessive accumulation of cartilage in the region of the notch. The remainder of the vertebral body was normal.

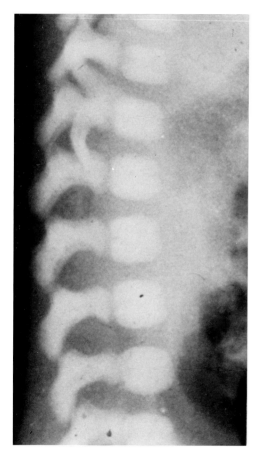
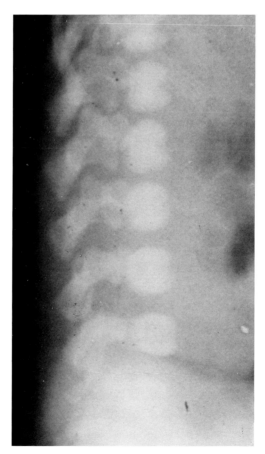

Fig. 8-19. Down's syndrome. Normal lumbar vertebra are shown in a newborn on the left. Note the increased vertical diameter and the anterior concavity in a newborn patient with Down's syndrome on the right.

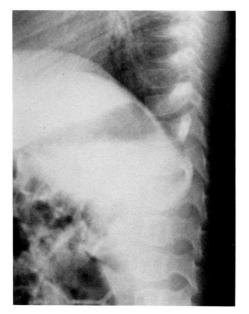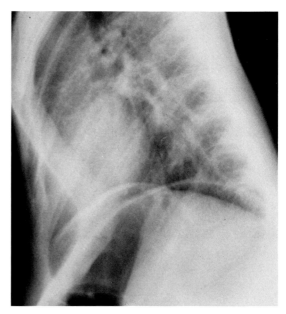

Fig. 8-20. Neuromuscular disease. Two patients with severe neuromuscular disorders. Note the tall vertebral bodies.

Disease Entities

Newborn
   Down's syndrome and other congenital anomalies
Infant and child
   Tall vertebrae in normal subjects
   Neuromuscular disorders

Differential Diagnosis

In newborns the presence of tall vertebrae is encountered in 85 per cent of patients with Down's syndrome (Fig. 8-19). In addition, an increased concavity is also present within the anterior margin of the vertebra. These alterations in size and configuration are best visualized in the upper lumbar region on the lateral projection. Despite its high incidence in Down's syndrome, the presence of tall vertebra is not diagnostic. However, it is a strongly suggestive, particularly when associated with other thoracic skeletal changes, such as a bifid manubrium.

Vertebral changes associated with Down's syndrome are prominent within the 1st 24 months. After this period the child begins to assume an upright, ambulatory status, and the vertical diameter of the bodies decreases relatively in height. However, they rarely resume a completely normal appearance.

Similar vertebral abnormalities are encountered in other trisomic anomalies (e.g., Trisomy 18 and Trisomy 15) but with far less frequency. In addition, we have observed tall vertebrae in a small percentage of cases of congenital heart defects without chromosomal abnormalities.

The presence of tall vertebrae in an older child should always suggest the presence of neuromuscular disease or other incapacitating diseases that prevent the patient from assuming a normal, upright position (Fig. 8-20). Occasionally, tall vertebral bodies are seen in normal individuals. The reason for their presence is not understood.

ABNORMALITIES OF THE INTERVERTEBRAL DISC

The nucleus pulposus and the surrounding annulus are rarely involved by a primary pathologic process. Rather, abnormalities of the intervertebral disc space are secondary to involvement of the contiguous vertebral body and have been discussed. Calcification of the intervertebral disc is occasionally seen in children as an isolated entity.

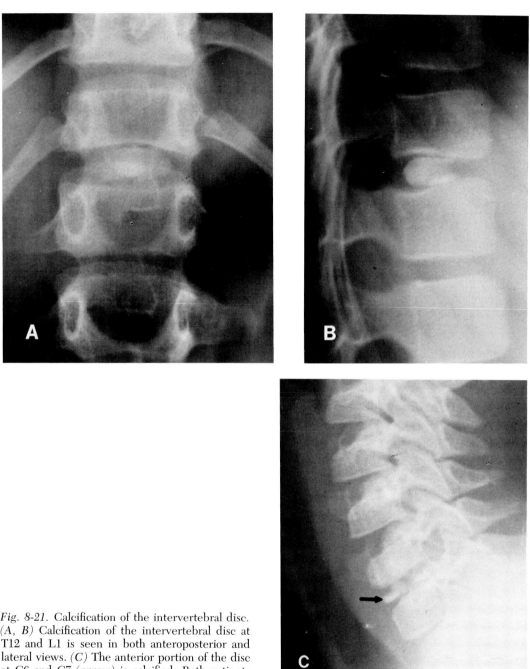

Fig. 8-21. Calcification of the intervertebral disc. (A, B) Calcification of the intervertebral disc at T12 and L1 is seen in both anteroposterior and lateral views. (C) The anterior portion of the disc at C6 and C7 (arrow) is calcified. Both patients were asymptomatic.

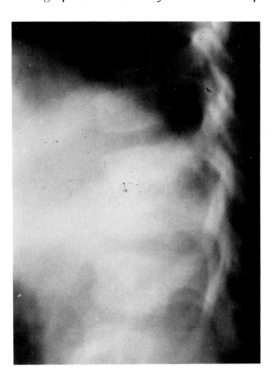

Fig. 8-22. Osteomyelitis. The intervertebral disc space is irregularly narrowed with some degree of sclerosis of the bony margins (not well outlined on this reproduction). The presence of bacterial osteomyelitis was proven.

Disease Entities

Calcification of the intervertebral disc

Narrowing of the intervertebral disc space

  Infection

  Trauma

  Discitis

Differential Diagnosis

Calcification of the intervertebral disc (Fig. 8-21) is usually an incidental and often insignificant finding, although pain is occasionally present when the cervical spine is involved. The process may be seen in patients of any age-group, including the neonate. The calcification is confined to the disc in most instances, but extension into the soft tissues has been described. The calcific radiodensity is usually fluffy and well circumscribed but may be fragmented and irregular. Multiple sites may be involved. The calcification is often absorbed over several months. Trauma has been implicated as a cause, but most often the process is idiopathic.

The intervertebral disc is secondarily involved in osteomyelitis (Fig. 8-22). The infection originates in the subchondral bone of the vertebral body, and then by erosion, pene-

trates the margins of the vertebral body and spreads into the intervertebral disc space. Narrowing or obliteration of the disc space and fusion may result. It is important to remember that a metastatic tumor does not involve the disc space. A chordoma is probably the only neoplasm that involves the disc space and thus mimics and infective process.

Fractures of the vertebral body may be associated with narrowing of the intervertebral disc space. The obvious changes and history of trauma make the diagnosis relatively easy.

A rather interesting lesion is discitis. This is believed to be the result of a mild infection within the intervertebral disc space that occurs in children approximately 5 years of age or younger. The most commonly involved level is L4 to L5, and the second most frequent level is L3 to L4. Hematogenous spread of microorganisms is the most likely explanation, since no direct entry can be demonstrated. The main radiographic feature is disc space narrowing, which may not be detectable until the 2nd to the 4th week after the onset of the disease. Vertebral end plate erosion producing a sawtooth appearance usually follows, and if a significant amount of erosion occurs, herniation of the disc into the vertebral body may result. Vertebral

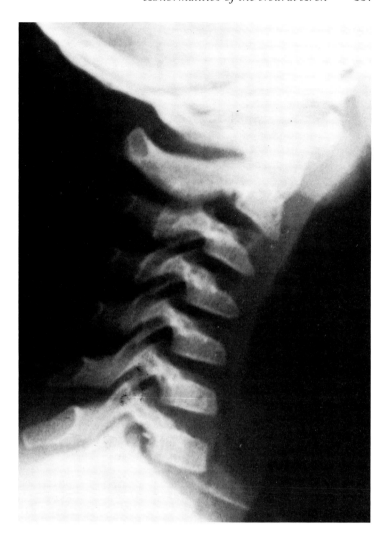

Fig. 8-23. Normal curvature of the cervical spine. The posterior margins of the second, third, and fourth vertebral bodies do not form a smooth curve, but rather are manifested by "step-offs." This is normal in children under 10 years of age.

body wedging or compression is not common. Marginal reactive bone proliferation is rare, as are paravertebral soft-tissue masses. Approximately 10 per cent of the cases demonstrate complete reconstitution. The remainder show persistent alterations, such as end-plate sclerosis.

ABNORMALITIES OF THE NEURAL ARCH

The neural arch is composed of the pedicles, the superior and inferior articular facets, the laminae, the transverse processes, and the spinous processes. The appearance of these structures varies in different parts of the vertebral column. An effort should be made to identify these structures on any radiograph which includes the spine. However, oblique views, special views with varying angulation, and tomography are often required to completely examine the neural arch.

Malformations of the neural arch have been discussed (see p. 320). Several diseases that involve both the vertebral body and the neural arch are described in the sections dealing with the vertebral bodies. However, some processes affect only the neural arch and others show major manifestations in the neural arch.

LYTIC DEFECTS OF THE NEURAL ARCH

A lytic defect of the neural arch is probably due to trauma if congenital malformations can be excluded. Other possibilities include tumors and osteomyelitis.

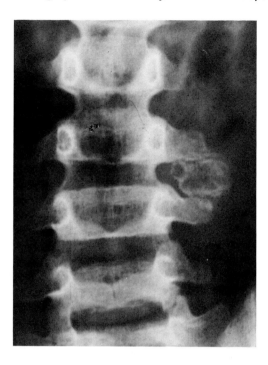

Fig. 8-24. Osteochondroma. The bony mass between the transverse processes of the third and fourth lumbar vertebrae on the left has an inner trabecular pattern and cortical margins, resembling normal bone. Such findings are characteristic of osteochondroma.

Disease Entities

Trauma
Osteomyelitis
Metastatic neoplasms
Primary neoplasms of bone
    Osteoid osteoma
    Osteoblastoma
    Osteochondroma
    Aneurysmal bone cyst
    Neoplasms originating within the
      spinal canal
    Neurofibroma
    Primary cord tumors
    Congenital tumors

Differential Diagnosis

Fractures of the neural arch are uncommon until the 3rd decade of life, and even then they are not as frequent as in older patients. In fractures of the lumbar region, the transverse processes are most often affected. The articular facets and their supporting structures and the atlanto-axial junction are the most frequent sites in the cervical region. Fractures in the thoracic and sacrococcygeal regions are less common than in other sites.

Radiographically a fracture is manifested by a radiolucent line. Demonstration of the fracture and differentiation from normal structures are often difficult. Oblique and angled anteroposterior views and tomography may be needed. Careful attention should be directed toward the articular facets to detect any misalignment. Subluxation and dislocation with fractures are more common in adults but may rarely be seen in the pediatric age-groups. These injuries are most common in the cervical region. Therefore, a frequent source of concern is the normal hypermobility of the upper cervical region in the child (Fig. 8-23). In forward flexion, the posterior portions of the vertebral bodies may not be manifested by a smooth line but rather by multiple "step-offs." This feature is not diagnostic for subluxation until it is demonstrated on carefully obtained flexion views. Actually, subluxation is quite rare in the first 2 decades of life.

Osteomyelitis of the vertebral column is primarily a disease of the vertebral body and the intervertebral disc space (Figs. 8-15, 8-22). The infection may involve the neural arch, producing bone destruction of a nonspecific type. Concomitant involvement of the vertebral body and disc space, as well as clinical signs and symptoms of infection, suggests a diagnosis.

A metastatic tumor is the most common neoplasm which affects any part of the ver-

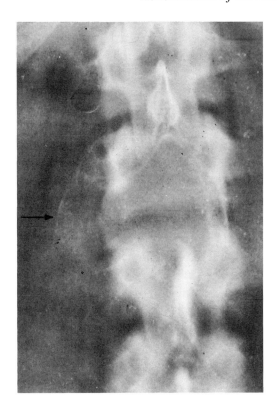

Fig. 8-25. Aneurysmal bone cyst. A large ballooned-out area of bone with a thin rim is seen to the right of L2 *(arrow)*. The transverse and spinous processes are destroyed, and the medial portion of the pedicle is faintly visible.

tebral column, including the neural arch. Most of such mestases arise from neuroblastomas, leukemia, and the soft-tissue sarcomas. Metastatic disease affects the vertebral body more often and to a greater degree than the neural arch.

Destruction of portions of the neural arch is more difficult to detect radiographically than destruction of the vertebral body, which is well outlined on a lateral view. No single view clearly outlines all portions of the neural arch. However, destruction of a pedicle is not difficult to detect on an anteroposterior projection. Loss of a spinous process or transverse process may also be seen on the same view. Involvement of the lamina and lateral masses may only be detected on oblique views or with tomography. Myelography may be required to outline the intraspinal component.

Primary tumors of bone are rare in the vertebral column and usually originate from the neural arch. These tumors may not be purely lytic; they frequently consist of a combination of lytic and sclerotic processes.

Osteoid osteoma is a common tumor and occurs most frequently in the lumbar region.

Chronic pain is the main presenting symptom. The radiographic appearance is manifested by bone sclerosis with a central radiolucent nidus. In some cases, the nidus is sclerotic, with a thin radiolucent zone and surrounding sclerosis. These findings may be difficult to detect and often require tomography. Any portion of the neural arch may be involved, but the pedicle is probably the most frequent site.

An osteoblastoma may be associated with pain, scoliosis, or even a palpable mass. The lesion is initially lytic with bone expansion. The cortex is thinned but usually intact. As the tumor heals, it calcifies and becomes sclerotic. It rarely extends into the spinal canal to compress the cord or nerve roots.

An osteochondroma (Fig. 8-24) occurs at sites of bone growth and most often originates from the spinous process. The tumor is broad-based with a bulbous distal portion. Irregular calcification may be seen in the cartilaginous cap. Ostechondromas may occur in the spine as part of the syndrome of hereditary multiple exostoses.

An aneurysmal bone cyst (Fig. 8-25) may develop in the spine and be associated with

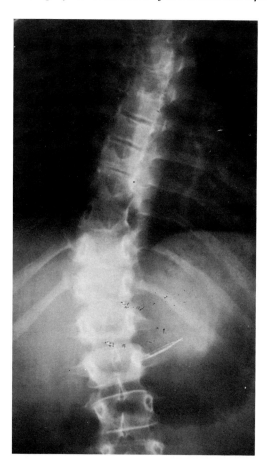

Fig. 8-26. Astrocytoma. The central and lower portions of the thoracic spine are curved to the right. The pedicles of T6 through T10 are flattened medially and thinned. The interpediculate spaces are widened at the same levels. An astrocytoma was confirmed at surgery after myelography.

pain or neurologic deficits if the mass expands into the spinal canal. These lesions are purely lytic and cause bone expansion. The overlying cortex may be penetrated by the tumor.

Lesions which originate in the spinal canal include neurofibromas and tumors of the spinal cord, primarily astrocytoma and ependymoma. The patients present with a number of neurologic abnormalities, depending upon the size and location of the mass. Meningioma, as frequent as neurofibroma in adults, is extremely rare in the pediatric age-group.

Neurofibroma occurs as either part of a generalized process, von Recklinghausen's disease, or as a single tumor. With von Recklinghausen's disease, neurofibroma is characterized by scalloping of the posterior margins of the vertebral bodies and neural arches. Such changes may occur in areas not directly affected with neurofibroma and are presumed to be due to dysplatic bone formation or herniated arachnoid cysts.

Single neurofibromas present as localized defects with widening of the intervertebral foramina. The tumor may reach a sufficient size to erode the pedicles and occasionally the laminae. The vertebral body is rarely involved. Myelography is usually required to accurately define the extent of the intradural tumor.

Intramedullary tumors, those originating within the spinal cord, usually consist of gliomas, with astrocytoma being most frequent, followed by ependymomas. Despite the large size of the tumor, neurologic findings may be minimal. Occasionally scoliosis may be the presenting symptom (Fig. 8-26). These tumors slowly erode the spinal canal, producing widening. This is manifested radiographically by thinning of the pedicles and widening of the interpediculate spaces. The widened canal may also be seen on lateral views, particularly in the cervical region. Standard radiographic measurements of the normal spinal canal in different age-groups are available and should be used if the changes are not ob-

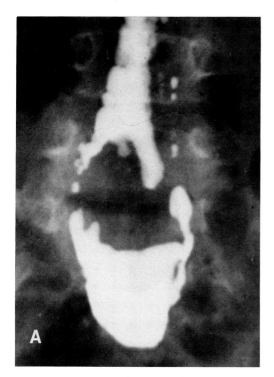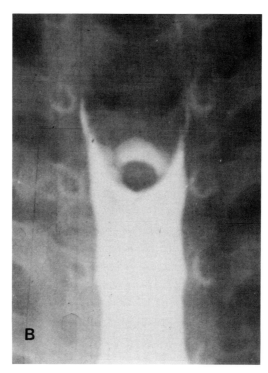

Fig. 8-27. Congenital tumors of the spinal canal. (A) A large lipoma was present that presented as an intradural, extra-axial mass. An abnormal collection of hair was present externally at the same level. (B) Dermoid. A complete block to the cephalic flow of Pantopaque is present. On the anteroposterior view, the spinal cord appears widened, simulating an intramedullary lesion, but on other views the column was shown to be flattened by an intradural, extra-axial mass. A skin dimple was present at the same level.

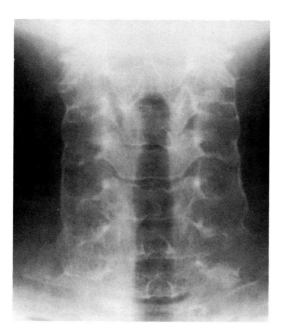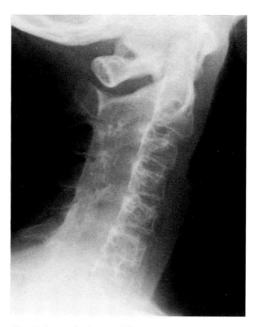

Fig. 8-28. Rheumatoid arthritis. Bony fusion involves all of the pedicles and laminae of the second through the seventh cervical vertebrae. The vertebral bodies are radiolucent and small.

vious. Myelography is usually required for accurate diagnosis and to determine the extent of the mass.

Congenital tumors include lipomas, dermoids, and teratomas (Fig. 8-27). These are usually associated with other malformations such as spina bifida, hairy nevus, sinus tracts, or external masses. Radiographic changes in the vertebral column are often minimal, although the tumor may erode portions of the neural arch. Again, myelography is required for accurate localization.

SCLEROTIC LESIONS OF THE NEURAL ARCH

Diseases producing local or diffuse sclerosis of the neural arch are few in number. Osteomyelitis may be associated with sclerosis late in the disease, but the other radiographic changes are far more impressive. The degenerative processes due to aging, so common in older adults, are not seen in children. An osteoid osteoma may have a sclerotic nidus, but more often the lytic component predominates. Metabolic diseases and hemolytic anemias are primarily lytic, although the remaining bony trabeculae may appear more radiodense than usual. Osteopetrosis, a dysplasia of bone, affects multiple sites, including the neural arch, producing dense but fragile bone.

Some degree of sclerosis of the neural arch is produced by juvenile rheumatoid arthritis (Fig. 8-28). The disease is more common in females than males and usually begins in the 1st decade of life. Peripheral joints are most often involved, but the cervical spine is involved in approximately 15 per cent of the patients. Unlike rheumatoid spondylitis, the process begins in the cervical spine and rarely involves the lumbar region. If splenomegaly, lymphadenopathy, and/or hepatomegaly are present, the process is referred to as Still's disease.

The initial radiographic examination in the symptomatic patient may be normal. Minimal decrease in bone density may be present but is difficult to recognize. The apophyseal joints are involved in the disease leading to destruction of the joint, adjacent sclerosis, and eventual fusion in more severe cases. Involvement of the ligamentous supports of the alanto-axial junction is frequent. Subluxation of the first and second cervical vertebrae may then occur with severe consequences.

Fusion may involve the neural arches and vertebral bodies of the upper cervical spine. The vertebral bodies may decrease in size and the intervertebral disc spaces become narrowed. These manifestations may resemble those of congenital fusion, but the clinical picture makes the correct diagnosis obvious.

REFERENCES

1. Caffey, J.: Pediatric X-Ray Diagnosis. ed. 6. Chicago, Year Book Medical Publishers, 1972.
2. Epstein, B. S.: The Spine. A Radiological Text and Atlas. ed. 3. Philadelphia, Lea and Febiger.
3. ———: The Vertebral Column. Atlas of Tumor Radiology. Chicago, Year Book Medical Publishers, 1974.
4. Gooding, C. A., and Neuhauser, E. B. D.: Growth and development of the vertebral bodies in the presence and absence of normal stress. Am. J. Roentgenol. Radium Ther. Nucl. Med., 93:388, 1965.
5. Rabinowitz, J. G., and Moseley, J.: The lateral lumbar spine in Down's syndrome-a new roentgen finding. Radiology, 83:74, 1964.
6. Rabinowitz, J. G., and Sacher, M.: Gangliosidosis (G.M.) Am. J. Roentgenol. Radium Ther. Nucl. Med. 121:155, 1974.
7. Schmorl, E., and Junghamns, H.: The Human Spine in Health and Disease. New York, Grune and Stratton, 1959.

9

Louis S. Parvey, M.D.

Radiographic Features of Joint Effusions and the Underlying Diseases

GENERAL COMMENTS

The clinical appearance of a swollen joint may be related to changes within the periarticular tissues or to actual distention of the joint itself. Occasionally, bony enlargement of the metaphysis or epiphysis may simulate joint enlargement. Radiographic distinction, however, is not difficult. Swelling of the periarticular tissues alone is usually the result of cellulitis or traumatic edema, and the joint space as well as the adjacent osseous structures is intact and normal. Fluid within a joint expands the joint capsule and causes an overall increase in soft-tissue opacity (Fig. 9-1). In the knee, the normally radiolucent infrapatellar fat pad is compressed and may be completely obliterated. The suprapatellar bursa becomes distended and displaces the quadriceps tendon and patella outward. Distention of the hip joint may be more subtle radiographically. Aside from widening of the joint space, the surrounding muscular structures, such as the iliopsoas and obturator muscles, and the gluteus medius and gluteus minimus, are displaced and present as masses of radiodensity around the joint (Fig. 9-2). It is often difficult to determine the nature of the effusion on radiographic criteria alone, although blood, because of its iron content, is generally more radiopaque than a transudate. Structural osseous abnormalities are quite obvious.

Disease Entities

Traumatic synovitis
Hemophilia
Juvenile rheumatoid arthritis
Septic arthritis
Tuberculosis
Acute transient synovitis
Acute rheumatic fever
Hypertrophic osteoarthropathy
Synovial sarcoma and other bone tumors

DIFFERENTIAL DIAGNOSIS

An isolated, swollen joint may be a diagnostic problem initially. However, a specific diagnosis can often be obtained when the radiologic and clinical manifestations are correlated.

For example, joint swelling following an episode of trauma with or without an obvious fracture may be the result of hemorrhage or an effusion due to traumatic synovitis. These two entities can be easily differentiated on a chronologic basis. Hemarthrosis occurs rapidly and is usually present within 15 minutes to 2 hours following injury, whereas a traumatic synovitis requires anywhere from 12 to 24 hours to appear. Hemorrhage is common in knee injuries and in children may be associated with a fracture of the tibial spine, often an anterior cruciate avulsion (Fig. 9-3). In

(Text continued on p. 346.)

343

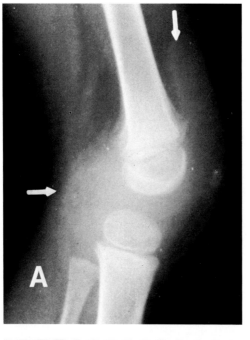

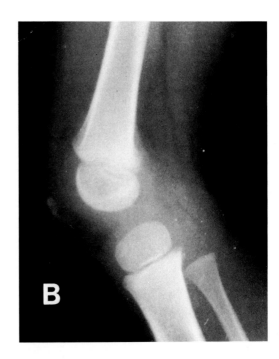

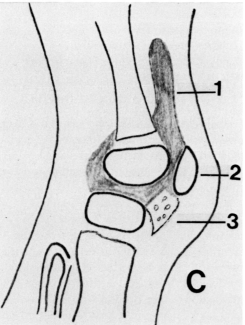

Fig. 9-1. Unilateral juvenile rheumatoid arthritis. *(A)* The left knee demonstrates effusion within the joint. In comparison to the right *(B)*, the left knee is markedly dense and the suprapatellar bursa *(upper arrow)* and posterior joint capsule *(lower arrow)* are distended. Both the patella and the infrapatellar fat pad are displaced, and the latter is almost obliterated. *(C)* A schematic drawing of a normal knee for comparison. *1*——Suprapatellar bursa. *2*——Patella. *3*——Infrapatellar fat pad. The darkened area represents the extent of the joint capsule.

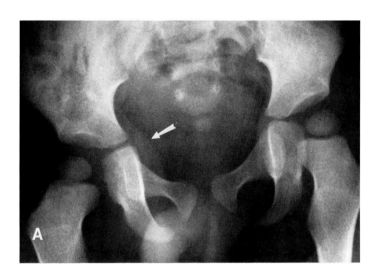

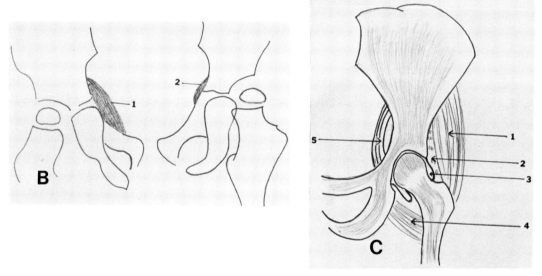

Fig. 9-2. Septic arthritis of the right hip. (A) The right femoral head shows minimal subluxation. The right obturator muscle is displaced and radiopaque *(arrow)*. Note the normal left side. *(B)* A schematic drawing of Fig. 9-2A better illustrates the difference in size between the normal *(2)* and the diseased *(1)* obdurator muscle. *(C)* A schematic drawing of a normal hip and its surrounding structures. *1*—gluteus medius and gluteus minimus muscles. *2*—Fat tissue. *3*—Joint space. *4*—Iliopsoas muscles. *5*—Obturator muscle.

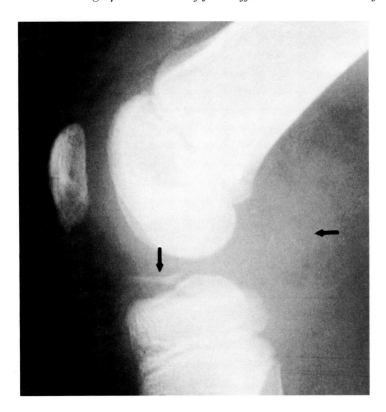

Fig. 9-3. Traumatic hemarthrosis. A lateral examination of a knee approximately 3 hours following injury reveals a swollen joint with posterior distention of the capsule *(horizontal arrow).* The anterior tibial spine is avulsed *(vertical arrow).*

many fractures that extend into the knee, a horizontal lateral film reveals a fat fluid level. This has been termed lipohemarthrosis and occurs following extrusion of marrow fat into the joint space.

Hemophilia is a well known cause of bleeding into a joint. The early radiographic appearance of an acute hemophiliac hemarthrosis is similar to traumatic hemorrhagic arthropathy, without evidence of gross trauma. However, hemophilia is associated with repeated episodes of hemarthrosis, and changes in the synovium, subchondral bone, and periarticular tissues eventually occur (Fig. 9-4). Such manifestations require a period of time to develop and become radiographically apparent well after the clinical diagnosis has been established. Continual hemorrhage into the joint not only injures the joint cartilage but also incites synovial hyperplasia, which produces a pannus that both erodes and destroys the articular surface (Fig. 9-5). Bleeding occurs not only into the joint space but also within the bone substance itself, and subchondral intraosseous cystic changes are subsequently produced. The entire process also stimulates dilatation of the capsular and epiphyseal blood vessels. The resulting hyperemia enlarges the epiphysis, accelerates

bone maturity, and produces osteoporosis. Chronic bleeding into the periarticular tissues results in the deposition of hemosiderin, and the soft tissues then look more radiodense than usual. When the extremities are severely affected, they are used less, and muscular atrophy as well as osteoporosis develops. Bony ankylosis is rarely encountered today.

Except for hemorrhaging, the pathologic and radiographic features of juvenile rheumatoid arthritis and hemophilia are remarkably similar. Joint effusion is the initial major manifestation in rheumatoid arthritis (Fig. 9-1). In this disease the synovium proliferates to form a pannus, which eventually destroys the cartilage and causes erosion of the articulating surface and loss of the joint space (Fig. 9-6). Massive erosion of the joint surface by the pannus may also occur in some individuals in whom the disease continues unabated. As a result, cystic excavations are produced that are associated with dissolution of the adjacent bony structures (Fig. 9-7). The joint space is markedly widened in this form of the disease. The accompanying vascular dilatation with its associated hyperemia also causes periarticular osteoporosis, epiphyseal enlargement, and accelerated bony mat-

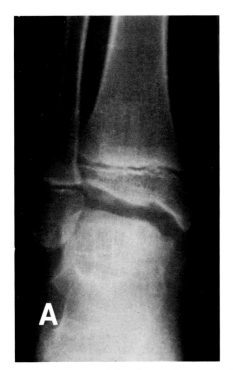 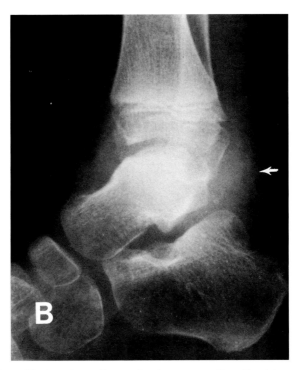

Fig. 9-4. Hemophiliac hemarthrosis. *(A, B)* The ankle joint is swollen and quite opaque. Considerable posterior distention is obvious *(arrow)*. In the frontal projection, joint surface irregularity and notching deformities exemplify some of the gradual changes that occur with hemophilia.

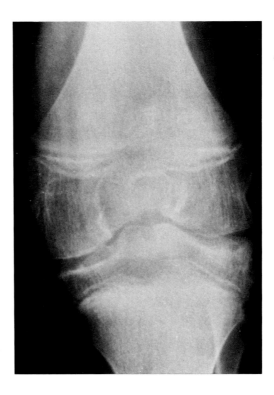

Fig. 9-5. Erosion of the joint in hemophilia. Many of the osseous changes characteristic of repeated hemorrhage are present. The joint space is narrowed and the surface irregular. The intercondylar notch is widened and eroded.

347

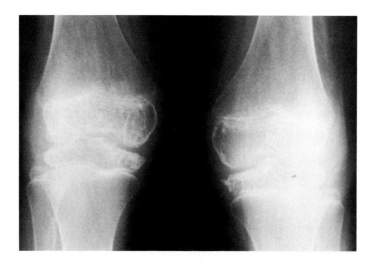

Fig. 9-6. Juvenile rheumatoid arthritis. Both knees contain fluid; an overall increase in tissue density makes this apparent. The joint surfaces are eroded. Note the decreased joint space bilaterally. The bones are noticeably osteoporotic.

uration. Since the inflammatory reaction extends into the periarticular tissues, muscular atrophy is present in advanced cases.

Although the radiographic features of juvenile and adult rheumatoid arthritis are similar, there are some differences. Monoarticular involvement occurs in 30 per cent of cases in the juvenile form, in contrast to the predominant polyarticular presentation in adults. The large joints are usually involved in monoarticular arthritis, and joint effusion within a knee or ankle in a young child 3 to 5 years of age is frequently the presenting finding (Fig. 9-1). Polyarticular involvement in children is similar to that in adults and affects mainly the smaller joints of the hands and feet. The proximal interphalangeal joints are most frequently involved, and periarticular swelling producing a fusiform appearance is the characteristic early manifestation (Fig. 9-8). A thin unilaminar periosteal reaction, surrounding the proximal phalanges, metacarpals, and metaphyses, occurs early in this disease. The spine, and more specifically the cervical vertebrae, is commonly affected in juvenile rheumatoid arthritis, in contrast to the adult form. In fact, many block cervical vertebrae encountered in the adult probably represent arrested juvenile rheumatoid disease. The inflammatory reaction also involves the surrounding ligaments and its attachments. As a result, joint loosening, particularly atlantoaxial subluxation, is commonly encountered (Fig. 9-9). In systemic rheumatoid disease associated hepatosplenomegaly, pericarditis, myocarditis (but not endocarditis), and/or subcutaneous nodules may be evident radiographically.

A pyogenic infection must be considered when high fever accompanies a hot, tender joint effusion. The effusion is an exudate and is due to bacterial invasion of the joint by way of a penetrating wound, extension from an adjacent osteomyelitis, or more commonly by way of a hematogenous spread from a distant focus. Pyogenic arthritis characteristically produces a periarticular edema that obliterates the surrounding fascial planes. This feature is not observed in most other joint effusions (Fig. 9-10). In certain joints (e.g., the hip or shoulder) destruction of the articular cartilage and the underlying bone occurs rapidly. Points of contact, such as the opposing articular surfaces, are initially destroyed. A flail joint, or fibrous or bony ankylosis may be the final result of inadequately treated pyogenic disease. Between the ages of 6 months to 2 years the causative organism is most often *Hemophilus influenzae.* In infants below 6 months of age, Staphylococcus, Pneumococcus, Gonococcus, Salmonella, and *Escherichia coli* may be responsible.

Tuberculous arthritis is manifested differently. Soft-tissue swelling is a major feature and may be present for a long time before bone destruction becomes obvious (Fig. 9-11). Enzymes capable of destroying cartilage do not exist in the tubercle bacillus. As a result, bone destruction is a slow process and the joint space is seldom narrowed. Characteristically, only a single peripheral surface is affected. Consequently, the major feature is an erosion of variable size within the outer margin of the joint. If the disease persists, the entire joint is eventually destroyed. In

(Text continued on p. 352.)

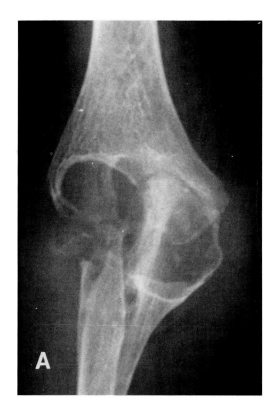

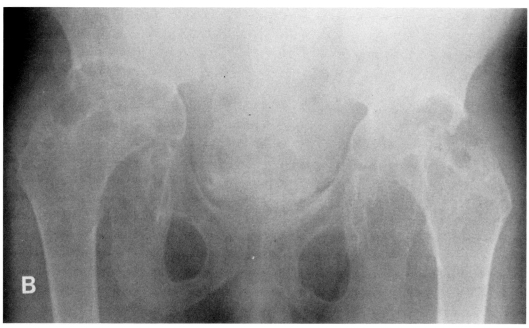

Fig. 9-7. Juvenile rheumatoid arthritis. (A) The elbow and (B) hips in this patient are destroyed. Huge cystic erosions are apparent.

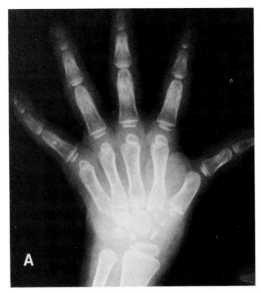

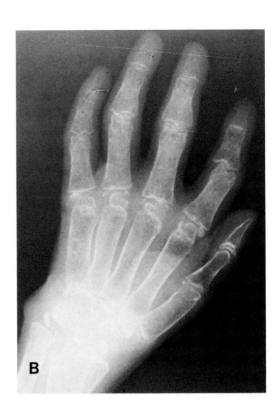

Fig. 9-8. Juvenile rheumatoid arthritis. (A) Relatively early findings in the hand are manifested by a periarticular swelling (fusiform appearance) that surrounds the proximal interphalangeal joints. Fluid within the wrist accounts for the increased radiodensity in this area. (B) Progressive changes are present in this child. All the joints are narrowed and irregular. Severe osteoporosis is present.

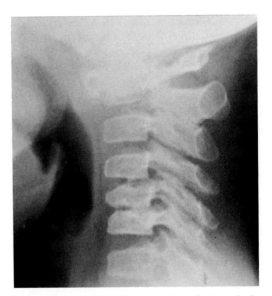

Fig. 9-9. Juvenile rheumatoid arthritis of the spine. Subluxation at the level of C1 to C2 is present, with C1 displaced anteriorly. All the articulating facets are irregular, and the joint space between C5 and C6 is decreased.

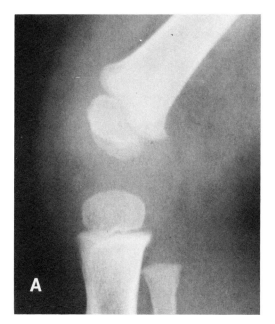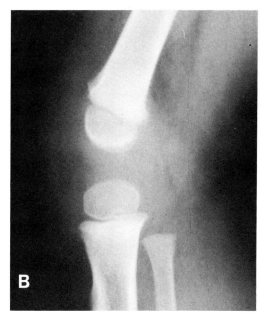

Fig. 9-10. Pyogenic arthritis. *(A)* The entire knee is swollen. The joint space is widened and distended diffusely. The infrapatellar fat pad is completely obliterated. The periarticular soft tissues are also inflamed, and as a result the joint capsule is not outlined. (Compare to Fig. 9-1.) *(B)* Following antibiotic therapy much of the inflammation has subsided. The infrapatellar fat pad and the joint capsule are now recognizable.

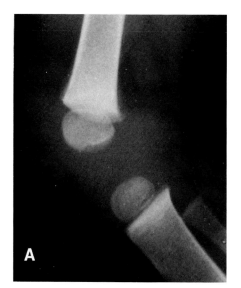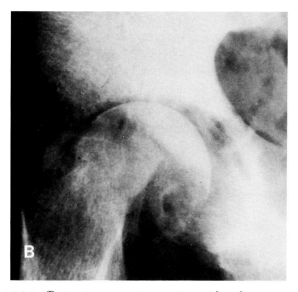

Fig. 9-11. Tuberculous arthritis. *(A)* Persistent joint effusion is present in a patient with miliary tuberculosis. Tubercle bacillae were cultured from the infusion. *(B)* Tuberculous changes in another patient demonstrate partial destruction of the inferior margin of the femoral head and neck. The lateral margin of the joint space is widened.

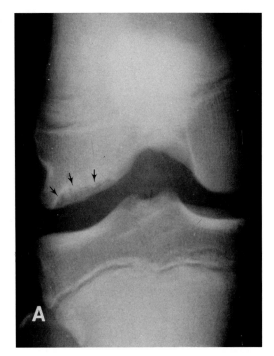 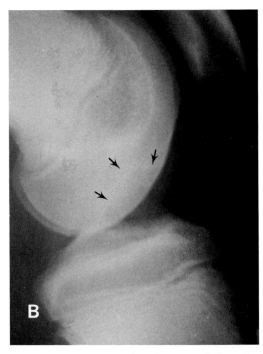

Fig. 9-12. Osteochondritis dissecans. *(A, B)* Examination of the knee reveals a large, oval-shaped, radiolucent defect within the posterior portion of the lateral condyle *(arrows).* The dense necrotic bone is not seen.

addition, if the infection arises in an epiphysis, the contact surface of the joint is involved. New periosteal bone formation is rarely encountered in children. Monoarticular involvement is strikingly frequent with an overall incidence of 90 per cent, and periarticular osteoporosis occurs early in the disease. These two features are important in distinguishing tuberculous arthritis from rheumatoid arthritis.

Clutton's joint, caused by congenital syphilis, is a rare, chronic joint effusion. The lesion arises between the ages of 8 to 16 years and is characterized by symmetrical knee effusions that persist for several years without causing any permanent joint sequelae.

Acute transitory synovitis of the hip is of clinical and radiographic importance. It is a benign, self-limiting process and should not be confused with any of the lesions above. The radiographic examination is most often normal, although the joint space may occasionally be widened. Swelling of the periarticular muscles surrounding the hip and obliteration of the fascial planes occurs occasionally. Complete resolution within a few days is the rule. The etiology of this lesion is unknown.

Acute rheumatic fever frequently begins with migrating polyarthritis and joint swelling. This lesion is recognized by the high incidence of associated cardiac disease. The effusion is a benign transudate that almost never involves the bones. However, periarticular fibrosis (Jaccoud's arthritis), a rare sequelae, is associated with severe joint deformity but with little or no radiographic bony alteration.

Polyarthritis is also a manifestation of an acute allergic reaction and is an infrequent complication following viral infection, such as rubella and mumps.

Osteochondritis dissecans is manifested clinically by pain and swelling due to an associated synovitis. The lesion commonly affects the knee, although other joints or bones may be involved. In the knee, the radiographic presentation consists of an area of radiolucency within the medial femoral condyle that in the early phase contains dense necrotic bone within its center (Fig. 9-12). The necrotic bone later sloughs into the joint, producing a joint mouse.

The benign tumorous neoplasms, such as chondromatosis, and pigmented villonodular synovitis, may be accompanied by an effu-

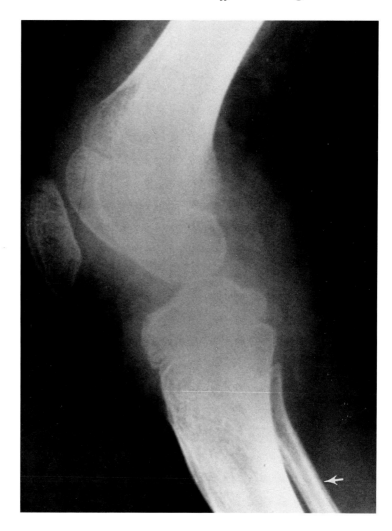

Fig. 9-13. Hypertrophic pulmonary osteoarthropathy. Some effusion is present within the knee. However, periosteal changes are present on all of the bones, best visualized on the fibula *(arrow)*.

sion; a patient with such a neoplasm may present with joint swelling. Radiographic manifestations are quite characteristic. Chondromatosis is a form of cartilaginous metaplasia within the synovial villi. The process produces small cartilaginous fragments that are extruded into the joint and subsequently calcify and/or ossify. Radiographically, the fragments look like round or ovoid calcified masses of varying sizes.

Pigmented villonodular synovitis also represents a benign overgrowth of synovium that produces nodular tissue masses. Both lesions are uncommon in children. Clinically and radiographically, villonodular synovitis resembles a chronic recurrent joint effusion. In the hip, however, the masses produce erosions on both sides of the joint that are manifested by sharply demarcated cystic lesions with sclerotic borders. This feature is quite distinctive. The knee is most frequently involved, but because of its distensibility, it

demonstrates fewer bony changes. Hemosiderin deposition accounts for the pigmented discoloration of the masses.

Persistent joint effusion in the hip is occasionally due to an underlying osteoid osetoma. This may be mistaken for pigmented villonodular synovitis, since many of the histologic and radiographic features are alike.

Hypertrophic osteoarthropathy should be considered when a synovitis which results in enlarged joints and effusion is associated with a periosteal reaction (Fig. 9-13). This lesion is usually secondary to chronic pulmonary disease with chronic bronchiectasis, such as cystic fibrosis and pulmonary metastases. Obviously, hypertrophic osteoarthropathy is sometimes confused with juvenile rheumatoid arthritis. However, the periosteal reaction is more pronounced and quite characteristic in osteoarthropathy.

Malignant neoplastic disease may also be

responsible for joint effusion or enlargement. Fortunately, the incidence of malignant joint disease is exceptionally low in children. Synovial sarcoma occurs during the 2nd through the 4th decade of life. Interestingly enough, despite the histologic origin of the tumor, the lesion is located primarily within the periarticular tissues and frequently demonstrates calcifications.

REFERENCES

1. Athreya, B. H., Barnes, P., and Rosenlund, M. L.: Cystic fibrosis and hypertrophic osteo-arthropathy in children. Am. J. Dis. Child., *129:*634, 1975.
2. Jaffe, J. L.: Tumors and tumerous conditions of the bones and joints. Philadelphia, Lea and Febiger, 1958.
3. Martel, W.: Cervical spondylitis in rheumatoid arthritis. Am. J. Med., *44:*441, 1968.

10

Louis S. Parvey, M.D.
Jack G. Rabinowitz, M.D., F.A.C.R.
Jeno I. Sebes, M.D.
Daniel Kirk Westmoreland, M.D.

Systematic Radiographic Evaluation of the Skeleton

PERIOSTEAL REACTION

Periosteal reaction refers to the deposition of new bone beneath the periosteum. Several types of reaction may be induced, each with a different dynamic and physiologic implication. The reactions may be unilaminar (single layer), multilaminar, cuffed (Codman's triangle), spiculated, or cloaked (Fig. 10-1). Each reaction should be evaluated with respect to the bone, joint, and soft-tissue manifestations, keeping the clinical presentation in mind.

The appearance of the periosteal reaction in many ways helps to specify the differential diagnosis of a particular lesion. A single, thin, unilaminar reaction is not distinctive and can be seen in association with benign or malignant disease. However, when such a reaction is localized to the metaphysis it is specifically related to inflammatory disease. A thick, uninterrupted (2 mms. long), unilaminar periosteal reaction almost always indicates a slowly progressing, benign process.

A multilaminar periosteal reaction develops in association with a cyclic process that intermitently induces new periosteal bone formation. There are many factors that stimulate this form of periosteal reaction: a tumor-elaborated humoral agent; vagus nerve stimulation; repeated displacement of the

periosteum by a dissecting tumor; pus or granulation tissue; and cyclic production of an osteoneogenic substance from the disease process itself.

A cuffed reaction indicates periosteal interruption due to a rapidly growing mass. It was originally described by Codman as a manifestation of a malignancy. However, benign but aggressive infections behave similarly. The periosteum is elevated from the shaft and is penetrated at one point by the expanding mass. The bone deposited by the periosteum then assumes a triangular appearance.

A spiculated reaction, often termed "sunburst" or "hair-on-end" reaction, is associated with aggressive, destructive bone lesions that rapidly elevate the periosteum. The long, thin spicules represent new bone which has been deposited along Sharpey's fibers in a reparative response. This form of reaction may be associated with aggressive, benign, or malignant processes. When the spicules are short and thick, the lesion is benign and the diagnosis is limited to a few entities, such as tuberous sclerosis, hypertrophic osteoarthropathy, thyroid acropachy, and hemangioma of bone.

A cloaked periosteal reaction is one in which new bone is deposited beneath a widely elevated periosteum; it is almost always associated with a benign process.

355

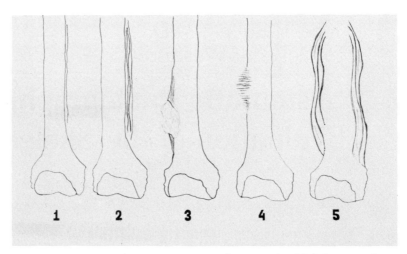

Fig. 10-1. Periosteal reactions. *1*—Unilaminar. *2*—Multilaminar. *3*—Cuffed (Codman's triangle). *4*—Spiculated. *5*—Cloaked.

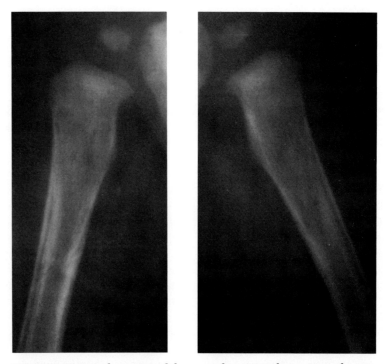

Fig. 10-2. Periosteal reaction of the normal, growing bone. Note the symmetrical, unilaminar periosteal reaction along the femoral shafts in a normally developing young infant.

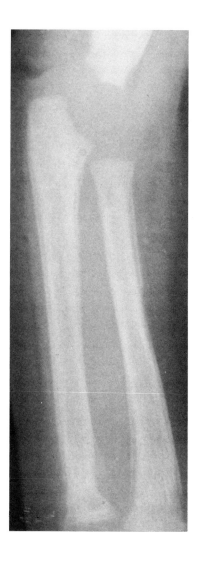

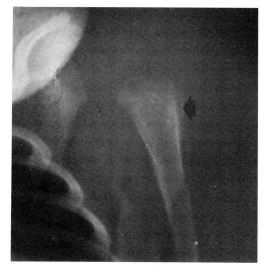

Fig. 10-4. Osteomyelitis and pyogenic arthritis. There is marked soft-tissue swelling surrounding the left shoulder as well as an effusion within the joint space. The latter is widened and the humerus subluxated. The lateral margin of the humerus shows evidence of dissolution, and a thick unilaminar periosteal reaction extends from this area along the humerus *(arrow)*.

←

Fig. 10-3. Congenital syphilis. The upper extremity in an infant with congenital syphilis reveals irregular metaphyseal changes in the distal radius and ulna. A generalized unilaminar and multilaminar periosteal reaction involves the bones visualized.

PERIOSTEAL REACTION IN NEWBORNS

Disease Entities

Osteomyelitis
  Congenital syphilis
  Pyogenic osteomyelitis
Infantile cortical hyperostosis
  (Caffey's disease)
Trauma
New periosteal bone formation in
  normal subjects

Differential Diagnosis

New periosteal bone formation, particularly unilaminar, is seen normally along the shaft of the extremities in a growing bone. This is particularly apparent in premature infants and is most pronounced in the 2nd and 3rd months of life (Fig. 10-2). The femur, humerus, and tibia are most frequently affected, and the reaction consists of a single layer of new periosteal growth of varying thickness. The remainder of the osseous structures are normal, and the infant is usually asymptomatic. Periosteum formation in growing bones should not be confused with that which occurs as part of an overall disease process.

Although the periosteal reaction is an important diagnostic feature of congenital syphilis, the initial changes in bone occur within the metaphysis. These consist of an irregular and serrated zone of provisional calcification and areas of bone destruction within the medial aspect of the metaphysis. The periosteal changes are unilaminar and multilaminar, forming a shell around the bone. The periosteal and diaphyseal changes may occur simultaneously, but frequently periosteal changes present sometime later (Fig. 10-3). The periosteal reaction, however, is an important feature in differentiating congenital syphilis from the congenital rubella syndrome. The metaphyseal changes in both diseases are strikingly similar. However, a periosteal reaction in the congenital rubella syndrome is rare. Both the periosteal and metaphyseal changes that occur in congenital syphilis resolve eventually, becoming incorporated into the bone.

Pyogenic osteomyelitis is an infection unusual in newborns. It is caused predominantly by Staphylococcus or Streptococcus. Being an acquired disease, pyogenic osteomyelitis differs from most congenital bone infections by its relatively late onset and high incidence of associated joint involvement. The radiographic findings are characteristic of osteomyelitis and consist predominantly of metaphyseal and periosteal changes (Fig. 10-4). The changes in the metaphysis begin with patchy, irregular areas of demineralization that quickly coalesce, forming larger osteolytic areas. The bone infection spreads rapidly, and periosteal changes, initially of unilaminar character, followed by multilaminar changes, become apparent. In newborns joint involvement is likely, since the vessels in the shaft communicate freely with the epiphyses. As a result the joint becomes swollen and enlarged, and frequently there is some degree of dislocation. If the infection progresses unabated, the entire joint may be destroyed.

Caffey's disease is recognized by its diffuse periosteal manifestations (see p. 364). It has a low incidence in the immediate neonatal period.

A localized, cloaked periosteal reaction that presents shortly after birth is usually related to a fracture which occurs as a result of trauma at birth. Fractures of the clavicle are frequent, although rib fractures are also common. Infants delivered in a breech position are more likely to sustain metaphyseal-epiphyseal fractures in the lower extremities. Such fractures are manifested by metaphyseal fragmentation; the periosteal reaction that develops during healing can be rather extensive. The radiographic features are similar to those of the battered child syndrome, seen in older children.

Discussion

Unilaminar new periosteal bone formation in newborns is seen in a high percentage of infants and is normal. The periosteum is loosely fixed to the shaft during this period, and the developing bone deposits underneath. The reaction was initially considered to be the result of normal manipulation. However, the same findings have been encountered in infants who received little or no manipulation.

Osteomyelitis in newborns is not common. It reaches the bones by way of the blood stream from a cutaneous focus or from an infected umbilical stump. The association of pyogenic arthritis with osteomyelitis is quite common. Pyogenic arthritis within the hip joint, however, may arise following femoral vein puncture.

PERIOSTEAL REACTION IN INFANTS AND CHILDREN

Disease Entities

Unilaminar reaction
  Osteomyelitis
  Metastasis
  Caffey's disease
  Hypervitaminosis A
  Rickets
  Crohn's disease
  Rheumatoid arthritis
  Hypertrophic osteoarthropathy
  Menke's syndrome
Spiculated reaction
  Osteosarcoma
  Ewing's sarcoma
  Metastasis
Multilaminar reaction
  Osteomyelitis
  Metastasis
  Caffey's disease
  Ewing's sarcoma
  Osteosarcoma
  Eosinophilic granuloma
Cuffed reaction
  Osteosarcoma
  Ewing's sarcoma
  Metastasis
  Osteomyelitis
Cloaked reaction
  Battered child syndrome
  Scurvy
  Caffey's disease

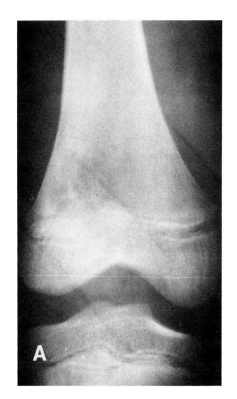

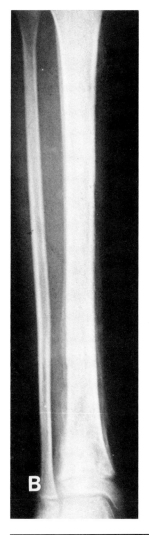

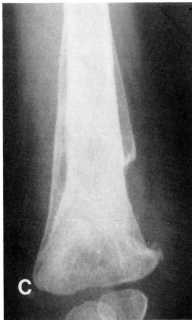

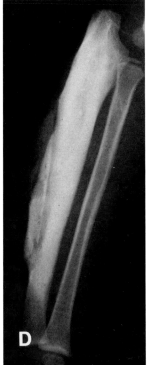

Fig. 10-5. Osteomyelitis. *(A)* Early staphylococcal osteomyelitis. Mottled areas of bone osteolysis are present within the femoral metaphysis. The surrounding bone is still intact and no obvious periosteal reaction is noted. *(B)* Active osteomyelitis. Staphyloccal osteomyelitis involves the entire tibial shaft. Destruction is noted mainly within the distal portion of the bone, although the entire shaft is surrounded by a thick, undulating, unilaminar periosteal reaction. *(C)* Chronic granulomatous osteomyelitis. Blastomycosis. Periosteal reaction in this patient is cuffed and unilateral. The cuffed reaction along the medial aspect of the humerus demonstrates the classic Codman's triangle. The lesion is well along in the process of healing. *(D)* Chronic osteomyelitis of the ulna is present, with a large sequestrum in the process of being extruded along the posterior surface. The remaining bone is thick and dense due to an extensive multilaminar periosteal reaction that is now being incorporated into the shaft.

359

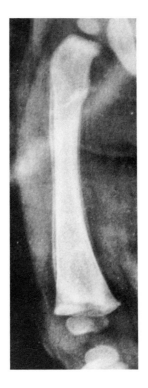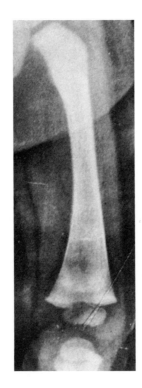

Fig. 10-6. Bone infarct in sickle cell disease. A dense, unilaminar periosteal reaction is present along the shaft of the right femur. This was associated with pain. However, no osteolysis occurred, and in a short time the child became asymptomatic.

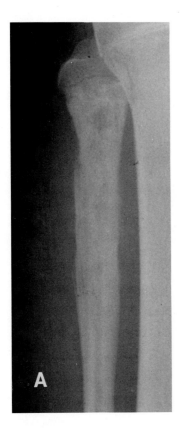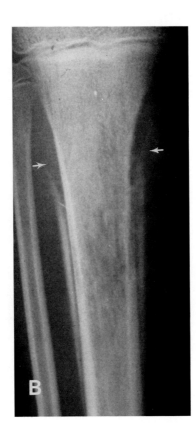

Fig. 10-7. Ewing's tumor. *(A)* Note the multilaminar, "onion skin" periosteal reaction in this bone. It is interrupted proximally by a soft-tissue mass. The entire metaphysis is involved with a diffuse permeative lesion. *(B)* The multilaminar periosteal reaction in this tumor is thick and interrupted. It presents as a bilateral, cuffed reaction *(arrows)*. The permeative nature of the lesion is obvious throughout the shaft.

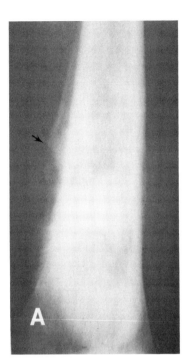
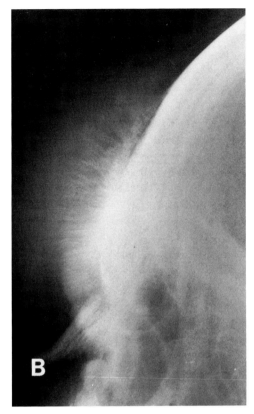

Fig. 10-8. Osteosarcoma. *(A)* A radiopaque mass is present within the distal femur. The surrounding periosteal reaction is interrupted by the tumor and produces a Codman's triangle *(arrow)*. A spiculated reaction is present within the tumor below. *(B)* The classical, spiculated periosteal reaction of an osteosarcoma is present within the frontal bone. Similar periosteal reactions can be produced by metastatic retinoblastoma or neuroblastoma. A large soft-tissue mass is also present. Note the dense new bone developing along the inferior aspect of the tumor.

Differential Diagnosis

Acute hematogenous osteomyelitis caused by pyogenic organisms most commonly begins in the metaphysis or epiphysis of a long bone. The earliest clinical and radiographic feature is deep, soft-tissue swelling adjacent to the metaphysis. The soft-tissue swelling is recognized radiographically by loss of the normal muscle planes and an overall increase in soft-tissue density. Pain is often present and can be localized with pinpoint precision. The bones at this time are essentially normal, although mottled areas of osteolysis begin to appear approximately 10 days later associated with periosteal reaction (Fig. 10-5A). The developing periosteal reaction may be varied, although unilaminar and multilaminar reactions are most frequently seen in the acute phase (Fig. 10-5B). A cuffed reaction in the form of Codman's triangle oc-

casionally occurs in infections that spread rapidly through the bone, causing cortical interruption (Fig. 10-5C). If the infection progresses to a chronic stage because of inadequate therapy, necrotic dead bone persists as a sequestrum and is surrounded by dense, reactive, proliferating periosteal bone, an involucrum (Fig. 10-5D). Sequestra look like islands of bone of greater density than the surrounding normal bone and are occasionally extruded through fenestrations, or cloacae, in the bone.

Patients with sickle cell disease have an increased incidence of osteomyelitis, caused predominantly by Salmonella. The appearance is similar to other forms of osteomyelitis, although the entire shaft is more commonly involved. It may be difficult to differentiate this form of osteomyelitis from a bone infarct (Fig. 10-6).

The radiographic and clinical patterns of

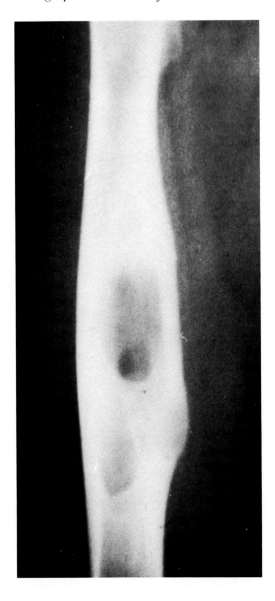

Fig. 10-9. Eosinophilic granuloma. A locular eosinophilic granuloma is present, with extensive multilaminar periosteal reaction. The margins of the lesion are sharp and beveled.

osteomyelitis and Ewing's sarcoma are also remarkably similar. Classically, Ewing's sarcoma is a permeative, destructive, medullary lesion that penetrates the cortex to induce a multilaminar periosteal reaction ("onion skin" reaction), as well as a soft-tissue mass (Fig. 10-7A). Consequently, it should be assumed that any osteolytic lesion associated with a soft-tissue mass is a Ewing's sarcoma, until proven otherwise. The metaphysis is most commonly affected, although the diaphysis can also be involved. The tumor itself does not produce bone, although bone formation may be stimulated within the lesion. Actually, any bone, including the flat bones, may be involved, and variations from the classical picture are frequent.

Osteogenic sarcoma can be associated with multiple periosteal reactions that may be either multilaminar, cuffed, or spiculated (Fig. 10-8). The spiculated reaction is the most characteristic. However, the same reactions are also found in Ewing's sarcoma, osteomyelitis, or even a metastasis. However, a soft-tissue mass is characteristic of Ewing's sarcoma and is not a feature typical of osteogenic sarcoma. The proximal tibia and distal femur are most frequently affected, although any bone may be involved. The tumor usually arises in the metaphysis and produces an osteosclerotic reaction in approximately 50 per cent of the cases. A combination of osteolytic and sclerotic lesions, or purely destructive, osteolytic lesions, are also frequent. New tumorous bone formation is characteristic of osteogenic sarcoma.

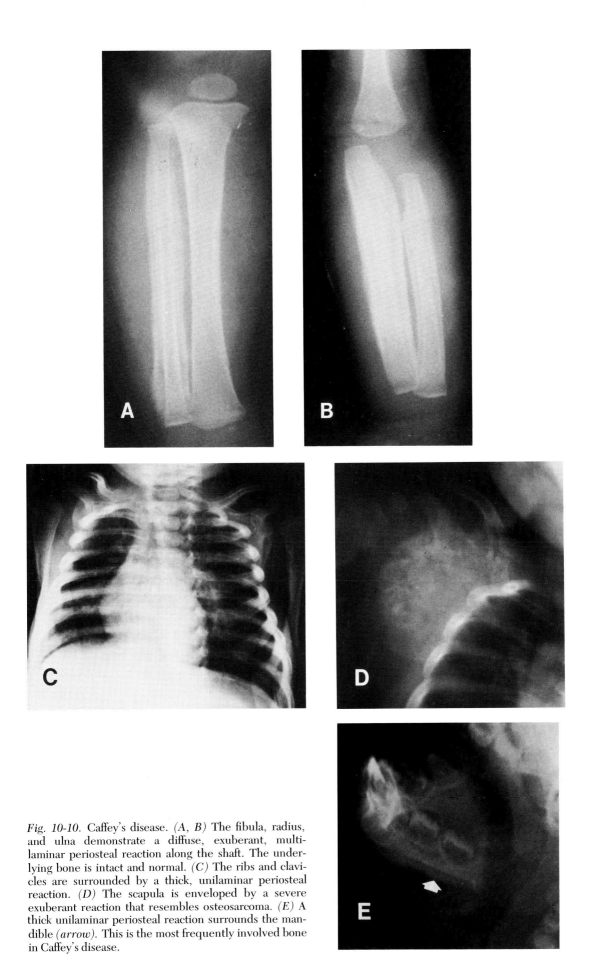

Fig. 10-10. Caffey's disease. (A, B) The fibula, radius, and ulna demonstrate a diffuse, exuberant, multilaminar periosteal reaction along the shaft. The underlying bone is intact and normal. (C) The ribs and clavicles are surrounded by a thick, unilaminar periosteal reaction. (D) The scapula is enveloped by a severe exuberant reaction that resembles osteosarcoma. (E) A thick unilaminar periosteal reaction surrounds the mandible (arrow). This is the most frequently involved bone in Caffey's disease.

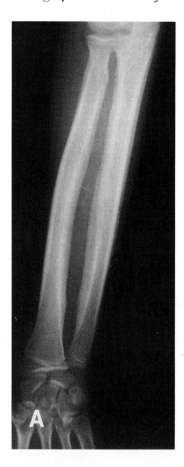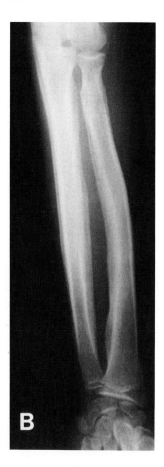

Fig. 10-11. Hypertrophic pulmonary osteoarthropathy. *(A, B)* A dense, multilaminar periosteal reaction surrounds both radii and ulnae in a symmetrical fashion.

Eosinophilic granuloma of bone is seen in older infants and children, usually under the age of 10 years. The lesion is located eccentrically within the bone, and therefore produces a thick unilaminar or multilaminar periosteal reaction along one side of the shaft. The underlying osteolytic lesion is well circumscribed and may have a well-defined or sharply demarcated border that often demonstrates a beveled edge (Fig. 10-9). Except in the skull, a soft-tissue mass associated with eosinophilic granuloma is unusual.

Metastatic disease is occasionally accompanied by a periosteal reaction. In children, neuroblastoma and leukemia are the most common lesions which produce metastasis. The cells lodge in the metaphyseal region, where they begin to destroy bone and produce patchy, osteolytic lesions. They eventually extend through the cortex to elevate the periosteum. Metastasis in many ways resembles osteomyelitis. However, simultaneous involvement in multiple areas and a definite delay in periosteal development is distinctive of metastasis.

In Caffey's disease, infantile cortical hyperostosis, the periosteal reaction is the only pathologic, radiographic feature. This entity is characterized by a radiodense, exuberant, unilaminar or multilaminar reaction that surrounds the shaft of the bone and spares the metaphysis and epiphysis (Fig. 10-10A, 10-10B). The underlying bone is always normal. The entire skeleton is affected, with the exception of the vertebrae and the small bones of the hands and feet. The mandible, clavicles, ribs and long bones are most frequently involved (Fig. 10-10C). Interestingly, when the disease involves the upper part of the body, the lesions tend to be symmetrical and bilateral. The scapula is the only bone in this region that can be affected unilaterally; occasionally, such an effect has been mistaken for a malignant osteosarcoma (Fig. 10-10D). The physician should bear in mind that Caffey's disease is rarely seen in infants beyond the age of 5 months, and a primary bone tumor at this early age is quite rare. The mandible is always affected at one time during the course of the disease and is

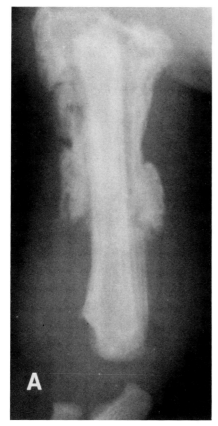

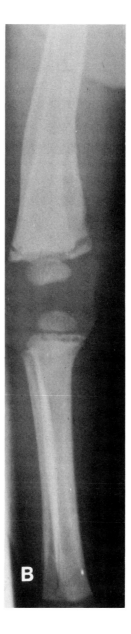

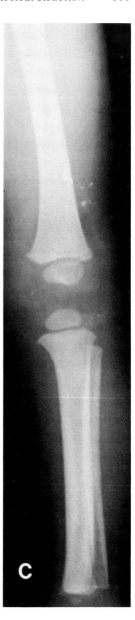

Fig. 10-12. Battered child syndrome. (A) An exuberant cloaked and multilaminar reaction surrounds the humerus. This appearance is the result of a severe subperiosteal hematoma that developed following a metaphyseal-epiphyseal fracture at the proximal end of the bone. (B, C) The lower extremities in another patient show multiple fractures in different stages of development. The right femur demonstrates a healing fracture through the distal metaphysis that is associated with a severe but well healing periosteal reaction. More recent fractures are present within the metaphyseal region of the right proximal and left distal tibia. Soft-tissue swelling is also present within the proximal left leg.

virtually pathognomonic (Fig. 10-10E). The prognosis is excellent, and complete resolution is the general rule despite the many bones involved. Occasional fusion of adjacent bones, such as the ribs, and the radius and ulna, occurs when exuberant periosteal reactions remain in contact with each other.

In infants, hypertrophic osteoarthropathy is usually secondary to cystic fibrosis, pulmonary metastasis, and severe liver disease due to biliary atresia. The periosteal changes range from a simple unilaminar reaction to a multilaminar reaction. The multilaminar reaction may appear wavy and undulating. The lesion is symmetrical and involves all of the extremities, including the small bones

(Fig. 10-11). The bones adjacent to the joints are affected mainly, although with severe disease the entire shaft may be involved. Such cases resemble Caffey's disease, although they occur at distinctly different ages. Soft-tissue thickening of the ungual tufts, as well as joint swelling and pain, completes the main features of this periosteal reaction.

A rare form of unilaminar periosteal reaction is excessive ingestion of vitamin A. The reaction is symmetrical, bilateral, and unilaminar, and it essentially involves the long bones. Hydrocephalus has been described as a very severe complication of this abnormality.

Occasionally, obvious periosteal changes

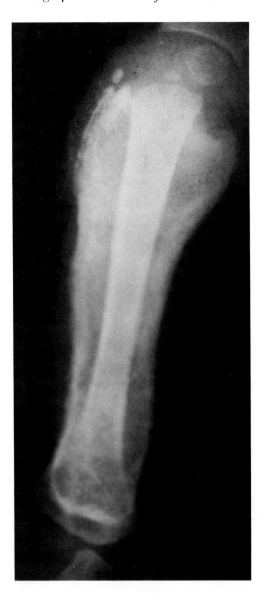

Fig. 10-13. Healing scurvy. A massive, cloaked periosteal reaction envelopes the entire humerus. This is the healing phase of diffuse subperiosteal hemorrhage. (Note the resemblance to the battered child syndrome.)

may be the first manifestation of the battered child syndrome. An exuberent, cloaked reaction is common. Although the periosteal reaction is apparently benign, it should alert the physician to the potential dangers inherent in this disease process. The prolific periosteal reaction is the result of extensive subperiosteal hemorrhage associated with an underlying fracture (Fig. 10-12A). The initial fracture may be subtle and is commonly overlooked. Such fractures are frequently metaphyseal-epiphyseal, and they characteristically present as small fragments arising from the distal part of a bone. The fractures are often multiple but significantly manifest an ostensible difference in their chronologic appearance and development (Fig. 10-12B).

Gross fractures also present along the shaft of the long bones. The battered child syndrome is known to occur in infants; therefore it should not be confused with infantile cortical hyperostosis or trauma at birth. Recently, Menke's syndrome has been described. It is manifested by symmetrical metaphyseal spurs in the long bones. These changes are usually encountered about the knee, and new periosteal bone formation commonly occurs along the medial femoral surfaces. Spurring and fragmentation usually indicate a fracture and to the casual observer are strikingly similar to the battered child syndrome. However, in Menke's syndrome the skull is small and thick and demonstrates excessive wormian bones.

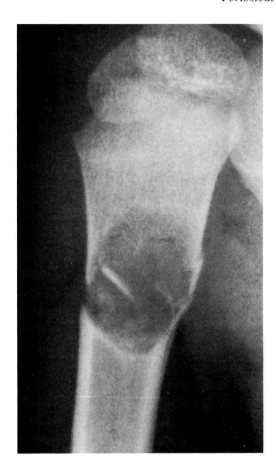

Fig. 10-14. Unicameral bone cyst with "fallen fragment." A large, well demarcated cyst is present within the proximal portion of the humerus. A pathologic fracture is present and fragments of bone are floating within the lesion. The inferior border of the cyst is sclerotic.

Today, use of daily vitamins and improved dietary habits have made scurvy almost nonexistent and vitamin D-deficiency rickets rare. The changes involving the metaphyseal region are distinctive in these diseases. Periosteal changes occur in both. Hemorrhage beneath the periosteum causes an exuberant reaction in scurvy (Fig. 10-13), and unilaminar as well as multilaminar changes occur during the healing phase of rickets.

Unilaminar reaction has been encountered in juvenile rheumatoid arthritis. This is a minor radiologic manifestation of the disease, but has been known to involve the fingers and other small bones. Rarely, Crohn's disease and diseases associated with hypoproteinemia have been associated with new unilaminar bone formation.

Discussion

Acute hematogenous osteomyelitis most often involves the rapidly growing bone and characteristically affects the metaphyses of long bones. The pattern of infection is related to the nature and development of the vascular network within the metaphyseal region, and therefore the infection behaves differently in various age-groups.

In infants below the age of 1, capillaries perforate the epiphyseal growth plate allowing the infection to spread rapidly from the metaphysis into the epiphysis. As a result, septic arthritis and destruction of the epiphysis are often concomitant. An analogous situation occurs in adults following resorption of the growth cartilage. Vascular anastomosis again develops between the metaphysis and the epiphysis, permitting rapid spread into the sub-articular tissues. In this age-group, however, the periosteum is firmly attached and subperiosteal abscess formation and intense periosteal proliferation are rarely seen. Between the age of 1 and puberty, there is no capillary communication across the epiphyseal plate. Therefore the infection begins and remains within the metaphyseal vessels. The epiphyseal plate prevents the infection from spreading into the epiphysis. Thus, the infection spreads laterally, perforates the cortex, and lifts the loose periosteum, producing a subperiosteal collection and a periosteal reaction. Since the epiphysis is protected from infection by the epiphyseal plate, normal growth is not usually impaired.

Staphylococcus aureus is the most common causative agent of osteomyelitis, although Salmonella osteomyelitis is far more common in patients with sickle cell anemia. There is growing evidence to suggest that the state of hemolysis is responsible for the high susceptibility of Salmonella infections by inhibition of the phagocytic activity of macrophages.

Clinically, infantile cortical hyperostosis resembles an infection, and it is conceivable that the disease may have a viral etiology. As in bacterial osteomyelitis, a soft-tissue swelling occasionally precedes the bone changes. However, the radiographic pattern and symmetry of the involved areas are distinctive.

Menke's syndrome is a new entity which has been found to occur in males. The disease is linked to an abnormal transport of copper through the gut wall.

SOLITARY OSTEOLYTIC LESIONS

The number of osteolytic lesions is large. Recognizing characteristic radiographic features of each and the response of surrounding bone are important in differentiating one lesion from another.

The response of the surrounding bone to the lesion is evaluated by the "zone of transition." This zone is defined as that portion of bone which is situated between the obvious pathological lesion and the obvious normal osseous tissue. It is an important feature; it describes the character of the process. For example, lesions which produce a wide and ill-defined zone of transition are characterized as aggressive. A sharp and narrow zone, and in some a sclerotic margin, is almost always associated with a slowly growing, benign lesion. This type of transition zone is produced when a chronic process progresses slowly enough to stimulate a strong reparative response within the surrounding bone. Brodie's abscess is such a process. Lesions without a sclerotic border which are surrounded by a narrow zone of transition are also benign but have either not been present long enough to induce new bone production

or do not elicit a host bone response, as in eosinophilic granuloma. Occasionally, a benign lesion grows faster than the rate of bone response, such as an aneurysmal bone cyst.

The expansile effect of a bone lesion is important. If the rate of expansion is slow, the surrounding cortex continues to produce bone and remains intact, as with a simple bone cyst. A rapidly growing lesion results in an interrupted and destroyed cortex.

The presence and the nature of calcification within the matrix of the lesion is a significant diagnostic feature. For example, an angular, radiopaque structure in the center of an osteolytic lesion may suggest a sequestrum, the sclerotic, dead bone of osteomyelitis. Finely stippled calcifications are typical of a chondroid matrix.

The location of the lesion within the bone itself must be considered. Some processes only affect the epiphysis, the diaphysis, or the metaphysis. Some are localized in the medullary cavity, and others in the cortex. The particular bone affected is also a significant factor.

Disease Entities

Lesions with a narrow transition zone
  Non-sclerotic border
    Bone cyst
    Enchondroma
    Aneurysmal bone cyst
    Eosinophilic granuloma
  Sclerotic border
    Fibrous dysplasia
    Chondroblastoma
    Abscess
    Chondromyxoid fibroma
    Non-ossifying fibroma
    Osteoid osteoma
    Bone infarct
    Epidermoidoma
Lesions with a wide transition zone
  Ewing's sarcoma
  Osteomyelitis
  Metastasis
  Early bone infarction

Differential Diagnosis

A simple bone cyst is manifested by a radiolucent lesion within the proximal metaphysis of a long bone. The lesion is ovoid, elongated, and expansile. It is centrally positioned within the medullary cavity

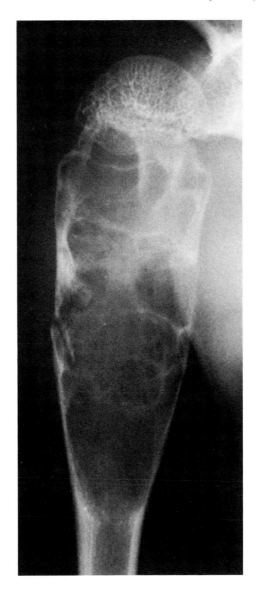

Fig. 10-15. Multilocular bone cyst with pathologic fracture. The entire proximal portion of the humerus is expanded by a large, multilocular, cystic mass. A pathologic fracture is also present. The expansile character of this cyst closely resembles an aneurysmal bone cyst.

close to the epiphysis and is surrounded by a sharply defined border (Fig. 10-14). A simple bone cyst is obviously benign and is quite distinctive radiographically, especially if a thin rim of intact cortex surrounds the expansile portion of the lesion and if no central calcification is present. A simple bone cyst is common, and the proximal humerus and femur are the most frequent sites. They are often asymptomatic and are discovered only following a pathologic fracture, when a displaced piece of cortical bone ("fallen fragment") may be detected within the lesion (Fig. 10-14). A periosteal reaction is encountered only after a fracture has been sustained. The lesion is most often unilocular, although irregular thinning of the cortex produces

what appears to be septations and multiple loculi within the cyst (Fig. 10-15).

A large solitary enchondroma is similarly radiolucent and expansile. The matrix of this lesion often contains calcifications and is therefore more radiopaque. In addition, solitary enchondromas are more likely to affect short tubular bones and are therefore common in the hand (Fig. 10-27).

Aneurysmal bone cysts are "blown out," cystic lesions that are located at the end of a long bone and abut upon the epiphyseal line (Fig. 10-16). The marked, expansile tendency of this lesion frequently results in cortical interruption and accounts for the term *aneurysmal.* Such tumors may also be multilocular. Clinically, pain, swelling, and limi-

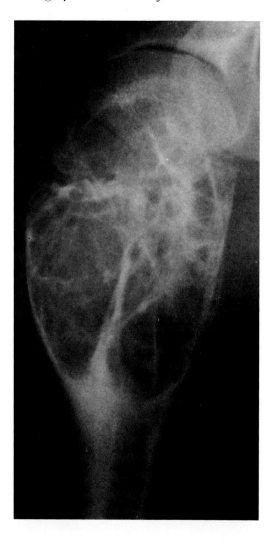

Fig. 10-16. Aneurysmal bone cyst. The marked expansile character of this lesion is well demonstrated. However, the cortex is still intact, and a sharp sclerotic transition zone is present along the inferior border of the lesion. (Aside from the degree of expansion, note the resemblance to Fig. 10-15.)

tation of motion have been associated with this lesion. Aneurysmal bone cysts differ from simple bone cysts by their extreme expansile character.

Eosinophilic granuloma occurs predominantly in the mid-shaft of a long bone, a location that is unusual for bone cysts. However, the metaphysis can also be involved. Characteristically, it occupies an eccentric position and occasionally arises in the cortex. The tumor as a result stimulates a unilaminar or multilaminar periosteal reaction that can be extensive. Initially the lesion is manifested by small areas of radiolucency that may or may not be well-defined. As the tumor grows, it eventually assumes a multilocular appearance, with multiple contours that produce a "hole within a hole" appearance (Fig. 10-9). The tumor rarely expands the medullary cavity of the bone.

Monostotic fibrous dysplasia is among the osteolytic processes that affect the metaphysis. This form of fibrous dysplasia usually occurs in the metaphysis and the shaft of the proximal femur (Fig. 10-17). Fibrous dysplasia is frequently surrounded by a well-defined sclerotic margin. Moreover, the tumor appears radiopaque because calcium and primitive bone are often formed within the center of the lesion. These features are quite characteristic although osteolytic, radiolucent forms of fibrous dysplasia also occur.

In addition, chondroblastoma, Brodie's abscess, chondromyxoid fibroma, nonossifying fibroma, and osteoid osteoma are surrounded by a sclerotic border, and several have a similar radiographic appearance. For example, an ovoid, non-expansile, osteolytic lesion located in the unfused epiphysis of the proximal tibia, surrounded by a narrow zone of

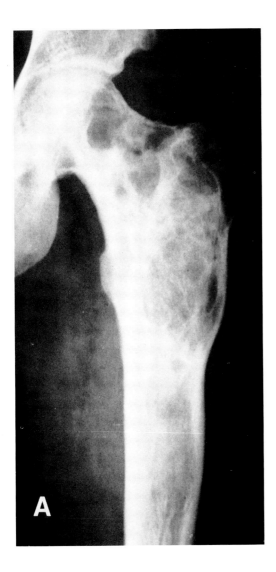

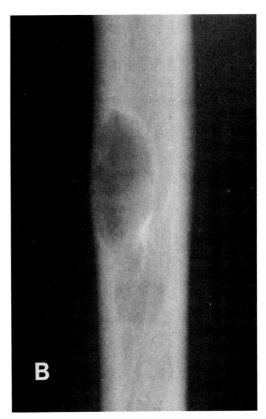

Fig. 10-17. Cystic fibrous dysplasia. *(A)* The femoral neck and proximal shaft are expanded and the cortex thinned. The lesion appears multiloculate and presents a somewhat hazy, "ground glass" appearance. *(B)* An osteolytic lesion within the medial portion of the mid-shaft of the femur is bordered by a thin sclerotic rim.

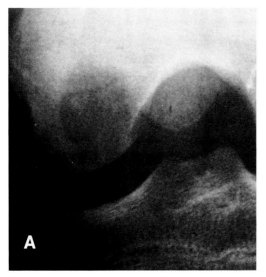

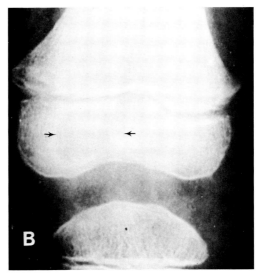

Fig. 10-18. Osteolytic epiphyseal lesions. *(A)* Chondroblastoma. A small osteolytic lesion with a well-defined margin is present within the condyle of the femur. The epiphyseal location is characteristic. No calcifications are apparent, although when present they demonstrate the chondroid origin of this lesion. *(B)* Brodie's abscess. A similarly located, radiolucent lesion proved to be an early Brodie's abscess. The location is somewhat atypical and the surrounding bone has not become sclerotic yet.

371

Table 10-1. Radiographic Characteristics of Cystic Lesions With a Non-sclerotic Border

Lesion	Zone of Transition	Expansile	Calcification	Location
Simple bone cyst	Sharp and narrow	Moderately		Prox. metaphysis long bone
Enchondroma	Sharp and narrow	Moderately	Mottled	Short tubular bone (e.g., hand)
Aneurysmal bone cyst	Sharp and narrow	Markedly		End of long bone
Eosinophilic granuloma	Sharp	("balloon effect")		Mid-shaft but eccentric (periosteal stimulation)

transition and a sclerotic margin, could represent either a chondroblastoma (Codman's tumor), Brodie's abscess (smoldering osteomyelitis), or focal fibrous dysplasia (Fig. 10-18). Chondroblastoma should be considered initially if the lesion involves the epiphysis, and even more consideration should be given if punctate calcifications are identified as a cartilaginous matrix. However, focal calcification may rarely be encountered in Brodie's abscess, and punctate calcifications also occur in fibrous dysplasia. The location within an unfused epiphysis is, nevertheless, far more characteristic of chondroblastoma (Fig. 10-18A), although chondroblastomas may extend across the epiphyseal plate to involve the metaphysis. A chondroblastoma is the only benign neoplasm that arises in an ossification center and commonly involves the proximal portions of the femur, tibia, and humerus.

A bone abscess may present in an acute, subacute, or chronic form (Fig. 10-18B). Brodie's abscess is identified as a subacute form of osteomyelitis that is characterized by focal bone necrosis and a surrounding area of bone repair that produces a thick and radiodense sclerotic border, which can be quite large. The lesion is customarily ovoid in shape and commonly located within the metaphysis. Occasionally, finger-like, radiolucent projections extend away from the main area of involvement. These represent tracts formed by the developing pus as it penetrates into the surrounding bone.

A non-ossifying fibroma probably represents the final stage in the development of a fibrous cortical defect that is in the process of being absorbed into bone (Fig. 10-19). Fibrous cortical defects occur in children over the age of 8, arise as an outgrowth of the periosteum, are primarily cortical in location,

and manifest a multilocular appearance (Fig. 10-20). Despite the cortical location and encroachment upon the medullary cavity, the lesions do not cause bulging of the outer cortex, in contrast to chondromyxoid fibroma. The latter is a rarely encountered, well-defined, elliptical and eccentrically located, benign bone tumor. Characteristically, the sclerotic border commonly involves only the medial aspect of the lesion. This tumor is not found in children; it presents within the 2nd and 3rd decades of life.

Most lesions with a sclerotic border are well-defined and have a narrow zone of transition. Ocasionally, the area of sclerotic bone around the lesion may be quite wide. This has been seen in forms of fibrous dysplasia showing a combination of lytic and sclerotic lesions, and in chronic osteomyelitis.

Osteoid osteoma (Fig. 10-21), a lytic lesion with a sclerotic border, is a benign bone tumor with a characteristic appearance that does not resemble any of the intracortical lesions previously discussed (see p. 376).

Epidermoidomas have a sclerotic border and a central radiolucency with a narrow zone of transition, and they almost exclusively involve the terminal phalanges. Epidermoidomas also have a characteristic expansile appearance. A glomus tumor of the phalanx may have the same affect.

Poorly defined lesions that have a wide zone of transition are either caused by an aggressive process with a growth rate which is greater than the rate of bone repair, or by a process that does not or has yet to elicit bone repair. A malignant lesion manifesting permeative destruction of bone results in trabecular absorption that produces a mottled radiolucency within the medullary cavity and a wide transition zone. Osteomyelitis and Ewing's sarcoma are classic examples. Unfor-

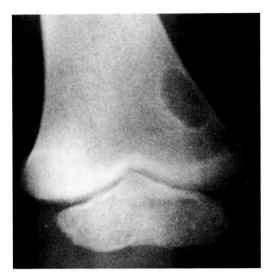

Fig. 10-19. Fibrous cortical defect. The defect presents as a small cystic lesion within the cortex of the distal femur. The margin is sharp and somewhat sclerotic.

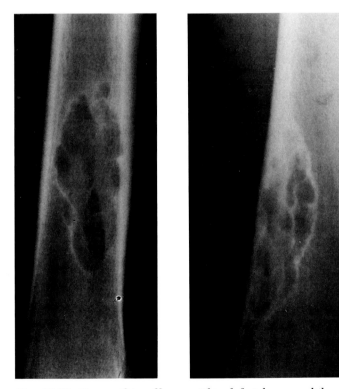

Fig. 10-20. Non-ossifying fibroma. This defect has a multilocular configuration, and the border is lobular and sclerotic. The location within the distal portion of the femur is typical. In addition, its origin from the cortical surface is well demonstrated, *although* the cortex remains unaltered.

Table 10-2. **Radiographic Characteristics of Cystic Lesions With a Sclerotic Border**

Lesion	Zone of Transition	Expansile	Calcification	Location
Fibrous dysplasia	Narrow (but occasionally wide)	Minimally	Hazy	Proximal metaphysis of long bone (or in ribs)
Chondroblastoma	Narrow		Mottled	Unfused epiphysis
Brodie's abscess	Sharp but thick		Sequestered	Metaphysis
Chondromyxoid fibroma	Sharp	Yes (eccentric sclerotic margin)	Yes	Distal metaphysis of long bone
Osteoid osteoma	Sharp but thick	Slightly, but eccentric	Nidus	Distal Metaphysis of femur and tibia
Epidermoidomas	Sharp and narrow	Minimally		Terminal digit, skull
Non-ossifying fibroma	Sharp			Distal metaphysis of long bone

tunately, both have many similarities. The lesions initially appear as multiple areas of demineralization that soon merge into larger areas of actual bone destruction. Although the cortex causes a periosteal reaction that may be quite pronounced in Ewing's sarcoma, both lesions extend into the surrounding bone to produce a wide transition zone. In osteomyelitis, however, with therapy and healing, this zone narrows and disappears. Metastases, massive osteolysis, and early bone infarction also produce bone destruction and wide zones of transition.

SOLITARY SCLEROTIC LESIONS OF BONE

The radiographic feature which is common to all sclerotic, or blastic, bone lesions is increased bone density. Sclerosis is the result of new bone production that originates from bone forming elements located either in the cortex, in the trabeculae, or in the periosteum. Infection, trauma, metabolic diseases, or neoplasm may stimulate production of osteoid by osteocytes. When mineralized this tissue looks like an area of sclerosis on the radiograph. It is of extreme importance to differentiate production of new bone due to a malignancy from the increased but orderly production of new reactive bone. New reactive bone looks like thickened but normal trabecular bone. New tumorous bone occurs as a result of a disordered proliferation of malignant osteocytes that produces a poorly organized matrix, upon which variable degrees and patterns of mineralization and bone are subsequently deposited. The result is a

radiographic appearance that is disorganized and does not conform to any consistent pattern.

In general, new bone forms either in an osteoid or chondrogenic matrix. Lesions associated with an osteoid matrix show degrees of mineralization that depend upon reaction of the underlying cells. The radiographic manifestations range from a somewhat cloudy reaction to completely dense sclerotic bone. Mineralization occurring within a benign chondrogenic matrix is seldom complete, and a radiolucent component is encountered in all benign cartilaginous lesions. When calcium is deposited it may be punctate and multiple or flocculent, with a "popcorn" appearance. Therefore, the pattern of mineralization observed in chondrosarcoma differs from that found in osteosarcoma. A neoplastic cartilaginous matrix consists of multiple, sharply defined collections of calcium that manifest a flocculent appearance and may be spread throughout or remain localized in the center of the lesion. Chondrosarcoma may form bone as well as cartilage and the radiographic appearance then displays matrix mineralization, reflecting changes of osteosarcoma and chondrosarcoma.

In general, a flocculent appearance strongly suggests a chondrogenic tumor, and sclerosis indicates lesions formed on a bony osteoid matrix. Cloudy or lumpy tumor mineralization indicates a less differentiated tumor with a relatively fast rate of growth. Reactive sclerosis associated with permeative bone destruction suggests a fast growing, malignant lesion such as Ewing's sarcoma or osteosarcoma.

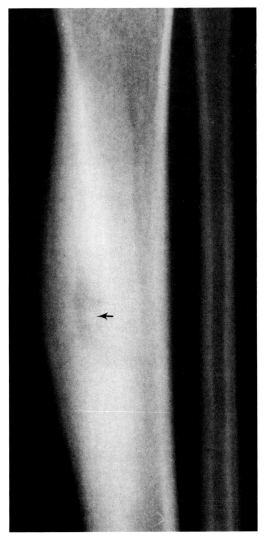

Fig. 10-21. Osteoid osteoma. The cortex in the mid-shaft of the tibia is markedly thickened due to an extensive periosteal reaction. The reaction surrounds a small, distinct, radiolucent central nidus that also contains a central deposit of calcification (*arrow*).

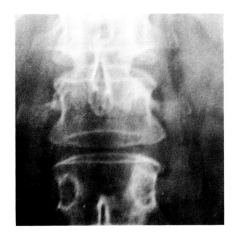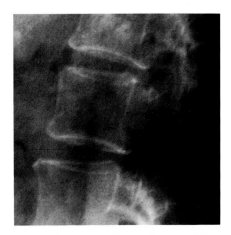

Fig. 10-22. Osteoblastoma of the spine. The posterior elements of L2 are destroyed by a radiolucent lesion resembling metastic disease.

Disease Entities

Lesions associated with an osteoid matrix
 Osteoid osteoma
 Osteoblastoma
 Chronic sclerosing osteomylitis (Garré's osteomyelitis)
 Localized fibrous dysplasia
 Stress fracture
Lesions associated with a chondroid matrix
 Osteochondroma
 Chondroma
 Chondromyxoid fibroma
 Benign chondroblastoma
Malignant sclerotic lesions
 Osteosarcoma
 Ewing's sarcoma
 Chondrosarcoma
 Lymphoma and leukemia

Differential Diagnosis

The majority of bone lesions containing an osteoid matrix are mainfested radiographically by dense sclerotic lesions that are sharply demarcated from surrounding normal bone. Many lesions are not always completely sclerotic and are also osteolytic. The appearance of both the radiolucent and surrounding sclerotic structures are often characteristic of each lesion. Nevertheless, striking similarities do exist. The most classic example of a sclerotic, benign bone lesion formed on an osteoid matrix is osteoid osteoma (Fig. 10-21). However, osteoblastoma, chronic osteomyelitis, and others have been mistaken for this lesion. The typical location of an osteoid osteoma is at the end of the shaft of the femur and tibia, although the humerus and fibula are sometimes affected. The calvarium is spared, and the vertebral column is only involved occasionally. By contrast, osteoblastoma most frequently occurs in the vertebral bodies. The early lesion contains a central nidus that consists of a osteoid matrix which is not mineralized and is radiolucent. The nidus subsequently undergoes calcification and at this stage may not be recognized on the conventional radiograph. Tomography, however, reveals the partially ossified structure. The surrounding bone is thick and sclerotic, a feature particularly noted when the lesion develops within the cortex. The periosteum also contributes to the thickness of the sclerosis and accounts for the asymmetric enlargement of the lesion.

The radiographic and pathologic appearance of osteoblastoma (Fig. 10-22) is remarkably similar to osteoid osteoma, and the term giant osteoid osteoma has been applied to this tumor. However, osteoblastoma is now considered a distinct entity, and the term giant osteoid osteoma is not used. Approximately 40 per cent of the tumors occur in the spine, a feature quite different from osteoid osteoma. It usually begins in the posterior elements (Fig. 10-22) and involves the vertebral bodies only when it extends anteriorly. Twenty per cent are found in the long bones, and the remainder are equally divided in a number of other locations. Radiographically the lesion manifests a slightly more variable appearance than osteoid osteoma and is therefore somewhat more difficult to diagnose. It is an expansile lesion that contains a central radiolucent zone, much larger than the nidus of an osteoid osteoma (Fig. 10-22). However, as the tumor matures the lesion becomes more and more calcified. A shell of periosteal new bone that is manifested by an extensive marginal sclerosis surrounds the central radiolucency. However, in peripheral lesions the uncalcified component of the tumor may predominate, and in some cases it is so irregular that it is thought to be a malignancy.

Chronic sclerosing osteomylitis also resembles osteoblastoma and osteoid osteoma; it too demonstrates not only surrounding bone sclerosis, but also central areas of mottled radiolucency (Fig. 10-23). The presence of a sequestrum, however, is often helpful in identifying this lesion. The latter, however, occurs relatively late and can be confused with the central calcified nidus of an osteoid osteoma. In addition, sequestered bone has also been found in other lesions such as eosinophilic granuloma and fibrosarcoma. Bony sequestra appear more radiodense than the surrounding infected bone because the infected bone becomes hypervascular and is continually demineralized. Sequestra vary in size and occasionally occupy the entire length of a long bone (Fig. 10-50). This has been observed in partially treated cases of pyogenic osteomylitis. In some cases, associated soft-tissue edema and a long history of recurrent or chronic pain in the affected area distinguishes a chronic infection from a rapidly growing malignant bone tumor.

On rare occasions monostotic fibrous dysplasia presents primarily as a sclerotic bone

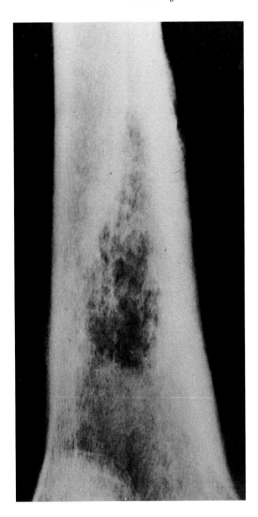

Fig. 10-23. Chronic osteomyelitis. The distal femur is dense, sclerotic, and somewhat wavy in appearance due to increased sclerosis and a periosteal reaction. The medullary cavity, however, is mottled and represents the site of active bone destruction.

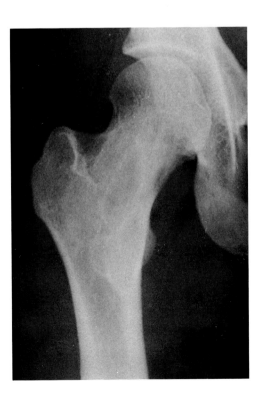

Fig. 10-24. Sclerotic fibrous dysplasia. A sclerotic lesion involves the medial aspect of the femoral neck. The neck is somewhat wide, and the lesion is sharply demarcated from the surrounding bone.

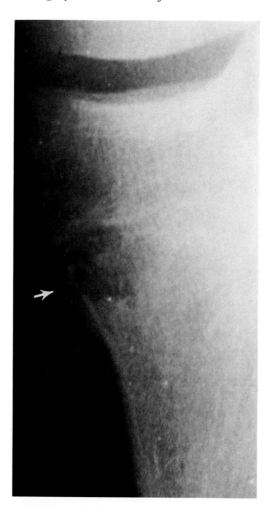

Fig. 10-25. Stress fracture. A radiolucent fracture line extends horizontally across the proximal tibial metaphysis for approximately 1 to 2 cms. A small periosteal reaction surrounds the medial cortical margin of the fracture *(arrow)*.

lesion (Fig. 10-24). More typically, the involved bone is expanded and the matrix manifests a "ground glass" appearance (Fig. 10-17B). The monostotic form usually involves the long bones and the majority of the lesions occur in the lower extremities, although the facial bones and ribs are frequently involved. The sclerosis present in monostotic fibrous dysplasia is due to an increased trabecular pattern. However, the undulating thickening or scalloping of the bone margin may be characteristic. When the sclerosis involves the entire medullary cavity, it may in fact resemble a sequestrum.

A stress fracture is manifested by a dense sclerotic lesion with a sharp zone of transition (Fig. 10-25). The location is so characteristic that confusion with other sclerotic lesions rarely occurs. Nevertheless, the radiographic resemblance to osteoid osteoma may be striking. A stress fracture is distinguished from os-

teoid osteoma by the absence of a central nidus. A recent stress fracture, however, may appear radiolucent when the surrounding bone undergoes rapid demineralization. The overall radiographic presentation of a stress fracture is characterized by the normal remodeling process of cortical and periosteal bone. Both small and large bones may be involved; the junction of the middle and distal third of the tibia or the distal shaft of the metatarsal bone are the most likely sites.

Lesions arising in a chondroid matrix are easily recognized. The benign lesions are less radiodense and the calcification is more or less spotty in nature. Osteochondroma, a prime example, is a form of exostosis (Fig. 10-26). An osteochondroma may be flat or pedunculated. The cortex and spongy portions of the normal bone are continuous with the base of the lesion. Calcification occurs within the growing cartilaginous matrix lo-

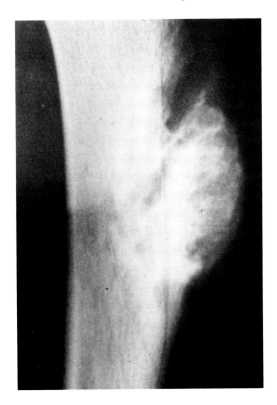

Fig. 10-26. Sessile osteochondroma. A radiodense, irregular calcified mass arises from the shaft of the bone. An increased area of sclerosis is present at the junction of the tumor with the normal cortex. The cartilaginous tip demonstrates punctate mineralization.

cated at the cap of the lesion. As a result the true size of the tumor may not be totally apparent on the radiograph. The configuration of adjacent bone is altered and appears wider than normal. The projection and direction of the osteochondroma is affected by the pull of adjacent muscle tendons.

A chondroma is another benign tumor composed of mature hyaline cartilage. These tumors may also occur in soft tissues. They are referred to as enchondromas when located centrally in bone. Radiographically, the tumor produces a well circumscribed, predominantly osteolytic lesion anywhere in the shaft of the bone, but most commonly in the hand (Fig. 10-27). There may be no calcification within this lesion, but more often there are prominent stippled or mottled deposits. Chondromas located in large tubular bones are more likely to demonstrate calcification. In the long bones the tumor may also cause irregular scalloping of the endosteal surface. A small percentage of tumors occur in the subperiosteum. These lesions produce cortical irregularities and erosion of the subperiosteal surface, as well as simultaneous expansion of new periosteal bone at its outer margin.

Radiographically, it is necessary to distinguish a chondroma from an epidermoid inclusion cyst in a phalanx and from a bone infarct in a long bone. An epidermoid inclusion cyst is predominantly osteolytic and occurs in the distal phalanx. A medullary bone infarct has a serpiginous appearance and is recognized by its radiodense, limiting outer margin and the absence of a flocculent central calcification (Fig. 10-28). The distinct rim seen in a bone infarct represents reactive bone repair. Although it may resemble an enchondroma, it never expands bone or demonstrates any degree of radiolucency. Chondromyxoid fibroma and chondroma may reveal chondrogenic calcifications, but these lesions are not blastic in nature (Fig. 10-29).

The malignant sclerotic bone lesions are easily recognized by the presence of underlying bone destruction, a poor transition zone, and an occasional soft-tissue mass. Osteogenic sarcoma is a prime example, and radiographically four distinct types are observed. Type I is the radiographic and histologic prototype. It is basically osteogenic and produces massive, new tumorous bone. This type is the least difficult to diagnose (Fig. 10-8A). Type II contains varying de-

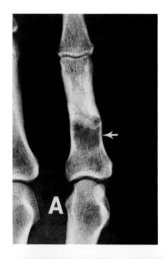

Fig. 10-27. Enchondroma. *(A)* A relatively radiolucent lesion is present in the proximal phalanx of the second digit *(arrow)*. There is a pathologic fracture through the distal aspect of the lesion. *(B)* Ollier's disease. Multiple enchondromas in the hands are present and demonstrate a high degree of mottled calcification within the chondroid matrix of each lesion. The larger lesions demonstrate endosteal scalloping.

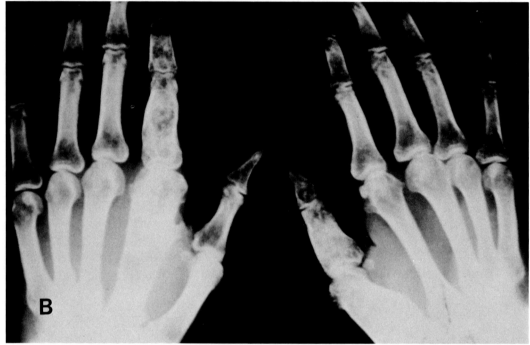

grees of cartilage formation within the tumor osteoid. At times only cartilage is produced, and the lesion resembles primary chondrosarcoma. Type III produces neither bone nor cartilage. It therefore appears radiolucent and is commonly mistaken for fibrosarcoma. However, if a sarcoma of Type III produces a metastasis, particularly in a lung, the metastasis often produces bone. Thus, the diagnosis in the later stages is simplified. In Type IV, the cells are so primitive and undifferentiated that no specific radiographic or pathologic features are present. Additional findings such as Codman's triangle, "onion skin" periosteal reaction, and other types of periosteal reactions are helpful but not distinctive.

Ewing's sarcoma may also be manifested by degrees of sclerosis and therefore must be differentiated from osteogenic sarcoma. In general, this tumor consists of a purely osteolytic, permeative process that is only partially sclerotic (Fig. 10-7). Ewing's tumor itself does not produce new bone. Reactive bone sclerosis and a laminated, "onion skin" periosteal reaction contribute to the increased radiodensity. However, the new reactive bone that occurs in Ewing's sarcoma may be extensive. This feature is commonly found when the tumor involves the flat bones

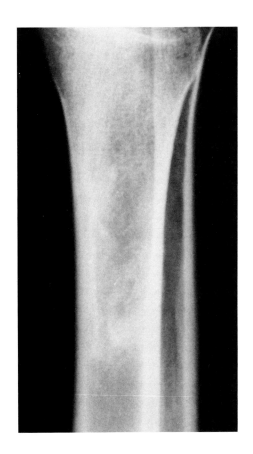

Fig. 10-28. Bone infarct. A bone infarct in the distal tibia is shown in a teenager with homozygous sickle cell disease. Sclerosis is most prominent at the periphery of the infarcted medullary bone.

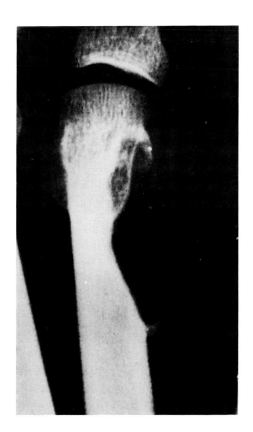

Fig. 10-29. Chondromyxoid fibroma. The elongated, predominantly osteolytic lesion shows no chondrogenic calcification. It is asymmetrically located and markedly expands the cortex.

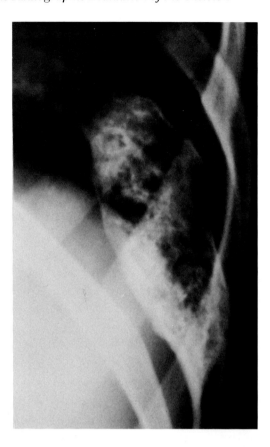

Fig. 10-30. Ewing's sarcoma of the rib. The tumor is predominantly blastic. The bone is expanded and almost appears benign. (This lesion had never been treated.)

such as the ileum, ribs, scapula, and mandible (Fig. 10-30). Consequently, the location of Ewing's sarcoma is more variable than osteosarcoma, which rarely involves the flat bones. In the long bones, Ewing's sarcoma may occupy the diaphysis or involve an entire shaft of the long bone. The tumor spreads by way of the haversian system and eventually penetrates the subperiosteal region, elevating the periosteum and causing the dramatic and characteristic periosteal changes.

Chondrosarcoma is decidedly rare in the pediatric age-group. It occurs in 3 to 5 per cent of cases and is typically located in the pelvis and the rib cage. It is a slowly growing tumor and may therefore be symptomatic for months or even years. Pain and swelling and a large soft-tissue mass are common initially. Radiographically, two distinct types are noted, central and peripheral. The central tumors arise from cortical or cancellous bone, whereas peripheral tumors originate either from the periosteum or from a pre-existing cartilaginous lesion. The central chondrosarcomas of long bones often produce slight fusiform expansion of the shaft with reactive scle-

rosis and thickening of the cortex. Calcific masses form the bulk of the matrix. The peripheral lesion is a tumor arising from the bone and consists of a cartilaginous matrix that varies from a well differentiated and distinct, radiodense cartilaginous mass to large calcified lobules of chondrogenic matrix. The adjacent bone may be destroyed.

The osseous manifestations of leukemia and lymphoma take several forms, with the osteolytic lesion predominating. Diffuse mineralization as well as periosteal reaction and metaphyseal bands may also occur. There are, however, a few reported cases of purely primary osteosclerotic lesions in leukemia. The majority occur following successful therapy and remission.

Discussion

Solitary unicameral cysts usually occur at the end of the long bones in the growing skeleton. However, a number have been found within the calcaneus, ribs, clavicle, and mandible. In most series of patients studied, a male predominance is noted, and the lesion is discovered most frequently between the ages of 3 and 14 years. The tumor grows slowly, and rarely, if ever, causes pain. Pain is noted only when the lesion has thinned the cortex to the point of pathologic fracture. A unicameral cyst begins in the spongy portion of the metaphyses and expands slowly until it occupies the entire width of the medullary cavity. The surrounding bone matures and grows away from the cyst, creating the illusion that the cyst is drifting toward the mid-diaphysis. The fluid within the cyst is most often amber in color, although occasionally it may be clear or even contain blood. There are no true pathognomonic features, although the cyst is lined by a definite wall that contains moderately young fibroblasts and a considerable amount of collagen material. Occasional giant cells may be scattered through the surrounding granulation matrix. The etiology of bone cysts is unknown. Defective bone formation in an area of the epiphyseal line has been suggested. Some physicians believe the cyst arises following trauma, with episodes of hemorrhage occurring within the growing metaphyses. Liquification and organization around the wall are eventually produced. However, since few patients with hemophilia develop bone cysts, this theory has not gained widespread acceptance.

The term aneurysmal bone cyst is used to describe cysts that demonstrate a marked expansile effect on the overlying cortex that in many ways resembles a saccular aneurysm of the aorta. It arises in the medullary structure at the end of the long bones, often very close to the epiphyseal line. This cyst never arises in a cartilaginous epiphysis, but may involve the epiphysis if the lesion continues to grow after the epiphyseal plate has fused. Aneurysmal bone cysts have been found in almost every age-group, although the majority occur in the 2nd decade. In contrast to the unicameral bone cyst, females are affected predominantly. The lesion usually causes pain of several weeks or months duration because of its expansile character. When a vertebral body is involved, muscle spasm or compression of the spinal cord or nerve roots are also responsible for causing pain. An aneurysmal bone cyst consists of an aggregation of thick-walled, vascular channels in which venous blood seems to flow freely through the cyst. Characteristically, there are no blood clots. As a result, a considerable hemorrhage often occurs at surgery, and the

bleeding may be difficult to control. A consistent microscopic feature is the presence of large fields of giant cells within a collagen-producing matrix, in which considerable quantities of hemosiderin have been deposited. This suggests that the lesion may represent an old intraosseous hematoma, the result of previous trauma in which one or more arteriovenous fistulas were formed. The possibility of an underlying congenital abnormality, such as hemangioma, or other pre-existing lesions associated with hemorrhage should also be considered; some studies have demonstrated a high association of either benign or malignant lesions in approximately 50 per cent of cases of aneurysmal bone cysts. This must be considered when curettage is planned as therapy, since serious complications may therefore arise. Recurrence has been reported in approximately 20 per cent of cases.

Eosinophilic granuloma is now considered to be a form of histiocytosis and is therefore related to Hand-Schüller-Christian disease and Letterer-Siwe disease. It differs somewhat from aneurysmal and unicameral bone cysts because it is a localized, benign granuloma of bone. Although a focal lesion is commonly encountered, 50 per cent of affected patients demonstrate two or more lesions. Most cases occur in childhood, adolescence, or early adult life. Almost any bone in the skeleton can be involved, although the frontal bones are the most common site. Eosinophilic granuloma is probably the most frequent cause of vertebra plana. The matrix of the tumor usually consists of a reticular mass of histiocytes infiltrated with eosinophilic leukocytes, which may be present in sheets of cells. In addition, Charcot-Leyden crystals have been reported within the cytoplasm of these cells. These type of crystals are usually associated with an allergic reaction, and such a pathogenesis has been suggested but not proven.

Osteoid osteoma comprises approximately 10 per cent of all benign bone tumors, and occurs more frequently in males in a ratio of 2 to 1. The majority of the lesions are discovered in the 1st 2 decades of life, with a peak of incidence occuring in the 2nd decade. The radiographic appearance and location of osteoid osteoma are characteristic. However, these tumors have also been found in the intra-articular areas of long bones. When they occur in the femoral neck, the adjacent bone may reveal areas of destruction. These changes are not caused by the osteoma itself but by an associated lymphocytic nodular synovitis. The occurrence of intra-articular osteoid osteoma with nodular synovitis is now recognized as a distinct radiographic entity. It resembles juvenile rheumatoid arthritis because of the accompanying swelling, inflammatory response, and bone changes.

Histologically, osteoid osteoma is composed of a nidus of partially mineralized osteoid. The young tumors are quite vascular, and angiography has been performed occasionally to distinguish this lesion from osteomyelitis and osteoblastoma. Pathologically, multinucleate giant cells, as well as fibroblasts and osteoblasts, are present. The adjacent sclerotic area reveals normal osteocytes, thickened trabeculae, fibrous tissue, and some blood vessels. The periosteum is also thickened, but usually not remarkably.

The clinical feature of this lesion is characterized by intense bone pain that is worse at night and often relieved by aspirin. Many patients reveal weakness and even wasting of the extremities. Patients who have intra-articular osteoid osteomas associated with nodular synovitis usually present with a limp or atrophy of the involved extremity. Resection of the lesion offers a cure. However, the central nidus must be removed in order to prevent recurrence.

Osteoblastoma, or giant osteoid osteoma as the lesion is sometimes still called, is a partially sclerotic tumor that produces osteoid. The tumor is relatively rare, comprising approximately 1 per cent of primary bone tumors and 70 per cent of tumors present in patients below the age of 20 years. It occurs more frequently in males in a ratio of 2 to 1.

Pathologically osteoblastomas are firm, usually well circumscribed, hemorrhagic tumors. A variable degree of calcification is present. The osteoid component of the tumor predominates, producing a sclerotic radiographic appearance. Serial examinations indicate that the lesions are at first predominantly osteolytic and undergo progressive ossification as they mature. The tumor is sclerotic in more than half the cases that involve the spine or ribs. Because the tumor is likely to occur in the axial skeleton, the presenting symptoms are usually vertebral or paravertebral pain or discomfort. Neurologic findings, such as muscular or sensory deficit, are also common presenting signs. Usually there is no significant difference in the duration of symptoms between patients with tumors of the spine and patients with tumors of the long or flat bones, although osteoblastomas of the spine, because of their location, are diagnosed earlier. Nerve root or cord compression may persist because of the continual local expansion of the tumor.

Chronic inflammatory lesions sometimes resemble bone tumors. The confusing clinical and radiographic picture often results in a misdiagnosis. This problem arises when an acute infection is only partially treated or not treated at all. Cases of subacute or chronic osteomyelitis may lack the characteristic findings of inflammatory disease. Consequently, differentiation between infection and tumor may be impossible on the basis of radiographic criteria alone, and a biopsy may be required. The diagnostic accuracy of the pathologist depends greatly upon the adequacy of the biopsy. A needle biopsy, which has the advantage of reduced surgical trauma, may not provide adequate sampling. Biopsy specimens should include sufficient material from the periosteum, bony cortex, and the medullary tissue.

The peculiar radiographic appearance of fibrous dyplasia is the result of a mixture of bony and cartilaginous elements within the tumor. Areas of bone islands and cartilaginous matrix are interspaced in what is presumed to be dysplastic collagen connective tissue. The dysplasia is caused by a defect in the proliferation of fibroblasts. The monostotic form usually involves long bones with the majority of the lesions occurring in the lower extremities. Facial bones and ribs are also frequently involved. Malignant degeneration very rarely occurs in the monostotic form of fibrous dysplasia. When this happens it is usually in the form of osteosarcomas, chondrosarcomas, or fibrosarcomas, occurring with or without associated radiation therapy.

A stress fracture represents a mechanical disturbance in the normal architecture of long bones. The defect develops over a period of several days, as opposed to traumatic fractures of long bones which occur almost instantaneously at the time of trauma. Stress fractures or fatigue fractures are not true fractures, since there is no structural discontinuity. They represent injuries which occur following repeated mechanical stress that causes weakening of bone at a specific site, where the remodeling of bone is either lagging or is delayed during skeletal growth. The accompanying symptomatology of sharp, localized pain and tenderness related to activity is also useful in distinguishing stress fractures from other benign sclerotic lesions.

Osteochondroma, also referred to as osteocartilaginous exostosis, is the most common benign bone tumor. Osteochondromas comprise approximately 45 per cent of all benign bone tumors. The actual incidence is not known because many of these tumors are asymptomatic and are never discovered. Nearly 90 per cent of patients have a single lesion. The majority of the tumors present in the 1st 2 decades of life, although approximately 45 per cent are discovered in the 2nd decade. The majority of osteochondromas have a predominantly osseous appearance, despite an origin from chondrogenic matrix. Enchondral ossification occurs within the cartilaginous cap, and the tumors grow at a rate which is proportional to bodily growth. The etiology is not clearly understood, but osteochondromas may be the result of a displaced focus of cartilage. As a result it can occur in any bone that develops by enchondral bone formation. The classical location is the metaphysis of long bones, particularly the femur and humerus. Nevertheless, flat bones such as the ileum can also be involved. The patients may complain of formation of a hard mass or pain of long duration. In some patients the pain is acute due to fracture of the tumor stalk. Rarely, the lesion may involve the spine and cause cord compression.

The cartilaginous matrix of the tumor is composed of hyaline cartilage, with apparently normal chondrocytes in the carilaginous cap. There are islands of cartilage embedded in the cancellous bone that may undergo degeneration of irregular calcification. Sudden growth or pain associated with the lesion implies the development of a chondrosarcoma. However, malignant transformation is extremely rare in the solitary tumor. Complete excision often results in cure. However, a very small number of tumors may recur anywhere from 1 to 25 years after excision, and the process is almost always benign. A peculiar lesion resembling an osteochondroma may occur in the distal humerus. It is a small spur that usually pro-

jects somewhat medially and is located about 5 cms. above the medial epicondyle. This is the supracondylar process and is not a true exostosis but rather an atavistic structure. Another unusual exostosis is located in the distal end of the terminal phalanges of the fingers and toes and most probably is the result of trauma with or without osteomyelitis.

A chondroma is another benign tumor composed of mature hyaline cartilage. Multiple chondromas may occur and tend to be unilateral. Such a presentation is called Ollier's disease and is probably a form of dysplasia, with failure of normal enchondral ossification. Single enchondromas comprise approximately 10 per cent of all benign tumors and are most frequent in the 1st 2 decades of life. This lesion is by far the most common tumor of the small bones of the hand. Some may arise within the pelvis. These have a greater tendency to undergo degeneration into secondary chondrosarcoma. Chondromas in general are asymptomatic, and a pathologic fracture may be the only presenting feature. Histologically, chondromas consist of chondrocytes that exhibit regular shapes and configurations. The cellular structures are not helpful in differentiating the benign chondroma from chondrosarcoma.

Osteogenic sarcoma is a primary malignant bone tumor consisting of malignant stroma, osteoid, tissue, and bone or cartilage formation. It is the classic example of a sclerotic malignant bone tumor and is the most common malignant bone tumor in the pediatric age-group. In fact, next to multiple myeloma, which is not encountered in children, it is the second most common primary malignant bone tumor. The etiology is unknown, although a combination of viral and genetic factors have been implicated. A viral etiology appears to be more acceptable, although reports in which siblings and first cousins have developed osteosarcomas in succession indicate some genetic factor. Males are affected predominantly; this may be related to the longer period of bone growth and greater bone mass found in most males. Not surprisingly, children with osteogenic sarcomas are usually tall. The tumor is likely to affect long bones, particularly prior to the age of 20. Approximately 60 per cent arise in the metaphysis of the lower femur, upper tibia, lower tibia, and upper humerus, but any bone in the body may be involved. The lesions are discovered because of the history of pain and swelling often associated with recent trauma. Most children, however, appear in good health with no significant weight loss or anorexia. The serum level of alkaline phosphatase is an excellent marker for tumor activity and is elevated in approximately 50 per cent of cases. It has also been used to determine the presence or abscence of recurrent tumor metastasis. The prognosis of osteogenic sarcoma is poor but varies somewhat according to the histologic grades. The osteoblastic type has the worst prognosis, with a survival of approximately 15 per cent over a 5 year period. The chondrogenic and fibroblastic types have a somewhat more favorable outcome. Radiographic features which indicate a poor prognosis include a pathologic fracture, a large tumor, and proximity to the axial skeleton.

Physicians should always be aware that the formation of a normal callus may resemble an osteogenic sarcoma and may be a difficult histologic problem. The radiographic diagnosis is vital in these situations.

Ewing's sarcoma is a primary malignant bone tumor that arises from primitive reticulum cells or undifferentiated mesenchymal cells within the medullary cavity, and not from endothelial cells as originally described. This tumor comprises approximately 7 to 10 per cent of all primary malignant bone tumors. It is rarely found below the age of 5 and has a peak incidence at approximately 15 years of age. It is far more common in males and is rarely, if ever, encountered in the black population. Unlike patients with osteosarcoma, patients with Ewing's tumor appear chronically ill. Fever, leukocytosis, and an elevated erythrocyte sedimentation rate suggesting an infectious process are often found. This is further complicated by the radiographic appearance of the tumor, which in many aspects closely resembles that of osteomyelitis, and by an initial positive clinical response to antibiotic therapy. On occasion, eosinophilic granuloma and osteogenic sarcoma may resemble Ewing's tumor radiographically.

Chondrosarcoma is a malignant cartilaginous tumor which may be primary or secondary, arising from pre-existing cartilaginous lesions (e.g., multiple hereditary exostosis, enchondromas). It is the third most common malignant bone tumor comprising approximately 10 per cent of all malignant bone tumors. Fortunately, the incidence of this tumor in children is quite low. The tumor grows slowly and symptoms usually persist for months or even years before the lesion is discovered. Large soft-tissue masses within the pelvis or ribs are the most common presenting physical features.

Acute leukemia, usually undifferentiated, and lymphoma are the most common malignant diseases in children. Skeletal involvement is common and important, since recognizing its presence may suggest a diagnosis of leukemia before the full blown clinical picture is apparent.

MULTIPLE OSTEOLYTIC LESIONS

Disease Entities

Metastatic tumors
  Neuroblastoma
  Leukemia, lymphoblastoma
  Reticulum cell sarcoma
  Rhabdomyosarcoma
  Retinoblastoma
Histiocytosis
  Letterer-Siwe disease
  Hand-Schüller-Christian disease
  Eosinophilic granuloma
Storage diseases
  Neimann-Pick disease
  Gaucher's disease
Inflammatory disease of bone
  Pyogenic osteomyelitis
  Fungal osteomyelitis
  Congenital syphilis
Brown tumor hyperparathyroidism
Fibrous dysplasia
Skeletal angiomatosis, lymphomatosis, and fibromatosis
Acro-osteolysis
Ollier's disease

Differential Diagnosis

Metastatic disease is by far the most frequent cause of multiple osteolytic lesions of bone. The lesions are often diffuse with irregular, ill-defined margins. However, some lesions demonstrate certain characteristics in appearance and presentation that suggest a specific diagnosis. Neuroblastoma is the most frequent metastatic neoplasm of bone in children. In neuroblastoma the bone lesions tend

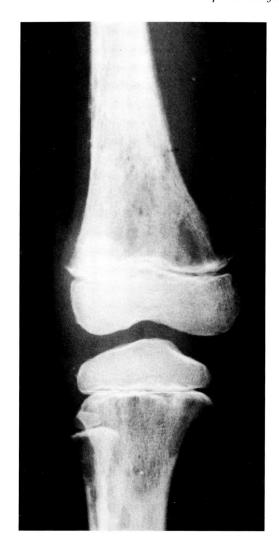

Fig. 10-31. Neuroblastoma. Multiple osteolytic lesions involve the metaphyses of all of the bones. The majority are ill-defined, vary in size, and involve both the spongiosa and the cortex. Note the periosteal reaction along the femoral shaft.

to be symmetrical in the extremities. The distal femur is the most common site. Cortical destruction occurs when the tumor penetrates the bone, and occasionally a periosteal reaction may be stimulated that resembles a "sunburst" reaction. This appearance, although typical of osteogenic sarcoma, is more indicative of neuroblastoma when multiple lesions are present. Multicentric osteogenic sarcoma is rarely observed. The osteolytic lesions in neuroblastoma are usually ill-defined and produce an irregular, mottled destruction of both the spongiosa and cortex (Fig. 10-31). These changes are at times radiographically indistinguishable from the osteolytic or mottled bone destruction of leukemia (Fig. 10-32). However, lymphocytic leukemia commonly presents with transverse metaphyseal bands; these are only occasionally

found in patients with metastatic neuroblastoma. The differential diagnosis of neuroblastoma includes Ewing's sarcoma with primarily destructive lesions. Metastases from Ewing's tumor occur predominantly between the ages of 5 and 30 years, while the greatest incidence of metastatic neuroblastoma is below the age of 5 years. Histiocytosis and other metastatic lesions such as rhabdomyosarcoma, retinoblastoma, and a multicentric reticulum cell sarcoma should also be considered. Reticulum cell tumor is encountered mainly in older patients but occasionally occurs in the pediatric age-group. A "moth-eaten," permeative, destructive appearance and an apparent absence of a noteworthy periosteal reaction are the main radiologic features of reticulum cell sarcoma.

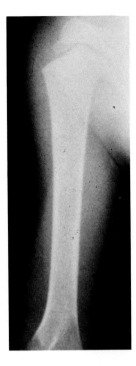 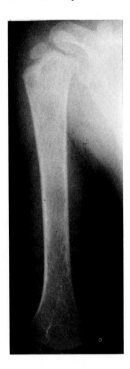 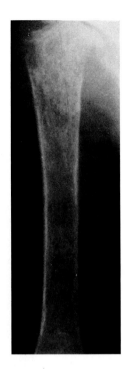

Fig. 10-32. Leukemia. Three studies demonstrate the progressive changes of leukemia over an 8-month period. Normal early metaphyseal mottling progresses to involvement of the entire shaft.

Lymphoblastomas of bone may involve multiple areas of the skeleton, with a "moth-eaten" pattern within the medullary and cortical portions. However, a superimposed periosteal reaction due to the stimulation by neoplastic cells also occurs.

Metastatic embryonic rhabdomysarcoma affects the extremities, as well as the pelvis, skull, and spine, with multiple destructive lesions. The lesions resemble metastatic neuroblastoma, retinoblastoma, and lymphocytic leukemia. Fortunately, the site of the primary tumor is almost always known. Three types of rhabdomyosarcoma have been described: embryonic, alveolar, and pleomorphic. The embryonic types comprises 50 per cent of the cases and affects infants and young children. The tumor usually arises in the orbit, head, neck, and retroperitoneum; only 5 per cent arise in the extremities. The alveolar form is more common in older children and adults and involves the extremities predominantly. The last form is rare and does not occur in children.

Retinoblastoma also produces osteolytic, destructive areas. Direct extention of the tumor through the orbit involves the frontal region. However, hematogeneous spread also occurs, producing multiple, nonspecific osteolytic areas of bone destruction. Retinoblastoma elicits a greater periosteal response than reticulum cell sarcoma or rhabdomyosarcoma. A "sunburst" appearance has also been associated with this lesion.

Eosinophilic granuloma, Hand-Schüller-Christian disease, and Letterer-Siwe disease all form part of a complex comprising histiocytosis. The severity ranges from the benign eosinophilic granuloma to the malignant Letterer-Siwe disease.

The peak incidence of eosinophilic granuloma occurs in the 1st 2 decades of life. However, only 30 to 40 per cent of the patients present with multiple osteolytic skeletal lesions. The flat bones such as the pelvis (Fig. 10-33A), the skull, and the vertebral bodies are most frequently involved, although the extremities are not spared (Fig. 10-33B). The basic radiographic finding is an area of bone destruction which may involve any portion of bone. The shaft and metaphysis are mainly involved in the long bones. The initial findings are small areas of radiolucency that may or may not be well-defined. As the lesions grow, endosteal scalloping occurs, and a multilocular appearance eventually develops. The lesion contains multiple contours and demonstrates what seems to be a "hole within a hole" appearance due to overlapping radiolucencies. The border of the lesion is sharply defined, and a narrow zone of transition is present. Small,

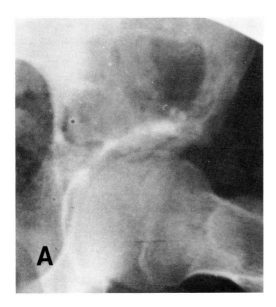

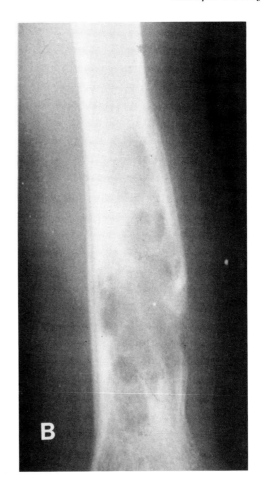

Fig. 10-33. Eosinophilic granuloma. *(A)* A sharply outlined and beveled rectangular lesion is present within the supra-acetabular area. This is a characteristic location for an eosinophilic granuloma. *(B)* The distal humerus reveals a multilocular lesion that slightly expands the bone. A well formed periosteal reaction is noted that is interrupted at one point by the expanding mass.

less osteolytic "satellite" lesions are often encountered in the long bones adjacent to the major lesion. Cortical destruction occurs readily. Some lesions actually arise in the cortex and stimulate an extensive periosteal reaction. True expansion of the involved bone is rare. In the flat bones, and especially in the skull, large areas of bone involvement can occur. The lesion heals with sclerosis and a "button sequestrum" may be seen. At this stage the lesion may resemble fibrous dysplasia. Eosinophilic granuloma is sometimes encountered in the mandible, with destruction of cortical and medullary bone. The lesion usually arises about the teeth, destroying the periodontal bone and giving the characteristic appearance of "floating teeth" in a seemingly completely destroyed bone. Other characteristic locations are the pelvis, particularly the supra-acetabular region (Fig. 10-33), and the ribs where bone expansion is frequently seen. Involvement of the vertebrae results in collapse (see Chapter 8,

p. 331). Partial destruction of the pedicle or the vertebral appendages is also noted in not only eosinophilic granuloma but in all forms of histiocytosis. The differential diagnosis of the lesion includes chronic osteomyelitis, tuberculosis, benign cystic bone tumors, and lipoid granulomatosis. Biopsy may be required in cases where the radiographic appearance is atypical or the lesions are discovered in the initial stages.

Letterer-Siwe disease is the most severe form of hystiocytosis and has its onset quite early in life with the symptoms of a rapidly progressive disease. Afflicted infants are usually anemic, present with fever, a skin rash, and bleeding from mucous membranes. Hepatosplenomegaly and pulmonary lesions may also be seen on the radiograph. In the most acute phase of the disease only soft-tissue changes are apparent. When present, the osteolytic areas are multiple and the borders poorly defined (Fig. 10-34). Letterer-Siwe disease has been known to change to a

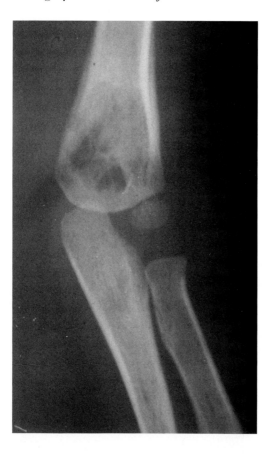

Fig. 10-34. Letterer-Siwe disease. Examination of the elbow in a patient with multiple skeletal lesions and mediastinal adenopathy reveals a conglomeration of lesions in the distal humerus. Some appear well-defined, although the main, large lesion is poorly outlined in comparison to the surrounding normal bone. Thick periosteal reaction is also noted.

more benign form of histiocytosis, Hand-Schüller-Christian disease, following corticosteroid and antibiotic therapy. In this stage a more advanced and chronic pattern may be observed. The patients may show retarded growth and sexual development. The multiple osteolytic skeletal lesions are widely disseminated and are much larger than in eosinophilic granuloma. The areas of bone destruction, particularly in the skull, may involve large areas of sharply outlined, round or slightly irregular, "punched-out," geographic defects that even include the floor of the skull (see Fig. 7-10). Involvement of the pituitary fossa completes the classic triad of Hand-Schüller-Christian disease, which consists of diabetes insipidus, exophthalmos, and the geographic skull pattern. The disease progresses slowly, and the defects in the bones may change little over a long period of time. Occasionally, patients develop a fulminating clinical course resembling Letterer-Siwe disease, and the osteolytic lesions become more prominent and numerous. Recognizing the presence of bone lesions in histiocytosis is important because the

frequency, number, and progression do have some prognostic significance. As a rule, the younger the child and the greater the number of bone lesions, the faster bone destruction occurs and the more serious is the prognosis.

Gaucher's disease is hereditary disorder characterized by deposition of the cerebroside kerasin in enlarged and abnormal reticuloendothelial cells, Gaucher's cells. Two clinical forms of the disease exist, infantile and adult. The infantile form is more acute, rapidly resulting in death, usually within several months. The form presents with predominantly visceral and central nervous system involvement (Fig. 6-24), and seldom exhibits obvious bone abnormalities. The adult form is more chronic and occurs over a wider age span. Although both sexes are equally affected, the typical patient is a Jewish teenager who presents with hepatosplenomegaly, anemia, thrombocytopenia, and a brown skin pigmentation. Symptoms affecting the skeleton include decreased range of motion in the hips and knees. The entire skeleton can be involved but the femur, hips,

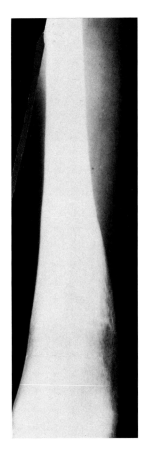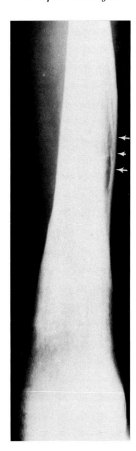

Fig. 10-35. Gaucher's disease. The distal end of the femurs are widened and resemble an Erlenmeyer flask. The trabeculae are thickened but somewhat cystic. On the lateral aspect of the left femur there is evidence of a cortical split in which a thin radiolucent line is visualized along the inner portion of the cortex *(arrows).*

shoulders, tubular bones, spine, and pelvis are more likely to be affected, particularly the lower extremities. The femur demonstrates the characteristic features, the most important being abnormal modeling. The distal portion of the bone becomes wide and resembles an Erlenmeyer flask (Fig. 10-35). Osteoporosis is characteristic and is due to resorption of trabeculae by infiltration of the bone marrow, caused by abnormal, lipid-distended histiocytes. A progression to multiple areas of osteolysis occurs, which is best seen peripherally in the long bones. Scalloping or an irregular endosteal margin is also observed. The appearance of long, thin, radiolucent lines in the inner portion of the cortex has been referred to as the "cortical split" (Fig. 10-35). Conversely, a long sclerotic area in the medullary aspect of bone or in the inner aspect of the cortex may also be observed, mimicking bone infarction. This manifestation, also commoonly seen in patients with sickle cell disease, is referred to as "bone within a bone" appearance and is secondary to repeated episodes of infarction

and reactive sclerosis within the bone. Aseptic necrosis of the femoral and humeral heads is the result of compression of vessels by Gaucher's cells. The lesion in the hip simulates Legg-Calvé-Perthes disease in the 1st decade of life. Less common findings include sacroiliac joint involvement, with sclerosis and actual bilateral obliteration of the sacroiliac joints.

Niemann-Pick disease demonstrates many of the bone changes of infantile Gaucher's disease. It is also an inherited abnormality involving abnormal deposition of lipids in histiocytes. In this entity a phospholipid, sphingomyelin, is deposited along with cholesterol. Enlarged histiocytes are most often found in the liver, spleen, and lymph nodes. Niemann-Pick disease chiefly affects children of Jewish ancestry. The clinical manifestations have been divided into four groups. The most severe form occur in early infancy, with hepatosplenomegaly, central nervous system involvement, and death within 1 or 2 years. The most benign form does not present until middle or late childhood, and moderate

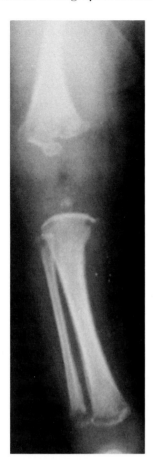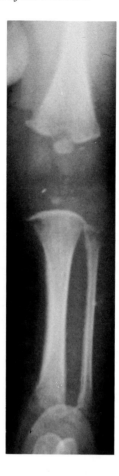

Fig. 10-36. Diffuse Salmonella osteomyelitis. Areas of mottling and obvious destruction, as well as periosteal reactions, are noted within all of the metaphyses of the lower extremities. The patient had Salmonella sepsis.

hepatosplenomegaly is the main clinical finding. These children do not succumb to the disease until the age of 15 or 20 years. The ribs, pelvis, and femurs are commonly involved. A peculiar characteristic of this disease is punctate calcific depositions in the sacrum and coccyx. The skull, as in Gaucher's disease, is spared. Development of the bones is usually retarded. Other radiographical manifestations include an interstitial nodular pattern in the lungs.

Both primary and secondary hyperparathyroidism affect the growing skeleton with an excessive secretion of parathyroid hormone. Long standing, untreated cases of hyperparathyroidism amy show a whole range of skeletal manifestations from diffuse demineralization to cystic areas of bone destruction by brown tumors. A brown tumor is an area of localized osteolysis due to a large accumulation of osteoclasts. Hemorrhage with hemosiderin deposition accounts for the brown coloration. The lesions may be single or multiple and appear anywhere in the skeleton. The usual sites, however, are the pelvis, ribs, and the long bones. Brown tumors are sharply demarcated and resemble simple cysts. When they occur in the epiphysis and are not diffuse, they can be confused with chondroblastoma. Fibrous dysplasia, chondromatous lesions of bone, and, in older patients, giant cell tumors all should be included in the differential diagnosis. However, other radiographic evidence of hyperparathyroidism, such as subperiosteal bone resorption, no lamina dura, soft-tissue calcification, and renal calculi, are frequently manifested.

Osteomyelitis most often affects a single area. However, multiple foci of infection may occur in patients with defective immune mechanisms or chronic debilitating diseases such as leukemia, diabetes, and tuberculosis. Multiple cystic lesions in newborns, particularly if they are localized in the medial, proximal metaphyseal region, are indicative of congenital syphilis. Additional findings such as metaphyseal irregularities and periosteal reaction are characteristic and almost always present.

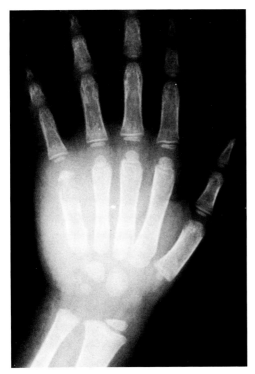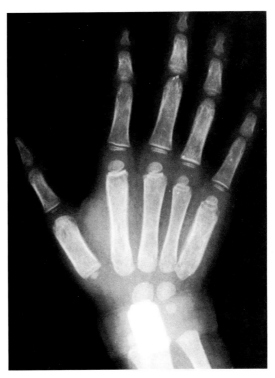

Fig. 10-37. Hand-foot syndrome in sickle cell disease. Bilateral palmar swelling is present and is quite prominent on the left. Both of the fifth metacarpals are surrounded by a periosteal reaction. The distal shaft on the left is destroyed and Salmonella was cultured from this region. This, in all probability, was a superimposed infection upon previously infarcted bone.

The radiographic development of osteomyelitis is basically the same regardless of distribution, consisting of diffuse soft-tissue swelling followed by periosteal reaction and bone destruction that begins as a small radiolucent focus in the metaphyseal area. The femur and proximal tibia are the bones most frequently involved (Fig. 10-36).

Patients with sickle cell disease demonstrate an increased susceptibility to infarction and to Salmonella osteomyelitis. In the young infant, the earliest clinical and radiographic manifestation of sickle cell disease is the hand-foot syndrome. This syndrome is the result of infarction and mainly involves the small bones, although the long bones are not always spared. Bilateral symmetrical involvement is a characteristic but unexplained feature. As in osteomyelitis, the earliest finding is a painful soft-tissue swelling. Periostial reaction and slow dissolution of the bone quickly ensue (Fig. 10-37). The bone undergoes fairly rapid separation, and new bone is formed that appears irregularly sclerotic. Occasionally the entire bone may

disappear. However, complete restitution is the rule. Distinguishing bone infarction from infection on a radiographic basis alone may be difficult. Radionuclide studies or actual bone biopsy to identify the causative agent are important and can be used to make a specific diagnosis.

Fungus infections are more likely to involve several bones. Some tend to involve a specific bone. Actinomycosis most often affects the mandible or the ribs and is sometimes accompanied by adjacent soft-tissue swelling and draining sinuses. Blastomycosis is likely to involve the long bones of the legs, such as the distal fibula and tibia. Most fungal infections are chronic and indolent and therefore differ from those caused by pyogenic organisms. The lesions are more sharply outlined and are surrounded by a sclerotic reaction (Fig. 10-38). This appearance is quite distinct, discernible from metastatic disease, retioculoendotheliosis, and other diseases producing multiple lesions with less distinguishable margins. Frequently, the primary site of infection is evident both ra-

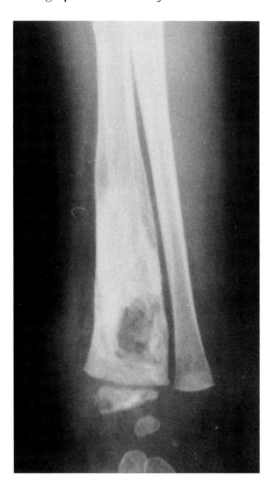

Fig. 10-38. Osteomyeletis (blastomycosis). A sharply demarcated lesion is present within the metaphysis of the radius. Note the extensive periosteal reaction and dense reactive bone. A similar lesion also involves the epiphysis.

diographically and clinically (e.g., pulmonary involvement in blastomycosis). Granulomatous osteomyelitis may be caused by other fungi such as *Histoplasma capsulatum* and *Cryptococus neoformans*. Radiographically the lesions are osteolytic, with a rather distinct sclerotic margin but with little or no periosteal reaction.

Tuberculosis may also involve multiple bones. The symptoms are rarely acute, and the radiographic findings do not reveal osteoporosis or new periosteal bone formation. Bone involvement may be seen in the epiphysis, metaphysis, or the shaft of long bones. The short tubular bones demonstrate a unique appearance. The phalanges are expanded, and the trabecular markings are destroyed, resulting in a "ballooned-out" appearance. Classically, this is called spina ventosa. Syphilitic dactylitis is less expansile and manifests a greater periosteal reaction. Tuberculosis of the ribs is rarely encountered today and consists radiographically of two forms, tuberculous chondritis and osteitis.

Both lesions develop somewhat differently but are eventually characterized by destructive bone lesions, a soft-tissue mass, and a periosteal reaction (Fig. 10-39). The lesion at the chondral junction begins as a soft-tissue mass, with a periosteal reaction, whereas bone destruction is encountered when the bone is initially involved. In small bones and flat bones tuberculous osteomyelitis produces cyst-like areas of destruction, with no reactive sclerosis. The most common site of involvement is the spine (Pott's disease), where the infection leads to destruction and collapse of the intervertebral disc space and corresponding vertebral body, with resultant gibbus deformity. A paravertebral or paraspinal abscess (calcified or not) is a helpful diagnostic feature.

Chronic granulomatous disease of childhood is associated with defective neutrophil function. Multiple abscesses occur throughout the body and the bones. The small bones of the hand and feet are frequently affected. An expansile lesion resembling tuberculous

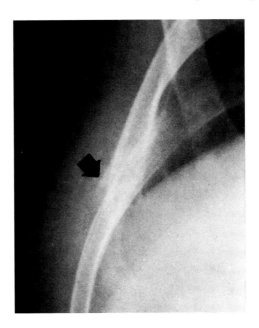

Fig. 10-39. Tuberculosis of the rib. The costochondral junction is destroyed and is associated with a small soft-tissue mass *(arrow)*.

spina ventosa, but without periosteal reaction, has also been produced.

The polyostotic form of fibrous dysplasia presents with various bone lesions but tends to be unilateral. The disease occurs in young individuals and on occasions may start in infancy. Abnormal cutaneous pigmentation consisting of irregular café au lait spots is seen in approximately one third of affected children. These spots have a rough "coast of Maine" appearance, in contrast to the smooth café au lait spots, "coast of California" appearance, characteristic of neurofibromatosis. Sexual precocity presents in approximately 30 per cent of the females but in only 6 per cent of the males affected. This feature is caused by the premature or early release of gonadotropin by the pituitary gland. Other associated, uncommon endocrine abnormalities include hyperparathyroidism, goiter, Cushing's syndrome, and parathyroid enlargement. Radiologically, the polyostotic form consists of cystic lesions with a sclerotic margin containing a "ground glass" or "soap bubble" appearance (Fig. 10-40). The involved bone is usually expanded. Individual lesions tend to have a variety of radiographic appearances. In some areas the bones are only diffusely expanded but gradually merge into the normal trabecular structure. This deformity is the result of structural weakness and is well exhibited in the femur. Pathologic fractures of the diseased bone occur commonly,

resulting in a varus deformity of the proximal femur, "Sheperd's crook" deformity. Fibrous dysplasia of the skull is predominantly sclerotic, although there are multiple areas of irregular radiolucency. At the time of sexual maturity the multiple lesions assume a stable radiographic appearance. Any change after puberty manifested by further expansion of the lesions with radiolucent areas represents a phase of cyst formation rather than malignant degeneration.

Cystic angiomatosis is quite different from isolated hemangioma of the axial skeleton, which is more common in the spine and somewhat less common in the calvarium. Cystic angiomatosis frequently presents in patients under the age of 20 years. Infants are also affected. The radiographic findings consist of multiple, oval, cystic lesions varying in size from a few millimeters to several centimeters in diameter. The initial manifestation is a conglomeration of small radiolucencies producing a mottled appearance. The lesions become more sharply demarcated as they coalesce to form single or multiple, round, oval, or lobular lesions. In fact, some may be surrounded by a fine sclerotic border. Some cortical expansion almost invariably occurs when the long bones are involved, but there is almost never an associated periosteal reaction. Angiomatosis is truly a systemic process and involves multiple organs. The general term *angiomatosis* is preferred, since

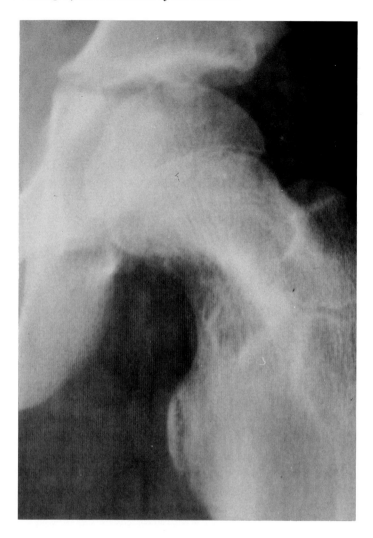

Fig. 10-40. Fibrous dysplasia. An osteolytic lesion is present within the inferior margin of the femoral neck. The matrix of the lesion manifests a "ground glass" appearance and is demarcated from bone by a thick and sclerotic margin.

the clinical features of cystic hemangiomatosis and lymphangiomatosis are the same in most patients and distinction between the two histologically may be difficult. The lesion must be distinguished from primary and secondary hyperparathyroidism, some forms of polyostotic fibrous dysplasia, and, on occasions, histiocytosis, fibromatosis, and neurofibromatosis.

Fibromatosis of bone involves the long bones with multiple osteolytic lesions and often with overgrowth of the involved extremity. The destructive lesions are usually subperiosteal, involve the cortex, and extend toward the medullary canal. They are often diffuse and involve the shaft rather than the metaphysis.

Osteolysis of bone, or acro-osteolysis, is a condition that is closely related to hemangiomatosis of bone. The disease may be famil-

ial and is seen in children and adolescents. Although it is usually associated with trauma, this is probably incidental. Most cases reveal associated angiomias.

Ollier's disease, or diffuse enchondromatosis, is rather unusual and affects several bones. The appearance of the cartilaginous tumors varies according to the amount of calcium present. The lesion may be radiolucent and expansile if no calcium is deposited (Fig. 10-41). However, the true nature of the lesion is revealed when stippled or amorphous deposits of calcium are present within the matrix of the lesion. The cortex is expanded but rarely destroyed, and no periosteal reaction occurs. The most characteristic feature is its predominant unilateral involvement. It is also known as Mafucci's syndrome when associated with cutaneous hemangiomas (Fig. 10-41C).

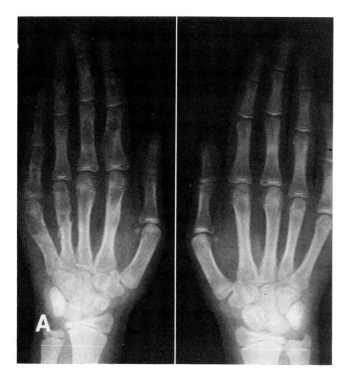

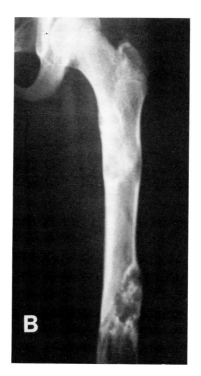

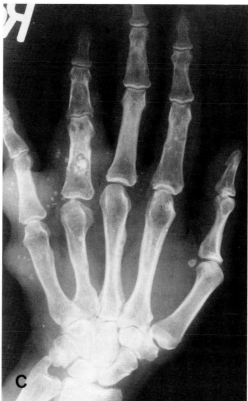

Fig. 10-41. *(A, B)* Ollier's disease. Diffuse unilateral changes are noted. In the hand multiple cystic lesions are present. In some areas the bones are markedly deformed by the lesions. The femur shows the more characteristic expansile lesions with a calcified cartilaginous matrix. *(C)* Maffucci's syndrome. This hand demonstrates multiple, soft-tissue hemangiomas and bony enchondroma. Note the multiply calcified phleboliths.

Discussion

Multiple radiolucent lesions throughout the skeleton are the result of either dissemination of malignant cells, inflammatory cells, or abnormal connective tissue cells. A complete radiographic survey is useful in evaluating these lesions. However, approximately 50 per cent of cancellous bone has to be destroyed in the spine before these defects are visible radiographically. Unless there is cortical involvement of long bones, medullary lesions 1 cm. long or slightly larger may not be detected on conventional radiographs. The multiple osteolytic lesions almost invariably start in the medullary cavity, with secondary involvement or invasion of cortical bone. In metastatic disease, such as neuroblastoma, rhabdomyosarcoma, or retinoblastoma, tumor growth may be too rapid for differentiation. This problem also arises in the very severe, rapidly progressive form of histiocytosis.

Cortical destruction is usually the result of erosion of bone by the tumor itself rather than by osteoclastic activity. The more aggressive is the neoplastic or inflammatory process, the smaller is the reaction elicited from the host bone, and the more prominent is the soft-tissue invasion or extension. Slowly growing processes which replace bone and result in a radiolucent appearance produce the characteristic expansile lesions that are seen in cystic lesions of bone such as angiomatosis, brown tumor of hyperparathyroidism, and tuberculosis.

Histiocytosis includes a group of disorders formerly described as individual entities. However, all are characterized by abnormal proliferation of histiocytes, with subsequent deposition of cholesterol and lipids within the cells, and in the advanced chronic stage, by fibrosis and scarring. All of these disease processes are now believed to be inflammatory rather than neoplastic. Eosinophilic granuloma is the least severe form of histiocytosis and often presents with single, well-defined bone lesions that disappear spontaneously in 1 or 2 years. Letterer-Siwe disease is the acute and most severe form and affects young infants, with a rapid clinical course that may result in death. Development into a more moderate course in the 2nd decade of life is known as the Hand-Schüller-Christian disease. All forms are closely related and most likely represent different stages of the same disorder. Males are more commonly affected than females. The age of onset is quite variable, although Letterer-Siwe disease usually occurs at 2 years of age or earlier.

MULTIPLE SCLEROTIC LESIONS

A number of conditions produce diffuse sclerotic lesions of bone. These include trauma, infection, tumor, and metabolic disease, as well as developmental abnormalities.

Disease Entities

Diffuse sclerotic lesions
  Developmental
    Osteopetrosis
    Pyknodysostosis
    Pyle's disease
    Engelmann's disease
    Ribbing's disease
    Melorheostosis
    Fibrous dyspasia
    Van buchem's disease (hyperostosis corticalis)
    Sclerosteosis
    Tuberous sclerosis
  Metabolic
    Renal osteodystrophy
    Fluoride intoxication
    Hemolytic anemias
    Mastocytosis
    Gaucher's disease
    Hyperphosphatasia
  Infectious
    Osteomyelitis
    Bone infarct
  Tumorous
    Chondrosarcoma
    Leukemia
    Reticulum cell sarcoma
Local sclerotic lesions
  Developmental
    Osteopoikilosis
    Osteopathia striata
    Heavy metal poisoning
  Infectious
    Osteomyelitis
    Bone infarct
  Metabolic
    Hyperparathyroidism (healing brown tumor)
  Tumorous
    Ewing's tumor
    Osteogenic sarcoma

A generalized increase in bone density may be more difficult to recognize than a localized lesion, since there is no surrounding, contrasting density. When the process involves both the medullary cavity as well as the cortex, the bone becomes homogeneously dense and distinction between cortex and medulla on the radiograph is no longer possible (Fig. 10-42A-D). Cortical thickening alone results in diffuse or selective areas of increased sclerosis as well as an increase in bone width. Increased bone density also results when the medullary trabeculae become thick and coarse for one reason or another. The overall bone size, however, remains the same. Diffuse sclerotic lesions may involve the entire skeleton, the extremities, or only portions of the bone. The following classification is based primarily upon the effect and distribution of a disease within a single bone and is divided into diffuse and local involvement.

Differential Diagnosis

Osteopetrosis, often referred to as marble bones or Albers-Schönberg disease, exemplifies best the diffusely sclerotic skeletal abnormality. It occurs in two forms, congenita and tarda. The congenital form is far more severe. All bones in the body are diffusely and homogeneously sclerotic, so that distinction between cortical and medullary cancellous bone is no longer possible in most cases (Fig. 10-42A, 10-42B). The metaphyseal ends of the long bones are frequently flared, and fine longitudinal or transverse radiolucent lines are often observed within this region. The epiphyses are not involved and a normal growth rate continues. The shafts of tubular and flat bones, particularly the ribs and the vertebral bodies, may show radiolucent centers early in the course of the disease. Other changes include squaring of the bodies and the anterior margins of the ribs. The skull is uniformly thickened. As a result the diploë are not distinguishable, the mastoids and paranasal sinuses appear dense, and the foramina are all narrowed. Hydrocephalus occasionally develops when the foramen magnum is involved. The chalky bones are very brittle, and an increased incidence of fractures of the long bones is another unfortunate complication of the disease. The fractures are characteristically transverse and frequently arise following minor injury (Fig. 10-42E). Healing occurs rapidly with the production of dense and extensive callus.

The clinical features in congenital osteopetrosis include anemia, jaundice, and hepatosplenomegaly. These findings are not strongly exhibited in osteopetrosis tarda, and as a rule, the axial skeleton is affected less. Sclerosis of the extremities is the only prominent feature. Occasionally the disease is episodic, and normal bone is produced during the remission. The resulting radiographic findings are unique and manifest alternating areas of normal and abnormal dense bone, the "bone within a bone" pattern (Fig. 10-42F).

Pyknodysostosis strongly resembles osteopetrosis, and at one time was considered a variant of the disease. The bones are also diffusely sclerotic, although the increased density is not as prominent, and the patients rarely manifest the clinical findings of anemia or hepatosplenomegaly. Patients with pyknodysostosis have hypoplastic or aplastic terminal phalanges, although some reveal clubbing of the fingers and enlarged nails as well (Fig. 10-43A). The mandible is typically hypoplastic, and the mandibular angle is almost completely flat (Fig. 10-43B). The fontanelles remain open for prolonged periods of time with the eventual development of wormian bones (Fig. 10-43B).

In Pyle's disease an accentuated splaying of the metaphyseal ends of tubular bones, associated with an overall increase in bone density, is characteristic (Fig. 10-44). The skull is part of the process and demonstrates marked thickening of the base and sclerosis of the cranial vault. The mandible is also thick and sclerotic. In addition, hypertelorism and underdevelopment of the paranasal sinuses may be encountered in newborns. Not surprisingly, the radiographic findings markedly resemble osteopetrosis, since metaphyseal flaring and sclerosis are common in both. However, the overall sclerosis of the skeleton is less prominent and less progressive in Pyle's disease. The vertebral bodies are also flattened as well as sclerotic.

Progressive diaphyseal dysplasia, Engelmann's disease, is a rare disorder associated with excessive periosteal activity that produces hyperostosis and periostitis. The resulting cortical thickening is restricted to the diaphysis and is found only in the long tubular bones. The epiphyseal and the metaphyseal areas are spared. Consequently, the major feature is an overgrowth of the normal

(Text continued on p. 403.)

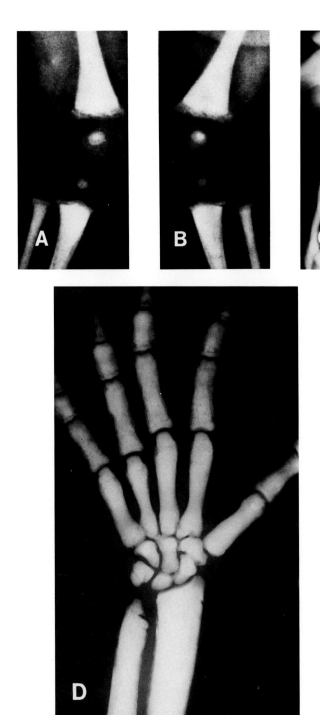

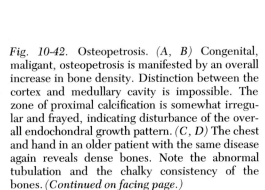

Fig. 10-42. Osteopetrosis. *(A, B)* Congenital, maligant, osteopetrosis is manifested by an overall increase in bone density. Distinction between the cortex and medullary cavity is impossible. The zone of proximal calcification is somewhat irregular and frayed, indicating disturbance of the overall endochondral growth pattern. *(C, D)* The chest and hand in an older patient with the same disease again reveals dense bones. Note the abnormal tubulation and the chalky consistency of the bones. *(Continued on facing page.)*

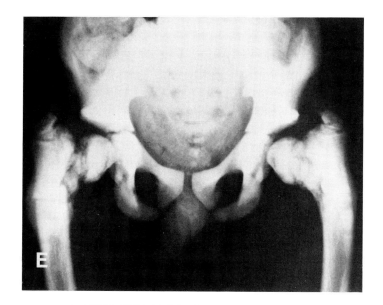

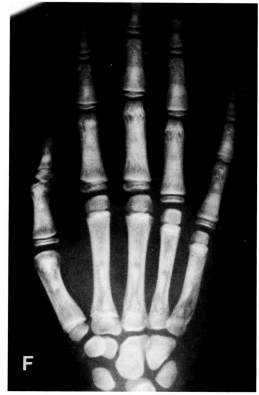

Fig. 10-42 (Continued). (E) The pelvis demonstrates coxa vara deformity and transverse fracture of the right femur. *(F)* The hand in a patient with osteopetrosis tarda shows dense but well formed bones. Dense enclosed bones are seen within the more developed structures.

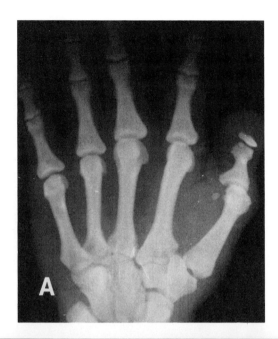

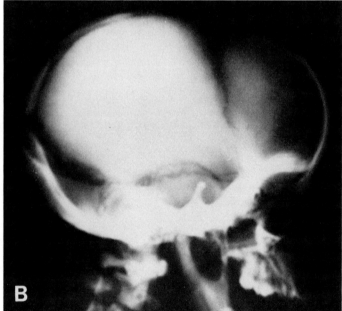

Fig. 10-43. Pyknodysostosis. *(A)* The bones of the hand are sclerotic, although the cortex and medullary canal and the normal outline of the bones are distinguishable. The distal ungual tufts are absent. *(B)* The entire cranial vault is dense. However, all the fontanelles remain open, despite the patient's age. Note the severely hypoplastic mandible, with complete loss of the angle.

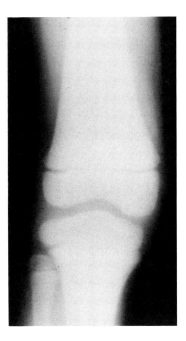 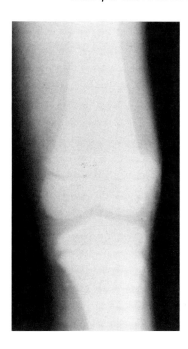

Fig. 10-44. Pyle's disease. Slight widening of the metaphysis is associated with increased bone density.

contour of diaphyseal bone, which results in a spindle-shaped shaft (Fig. 10-45). This finding distinguishes Englemann's disease from osteopetrosis, pyknodysostosis, and Pyle's disease. The extremities are also somewhat elongated in relationship to the overall size of the patient (Fig. 10-45C, 10-45D). Moreover, the skull, vertebral bodies, and flat bones are not usually involved, although the base of the skull and the pelvis are sometimes affected. Calcification in vertebral ligaments as well as other ligaments, such as the ischiosacral ligaments, also occurs. The clinical symptomatology is dramatic, since the incidence of generalized wasting and muscular atrophy is high. The patients are not anemic and have no leucocytosis.

Somewhat akin to Englemann's disease is Ribbing's disease, which is also referred to as hereditary multiple diaphyseal sclerosis. The lesion is familial and seemingly does not occur before adolescence. The main radiographic feature is diaphyseal osteosclerosis and hyperostosis (Fig. 10-46). This strongly resembles Englemann's disease but may be limited to only one or more of the long bones. Symmetrical involvement of the proximal tibial shaft almost always occurs, despite the strong tendency for isolated bone involvement. Pain is a common symptom and originates at the time of puberty. This symptom may be related to the activity of the disease, since individuals who show no symptoms have a corresponding absence of radiographic progression.

Flowing hyperostosis or melorheostosis is a rare disease in which the long bones of a single extremity or an entire side of the body are affected by a unique form of sclerosis. It has, nevertheless, also been reported in flat bones, such as the ribs and pelvis, as well as the spine and the skull. Clinically, the findings of swelling and atrophy of the overlying soft tissues are found, associated with pain and stiffness of the extremity and the adjacent joints. The diagnosis is made by the radiographic demonstration of longitudinal zones of cortical thickening that produce zones of sclerosis. The sclerotic zones are characterized by an undulating, continuous, and eccentric appearance. The eccentric zones are produced rather late in the disease and have been likened to "flowing candle wax." Inner cortical sclerosis occurs much earlier (Fig. 10-47). Medullary sclerosis is also observed and results in some obliteration of the endosteal medullary space.

Van Buchem's disease, or hyperostosis corticalis, is a rare and unusual disorder that may represent a form of juvenile Paget's disease. This disease affects the entire skeleton, with cortical thickening of the ribs and clavicle (Fig. 10-48). The diaphyseal cortices are wide, and there is sclerosis of the skull.

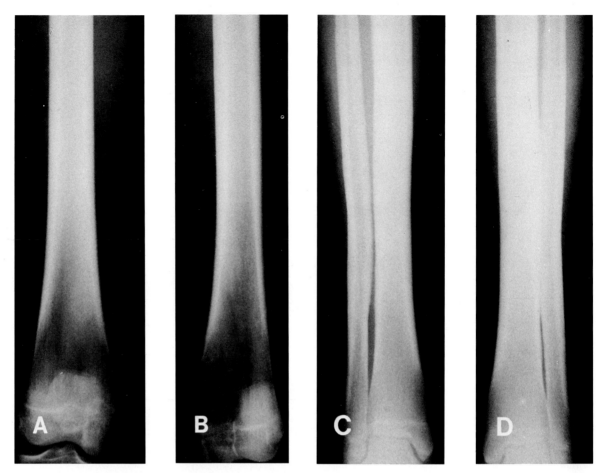

Fig. 10-45. Engelmann's disease. *(A, B)* Both femurs reveal subtle cortical widening of the diaphysis. The metaphyses are completely normal. *(C, D)* The tibias and fibulas in another patient show obvious widening of the central portion of each bone. The widening is caused by increased cortical thickening. The overall increase in bone length is quite apparent.

Extremely similar to Van Buchem's disease is sclerosteosis. This is a genetic disorder in which syndactyly is associated with thickening and overgrowth of the bones. Generalized bony overgrowth and progressive enlargement of the mandible and forehead are usually noted after the age of 4 years. Gigantism is apparent in childhood. Increased bone density is particularly obvious in the pelvis and skull. The cortices of the tubular bones are dense and the diaphyseal constriction is absent. Alkaline phosphatase is also elevated. The difference in the two diseases is slight. The bones tend to bulge more, and the entire bone is involved in sclerosteosis. In addition, deafness and facial palsy are common complications.

Mastocytosis is a generalized disease that has been associated with diffuse bone sclerosis. The bone changes vary from well-defined, blastic lesions to an overall diffuse increase in bone density due to thickening of the trabeculae. Urticaria pigmentosa and other manifestations of gastrointestinal disease better define the syndrome.

Excessive intake of flourine is another known but rare cause of bone sclerosis. This is also associated with ligamentous calcification.

The anemias, particularly Cooley's anemia and sickle cell anemia in the later stages, may produce sclerotic bone. However, in the 1st decade of life the reverse is usually found, and radiolucent bones with thinning of the cortex and widening of the spongiosa due to erythropoetic marrow proliferation is the general rule. Increased bone density develops slowly as a result of multiple fac-

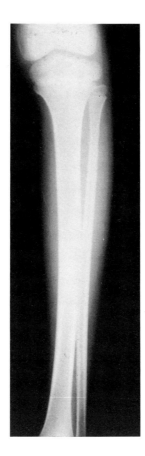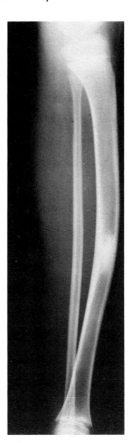

Fig. 10-46. Ribbing's disease. Note the sclerosis and thickening within the mid-shaft of the tibia. No other abnormalities are noted in this extremity.

tors. Repeated episodes of bone infarction probably account for many of the changes noted in the extremities. In a large percentage of the cases, particularly with homozygous sickle cell disease, diffuse as well as localized cortical thickening is the result not only of bone infarction but of an associated osteomyelitis. Moreover, the weight-bearing or stress trabeculae of the bones become accentuated and more prominent with time after other trabeculae have been absorbed (Fig. 10-49).

Localized areas of irregular sclerosis and deformity due to aseptic necrosis are encountered in the epiphysis of the proximal femurs and humeri, in both the homozygous and heterozygous forms of sickle cell anemia. The skull is quite commonly involved in thalassemia and to a lesser degree in sickle cell disease. The diploic space is widened and in extreme cases the outer table of bones of the skull is replaced by long, vertical, bony spiculations that produce the so called "hair-on-end" appearance.

In some cases of renal osteodystrophy, the bones throughout the body demonstrate osteosclerosis, or an increased density in bone that is manifested as coarsening of the trabecular pattern. The ribs, spine, pelvis, and long bones are commonly affected. The disease is easily distinguished from other sclerotic lesions by the presence of other manifestations of hyperparathyroidism and rickets, such as subperiosteal resorption of the phalanges and bones, associated with a widened and frayed distal metaphysis.

Children with hyperphosphatasia display a large head with overhanging frontal bones, a short neck and thorax, long extremities, lateral bowing of the femurs, and anterior bowing of the tibias. The cortices are thick and the skull is dense. The spine may show collapsed vertebrae.

Gaucher's disease produces many of the radiographic features of sickle cell disease. Basically, the large Gaucher's cells replace the bone marrow and lead to patchy or diffuse demineralization. However, superimposed infarction and hypertrophy of secondary trabeculae eventually produce a

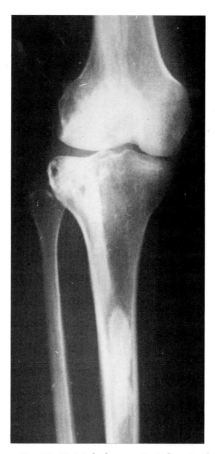 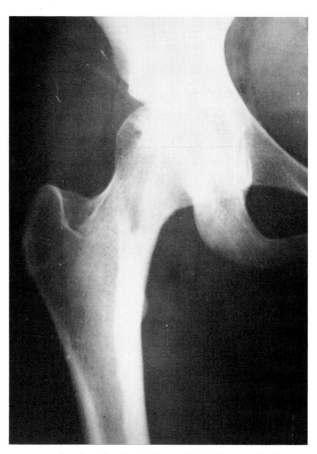

Fig. 10-47. Melorheostosis. Sclerotic changes are noted within the distal tibia and the femur. The lesion at this stage affects only the endosteum.

generalized increase in bone density (Fig. 10-35). Localized aseptic necrosis of the femoral heads is also characteristic. The vertebral bodies may be collapsed. Massive splenic enlargement, however, is the rule, in contrast to the small infarcted and occasionally calcified spleen in sickle cell disease.

Diffuse sclerosis has been encountered with diffuse leukemic infiltration of the bones. This most commonly follows remission due to a successful therapeutic regimen but may rarely be seen in patients with acute disease.

An important disease producing diffuse or localized areas of sclerosis is fibrous dysplasia (Fig. 10-50). Cystic lesions have also been described. In the extremities, the sclerotic lesions present as waxy, linear striations of varying thickness that simulate melorheostosis (Fig. 10-50A). Localized lesions are circular or oval, homogeneous, or lined by a thin ring of sclerosis (Fig. 10-50B). Fusiform thickening of the rib with increased areas of

bone density is another common manifestation of the disease (Fig. 10-50C). In the local lesions, the sclerosis is limited to only one part of the bones.

In osteopoikilosis, stippled areas of increased bone density involve the ends of long bones. The dense sclerotic lesions are round or oval and resemble individual bone islands (Fig. 10-51). The growth or shape of the involved bones are not affected, and the development of the lesion is variable. Some regress and completely disappear, whereas others become denser. In flat bones the areas of density occur primarily in periarticular regions such as the superior acetabulum and the iliac side of the sacroiliac joints. There are no significant clinical features associated with this entity. However, approximately 10 to 15 per cent of the patients reveal skin lesions consisting of small, whitish-yellow, cutaneous and subcutaneous nodules.

Osteopathia striata, or Voorhoeve's disease, is closely related to osteopoikilosis.

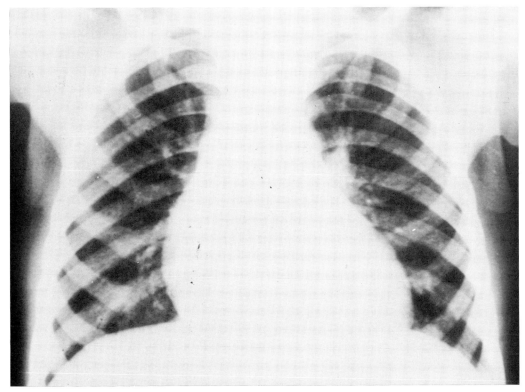

Fig. 10-48. Van Buchem's disease. This chest film reveals thickened ribs. The clavicles are not well-defined.

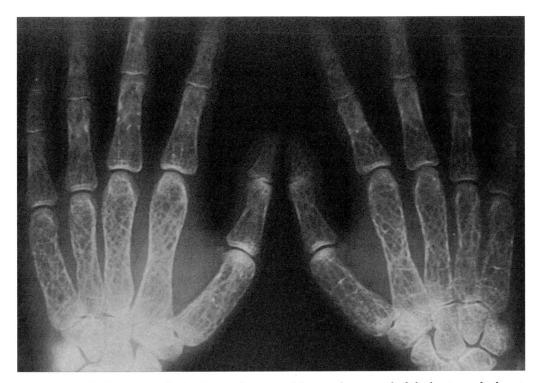

Fig. 10-49. Cooley's anemia. The hands reveal increased density due to marked thickening and sclerosis of the remaining trabeculae, most of which have been previously destroyed.

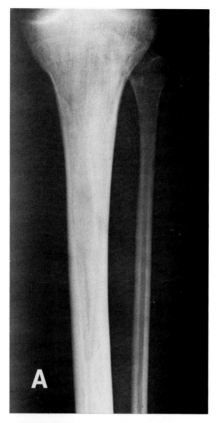

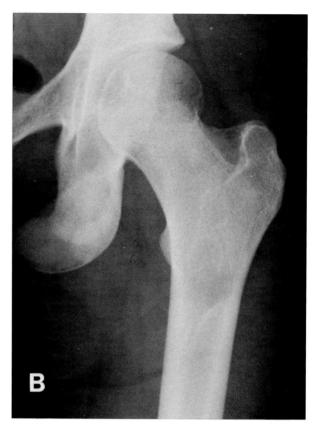

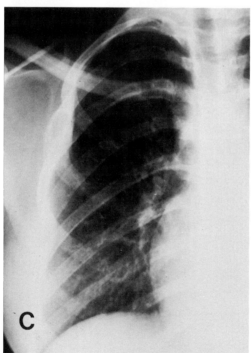

Fig. 10-50. Fibrous dysplasia. *(A)* The tibia is diffusely involved with linear, wavy, sclerotic bands of varying thickness which affect the entire shaft. *(B)* Localized sclerotic lesions of varying sizes, configuration, and appearance are present in the proximal femur and ischium. *(C)* On the right, the third, fourth, and fifth ribs are expanded and thickened.

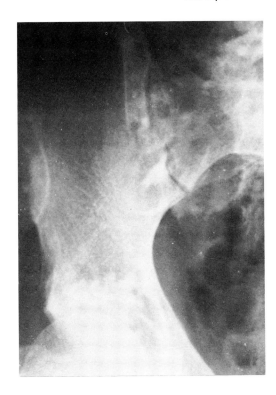

Fig. 10-51. Osteopoikilosis. Multiple, dense bony islands are noted in the immediate juxta-articular regions. These are sharp and well-defined.

However, in this condition the radiopacities, rather than being circular or ovoid in configuration, form vertical patterns consisting of relatively thin, parallel sclerotic lines. It is not difficult to recognize osteopathia striata although it is frequently combined with other diseases which produce increased areas of bone density, such as osteopoikilosis or melorheostosis.

Chronic intake of lead during childhood leads to deposition of the metal and increased calcium in the zone of provisional calcification, adjacent to the epiphyseal line. The lead therefore contributes to but is not totally responsible for the production of the increased dense metaphyseal band known as the "lead line." The histologic picture of the lead line consists of an increased *number* of bony trabeculae and amount of calcified cartilage (which contains some lead). In some cases, widening of the ends of the long bones with cortical thickening simulating metaphyseal dysplasia has resulted following lead poisoning. If the lead is intermittently ingested, multiple parallel transverse bands within the diaphysis are produced. The heavy, dense, wide lines are not pathognomonic of lead intoxication, since they have been produced by overdosage of phosphorus

and bismuth as well. The transverse lines of Park are similar but much thinner.

Tuberous sclerosis is another fairly well known cause of bone thickening due to periosteal stimulation. These are typically encountered in the small bones and are frequently associated with cystic alterations of the trabecular pattern (Fig. 10-52). The ribs are rarely involved but can resemble fibrous dysplasia. The changes here, however, are the result of periosteal reactions.

Ewing's sarcoma and osteogenic sarcoma rarely involve multiple bones. Whether this represents multicentric tumor growth or metastatic disease is unimportant, since the outcome is the same in both. Brown tumors in patients with hyperparathyroidism are basically osteolytic during the active stage of the disease. However, if and when the primary stimulus, elevated levels of parathyroid hormone, is removed, the lesions heal with the deposition of calcium and eventual bone formation. As a result they convert from osteolytic to osteoblastic lesions.

Discussion

Many of the disease entities discussed in this chapter are the result of errors in bone formation. Since osteogenesis is a complex

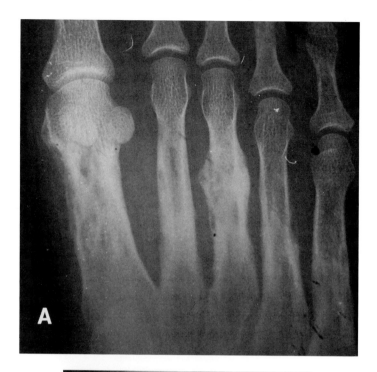

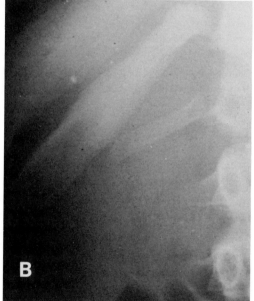

Fig. 10-52. Tuberous sclerosis. *(A)* The metatarsals demonstrate thick wavy periosteal changes associated with cystic changes in the bones. *(B)* Diffuse thickening of the tenth and eleventh right ribs is shown. The thickening is formed by a massive periosteal reaction.

process, multiple factors may interrupt or arrest normal bone formation at any stage of its development. Bone develops by two mechanisms. In intramembranous formation, osteoid is formed without the presence of previous cartilage. The bone salts are deposited directly in the osteoid tissue. Almost all the compact bone of the shafts of long bones and nearly all of the flat bones are formed by this method. The second mechanism is enchondral bone formation. The osteoblasts deposit bone in osteoid tissue formed essentially on calcified chondroid tissue that resembles preformed primary bone. In general, bone mass is usually the result of intramembranous bone formation, and bone growth is accomplished by enchondral bone formation. Both types of bone formation may be disrupted, resulting in sclerotic lesions.

Bone is always in an active state of remodeling, even after the closure of the secondary ossification centers. The term *bone flow* has been introduced to explain some newer concepts of bone modeling. The new trabeculae formed in the metaphysis do not remain perpendicular as the epiphyseal plate grows away from them but tend to flow or orient themselves toward the center of the diaphysis. As a result, the trabeculae at the periphery of the metaphysis show the greatest change in direction. Bone modeling, constriction, is the result of trabecular osteolysis proceeding at a greater rate at the flaired end of the metphysis than at the center of the metaphysis. Osteolysis is related to osteocytic function, and the osteoclasts remove the debris resulting in a funneling of the metaphysis. In most forms of dysplasia the modeling error occurs in the initial stages of bone formation, related to either a disturbance or maldevelopment of the primary center of ossification, a malfunction of osteoblasts, as in osteosclerotic diseases, or an overproduction or a failure of resorption of primitive dense primary cartilaginous bone, as in osteopetrosis and probably in pyknodysostosis as well.

The primary defect in osteopetrosis is the persistence of calcified primary cartilaginous spongiosa. The proliferation of osteoid is normal up to this point. However, there is no resorption of the very dense primary spongiosa which, because of its compactness, is radiopaque. Overall, the cartilage, calcification, and vascular supply of primitive bone are all normal. No satisfying explanation has been given for the failure of bone resorption.

Osteopoikilosis is mainly due to an error in the modeling of the spongiosa. The areas of increased bone density vary in number throughout childhood. In adults, the radiographic picture is usually stable. There are many reports of complete disappearance of the lesions when skeletal maturity is reached. Reports demonstrating the association of osteopoikilosis and melorheostosis in the same patient have been described. As a result, the possibility of a similar pathogenesis in both entities has been postulated.

Several physicians have suggested that osteopathia striata is a variant of osteopetrosis. However, there is no evidence to support this theory, since many of the radiographic changes of the two are different, such as flaring of the metaphysis of long bones in osteopetrosis. In addition, patients with osteopathia striata are usually asymptomatic and have a normal life span. Osteopetrosis has a familial occurrence.

Pyle's disease is unusual and peculiar. It is often referred to as familial metaphyseal dysplasia or metaphyseal dysplasia, and it is presumably the result of an inability to absorb secondary spongiosa due to inadequate osteoclastic activity. This process, however, is restricted to the metaphyseal regions of long bone. Although many physicians consider the associated cranial changes to be part of the same process, some regard them as separate diseases.

Since Ribbing's disease may represent a delayed or adult form of Engelmann's disease, it is somewhat ineffective to discuss each as a separate entity. In both, the overproduction of intramembranous periosteal bone may be a reactive process due to some inflammatory agent, although no such agent has been isolated to date. However, unlike Englemann's disease, in Ribbing's disease muscular development is normal and there is a distinct paucity of systemic manifestations.

Sclerosis encountered in renal osteodystrophy is the result of secondary hyperparathyroidism. The cause of sclerosis is not well understood; osteomalacia is encountered far more often (see p. 417).

Hyperphosphatasia, an interesting disease, demonstrates many features which suggest that it may represent juvenile Paget's disease. The serum level of alkaline phosphatase is comparably elevated, and the microscopy appears similar to that of florid Paget's disease. High serum levels of alkaline phoshatase are also found in Van Buchem's disease, which suggests some relation to both Paget's disease and hyperphosphatasia.

OSTEOPENIA

Osteopenia ("bone poverty") is reflected radiographically by diminished bone density. Osteopenic bone disease may be classified under two broad headings, osteoporosis and osteomalacia. Bone remodeling continues throughout life as a combination of simultaneous bone resorption and bone production. The rate of remodeling may increase or decrease at various ages and in certain disease states. However, when resorption proceeds at a relatively faster rate than bone production, the net result is loss of bone mass or *osteoporosis*. Generally, the bone present, although diminished in quantity, is qualitatively normal. A generalized increase in pre-osseous matrix (osteoid) associated with poor mineralization characterizes osteomalacia. This entity may be summarized as a derangement of the *quality* of existing bone. Mature lamellar bone gradually replaces immature woven bone in the normal growing process. When malacic disease involves woven bone primarily (the first type of bone produced in linear growth), the term *rickets* is used. When it involves lamellated or haversian bone, the term *osteomalacia* is used. Therefore, it is understandable why rickets and osteomalacia are both present in growing individuals, and why osteomalacia alone is present when skeletal growth is complete.

Osteopenia results in diminished bone density. Thirty percent of the bone mass (50 percent in the spine) must be lost before a decrease in bone density can be recognized radiographically. The actual detection of decreased density varies with the individual and may be related to the patient's age or the type of disease in question. The size of the bone or its initial state of mineralization may also influence radiographic appearance. Localized areas of decreased density afford earlier recognition than generalized disease because of relative differences in density of adjacent bone. Unfortunately, differences in exposure and processing factors alter film quality and limit the ability to detect subtle changes in mineralization or bone mass.

Various techniques have been used to measure bone density. Densitometry is one method by which a calibrated beam of light is passed through a radiograph of the bone, and the amount of transmitted light is measured by a photoelectric cell. The amount of transmitted light is proportional to the amount of mineral content of the bone. A technique of nuclear medicine, utilizing a monochromatic energy source coupled to a detector, may also be used. The extremity is scanned and the amount of radionuclide absorption is proportional to the quantity of mineral present within the bone.

In the presence of complicated disease states, such as renal osteodystrophy, these techniques are limited. Changes of osteomalacia due to altered vitamin D metabolism cannot be distinguished from changes of osteoclastic resorption due to superimposed hyperparathryoidism. Higher than normal quantitative mineral values may also be present when osteosclerosis and florid osteitis fibrosa cystica are concomitant.

Biopsy is the most accurate method of diagnosis. Care must be taken regarding the site of biopsy, processing of the specimen, and standardization of interpretation.

Much has been written on the radiology of osteoporosis and osteomalacia. Some confusion persists. The lack of absolute diagnostic criteria and increased concomitance have been major impediments. Moreover, the individual variations of host response, diet, and geography, as well as the subtle histochemical or physiologic variations of each disease, can cause distinct differences in radiographic presentation. For example, primary hyperparathyroidism may present as exaggerated osteoporosis, while secondary forms of the same disease may at times be overshadowed by the initiating malacic process.

Radiographic examination alone may afford a specific diagnosis in some instances and many times indicates the basic or underlying process affecting the skeleton. The involvement of interrelated systems, hormones, vitamins, and electrolytes, however, accen-

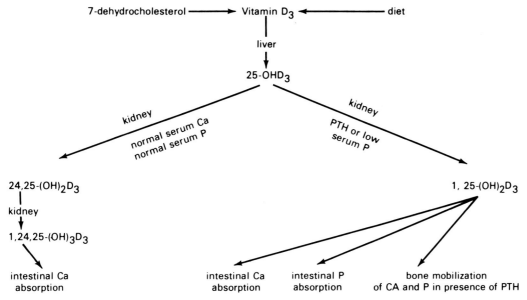

Fig. 10-53. Vitamin D metabolism.

tuates the need for a combined clinical, radiographic, and laboratory analysis of the individual case.

RICKETS AND OSTEOMALACIA

Historically, rickets and osteomalacia have been viewed fundamentally as the result of a deficiency of vitamin D. However, recent attention has focused upon the aberrations of vitamin D metabolism. In addition, knowledge of direct and indirect effects of abnormal phosphate metabolism has expanded our ability to separate and classify many closely related and hitherto poorly understood conditions. While many interactions of vitamin D, parathyroid hormone, thyrocalcitonin, and inorganic ions remain the subject of intense research and some controversy, an understanding of acknowledged interactions helps to explain some of the underlying disease entities (Fig. 10-53).

Parathyroid Hormone (PTH) is a polypeptide hormone secreted by the parathyroid gland. Secretion of this hormone is regulated, for the most part, by prevailing serum levels of ionizable calcium or the combined serum concentration of magnesium and calcium ions. It promotes movement of bone mineral into extracellular fluid, probably by inhibiting osteoblasts lining the bone en-

velope and stimulating osteoclastic resorption. In the kidneys the hormone promotes calcium resorption and decreases tubular resorption of phosphate. Studies also indicate that parathyroid hormone increases calcium absorption from the gut by stimulating the renal production of the active vitamin D metabolite.

Vitamin D is converted to the active metabolite in the kidney, where the enzyme 25-hydroxycholecalciferol-1-alpha-hydroxylase changes the inactive presursor 25-hydroxycholecalciferol to 1-25-dihydroxycholecalciferol, which is active in the mobilization of mineral from bone. The metabolites of vitamin D may act preferentially at different sites. This depends upon the electrolytic state and hormonal balance of the individual. Vitamin D may also influence synthesis and maturation of collagen substrate, as well as facilitating mineralization of pre-osseous matrix.

Hyperphosphatemia, even when present in patients with normal renal function, may induce hyperparathyroidism. High blood levels of phosphate inhibit the mineral-mobilizing system and produce hypocalcemia. Increased parathyroid activity may compensate for the hypocalcemic state. Bone turnover rate and bone formation are both enhanced.

Disease Entities

Vitamin D deficiency
Vitamin D dependency
Gastrointestinal abnormalities
    Malabsorption of vitamin D
        Postoperative states
            Gastrectomy (gastroenterostomy)
            Ureterosigmoidoscopy
            Intestinal bypass or small bowel resection
        Gluten sensitive enteropathy
        Regional enteritis
        Diverticulosis of the small intestine (blind loop syndrome)
        Lymphosarcoma
        Intestinal lymphangiectasia
        Rickets of premature infants
    Pancreatic insufficiency (cystic fibrosis and pancreatitis)
    Hepatic and bilary diseases
        Chronic parenchymal disease (cirrhosis)
        Chronic or congenital bilary obstruction
        Long-term anticonvulsant therapy
Renal diseases
    Decreased glomerular filtration in renal osteodystrophy
    Tubular disorders
        Renal tubular acidosis
            Type I (acidosis of the distal tubule, potassium wasting)
            Type II (acidosis of the proximal tubule, bicarbonate wasting and Fanconi's syndrome)
            Fanconi's syndrome (multiple tubular defects)
            Acquired (heavy metal poisoning and effect of tetracyline degradation products)
            Hereditary
                Cystinosis
                Wilson's disease
                Oculocerebrorenal syndrome
        Hypophosphatemia
            Familial hypophosphatemic vitamin D-refractory rickets
            Sporatic hypophosphatemia
Tumor dependent disorders
    Tumors with endocrine effects
        Malignant tumors with parathyroid-like activity
    Nonendocrine tumors
        Giant cell tumors
        Mesenchymal tumors
        Hemangiopericytoma
        Neurofibromatosis
Hypophosphatasia

The inhibition of an active renal metabolite of vitamin D may tend to decrease intestinal absorption of calcium. However, this may be overshadowed by the effects of parathyroid hormone on maintaining or elevating serum levels of calcium.

Hypophosphatemia impairs the phase of bone formation of the bone turnover process and probably impairs osteoblastic function of substrate synthesis and mineralization. Stimulation of the active renal metabolite of vitamin D may serve to increase calcium absorption and phosphate from the gut.

Thyrocalcitonin is secreted from the C cell of the thyroid gland and functions mainly by inhibiting parathyroid-stimulated bone resorption, thereby decreasing plasma calcium levels. Blood calcium is therefore regulated by the dual action of parathyroid hormone and thyrocalcitonin, with the two hormones functioning antagonistically. However, it has been difficult to obtain convincing evidence that calcitonin plays a role in renal osteodystrophy.

Differential Diagnosis

Rickets is characterized by diminished or no calcification of the cartilage at the growth plate. This is due to lack of mineral and probably abnormal cartilage substrate. Radiographically rickets is manifested by abnormal widening of the epiphyseal plate and irregular mineralization of the provisional zone of calcification. The distal end of the bone shaft becomes irregular and frayed and assumes a cupped or transversely straight appearance (Fig. 10-54). Areas of increased density may appear in the provisional zones of calcification if the patient received some vitamin D, or once regular therapy begins. Pseudofractures (Milkman's syndrome or Looser's lines), when observed, are almost pathognomonic of osteomalacia and are almost always accompanied by pain and tenderness. They present as radiolucent defects that extend perpendicular to the cortex and are frequently symmetrical. The defects are more prominent in the outer areas of the cortex but can extend to the endosteal surface in many cases. The most frequent bones affected are the scapula, femoral neck, ischia, pubic rami, and the ribs. In many aspects, they are similar to stress fractures, and in some cases true fractures develop.

In forms of rickets and osteomalacia characterized by low serum levels of ionizable

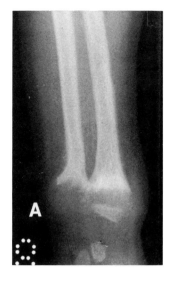 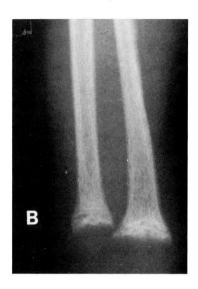

Fig. 10-54. Rickets. *(A)* Active stage. The distal portions of both the radius and the ulna are markedly cupped and splayed. The zone of provisional calcification is no longer apparent. Unmineralized osteoid is accumulating between the metaphysis and the epiphysis, with irregular zones of ossification present within. The trabecular pattern of the remaining portion of the bone is somewhat coarsened. *(B)* Healing stage (in a different patient). The cupping deformity is still apparent. However, the zone of provisional calcification is reappearing, with reossification of previously unossified osteoid.

calcium, hyperparathyroidism is initiated. When superimposed hyperparathyroidism complicates rickets or osteomalacia, radiographic evidence of increased parathyroid activity is found. Parathyroid hormone activates osteoclastic resorption of bone and therefore manifests its greatest effect in areas where bone remodeling occurs most rapidly, and where these cells are in greatest abundance. The radiographic findings are dependent on the age of the patient and the severity of the underlying process. Areas of resorption are frequently noted along the radial surfaces of the second and third middle phalanges of the hand (Fig. 10-55A). Concavities within the metaphyseal surfaces of long bones, the skull, acromioclavicular joints, the symphysis pubis, and the lamina dura of the teeth are also common (Fig. 10-55B). When resorption is active within the central portion of a bone, a defect is created which is filled with highly vascularized connective tissue and many interspersed osteoclasts. These are osteoclastomas. When bleeding occurs in the cystic lesions, brownish, oxidized blood elements predominate. The lesions are then referred to as "chocolate cysts" or brown tumors. Such tumorous or cystic lesions are more common in patients with primary hyperparathyroidism, and most heal by sclerosis following removal of the parathyroid adenoma. They also occur in severe forms of secondary hyperparathyroidism, such as renal osteodystrophy.

As hyperparathyroidism becomes more severe, patients become predisposed to transverse fractures near epiphyseal plates. Secondary epiphyseal slippage is common (Fig. 10-56). This occurrence is usually a late manifestation of severe hyperparathyroid activity, and other bone changes are almost always present. Sites of involvement include both proximal and distal femoral epiphyses and proximal humeral growth centers. Slippage is also found in the metacarpal and metatarsal heads, and the distal radial and ulnar epiphyses.

Premature closure of cranial sutures (usually involving at least the sagittal suture) is particularly frequent finding in hypophosphatemic renal rickets. A resultant dolichocephalic or scaphoid calvarial shape is common.

Diet, sunlight, intestinal absorption, hepatic and renal metabolism, and organ system interaction all determine the sequence of proper utilization of vitamin D. An error at any point in this sequence results in similar disease processes that are characterized by lack of or increased need for the vitamin or its metabolites. Loss of vitamin D or its metabolites may promote defects in intestinal calcium absorption. A fall in blood levels of ionizable calcium initiates increased parathyroid activity. The persistence and degree of hypocalcemia determines, in part, the type and severity of hyperparathyroidism.

In the event of renal insufficiency (a glomerular filtration rate of less than 25 to 30 mls./min.) hyperphosphatemia ensues, and the hypophosphatemic stimulus for production of vitamin D metabolite is lost. While demineralization may continue, areas of increased mineralization are promoted. This

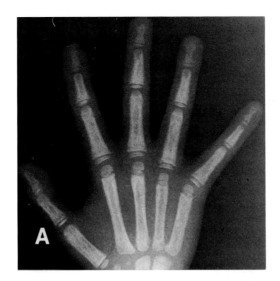

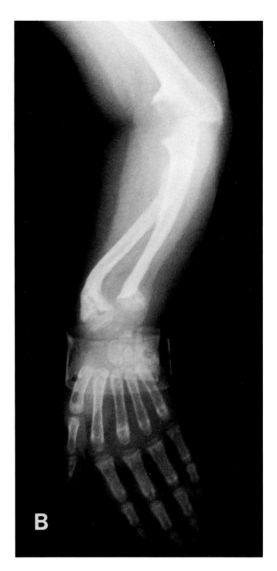

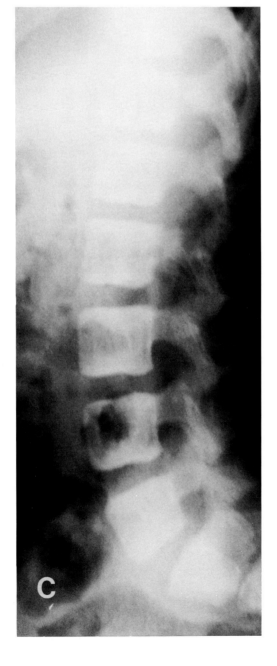

Fig. 10-55. Renal osteodystrophy. (A) Superiosteal erosion is present in the medial surface of the middle phalanges. Bone trabeculation is markedly coarsened. (B) Rachitic changes consisting of cupping and widening of the epiphyseal plate are present in the radius, ulna, and distal humerus. Severe deformities are apparent because of previous fractures through Looser's lines. (C) Osteomalacia of the spine. A "rugger jersey" configuration is noted. The trabecular pattern is coarsened.

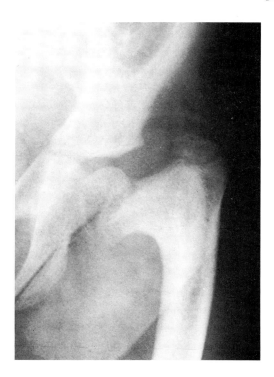

Fig. 10-56. Renal osteodystrophy with epiphysiolysis. The left hip shows coxa vara deformity. Note the peculiar relationship of the femoral epiphysis to the neck. This is due to previous slippage.

may be partially responsible for areas of osteosclerosis that occur in renal osteodystrophy. Hyperphosphatemia inhibits calcium mobilization, thereby resulting in hypocalcemia. Even when the kidneys are normal, this may cause hyperparathyroidism. It is not surprising then that in renal failure with hyperphosphatemia, the combined stimulus of hypocalcemia and hyperphosphatemia are responsible for the most severe hyperparathyroid state. In this situation, the bone changes may be more severe than in any other form of rickets or osteomalacia, and even more severe than in primary hyperparathyroidism. The bone texture is not homogeneous and of variable density. This is particularly prominent in the vertebral bodies and the metaphyseal portions of long bones. Such patterns of patchy density are only seen with this form of osteomalacia and rickets in untreated patients. In the vertebral bodies, areas of sclerosis parallel the end plates and the central portions of the vertebral bodies appear relatively radiolucent. This results from secondary hyperparathyroidism combined with inhibition of bone mobilization caused by hyperphosphatemia, superimposed on malacic bone. The resultant appearance has been called "rugger jersey" spine (Fig. 10-55C).

Vitamin D therapy in the early phases of renal failure (before hyperphosphatemia is present) is effective in retarding the effects of parathyroid activity. In renal failure of this type, soft-tissue calcification is prevalent. It may occur in the tips of fingers, salivary glands, abdominal viscera, eyes, subcutaneous tissue, and in or around joints. These changes consist of hydroxyapatite crystals and pyrophosphate dihydrate crystals. Deposition of pyrophosphate crystal is more common in primary hyperparathyroidism, and deposition of calcium hydroxyapitite (in the form of tumoral calcinosis or peritendinitis calcarea) is more prevalent in secondary forms of the disease. When these types of soft-tissue depositions exist, they are almost always accompanied by underlying osteitis fibrosa cystica.

In patients with only a slight degree of hypocalcemia, hyperparathyroidism is not a factor. This is exemplified by isolated, single renal tubular defects that result in moderate to severe hypophosphatemia. Hypophosphatemia stimulates calcium mobilization from bone and intestinal absorption of calcium, in part, by stimulation of renal production of the vitamin D metabolite which specifically acts on the gut. Hyperparathyroidism and its radiographic findings are therefore

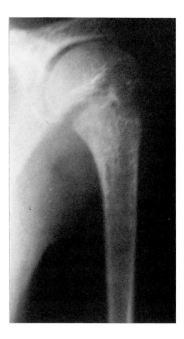 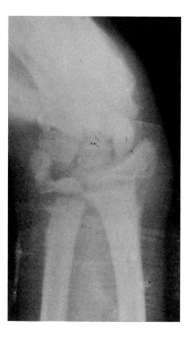

Fig. 10-57. Rickets due to anticonvulsive therapy. This 12-year-old patient had been on anticonvulsive therapy because of epileptic seizures since early childhood. Bone growth is severely retarded, and marked rachitic changes are present. The epiphyseal line is irregular and is accompanied by increased width between the shaft and the epiphysis. Epiphyseal separation is apparent in the distal radius.

not significant. There are no clinical signs of hypocalcemia; muscular weakness, abnormal sweating, irritability, and tetany are not present.

Familial hypophosphatemic vitamin D-refractory rickets is an X-linked, dominant disease. Despite its overall radiographic similarity to vitamin D-deficiency rickets, certain characteristic differences are present that may afford a specific diagnosis. This may be difficult in the early stages of the disease. However, as patients reach ambulatory age, anterior and lateral bowing of the femur and genu varum become predominant. Coxa vara is always present, but, unlike renal osteodystrophy, epiphyseal slippage is uncommon. Growth retardation is marked and a height of 5 ft. is seldom reached. The bones are widened and cortices are thick and often poorly demarcated. About half of these patients have sclerotic bones. (This is the only type of rickets and osteomalacia without parathyroid activity with this characteristic.) The skull is often dolichocephalic and craniosynostosis of the sutures, particularly the sagittal suture, is common. Frontal bossing may be present, and the condition is frequently mistaken for a form of chondrodysplasia or rhizomelic dwarfism. Near puberty, accessory ossicles are noted and are particularly common in the wrist. These are characteristic of the disease when found in

the radio-ulna-carpal space. Stress remodeling may be manifested by bony overgrowths, and ossification of periarticular tendinous and capsular insertions is noted. When vertebral end plates are affected, ankylosing spondylitis or fluorosis may be simulated. Sacroiliac fusion has been observed. Hypophosphatemia is constant, and its effect on bone remodeling and turnover rates may, along with stress, account for growth retardation and deformities. The severity varies with the individual. The activity of the disease frequently subsides when epiphyseal closure is complete, but recurrence in adults has been noted. If treated early, bone pain and deformities can be slowed. Although less successful, some progress in abating longitudinal growth disturbances has been reported.

Certain diseases are manifested by an increased need for vitamin D and therefore appear refractory to treatment with vitamin D. This has been observed in patients undergoing long-term anticonvulsant therapy and in congenital vitamin D-dependent rickets.

Epileptic children undergoing anticonvulsant therapy frequently have significant hypocalcemia and elevated serum levels of alkaline phosphatase. Some develop frank rickets and osteomalacia. The disease appears to be related to dose and length of therapy (Fig. 10-57). Phenobarbitone, Pheneturide, and primidone have been implicated. Barbiturates may induce synthesis of microsomal hepatic enzymes, which speed or alter metabolism of vitamin D within the liver.

Vitamin D-dependent rickets is a form of rickets in which no real vitamin D deficiency exists. It can be cured by administration of inordinately large doses of vitamin D. The entity is uncommon and most likely transmitted as a recessive trait. It occurs as a result of deficiency of 25-hydroxycholecalciferol hydroxylase. It is the most severe and deforming rickets known; significantly, this form of rickets is completely curable if recognized and treated. Bone age may be severely retarded and muscular weakness marked. Walking is noticeably delayed. Concomitant bone deformities are similar to those of other severe rachitic diseases.

Hypophophatasia is a hereditary abnormality characterized by retardation and diminished concentration of alkaline phosphatase within the body. Osteoid is poorly formed and poorly ossified. The abnormality may be a form of osteomalacia or rickets. Ossification defects are similar, with an overabundance of uncalcified osteoid. The disease varies in severity and onset. The diagnosis may be difficult in a given instance. The disease may resemble rickets, enchondromatosis, or metaphyseal dysplasia. In older age-groups, a characteristic central diaphyseal defect is seen and phosphorlyethanolamine may be found in the urine. Nephrocalcinosis and deposition of calcium pyrophosphate crystal also occur.

Summary of Common Findings in Rachitic and Malacic Disease

Dietary and malabsorptive deficiency states
  Rickets and osteomalacia (prevalent)
  Looser's lines (common)
  Secondary hyperparathyroidism (common) with subperiosteal resorption; thin cortices
  Brown tumors (uncommon)
Familial hypophosphatemia vitamin D-refractory rickets and osteomalacia
  Sclerotic bones (present in 50% of the cases)
  Thick cortices
  Accessory ossicles
  Looser's lines (rare)
  Craniosynostosis of sagittal suture (common)
  Rickets (more prevalent in lower extremities)
  Ossification of tendinous attachments
  X-linked dominant transmission
  Essentially nonexistent in the black race

Renal failure (glomerular failure and hyperphosphatemia)
  Rickets and osteomalacia (early)
  Patchy sclerosis, "rugger-jersy" spine (late)
  Soft-tissue calcification (common)
  Slipped epiphysis (common; late)
Vitamin D-dependent rickets
  Similar to deficiency rickets (but frequently more severe and deforming)
  Fractures (common)
  Severe growth retardation
  Curable with large doses of vitamin D
Rickets associated with hepatic disease or infantile biliary atresia
  Clubbing of the fingers (may be associated)
Rickets related to long-term anticonvulsant therapy
  High serum levels of alkaline phosphatase
  D-glutaric acid in urine
Hypophosphatasia
  Manifested by rickets in newborns
  Abnormally low levels of alkaline phosphatase
  Phosphorylethanolamine in urine
  Characteristic mid-metaphyseal ossification defect
  Craniosynostosis (common)
  Premature loss of deciduous teeth
  Lack of osteoid mineralization of cranial vault and skull base

---

OSTEOPOROSIS

Osteoporosis, as noted earlier, results primarily from loss of bone mass. Bone formation and resorption are dynamic processes occurring continually throughout life. At different ages, and in certain diseases, the rate of these ongoing processes (remodeling rate) changes. If individual processes occur proportionally, the quantity of bone or bone mass remains constant and only the structural aspects and strength of existing bone is altered. When resorption proceeds at a relatively greater rate than production osteoporosis results. This happens normally, beginning at ages 35 to 40 depending on race or sex and, to some extent, heredity. In some congenital forms of osteoporosis, actual formation of bone (and probably bone precursors) is diminished. Aside from some local transient forms of osteoporosis that have not become well established, complete reversal or healing is not possible with presently available modes of therapy.

The number and thickness of bone trabeculae are decreased as resorption takes place. The trabeculae along lines of stress tend to be preserved and may be accentuated as surrounding trabeculae are resorbed (Fig. 10-49). In generalized forms of osteoporosis, resorption takes place along all bone surfaces. Bone turnover rates for cortical bone are less than that of cancellated bone. The surface area of cancellated bone is reported to be 10 times that of cortical bone. These combined effects make osteoporosis more pronounced and therefore more easily detected in areas where cancellated bone predominates. This type of bone is found in the femurs, tibias, humeri, and vertebral bodies, and it is most prevalent in the subchondral and juxta-articular locations. Fractures often involve these areas when they have become structurally weakened by osteoporosis. The vertebral bodies of the spine frequently are radiographically diminished in density with accentuated end plates. Compression fractures are manifested by an overall loss of vertebral body height or concavity of vertebral end plates due to subchondral fractures. Symptoms may be present without initial radiographic evidence of compression and may precede gradual collapse by as much as 2 months. The complex of delayed symptoms of compression fractures is known as Kümmell's disease. Cortical bone is gradually thinned due to resorption along both endosteal and periosteal surfaces.

Forms of osteoporosis associated with increased remodeling rates result in bone which is usually structurally superior to osteoporotic bone associated with decreased remodeling rates, in which fractures are more common. Such bone tends to be older and more brittle. When fractures do occur, healing is much faster when the remodeling rate is increased. Forms of osteoporosis with a decreased rate of bone remodeling include Cushing's disease, osteogenesis imperfecta, congenital neuromusculature wasting, and gonadal dysgenesis. Forms with an increased remodeling rate include local hyperemia, thyrotoxicosis, and immobilization.

Differential Diagnosis

Osteogenesis imperfecta is an inherited form of generalized osteoporosis, with autosomal dominant transmission. The trabecular pattern is not apparent, and the bones appear homogeneously clear with an exquisitely thin cortex. Two types, with variable severity, have been described, the congenital and tarda form. The basic abnormality is defec-

Disease Entities

Congenital diseases
  Osteogenesis imperfecta
  Gonadal dysgenesis
  Trisomy 18
  Progeria
  Ehlers-Danlos syndrome
  Homocystinuria
  Neuromuscular diseases
    Werdnig-Hoffman disease
    Muscular dystrophy
    Myotonia congenita and myotonia dystrophica
    Arthrogryposis
    Acquired paralysis
  Hypophosphatasia
  Achondrogenesis
Endocrine related disease states
  Hyperthyroidism
  Primary hyperparathyroidism
  Cushing's syndrome (iatrogenic, adrenocortical hyperplasia, adrenal carcinoma)
  Diabetes mellitus
  Hypogonadism
  Addison's disease
Acquired nonendocrine disease
  Dietary
    Protein deprivation or catabolic states starvation, malabsorption, regional enteritis)
    Vitamin C deficiency
  Immobilization
Acute Sudeck's atrophy
Idiopathic juvenile osteoporosis

tive formation of collagen, and as a result multiple systems are involved. The remodeling rate of bone is markedly reduced, which makes the bones highly susceptible to stress and to frequent fractures. Fractures are the hallmark of this disease. They appear either at birth or later in life, depending upon the form of the disease. Severe deformities may be present at birth as a result of multiple intrauterine fractures (Fig. 10-58). In the tarda form the long bones are frequently thin, gracile, overtubulated and have a tendency to fracture and to heal with an inordinate amount of callus (Fig. 10-59). Shortening of the limbs is frequent and felt to be due to previous or repeated fractures. Osteogenesis imperfecta is the only form of osteoporosis associated with bowing of bones. The skull also

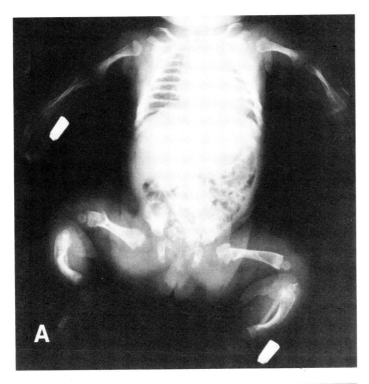

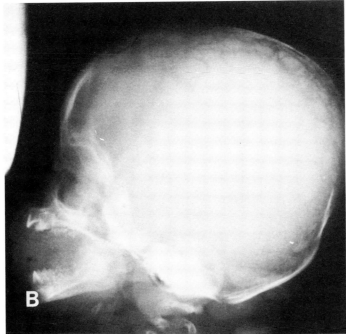

Fig. 10-58. Osteogenesis imperfecta in a newborn. *(A)* Marked deformities involve all the extremities. The bones are foreshortened and curved due to previous multiple fractures. Recent fractures are noted within the right distal and left proximal femurs. *(B)* Irregular bone formation is manifested by multiple islands of bone (wormian bones).

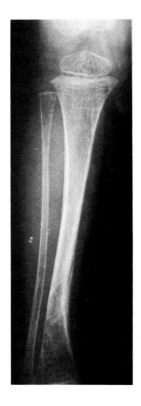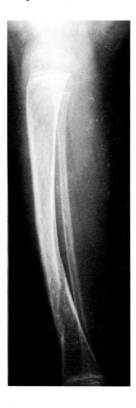

Fig. 10-59. Osteogenesis imperfecta tarda. The tibia and fibula in this patient are markedly osteopenic. The trabecular pattern is completely gone and the surrounding cortex is well-defined but thin. The configuration of the bones is slightly distorted due to previous multiple fractures. A large spiral fracture through the lower third of the tibia is present, with evidence of healing.

has a characteristic appearance. In the severe congenital form, almost no calvarial ossification is noted and only small islands of bone within unossified connective tissue cover the brain. In older patients, the calvarium is markedly thin and dolichocephalic, with numerous wormian bones, excessively aerated sinuses, and basilar impression (Fig. 10-58B). Anomalies of the teeth are also common. Other main features of the disease are deafness secondary to stapedial or cochlear abnormalities and blue sclera due to thin, transparent occular tissue. Osteogenic manifestations of the disease subside with age but the bones are never normal.

Trisomy 18 is a condition associated with 47 chromosomes, an extra chromosome 18. All affected infants are of low birth weight. Increased maternal age and polyhydramnios are common. Females are reported to be affected more frequently than males, in a ratio of about 3 to 1. Multiple skeletal abnormalities are noted, and muscular and soft-tissue wasting account for marked hypotonia, which may contribute to osteopenia (Fig. 10-60). Cardiac anomalies are common, particularly ventricular septal defects, which occur in 89 per cent of cases of Trisomy 18,

and patent ductus arteriosus, which occurs in 63 per cent (63%). Clinical diagnosis is usually made without difficulty. Only one of ten individuals survive the 1st year of life.

In gonadal dysgenesis, the gonads never develop and fetal castration syndrome is present. Lymphedema of the ankles and feet may be present in infancy (Fig. 10-61), and webbing of the neck is seen in approximately 30 per cent of these individuals. Abnormal skeletal growth is present, with diminished stature. Osteopenia is mild in juvenile patients, reflecting hormonal and maturation imbalance. Gonadal dysgenesis may not be clinically or radiographically apparent during the neonatal period, except for the presence of pedal and palmar edema. Chromosomal confirmation is necessary.

Progeria occurs spontaneously and is characterized by premature aging and growth disturbances resulting in symmetrical dwarfism. Affected individuals are essentially normal at birth, other than a possibly diminished size. The disease becomes clinically apparent between 24 and 30 months of age. Complete alopecia, a hypoplastic mandible, and a beaked nose give the appearance of advanced age. The musculature, skin, and subcutaneous tissues are atrophied. Early death

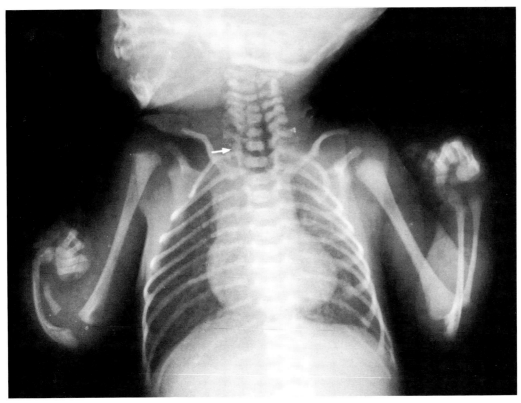

Fig. 10-60. Trisomy 18. Multiple anomalies are noted on this chest radiograph. The bones are thin and osteopenic. Radial hypoplasia and deformed phalanges are present. Other anomalies present include esophageal atresia *(arrow),* with no tracheoesophageal fistula, and cardiomegaly.

is common due to myocardial or cerebral infarction as a result of advanced and accelerated atherosclerosis (Fig. 10-62). Radiographically, muscle and soft-tissue loss are apparent. Skeletal osteopenia is present and fractures common. Progressive osteolysis of the ribs, clavicles, and fingertips may be noted. Delayed closure of the cranial sutures is common, as are calvarial wormian bones (Fig. 10-62C). Skeletal osteopenia is likely, due to a combination of abnormal bone formation and muscular atrophy with loss of stress.

The Ehlers-Danlos syndrome is a hereditary disease transmitted by an autosomal dominant trait. It is characterized by derangement of collagen, manifested by abnormal and structurally weak connective tissues. Affected patients demonstrate inordinate laxity of soft tissues which are susceptible to trauma. The disease may be associated with recurrent articular dislocations and hyperextensibility of synovial joints. Gastrointestinal diverticulosis and spontaneous rupture of the bowel may be observed in young patients

due to poor intestinal wall integrity. Other associated abnormal entities include aortic aneurysms and/or aortic rupture, soft-tissue nodules, spondylolisthesis, spontaneous pneumothorax or pneumomediastinum, and acro-osteolysis. Joint subluxations may be associated with secondary degenerative osteoarthritis. Osteopenia can result from abnormal collagen substrate and lack of normal musculotendinous stress.

Arthrogryposis multiplex congenita represents a group of abnormalities characterized by fibrosis of structures in and around joints. Many, but not all, are associated with abnormal muscular development, and the bones may be osteopenic as a result of fixation and disuse or absence of stress when primary musculature development is impaired.

The neonatal presentation of hypophosphatasia is characterized frequently by a severely ossified skeleton, with shortened and deformed extremities. Early death is the rule (Fig. 10-66A).

Another congenital disease associated with

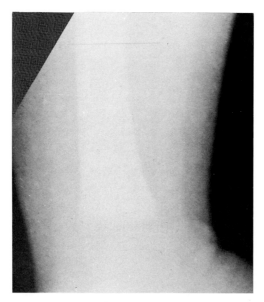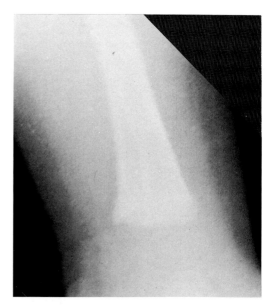

Fig. 10-61. Gonadal agenesis. Bilateral pedal edema is present. This infant also demonstrated webbing of the neck.

a marked decrease in mineralization and early death is achondrogenesis. It is characterized by markedly shortened limbs and affected patients have been mistaken for achondroplastic dwarfs. However, achondrogenesis produces almost complete hypoplasia of bone.

Osteoporosis may be associated with a number of neuromuscular disorders, as well as immobilization of a portion of the skeleton. Such forms of osteoporosis have a high rate of bone remodeling. Simple casting, with or without a fracture, may result in local demineralization. Children immobilized by body casting or secondary to burns are particularly susceptible. In general, younger patients are affected to a greater degree. If extremities are involved, demineralization begins at the ends of the bone and may eventually involve the entire bone, as in poliomyelitis. The spine is rarely affected. Carpal or tarsal bones frequently show early changes. A patchy, rapid osteoporosis is present in 50 per cent of cases and may resemble reflex sympathetic dystrophy. Wide transverse bands of radiolucency may be noted in the metaphyses. Some cortical subperiosteal resorption and endosteal scalloping may be observed as the disease progresses. A sustained hypercalcemia is usually not present, although initially it may be sig-

nificant. Clinical symptoms of hypercalcemia are rare. However, renal calculi may cause significant morbidity, particularly in patients who are paraplegic or who suffer from bulbar poliomyelitis. Stasis and high urinary pH contribute to this problem.

Steroid-induced forms of osteoporosis are similar regardless of the type or origin of the glucocorticoid responsible for the abnormality. There is a temporal variance of bone response to steroids. Initially increased numbers of osteoclasts are seen and bone loss is very rapid. Over a period of time, this rate decreases and a relative state of equilibrium is subsequently reached. The overall effect is a diminished remodeling rate with a variability of actual rate of bone loss.

Cushing's syndrome is an excellent model for steroid-induced osteoporosis. This condition is produced by either adrenal hyperplasia, carcinoma of the adrenal gland, or exogenous steroid therapy. Poor protein assimilation for the production of pre-osseous matrix may, in part, be responsible for diminished remodeling rates. As in other forms of osteoporosis with diminished remodeling rates, fractures are common. These may be apparent in the anterior ribs, pubic and ischial rami, and vertebral bodies. Aseptic necrosis of the femoral and humeral heads is common. The dental lamina dura may be

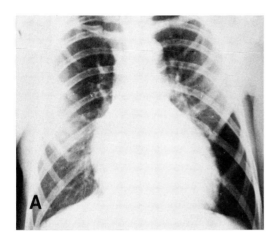

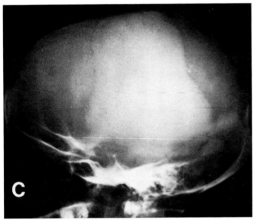

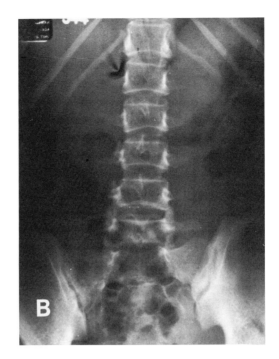

Fig. 10-62. Progeria. *(A)* The ribs are thin and the heart enlarged. *(B)* The vertebral bodies are osteoporotic with compression deformities. *(C)* The calvarium is poorly mineralized, and a large defect is noted posteriorly.

lost. A patchy, almost destructive mottling of the calvarium is often present, which is not common in any other form of osteoporosis but may be seen in hyperparathyroidism. The sella turcica may be abnormally small. Decreased bone production may be reflected by abnormally thin epiphyseal plates. Once the excess steroid stimulus is removed, accelerated growth occurs that slows to normal as the skeleton approaches the size which corresponds to the age of the patient. In general, steroid-induced osteoporosis is the most reversible type, other than mild transient regional osteoporosis.

Dietary osteoporosis may result from inadequate intake of calcium, protein, or vitamin C. Malabsorption processes may result in osteoporosis as well as osteomalacia. The poorly understood protein catabolic state seen in regional enteritis may, in part, account for the diminutive stature and failure to thrive seen in many younger patients with the disease. In starvation and protein depri-

vation states, osteoporosis is noted, but loss of muscle mass and disuse may be contributory factors.

Scurvy results from an inadequate intake of vitamin C, which plays a role in many metabolic systems and is, in part, responsible for the hydroxylation of proline, an amino acid integrally associated with the production of collagen and intracellular cement. Deficiency of vitamin C results in abnormalities of the pre-osseous matrix, connective tissue, capillary integrity, and cartilage. The pre-osseous matrix of bone (osteoid) is poorly formed, with resultant poor ossification.

Scurvy is distinctly rare before 3 months of age and is most frequently seen between 6 and 18 months. It is uncommon after the age of 2 years. When seen in adults, bone changes are not obvious, and capillary fragility and bleeding are the dominant features.

Normally, the provisional zone of calcification at the end of a long bone receives deposits of calcium salts. With growth and

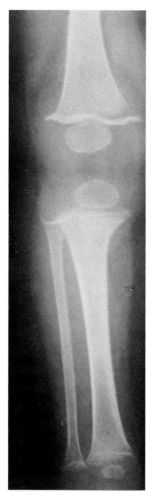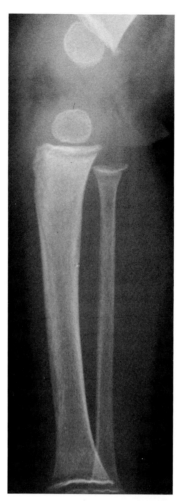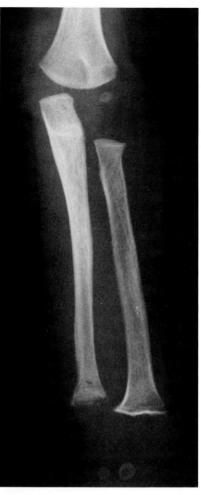

Fig. 10-63. Scurvy. Minimal cupping is encountered in the metaphysis of the bones. The zone of provisional calcification is thick, dense, and irregular, and extends into the soft tissues (Pelken's spur). Immediately proximal is an area of increased radiolucency (Trummerfeld zone). The epiphysis shows similar findings. The bones are demineralized and surrounded by a thin but dense cortex (Wimberger's sign).

maturity, vascularized connective tissue invades this portion of the metaphysis and removes these salts from the cartilaginous matrix in preparation for laying down osteoid matrix. In scurvy, cartilaginous growth in this area slows, but preliminary calcification continues. The invading vascularized connective tissue is defective, and there is failure to remove calcium salts. Radiographically this area presents as a dense, white band (Fig. 10-63). This radiodense zone, as it surrounds the epiphyses and small bones, is referred to as Wimberger's sign. Lateral extension of the band may be manifested by small spurs projecting laterally from the end of long bones.

This, coupled with possible early healing of small fractures and hemorrhage, is called Pelken's spur.

Beneath this dense zone is a wide, radiolucent, metaphyseal band which is sometimes called the Trummerfeld zone. Osteoblasts fail to develop in this zone and calcification is therefore replaced by fibrous tissue. Hemorrhage usually begins here and then appears beneath the periosteum. Bone infractions may occur in this zone, and also the "corner" sign may be manifested.

Reflex sympathetic dystrophy and Sudeck's atrophy represent special forms of regional osteoporosis. The former is characterized by severe local pain at the site of previous trauma, with or without fracture. The pain is often exaggerated, and at times no pertinent history is present. Sudeck's atrophy is used to describe the associated osteoporotic demineralization of bone and is present in 30 to 50 per cent of cases. If the disease is untreated and allowed to persist, the joints may become rigid and ankylosed. Pain becomes intractable.

Variants of Sudeck's atrophy seen in adults may be associated with degenerative cervical spine disease, prolonged bed rest, and coronary heart disease. These collectively constitute the shoulder-hand syndrome. A combination of hyperemia, immobilization, edema, and stasis, may be of etiologic significance. Osteoporosis, when present, is similar to that of sympathetic dystrophy.

A rare but often self-limited form of osteoporosis affecting children between 8 to 10 years of age is idiopathic juvenile osteoporosis. The diffusely demineralized skeleton is susceptible to fractures, and pain is frequent. Impaired intestinal absorption of calcium is thought to be the cause. The disease usually regresses without treatment.

Homocystinuria is an error in metabolism caused by a deficiency of cystathionine synthatase. It is characterized by abnormal accumulation of homocystine and homocysteine in the body, and by homocystinuria. The importance of a diagnosis lies in differentiating the disease from Marfan's syndrome, which is genetically unrelated, and in the institution of proper therapy to possibly reduce venous and arterial thrombosis commonly associated with this entity. Although some clinical manifestations of Marfan's syndrome and homocystinuria may be similar, osteoporosis occurs only in homocystinuria. The vertebral bodies often show end plate compression and are biconcave, as in other forms of osteoporosis. The vertebral bodies in Marfan's syndrome are typically tall and show posterior scalloping. Both are associated with high, arched palates, ocular lens dislocations, genu valgum, and pectoral deformities of the chest. Arachnodactyly and scoliosis may be seen in either abnormality, but are more common in Marfan's syndrome. Widening of the epiphyses of long bones is more common in homocystinuria. Vascular thromboses are seen in patients with homocystinuria, and

aortic aneurysms typical of cystic necrosis frequently complicate Marfan's syndrome. Features of the two diseases may vary but radiographic, clinical, and laboratory analysis are usually sufficient for differentiation.

Summary of Findings in Diseases Associated With Osteoporosis

Osteogenesis imperfecta
  Calvarial demineralization with multiple wormian bones
  Multiple fractures with inordinate callus production
  Blue sclera and postpuberal deafness
  Defective dentition
  Overtubulation of bones
Steriod excess
  Severe mottling of the calvarium
  Spontaneous anterior rib fractures
  Subchondral and juxta-articular fractures
  Biconcave vertebra, end plate compression
Scurvy
  Osteopenia
  Widened sclerotic zones of provisional calcification
  Metaphyseal radioluceny (late)
  Subperiosteal hemorrhage
  "Corner" sign
  Lateral distal spurring of the provisional zone of calcification
  Fractures of the provisional zone of calcification
  Fractures of the metaphyseal radiolucent zone
Reflex sympathetic dystrophy and Sudeck's atrophy
  Patchy rapid osteoporosis
  Localized pain
  History of local trauma
  Inordinate causalgia
  Tropic skin changes and edema
Primary hyperparathyroidism
  Osteitis fibrosa cystica
  Osteoclastomas (brown tumors)
  Subperiosteal resorption
  Pyrophosphate crystal deposition
Homocystinuria
  Marfan-like changes
  Osteoporosis (uncommon in Marfan's syndrome)
  Arterial and venous vascular thromboses (common)
  Thoracic aortic aneurysm (uncommon)

METAPHYSEAL ABNORMALITIES

The metaphysis is that part of bone where growing cartilage is transformed into bone and where the primary spongiosa and medullary cavity is formed. The blood supply to the metaphysis arises from nutrient arteries. In infancy, these vessels cross the epiphyseal

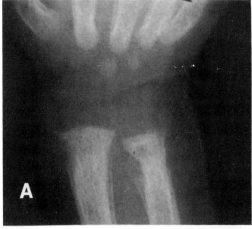

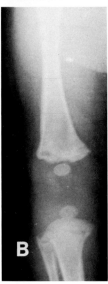 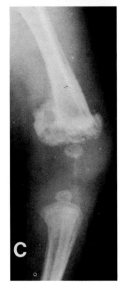

Fig. 10-64. Congenital syphilis. *(A)* The zone of provisional calcification is no longer apparent. The margin is irregular and dentate. A dense, unilaminar periosteal reaction is noted in all the bones. *(B, C)* Extensive changes are present in this case. The entire metaphyseal regions are irregular. Epiphyseal-metaphyseal separation is present on the left, associated with a large subperiosteal hematoma.

plate to mingle with the epiphysis. However, by the 8th month they no longer traverse the plate but perfuse the metaphysis as ascending terminal arteries.

The zone of primary spongiosa in the metaphysis is the area where new bone is formed by the deposition of osteoid onto cartilage cores. This then ossifies to become the zone of provisional calcification. The zone of secondary spongiosa is that region of the metaphysis where the primary trabeculations are transformed into the mature trabeculae of the medullary cavity. The zone of provisional calcification in early infancy is only manifested by a thin radiopaque line at the distal end of the metaphysis. This zone is most thick and compact between the 1st and 3rd years of life.

There are a number of changes that result when this process is altered. These rarely occur singly and are usually associated with a combination of abnormalities that occur in the bone or the surrounding tissues.

Categories of Metaphyseal Abnormalities

Splayed and frayed metaphysis
Sclerotic and radiolucent bands
Breaks and fragmentations
Erosions and dissolutions
Overtubulation and undertubulation
Cupped metaphyses

SPLAYED AND FRAYED METAPHYSIS

Splaying refers to the formation of a mild concave deformity at the margin of the metaphysis. This deformity is due to a growth disturbance in the metaphysis or to impaction of the epiphysis into the metaphysis when the surrounding bone is softened. Fraying is also the result of altered bone development. The zone of provisional calcification becomes irregular. The border loses its sharp margin, becomes less radiopaque, and assumes a spiculated or serrated appearance. The latter may be fine or coarse and in severe cases is grossly deformed.

Disease Entities

Newborns
    Infection
        Syphilis
        Rubella
        Cytomegalic inclusion disease
        Viral disease
    Metaphyseal chondrodysplasia (Jansen's disease)
    Metabolic diseases
        Rickets in the premature infant
        Scurvy in the premature infant
        Hypophosphatasia
Infants and Children
    Rickets
    Scurvy
    Hypophosphatasia
    Metaphyseal chondrodysplasia
        Cartilage-hair hypoplasia
        Schwachman's syndrome
        Schmidt type
    Spondylometaphyseal dysplasia (Kozslowski type)

Differential Diagnosis

Skeletal involvement in congenital syphilis is common. The abnormalities range from simple metaphyseal trophic bands of radiolucency to metaphyseal destruction and fracture. The frayed metaphyseal border, which presents as sawtooth serrations, is characteristic of congenital syphilis (Fig. 10-64). These changes may represent a generalized disturbance of enchondral bone growth due to a vascular or immunologic reaction. Inflammatory changes within the bone have also been confirmed. Most of the bone alterations are present at birth, although the most florid changes are encountered at 3 weeks of age. Occasionally a delayed onset results at 2 months postpartum due to late transmission of the organism. All of the lesions heal by about 6 months regardless of treatment. Ninety per cent of newborns with congenital

syphilis manifesting skeletal involvement will also have a unilaminar or multilaminar periosteal reaction (Fig. 10-64). This is an important finding; when associated with the metaphyseal changes, it is disgnostic.

Metaphyseal fraying is a significant radiographic feature in the congenital rubella syndrome. Although all the bones may be involved, the changes are most evident in the knees. The zone of provisional calcification is replaced by an irregular dentate margin. In addition to metaphyseal fraying, some cases manifest alternating bands of radiolucency that are perpendicular to the epiphysis (Fig. 10-65). Nonspecific, horizontal radiolucent stress lines are also apparent. The changes encountered in the metaphysis in many respects are not unlike congenital syphilis or the neonatal form of hypophosphatasia. However, rubella rarely, if ever, presents with a periosteal reaction, and most of the bone changes regress spontaneously within 4 to 8 weeks. In some cases the changes have been known to persist for several months, and residual metaphyseal sclerotic bands have remained for years. Congenital syphilis and congenital rubella both present with hepatosplenomegaly, rash, and anemia. However, the ocular funduscopic changes, the presence of cataracts and cardiac lesions (e.g., patent ductus arteriosus, pulmonary stenosis), laboratory data, and a maternal history of a rubella infection in the first or second trimester suggest the diagnosis.

Cytomegalic inclusion disease should be considered when metaphyseal fraying occurs, since occasional reports of this disease have shown metaphyseal alterations identical to those of rubella. Other viruses have been implicated in metaphyseal fraying and longitudinal streaking.

Splaying and fraying of the metaphysis in a rachitic fashion is also seen in hypophosphatasia. This is a hereditary disease transmitted by an autosomal recessive trait and is manifested by an inability of osteoblasts to elaborate alkaline phosphatase. The result is defective bone mineralization. The serum calcium and phosphorous are usually normal, although a transient, and occasionally persistent, elevation of serum calcium level occurs. The disease presents in various forms. The neonatal form is usually the severest, and stillbirth or early death is the rule. The skeleton is poorly ossified, and extreme shortening with multiple prenatal fractures and bowing

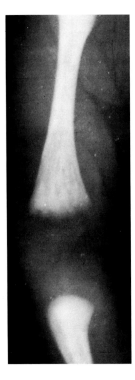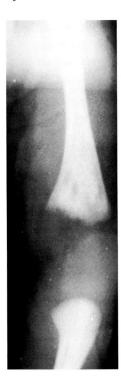

Fig. 10-65. Congenital rubella. The changes in these bones are characteristic. The zone of provisional calcification is absent and is replaced by areas of uncalcified osteoid. The metaphysis is irregular and dentate. Retained cartilage is also present within the distal portions of the bone, resulting in linear radiolucent areas extending into the shaft.

of the extremities is present (Fig. 10-66A). The metaphyses are markedly frayed and cupped, with streak-like bands of irregular ossification alternating with areas of unossified osteoid. The skull and entire skeleton are soft.

The infantile presentation becomes evident during the 1st 6 months of life. Constitutional signs, such as failure to thrive, vomiting, and convulsions, are present. Radiographically, the metaphyses become osteopenic and rarefied. As the disease progresses, the zone of provisional calcification diminishes, and the margins of the metaphyses become cupped and frayed. Again, the bones are prone to fracture. Death may occur in the latter part of the 1st year of life. If the child survives, the lesions slowly heal, leaving residual changes or a unossified notch in the femoral metaphysis (Fig. 10-66C, 10-66D). Similar notching may be seen in the proximal tibial and proximal humeral metaphyses. Fractures are common. The space between the cranial sutures is wide, but as the child grows there may be premature fusion with crainostenosis and signs of increased intracranial pressure. Shortness of stature and rachitic deformities develop.

The mildest form of the disease presents in late childhood or in young adults. These patients usually have a diminutive stature with genu valgum. Kyphoscoliosis is common and Looser's lines may be noted. Fractures are seen with minimal trauma.

Recognizing the neonatal form of hypophosphatasia should not be difficult. It must be distinguished from osteogenesis imperfecta and other severe forms of short-limbed dwarfism. Distinguishing the infantile form of hypophosphatasia from vitamin D-deficiency or vitamin D-refractory rickets may be more difficult. However, low serum levels of alkaline phosphatase, increased urinary phosphorylethanolamine, and a positive family history are diagnostic of hypophosphatasia.

Metaphyseal chondrodysplasia may also result in frayed and splayed metaphyses. Several forms of metaphyseal chondrodysplasia with varying degrees of severity are recognized.

Metaphyseal dysplasia occurs in two main forms, a severe form (Jansen type) and a moderate form (Schmidt type). In the Jansen type, the metaphyses show osteopenia, severe cupping, and irregularity. Metaphyseal dysplasia becomes more severe as the infant grows older.

The Schmid type is far more common (Fig. 10-67). It begins around the 2nd year of life and is manifested by small stature, lumbar lordosis, and bowing of the lower extremities. The metaphyses are ragged and flared. Metaphyseal fraying and shortened bones resemble that of hypophasphatemic rickets (familial rickets or vitamin D-refractory rickets). The skull is essentially normal. An interesting feature is the presence of fine spurs of bone that extend the whole width of the metaphysis into the widened epiphyseal cartilage. Coxa vara also develops. The absence of other osseous features of osteomalacia helps to differentiate Schmid type of metaphyseal chondro-dysplasia from the other forms of rickets. Another form of metaphyseal dysplasia in which only a few joints are affected was described by Kozlowski (Fig. 10-68).

Cartilage-hair hypoplasia is a type of metaphyseal chondrodysplasia characterized by shortness of limbs and fine sparse hair. The bone changes are mainly in the ribs, hip, and knees. Coxa vara and changes simulating Perthe's disease have been noted. The disease is common among the Amish population.

Pancreatic insufficiency has been reported in patients, with neutropenia and irregular and sclerotic changes which affect all of the metaphyses, particularly the upper end of the femur.

Spondylometaphyseal dysplasia described by Kozlowski is a form of dwarfism in which patients have a shortened trunk; it is usually manifested after the 2nd year of life. Waddling gaint is noted in early childhood, with restricted joint mobility. Scoliosis and kyphosis are frequent in adolescence. Radiographically, generalized platyspondylisis is noted (Fig. 10-69). The major feature is irregular metaphyseal ossification, most marked in the proximal femurs where coxa vara is common. The epiphyses may be deformed.

Splaying and fraying of the metaphyses in premature infants may be the result of copper deficiency, although a combination of deficiencies is probably present. Menke's syndrome (the kinky hair syndrome), a degenerative disease of the nervous system related to abnormal copper metabolism, demonstrates an increase in osseous fragility and metaphyseal fractures that may mimic purposeful trauma. It is transmitted by an X-linked recessive trait and is therefore found predominantly in males. The hair is coarse and kinky, as well as sparse. Systemic arteries are tortuous and may show amputation. The bones are osteoporotic. In addition, the metaphyses show symmetrical spurring at the lateral margins of the distal femoral metaphyses. The changes resolve by the end of the 1st year of life.

Phenylketonuria may produce lateral beaking of the distal femoral metaphyses, similar to the findings of Menke's syndrome. This may be a normal variation in young infants and has also been reported in infants with homocystinuria.

Classically, rickets is known to produce metaphyseal ends which are splayed and frayed. Rickets refers to a complex of disorders of deposition of calcium hydroxyapatite crystal in osteoid, which results in osteomalacia and a loss of the zone of provisional calcification (Fig. 10-54). Rickets can result from the lack of vitamin D in the diet (nutritional rickets). In such cases the skeletal manifestations are usually not seen in infants under 6 months if they have received an adequate intrauterine vitamin supply. Exceptions include premature infants and infants whose growth requirements exceed what is provided by parenteral feedings.

Rachitic changes also result from renal failure where tubular function is destroyed or inadequate. Renal osteodystrophy is manifested by a combination of rachitic changes and changes of hyperparathyroidism, depending upon the etiology and the degree of glomerular insufficiency. In our experience, renal osteodystrophy is now more commonly encountered than nutritional rickets.

The radiographic changes in rickets are not difficult to detect when the changes are well advanced. Rarefaction and fraying of the margins of the metaphysis at the epiphyseal plates, with loss of the normal zone of provisional calcification, are the most prominent findings (Fig. 10-54A). The continually forming osteoid does not become crystalized, resulting in an increase in the width of the epiphyseal plate. The trabeculae in the metaphysis become coarse in appearance and

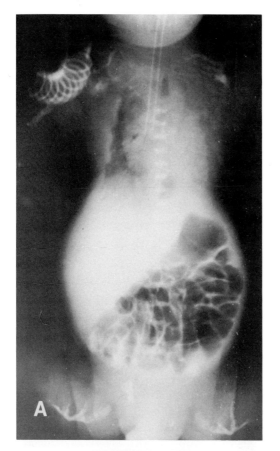

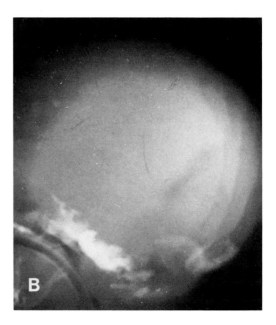

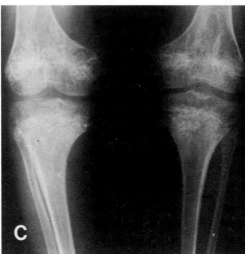

Fig. 10-66. Hypophosphatasia. (A) The entire skeleton is poorly ossified and the limbs are extremely short, distorted, and bowed. The distal ends are grossly irregular. (B) The cranial vault is devoid of any obvious bone. (C) Residual changes in a patient with hypophosphatasia demonstrate irregular ossification in the region of the metaphysis. (Continued on facing page.)

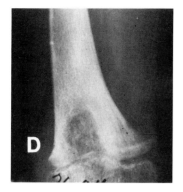
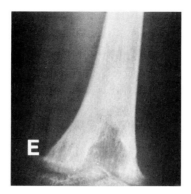
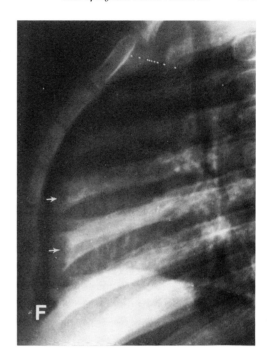

Fig. 10-66 (Continued). (D, E) In this young patient deep notches are are noted within the central portion of both femurs. (F) A lateral film of the ribs demonstrates a rachitic rosary. Note the frayed and cupped margins (arrows).

less distinct due to the incomplete saturation of the available sites of crystal deposition on osteoid. Cup-like, central depressions in the metaphyses are created by the epiphyses, compressing the softened metaphyses. This finding is more likely to be seen in active or weight-bearing infants. When treated with vitamin D, normal bone is produced with the reappearance of the zone of provisional calcification and a periosteal reaction (Fig. 10-54B).

In rickets complicated by diminished protein metabolism, as might be seen in combined nutritional deficiencies, not only is there insufficient mineral to deposit on the osteoid, but there is a diminished production of osteoid. The result is a combined of osteomalacic and osteoporotic bone, with greater rarefaction of bone than is seen with rickets alone. This is seen in neonates who have been on parenteral nutrition and who have been immobile becuase of pulmonary complications requiring long-term assisted ventilation or oxygenation.

Scurvy also results in splaying of the metaphysis and is the result of vitamin C deficiency. This disease is now uncommon in its classical form, although it is being seen with increasing frequency in nutritionally crippled, premature neonates on long-term parenteral nutrition (Fig. 10-70). More commonly, such infants have a combination of

nutritional deficiencies manifested by generalized osteopenia and a combination of malacic and porotic bone changes. Fraying is not *usually* a feature in these infants, despite other alterations of bone structure which suggest osteomalacia.

The basic bone pathology in scurvy is osteoporosis (see p. 425). The zone of provisional calcification becomes thin and brittle. Metaphyseal infractions occur, producing the characteristic Pelken's spurs. The epiphyses may become impacted, extending into the brittle metaphyses with resultant cupping. Defects in the cortex and spongiosa beneath the zone of provisional calcification may permit incomplete separation of the epiphyseal plate from the metaphyses, resulting in the "corner" sign. With healing, deep cupping may persist in the knee metaphyses and resemble residual changes of hypervitaminosis A. Improvement may continue, resulting in an almost normal metaphysis by adulthood.

SCLEROTIC AND RADIOLUCENT BANDS

Metaphyseal bands may be horizontal or vertical in direction, and radiolucent or sclerotic in appearance. The most commonly encountered metaphyseal band is the radiolucent, trophic line produced by enchondral bone growth arrest (Fig. 10-71). In general, bone growth in the region of the metaphysis is dependent upon a balance of osteoneogenesis and osteolysis. A slowing of enchondral bone formation at the zone of provisional calcification allows for excessive osteolysis, which results in rarefaction of the metaphysis. These metaphyseal bands are best seen in the long bones and are transverse and symmetrical. As growth resumes, calcifium is redeposited in the compact osteoid at the zone of calcification and migrates toward the diaphysis as a growth restitution line. The radiopaque, transverse lines that result are called post-arrest lines or the transverse lines of Park. The transverse radiopaque lines are produced by a resurgence of osteoblastic activity during the period of recovery. During the stage of growth arrest, osteoblasts form a thin, transverse, bony template under the zone of proliferating cartilage, and as a result of increased activity the zone becomes several times thicker than normal.

Disease Entities

Horizontal radiolucent bands
  Newborns
    Hyaline membrane disease
    Neonatal infection
    Meconium peritonitis
    Volvulus
  Infants
    Stress
    Leukemia
    Scurvy
Horizontal sclerotic bands
  Growth restitution lines (lines of Park)
  Chronic lead poisoning
  Hypervitaminosis D
  William's syndrome (idiopathic hypercalcemia)
  Irradiation (osteonecrosis)
  Atypical osteopetrosis
  Dialysis
Longitudinal sclerotic and radiolucent bands
  Rubella
  Cytomegalic inclusion disease
  Atypical syphilis
  Neonatal hypophosphatasia
  Other congenital viral infections
Irregular metaphyseal bands
  Dygvve-Melchior-Clausson syndrome
  Ollier's disease
  Parastremmatic dwarfism

Differential Diagnosis

Almost any form of stress results in radiolucent metaphyseal bands or stress lines in newborns (Fig. 10-71). The finding is therefore not distinctive. The transverse radiolucent metaphyseal band has been noted early during the course of hyaline membrane disease and in other diseases arising during the neonatal period. The radiolucent stress line may be the only manifestation in some cases of congenital syphylis or rubella. It is often overshadowed by other characteristic bone changes. A combination of radiolucent and sclerotic lines occurs in newborns with meconium peritonitis and probably represents some form of intrauterine growth arrest (see Fig. 2-45).

Irregular calcification and widening and distortion of the metaphyses are important features of the Dygvve-Melchior-Clausson syndrome and parastremmatic dwarfism. Other findings in the bones are more diagnostic.

In older infants, in addition to a host of infectious diseases, chronic debilitating diseases that are accompanied by recurrent exacerbations and remissions, such as cystic fibrosis, cause stress lines to appear.

The metaphyseal line accompanying leukemia is significant. It is a transverse and radiolucent, and characteristically it is thin and separated from the zone of provisional calcification by an area of normal bone, which distinguishes it from the usual stress line (Fig. 10-72). Areas of adjacent rarefaction may also be apparent (Fig. 10-73).

Sclerotic metaphyseal bands, aside from the transverse lines of Park, generally suggest an underlying pathologic process. Chronic lead intoxication is frequently manifested by the presence of a dense zone of bone that merges with the zone of provisional calcification (Fig. 10-74). The zone can vary in appearance and is best seen within the long bones. At times it may be thick or assume a wavy, undulating appearance or consist of multiple and parallel lines. The dense line does not reflect the amount of lead deposited but relates to an impeded rate of bone mineralization. Histologically, an excessive amount of ossifying, cartilaginous primary spongiosa is present. Since the zones of provisional calcification are normally dense and thick in the older child, it may be difficult to appreciate the abnormal findings. However,

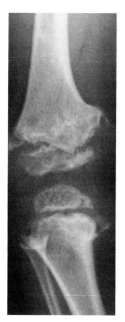
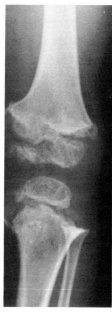

Fig. 10-67. Metaphyseal dysplasia (Schmidt type). The metaphyseal area is distinctly irregular and splayed. The zone of provisional calcification is poorly defined.

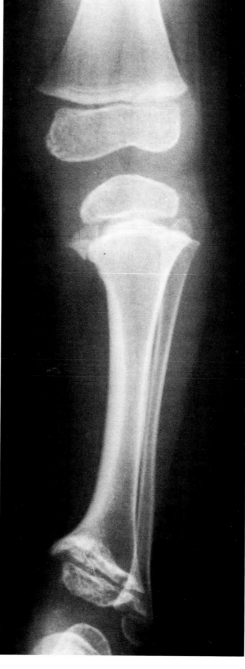

Fig. 10-68. Metaphyseal dysostosis (Kozlowski type). The distal tibial metaphysis in a young infant is splayed, irregular, and deformed. The zone of provisional calcification is somewhat sclerotic and thickened and distinctly irregular. A similar finding is noted along the medial aspect of the proximal tibial plateau. The distal femur is completely normal.

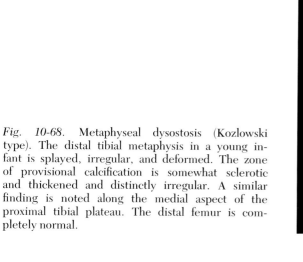

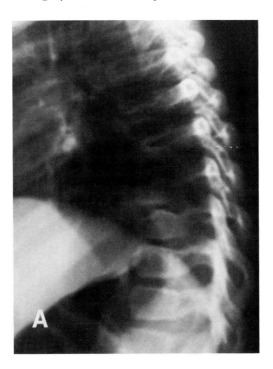

Fig. 10-69. Spondylometaphyseal dysplasia (Kozlowski type). *(A)* Spine. Evidence of platyspondylisis is noted in the thoracic spine. *(Continued on facing page.)*

certain bones (e.g., the ends of ribs, tips of the scapulas, fibulas) normally contain exceptionally thin zones of provisional calcification, and when these bones demonstrate sclerotic lines the probability of lead intoxication is high. Elevated serum levels of lead confirm the diagnosis in questionable cases.

Bismuth and phosphorus are other mineral intoxicants that produce similar alterations but are presently only of historical significance.

Chronic and excessive ingestion of vitamin D also thickens the zone of provisional calcification. Eventually, alternating bands of sclerosis and radiolucency may be seen running parallel to the margin of the metaphysis. Fortunately, hypervitaminosis D is only encountered infrequently. Similar bands of sclerosis are noted in idiopathic hypercalcemia, William's syndrome. In addition to sclerotic skeletal changes, metastatic calcifications in soft tissues, craniostenosis, stenosis of the supravalvular aortic and pulmonary artery, and undertubulation of the extremities are major findings in this syndrome.

Alternating bands of radiolucency and sclerosis orientated parallel to the epiphyseal plate can develop in infants on dialysis. Sclerotic, irregular metaphyseal bands following radiation can occur, in association with flaring and sometimes overtubulation.

Perpendicular bands of radiolucency or sclerosis are difficult to explain on a pathophysiologic basis. It is conceivable that alterations in the ascending terminal arteries result in a nonuniform blood flow that may affect the rates of growth and crystal deposition in the metaphysis. Such bands are mainly produced by rubella (Fig. 10-65), cytomegalic inclusion disease, syphilis, and neonatal hypophosphatasia. In rubella the vertical radiolucent stripes are thought to represent retained zones of cartilage that are not mineralized.

Irregular areas of radiolucency intermixed with bands and streaks of cartilage characterize Ollier's disease. This anomaly is also accompanied by bone widening. The abnormal areas are predominantly unilateral.

BREAKS AND FRAGMENTATIONS

Disease Entities

Newborn
    Trauma at birth
Infants and children
    Purposeful trauma
    Neuromuscular abnormalities
    Scurvy
Blount's disease

(Text continued on p. 441.)

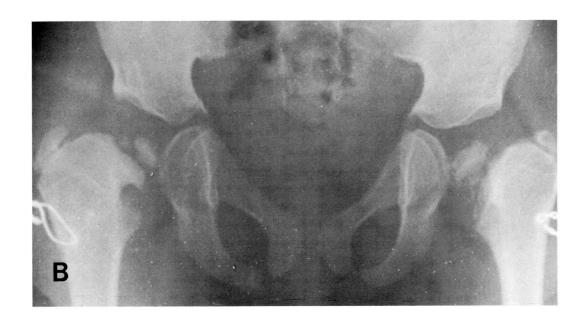

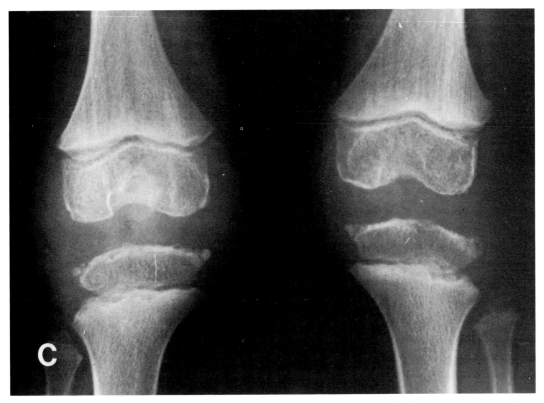

Fig. 10-69 (Continued). (B) Pelvis. Short, broad iliac bones and coxa vara deformity are present. The epiphyses are also small and irregular. (C) Knees. Ossification in the metaphysis is irregular, producing an overall mild deformity in the knee.

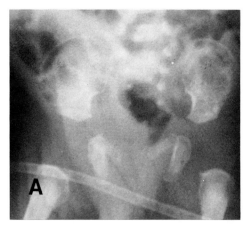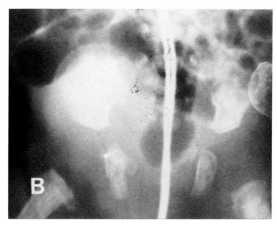

Fig. 10-70. A combination of rickets and scurvy. *(A)* This is the pelvis of a newborn maintained on parenteral feedings because of severe respiratory distress followed by necrotizing enterocolitis. Radiolucent metaphyseal lines and increased density in the zone of provisional calcification are apparent on the initial study. *(B)* One week later metaphyseal-epiphyseal fractures occurred through this area. The findings resemble those of scurvy.

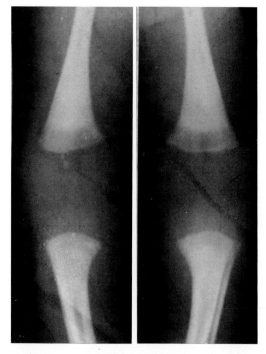

Fig. 10-71. Radiolucent stress line. A large, transverse radiolucency is located just proximal to the zone of provisional calcification in a newborn with toxoplasmosis. Similar findings can be seen in the congenital rubella syndrome and congenital syphilis.

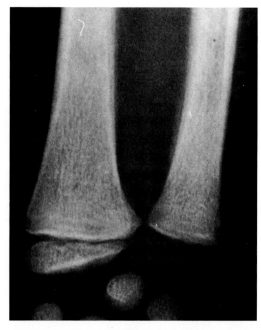

Fig. 10-72. Acute lymphatic leukemia. Note the thin, transverse, radiolucent line that is separated slightly from the zone of provisional calcification by normal bone. This is a characteristic appearance.

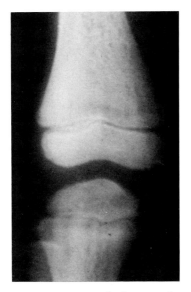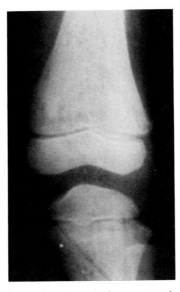

Fig. 10-73. Acute leukemia. The radiolucent line is well demonstrated. Multiple areas of rarefaction are also present throughout the metaphyses.

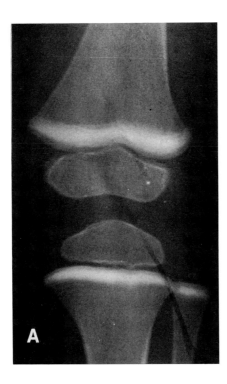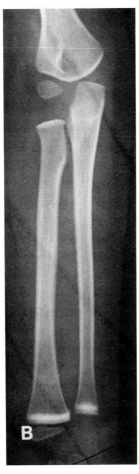

Fig. 10-74. Lead intoxication. (A) Dense, sclerotic, metaphyseal lines are present that merge with the zone of provisional calcification. (B) Within the distal radius and ulna multiple, dense lines are visualized that are separated slightly from each other by a radiolucent area. The proximal portion of the radius is also densely sclerotic.

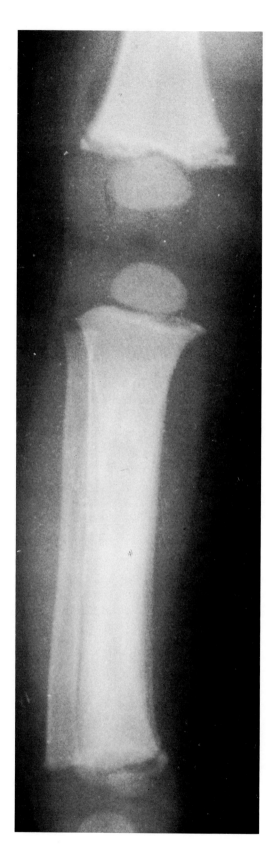

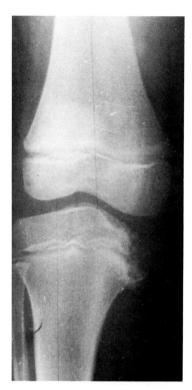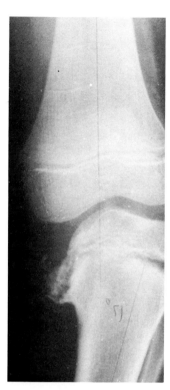

Fig. 10-76. Blount's disease. The metaphyseal region of the medial tibial plateau is markedly irregular. The area is irregularly calcified and depressed. The adjacent epiphysis is also abnormal and the medial femoral condyle is elongated.

Fig. 10-75. Purposeful trauma. Multiple fractures are present within the lower extremity. The fractures are predominantly metaphyseal-epiphyseal and manifest different stages of development. A relatively new injury is in the distal femur and an older injury with a large periosteal reaction is in the tibia.

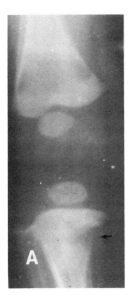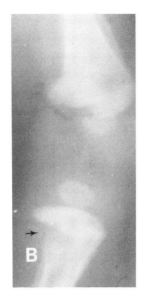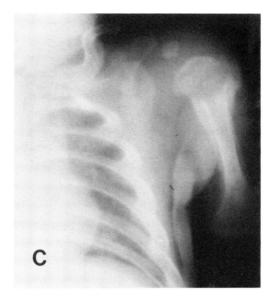

Fig. 10-77. Congenital syphilis (Wimberger's sign). *(A, B)* The proximal medial aspect in both tibias demonstrates notch deformities *(arrows)*. The metaphyses, however, are intact. Periosteal reactions are also evident. *(C)* Parrot's pseudoparalysis. The left shoulder in another patient shows subluxation. A large periosteal reaction and medial notch defect are present.

Differential Diagnosis

The newborn infant delivered by breech presentation is prone to injury. Metaphyseal-epiphyseal fragmentation associated with subperiosteal hemorrhage and a diffuse periosteal reaction are not uncommon (see p. 491).

Fortunately, the bones of an infant are resilient and resistant to the effects of trauma. After the neonatal period, the presence of metaphyseal fractures is most significant, since such an injury is frequently associated with and therefore diagnostic of purposeful trauma (Fig. 10-75). Fractures at the edges of the metaphysis and are due to the stress of traction and shearing that occur at this region where the pereostium is attached tightly to the metaphysis. These corner fractures are similar in appearance to the lateral corner fractures seen in scurvy (Fig. 10-63). In more severe shearing injuries the infraction seen in scurvy (Fig. 10-63). In more severe shearing injuries the infraction may extend across the entire metaphysis, resulting in a "bucket-handle-like" deformity. In this lesion a transverse fracture through the metaphysis allows separation of a horizontal bar of the metaphysis from the remainder of the bone. Hemorrhage under the periosteum with calcification, new bone deposition, and ossification complete the picture (Fig. 10-75).

Displacement of the epiphysis occurs in cartilage plate fractures. Purposeful trauma should be considered in all cases where multiple bone injuries in varying stages of healing and development are observed. The examination of the infant should include a radiograph of the entire body, not only to look for other bone lesions but also for injuries that might be life threatening, such as a subdural hematoma, hemoperitoneum, and a ruptured spleen.

Despite the relative specificity of the radiographic findings in purposeful trauma, there are other diseases that present with similar manifestations, most of which are neuromuscular disorders: cerebral palsy; meningomyelocoele-myelodysplasia; muscular dystrophy; spinal cord injury; arthrogryposis; Werdnig-Hoffman syndrome; Larsen's syndrome; chrondystrophia calcificans congenita (congenital stippled epiphyses); caudal regression syndrome; congenital insensitivity to pain (congenital analgesia); myositis ossificans progressiva; Riley-Day syndrome (familial dysautonomia); and oculo-cerebrorenal syndrome (Lowe's syndrome).

Infants who have congenital insensitivity to pain may fracture their bones in the same fashion as those injured by purposeful traction and stress. Subperiosteal hemorrhage may also occur.

Myositis ossificans progressiva is not

difficult to recognize once the soft-tissue bone becomes obvious. This is usually preceded by inflammatory, painful swellings in the back and neck that gradually convert to ossified tissue in a linear pattern between the muscle bundles. Eventually all the connective tissue and muscles in the body are involved. The diagnosis of the disease may be suggested early if the associated deformity of the big toe and thumb is present.

Patients with Riley-Day syndrome also have a degree of pain insensitivity and are therefore subject to similar bone injury.

Diseases which are not neuromuscular and which produce fractures similar to those of purposeful trauma include scurvy, rickets, hypophosphotasia, osteogenesis imperfecta, syphilis, copper deficiency, hyperparathyroidism, and steroid-induced, osteoporosis.

In addition, Blount's disease is presently considered to be a form of stress injury and not osteonecrosis. The disease may have its onset during the 1st 2 years of life and is also known as *tibia vara*, a term that describes the resultant deformity. The lesion is thought to result from unusual stress placed upon the proximal tibial metaphysis in active older children or in infants that walk early. The medial tibial metaphyses develops a beaked appearance. The margin at the zone of provisional calcification becomes progressively depressed until the metaphyseal flare becomes angular, sclerotic, and often appears fragmented (Fig. 10-76). According to Caffey, the primary spongiosa is not truly fragmented but replaced by unossified cartilage.

EROSIONS AND DISSOLUTION

Disease Entities

Osteomyelitis
  hyperparathyroidism (primary or secondary)
Metaphyseal chondrodysplasia (Jansen type)
Primary and secondary neoplasm
Congenital fibromatosis
Syphilis
Gaucher's disease
Farber's disease
Neurofibromatosis
Angiomatosis

Differential Diagnosis

Osteomyelitis was discussed in the section on periosteal reactions (see p. 361). Acute pyogenic osteomyelitis in newborns is the result of a hematogenous spread of bacteria. Many times the portal of entry is not determined, although the umbilicus (omphalitis) and skin (pyoderma) are common sites.

The bones most frequently involved in newborns are the distal and proximal femurs, humeri, and tibias. The infection spreads early into the joint space and through the cortex into the subperiosteal tissues. Septic arthritis is therefore frequently associated with neonatal osteomyelitis, and subluxation of the involved joint may result. The radiographic signs progress in a similar fashion, as in older children, with deep soft-tissue swelling antedating the radiographic evidence of osteolysis and periosteal reaction. Poorly marginated areas of radiolucency develop within the metaphysis proximal to the zone of provisional calcification. A single bone is involved in 90 per cent of the cases, although multiple bone involvement also occurs. As opposed to older children and infants, healing of osteomyelitis progresses more rapidly, and only rarely is sequestration encountered in newborns. Metaphyseal pathologic fractures may occur but often heal without complication.

Skeletal tuberculosis, as seen today, is primarily an articular process that is usually limited to one joint. The changes are preceded by a persistent joint effusion that may last several weeks before obvious bone lesions develop (see Fig. 9-11). The osteolytic lesions eventually become more circumscribed and demonstrate sharper zones of transition than those of pyogenic osteomyelitis.

Syphilitic osteitis has been discussed (see p. 429). However, varying degrees of metaphyseal destruction are manifested, in addition to fraying and periosteal reactions. There are large, notch-like defects that occur symmetrically within the medial proximal metaphysis (Wimberger's sign) (Fig 10-77). The proximal tibias, distal and proximal femurs, and the proximal humeri are frequently involved. The granulation tissue produced within the defects occasionally grows into the joint and displaces the epiphysis, producing a limp extremity (Fig. 10-77C).

Poorly marginated areas of destruction presenting as mottled rarefaction in the metaphysis should always suggest the presence of neoplastic disease. In infants, diseases which most often produce this feature

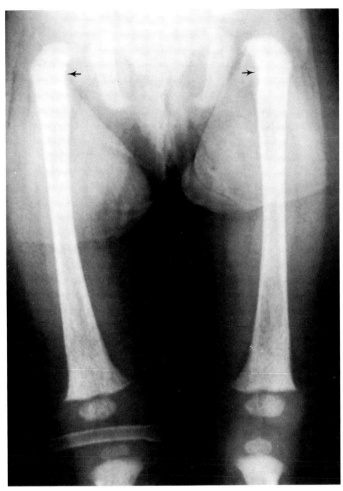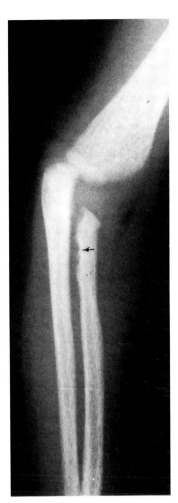

Fig. 10-78. Secondary hyperparathyroidism. Subperiosteal erosion is noted within the proximal portion of the femurs and ulna *(arrows)*. The trabecular pattern is markedly coarsened. This patient is only 8 months old and has adequate vitamin D storage. As a result, no rachitic changes are visualized.

include leukemia, neuroblastoma, retinoblastoma, and rhabdomyosarcoma. The poorly marginated areas do not distinguish each disease, although in our experience the defects produced by rhabdomyosarcoma are usually better defined and easier to detect than the subtle mottled areas produced by leukemia or neuroblastoma (Fig. 10-73). A diagnosis of rhabdomyosarcoma is usually obvious; in most cases the patient is in the process of being evaluated for a primary tumor mass. However, in leukemia the initial complaints are more variable. The metaphyseal changes are frequently associated with characteristic metaphyseal radiolucent lines, a unilaminar or multilaminar periosteal reaction, and hepatosplenomegaly.

Gaucher's disease also presents with poorly marginated, mottled areas of spongiosa in the metaphysis, but it is recognized mainly by the expanded and poorly tubulated metaphyses. Hepatosplenomegaly is almost always present. The changes in the spongiosa are the result of an excessive accumulation of kerasin in reticulendothelial cells, which also results in expansion of the shaft and thinning of the cortex. Focal areas of sclerosis and radiolucency may develop in the metaphysis in older children as a result of bone reparative response. However, some infants with Gaucher's disease may present with only an enlarged liver and spleen and interstitial pulmonary involvement.

Similar radiographic findings are occasionally noted in Nieman-Pick disease.

Generalized osseous rarefaction associated with endosteal and subperiosteal bone resorption is the principal feature in hyperparathyroidism. This disease occurs in both a primary and secondary form. The primary lesion is rare in the pediatric age-group but can be rapidly fatal when it has its onset in the 1st weeks of life. The familial form of hyperparathyroidism is likely to be transmitted by an autosomal recessive trait. Secondary hyperparathyroidism is usually the result of renal failure. The radiographic features of hyperparathyroidism are essentially the same regardless of origin (Fig. 10-78). Osseous rarefaction results in indistinct corticomedullary junctions and poorly defined trabeculae. Subperiosteal surface is resorbed, producing a frayed margin to the shaft of the bone. Longitudinal fissuring of the cortex is also present. The most striking abnormalities in the metaphysis are erosions that penetrate deep into the medial aspects of the bone. The erosions are poorly marginated and extend as far as the zone of provisional calcification. Because this bone is weaker than normal, bone infractions of the metaphysis can occur, resulting in angulation of the flaired ends of those bones.

Metaphyseal fraying is not seen in primary hyperparthyroidism. However, in renal osteodystrophy the combination of rickets and hyperparathyroidism is expected after the 1st few months of life. As a result, subperiosteal bone resorption accompanies widening of the epiphyseal plate and fraying of the metaphysis.

OVERTUBULATION AND UNDERTUBULATION

Tubulation is the result of osteolysis in the metaphysis. Bone modeling and growth occurs at the metaphysis as growing bone is removed and replaced. Appositional bone growth occurs as the periosteum adds bone to the diaphysis allowing for circumferential growth. Motor activity is a stimulus to bone growth. Bone atrophy and overtubulation result from immobilization or disuse. Undertubulation results when the normal process of osteolysis has been impaired, or when appositional bone growth proceeds at a faster rate. The resulting configuration is that of an expanded bone.

Differential Diagnosis

Gaucher's disease is usually recognized by an undertubulated femoral shaft in the region of the metaphysis. The shaft is slightly expanded and the trabecular pattern is coarened, with cortical thinning (Fig. 10-35).

Disease Entities

Undertubulation
  Newborns
    Osteopetrosis
    Metatropic dwarfism
    Kniest sydrome
    Parastremmatic dwarfism
  Infants and children
    Gaucher's disease
    Hyperphosphatasia
    Pyle's disease
    Osteochondromatosis
    Ollier's disease
    William's syndrome (idiopathic hypercalcemia syndrome)
    Healed infantile cortical hyperostosis
    Homocystinuruia
Overtubulation
  Neuromuscular disorders
  Arthrogryposis
  Arachnodactyly
  Myotonia congenita
  Cockayne's syndrome
  Winchester-Grossman syndrome
  Kinney-Caffey syndrome
  Aminopterin embryopathy
  Marshall's syndrome

Pyle's disease and craniometaphyseal dysplasia refer to the same disease or to variations of the same disease. The main feature is a lack of modeling of the metaphyses of tubular bones (Fig. 10-44). In neonates osteosclerosis is present. As skeletal development progresses, the sclerosis regresses and is replaced by an abnormal tubulation process that produces an appearance of metaphyseal bulbous swelling with rarefaction. When cranial hyperostosis is present, the disease may be referred to as craniometaphyseal dysplasia. The calvarial thickening includes the frontal bone, mandible, and occiput. The dysplasia also manifests enlarged supraorbital ridges, a lack of frontal sinuses in the skull, and "coat hanger" ribs in the thorax.

Osteopetrosis occasionally demonstrates undertubulation of the metaphysis and is distinguished from Pyle's disease by the extreme radiopacity of the bones (Fig. 10-42). Infants who have idiopathic hypercalcemia may be osteosclerotic as well and show some degree of poor bone modeling. As a result, this entity could be confused with osteope-

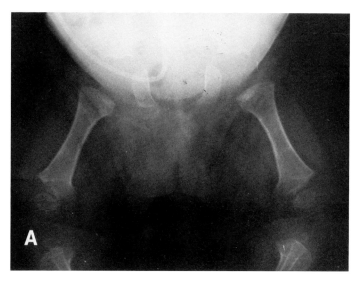

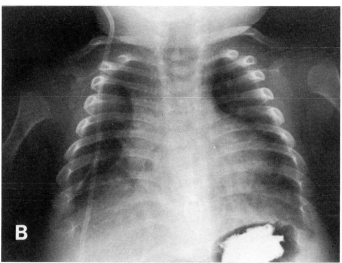

Fig. 10-79. Kniest syndrome. (*A, B*) Note the short extremities with dumb-bell flaring of the metaphysis and the broad thorax.

trosis or even infantile Pyle's disease, were it not for the characteristically elevated serum calcium levels.

Metatropic dwarfism and the Kniest syndrome are both characterized by a bulbous, flaring (dumbell-shaped), metaphysis (Fig. 10-79). They have been confused with each other but are separate and distinct conditions. In metatropic dwarfism, the infant is at first disporportionately short-limbed, but vertebral anomalies and the subsequent development of scoliosis also leads to a short trunk. The vertebral bodies are defectively ossified and small in both lesions, but may be diamond-shaped in the metatropic dwarf. The thoracic cage is small in the latter disease and resembles asphixiating thoracic dystrophy (Fig. 10-80). This is different from the broad thorax with a protuding sternum found in the Kniest syndrome. In both the pelvis is short with a horizontal acetabular roof. The patient with Kniest syndrome also manifests cleft and depressed palate, myopia, and hypertelorism.

Parastremmatic dwarfism is an extremely rare severe form of dwarfism, with bizarre asymmetrical deformities of the lower leg in which the bones appear to have twisted around their axis. Radiographically, the epiphyses and metaphyses are distorted. The metaphyses are characterized by irregular stippling and streaks, producing a floccular appearance in the bones.

The metaphysis in homocystinuria is also widened, with general failure of bone modeling being most obvious in the knee.

Familial hyperphosphatasemia is defined as a disorder of growing membranous bone in

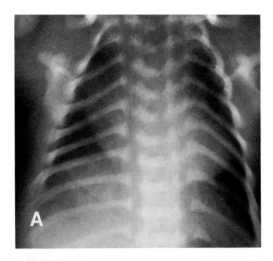

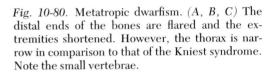

Fig. 10-80. Metatropic dwarfism. *(A, B, C)* The distal ends of the bones are flared and the extremities shortened. However, the thorax is narrow in comparison to that of the Kniest syndrome. Note the small vertebrae.

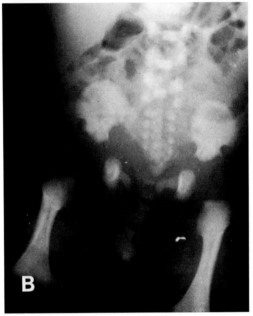

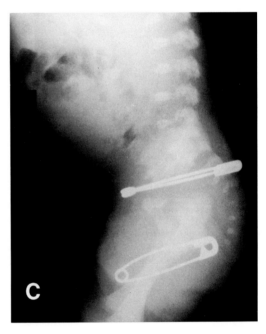

which primitive fibrous bone fails to mature into compact bone, with a concurrent increased turnover of bone. In the infantile form of this disease, the extremities are swollen and the patient has difficulty walking. There is lack of normal tubulation of the bones, and they are more radiolucent than normal. The cortex is not formed normally but is thin throughout the entire shaft. The trabecular pattern and the shaft of the bone is coarse, the shaft itself becoming bowed as well as dilated. The zone of provisional calcification is intact. Macrocrania accompanies this disease and calvarial changes similar to those seen in adult Paget's disease may be present. The entity is probably autonomal recessive, with onset usually between the 3rd and the 18th months of life. Laboratory findings consist of increased levels of alkaline and acid phosphatase.

Osteochondromatosis (multiple hereditary exostosis) results in inadequate modeling of the metaphysis of the long bones (Fig. 10-81). These exostosis is not present in neonates but may be seen after the 1st year of life. As the child ages an abnormality in tubulation develops as a result of a primary defect in modeling. The epiphyseal plate and zone of provisional calcification are normal. The most severe form of the disease results in dwarfism and poor tubulation as well as a spurious form of Madelung's deformity of the wrist.

In Ollier's disease, characteristically unossified areas of cartilage remain in the metaphysis and diaphysis which sometimes expands to form huge tumor masses (Fig.

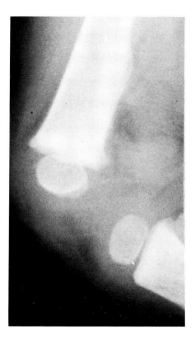 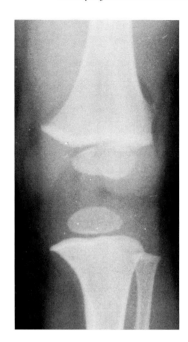

Fig. 10-81. Undertubulation in multiple exostosis. A small exostosis is present within the distal portion of the femur, resulting in a distinct widening of the metaphysis.

10-41). As a result, the presenting clinical finding is often swelling of the metaphyseal region, commonly around the knee and at the end of the radius and ulna. Radiographically, irregular translucent areas and streaks of cartilage are characteristic. As the child grows these may extend into the shaft. Other deformities may present as a result of the bone changes such as shortening, genu valgum, and Madelung's deformity. The disease manifests a striking propensity for unilateral involvement.

Healing subperiosteal hemorrhage in scurvy results in temporary undertubulation until modeling has rendered the bone normal. A similar phenomenon takes place in infantile cortical hyperostosis. Again, the tubulation abnormality is transient and is due to the proliferative, new periosteal bone that takes time to resorb and remodel.

Overtubulation and undertubulation are difficult to detect when there is only a slight degree of abnormality. This is particularly true of patients whose bones are overtubulated.

The number of diseases that produce overtubulation or undertubulation is far more extensive than indicated here. We have noted that activity and muscular pull are necessary stimuli for appositional bone growth. It follows, then, that if activity is diminished or if muscular tension and/or muscular mass is not normal, appositional bone growth will be affected negatively. This can result in overtubulation or gracile bones, well demonstrated in patients with diseases of neuromuscular origin.

In infancy, arthrogryposis is a typical example. The disease is also called amyoplasia congenita, and as the name implies the muscles are small and contracted. Excess subcutaneous fat is present, reversing the normal muscle cylinder ratio. The bones are thin and gracile and with time overtubulation becomes evident (Fig. 10-82). There is a limitation of movement of all of the joints due to muscular contractures. Most of affected infants have club foot deformities and dislocated hips. Micrognathia is commonly present. It is not known if the disease originates in the central nervous system or is a primary muscular abnormality.

Excessive fat and diminished muscle mass is a feature of Werdnig-Hoffman disease, in which primary anterior horn cell degeneration in the spinal cord is the basic abnormality. Thin, gracile bones and diminished muscle mass are evident soon after birth, and as the infant ages overtubulation of the metaphysis and diaphysis becomes evident. Similar radiographic findings are present in the infantile form of a myotonia congenita (Fig. 10-83).

Overtubulation of the metaphysis and diminished muscle mass are found in infants with cerebral palsy. Infants with perinatal as-

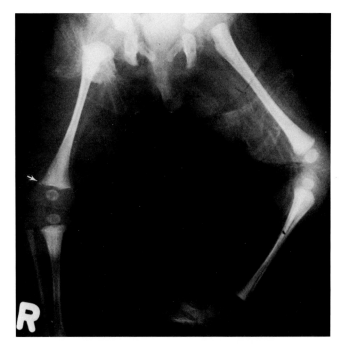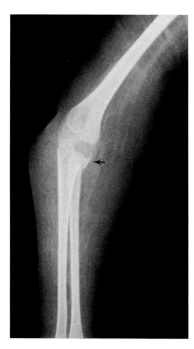

Fig. 10-82. Arthrogryposis. The bones are elongated and gracile. The subcutaneous fat tissue is increased and little muscle mass is evident. The proximal radius and the distal right femur show corner fractures *(arrows)*, and the left hip is dislocated.

phyxia and cerebral damage who are unable to walk may develop the same skeletal configuration. Cerebral damage due to asphyxia, as in cerebral palsy, is the most common cause of undertubulation of bones.

Other well recognized but rare disorders associated with overtubulation at the metaphysis include Cockayne's syndrome and progeria, Hutchinson-Gilford disease (Fig. 10-84).

CUPPED METAPHYSES

Cupping is radiographically manifested as central shaft depression, associated with spreading of the metaphysis and an overall shortening of bone. The depression is deepest in the central part of the metaphysis and is best manifested in the distal femur, where marked deepening of the intercondylar notch occurs. The contiguous epiphyseal ossification center enlarges and grows into the depression, producing a ball-and-socket pattern (Fig. 10-85). The adjacent epiphyseal plate becomes thin, resulting in premature fusion of this immediate segment. Longitudinal growth continues at a slightly more rapid

pace at the margins of the bone. Although the distal ends of the femur demonstrate these findings best, other metaphyses show similar abnormalities but are much more shallow.

Disease Entities
Achondroplasia
Sickle cell anemia
Trauma
Rickets
Scurvy
Ellis-van Creveld syndrome
Peripheral dysostosis
Tricho-rhino-phalangeal syndrome
Osteopetrosis
Vitamin A posioning
Infection

Differential Diagnosis

In achondroplasia, the metaphysis characteristically manifests a V-shaped notch into which the epiphysis fits (Fig. 10-85). This feature, however, is not obvious in newborns with achrondroplasia but develops as the child matures. In newborns, the proximal

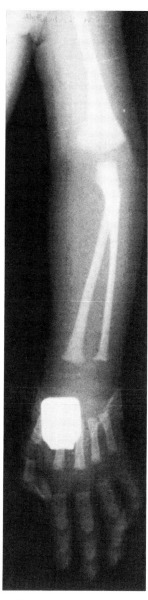

Fig. 10-83. Amyotonia congenita. Little muscle mass is evident. The extremity consists mostly of subcutaneous fat tissue. The bones are thin and elongated.

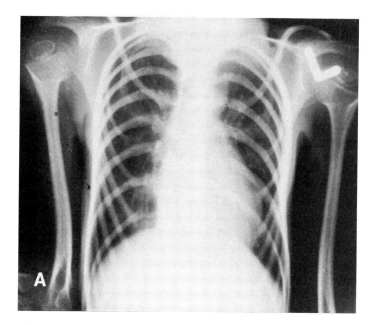

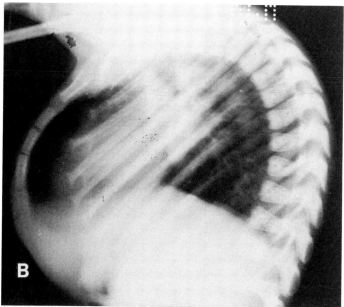

Fig. 10-84. Cockayne's syndrome. *(A)* The chest shows remarkably thin and gracile ribs. The clavicles are markedly curved and elongated. The humeri appear long and thin. *(B)* The lateral projection demonstrates a large anteroposterior diameter.

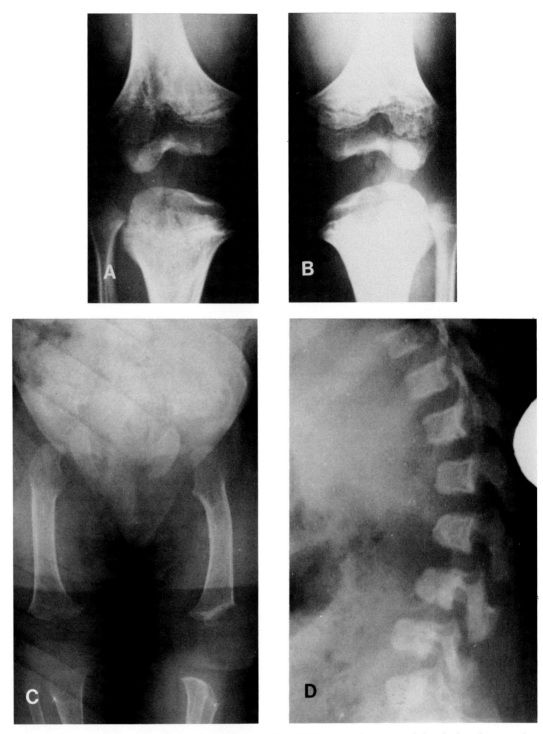

Fig. 10-85. Cupped metaphysis in achondroplasia. *(A, B)* The central portion of the shaft is depressed, producing a notch in the intercondylar region. The adjacent part of the epiphysis is enlarged and lodges in the depression. *(C)* Newborn with achrondroplasia. Note the short limbs and the relatively straight distal ends of the femurs. In fact, there is a characteristic lateral angulation distally. *(D)* The spine of an achondroplastic patient. Box-shaped vertebrae, with mild wedge deformity in the upper lumbar bodies, are shown.

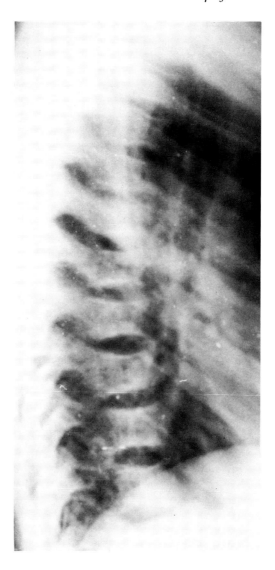

Fig. 10-86. The vertebrae in sickle cell anemia. Note the central cup deformity producing an H shape.

ends of the femur are relatively square and the distal ends are ossifed laterally (Fig. 10-85C). In infants with achondroplasia the extremities are short and thick, producing short-limbed dwarfism. A bulging cranium is also characteristic. This is the result of a normal vault developing on a short base that manifests growth retardation. As a result, the diameter of the foramen magnum is reduced, and some degree of obstruction and hydrocephalus results. The interpedicular distance in the lumbar spine remains narrow in comparison to the gradual widening noted in the normal lumbar spine. In addition, the vertebral bodies are small and box-shaped and demonstrate anterior wedging at the thoracolumbar junction (Fig. 10-85D). The pelvis is smaller than normal. The inferior

margin of the ilium is horizontal, and the iliac wings are square. As a result, the acetabular angle approximates zero and the sacrosciatic notch is slit-like.

Metaphyseal cupping is not infrequent in patients with sickle cell anemia. This is commonly found in the metatarsals of African children. In American children it is more frequently encountered in the central segment of the vertebral bodies (Fig. 10-86). The peripheral end plates remain normal, and as a result the central portion of the body is depresssed, producing and H or fish-shaped vertebral configuration. This deformity is characteristic, although it has also been sometimes noted in thalasemia and Gaucher's disease.

Metaphyseal cupping within the distal

femurs has been observed following trauma. The changes are not directly related to the injury, since several months or even a year of bone growth must occur before these alterations become apparent. Similar metaphyseal changes have been known to follow bouts of poliomyelitis, osteomyelitis occurring in other parts of the bone, or paralysis of the leg muscles.

Permanent deformity as a sequel to vitamin A poisoning has been found in a number of patients. The affected bone grows poorly and manifests a severe and permanent shortening. A shortened extremity associated with cupping and premature fusion of the central part of the epiphysis is the main radiographic finding. Manifestations of acute hypervitaminosis A are different and consist basically of a bilateral symmetrical periosteal reaction that involves the shaft of the tubular bones. The ulnae and some metatarsals are consistently affected, with a wavy and thick external cortical wall.

Although mild cupping abnormalities accompany osteopetrosis and Ollier's disease, the overall bone changes are characteristic. Osteopetrosis demonstrates a marked sclerosis of the entire skeleton, in which distinction between the cortical and medullary structures are no longer possible. In Ollier's disease, calcified cartilaginous lesions, which are mostly unilateral, are present throughout.

Metaphyseal cupping is also characteristic of either the Jansen or Schmidt types of metaphyseal dysplasia. The metaphysis is expanded, cystic, fragmented, and more severely distorted in the Jansen type. In both types, the epiphyses are well formed and normal, although they may develop late. The Jansen type is extremely rare and affected patients are severly deformed, with a short-limbed type of dwarfism, contractures of the hip, and expanded knees. The Schmidt type is far more common and the bones are less deformed, this type results in short-limbed dwarfism and effects the hip to a greater extent than the knee. Patients manifest an extreme degree of shortness, lumbar lordosis, and a waddling gait. In both types the skull is normal.

Discussion

Regardless of the cause of metaphyseal cupping, the major pathogenesis is believed to be interference with the vessels supplying the proliferating rows of cartilage in the central portion of the epiphyseal plate. These vessels are made up of metaphyseal arteries, and interruption of flow, for one reason or another, is associated with reduced growth. The external portion of the metaphysis is supplied by additional penetrating metaphyseal arteries and is, therefore, wholly unaffected. Thrombosis and stasis in these vessels occur easily in sickle cell disease. It appears that most patients with cupping following trauma have been immobilized for long periods of time. Immobilization apparently results in local oligemia due to thrombosis secondary to stagnation of blood and slow flow in the internal epiphyseal arteries. Impeded perfusion may also underlie the changes that occur in achondrophasia and some of the other forms of dysostosis. Osteopetrosis, for example, is primarily the result of failure to fully absorb the calcified metaphyseal cartilage and primary spongiosum, which may be related to decreased blood flow. Failure to resorb large areas of calcified cartilage could also well explain the findings in Ollier's disease.

EPIPHYSEAL ABNORMALITIES

The epiphysis is composed primarily of cartilaginous tissue with one or more centers of ossification during the growth period. A number of disease entities alter the development of these centers and changes in appearance, structure, and configuration occur. These alterations are manifested by irregular ossification (or calcification), a lack of or delayed epiphyseal ossification, a cone-shaped appearance, a ringed epiphysis, and an ivory epiphysis.

IRREGULAR
OSSIFICATION OR CALCIFICATION

Under normal conditions the epiphysis has a distinct structure and overall appearance. The ossification center normally looks like a spherical structure within the cartilaginous epiphysis. The center gradually enlarges and eventually assumes the shape of the bone it forms. Occasionally, multiple centers appear and a stippled appearance is produced. This presentation is not unusual during periods of growth and is commonly limited to a single epiphysis. However, it is distinctly abnormal if multiple epiphyses are involved and if the epiphysis appears grossly exaggerated and irregular.

Disease Entities

Multiple Epiphyses
    Chondrodystrophia calcificans congenita
    Hypothyroidism
    Pseudoachondroplasia
    Multiple epiphyseal dysplasia
    Trisomy 18
    Cerebro-hepato-renal syndrome
    Ollier's dyschondroplasia
    Hurler's syndrome
    Familial spotted epiphysis
    Parastremmatic dwarfism
    Dyggve-Melchior-Claussen syndrome
    Prenatal infections
Single Epiphysis
    Osteochondrosis
    Gaucher's disease
    Sickle cell disease
    Acute pancreatitis
    Morquio's syndrome

Differential Diagnosis

Conradi originally described the entity chondrodystrophia calcificans congenita in apparently normal individuals manifesting large, calciferous stippling of the growing cartilage. Presently, it appears that this disease consists of a heterogeneous group of conditions; the severe form may be accompanied by a short-limbed type of dwarfism or by asymmetrical shortening of a limb. The patients generally have a flattened nose, a high, arched palate, frontal bossing, a short neck, and short stature. Stippling is distributed throughout most of the primary and secondary ossifications centers in newborns (Fig. 10-87). The epiphyses also appear wider and more bulbous. The abnormality is not only confined to the long tubular bones but is also seen in the sternum, scapulas, vertebrae, ribs, and synovial tissues (Fig. 10-87B). The tracheobronchial tree may also be abnormally calcified, resulting in respiratory difficulties. Craniostenosis is apparently another important radiographic feature.

Irregular, stippled epiphyses are frequently encountered in hypothyroidism. These appear late and may not be seen until the 2nd or 3rd year of life. Ossification in this entity begins not from a single center but from numerous, small, irregular zones that ultimately fuse to form a single center of uneven density. This phenomenon has been called cretinoid epiphyseal dysgenesis. In patients with hypothyroidism the femoral heads are not only irregular but appear to be flattened, and the femoral neck may show evidence of coxa vara.

The basic defect in multiple epiphyseal dysplasia is mainly in the extremities. The epiphyses appear late and are variable in shape. They can be small, rough, or irregularly calcified (Fig. 10-88). Some are merely flattened, others are square in outline. The majority, however, are grossly irregular and fragmented. Although the epiphyses improve with growth, they still manifest some degree of deformity in adult life. The femoral capital epiphysis is nearly always involved and changes strongly resembling Legg-Calvé-Perthes disease are produced. Slippage of the epiphysis also occurs, and a slanting mortise in the lower tibial epiphysis is a common and characteristic finding (Fig. 10-88F).

Pseudoachondroplasia is a form of short-limbed dwarfism that resembles multiple epiphyseal dysplasia, but with associated vertebral and metaphyseal changes. In infancy, the vertebral bodies are flat with a distinctive anterior, tongue-like protrusion present in the center of the body (Fig. 10-89A). The metaphyses are flared, and the epiphysis are small and irregular (Fig. 10-89B). However, by the time the patient reaches adolescence, differentiation from multiple epiphyseal dysplasia may be almost impossible, since the vertebral aberration described in pseudo-achondroplasia approaches a normal appearance with growth.

Irregular stippling and calcific streaks within the epiphysis and metaphysis characterize some of the changes noted in the parastremmatic dwarf. The main radiographic feature, however, is a bizarre, twisted appearance of the limbs. The skull is normal, but the vertebrae are flat with irregularly ossified end plates.

The Dyggve-Melchoir-Claussen syndrome manifests irregular calcification in both the epiphysis and metaphysis, but often of a lesser degree than pseudoachondroplasia. The epiphyses are also cone-shaped. The vertebral bodies are flat, with a characteristic

(Text continued on p. 458.)

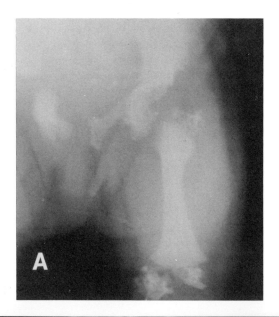

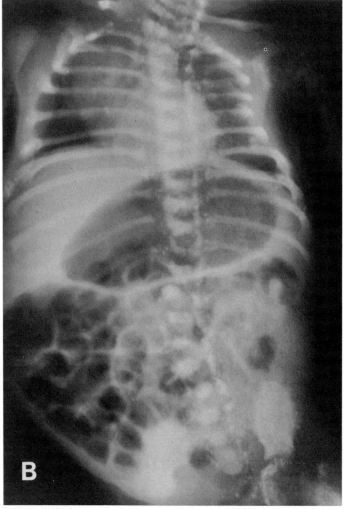

Fig. 10-87. Chondrodystrophia calcificans. *(A)* This radiograph of a newborn shows irregular calcifications within the epiphyses. The epiphyses are also deformed, bulbous, and irregular. *(B)* Irregular calcifications are present in the vertebral bodies and the ends of the ribs. *(Continued on facing page.)*

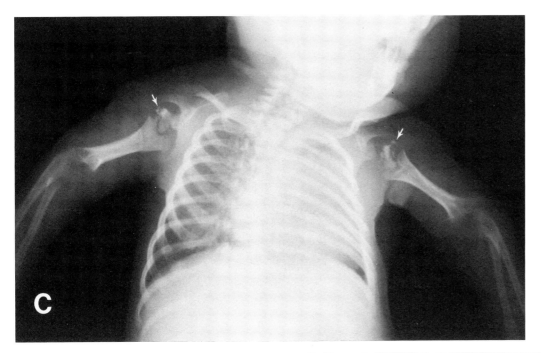

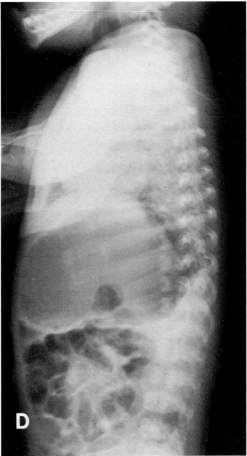

Fig. 10-87 (Continued). (C) Rhizomelic form. Note the markedly irregular calcified epiphyses in the proximal humeri (arrows). Both humeral bones are small, and the metaphyseal margins are irregular and cupped. (D) Coronal clefts. Note the vertical radiolucent defects dividing the vertebral bodies.

455

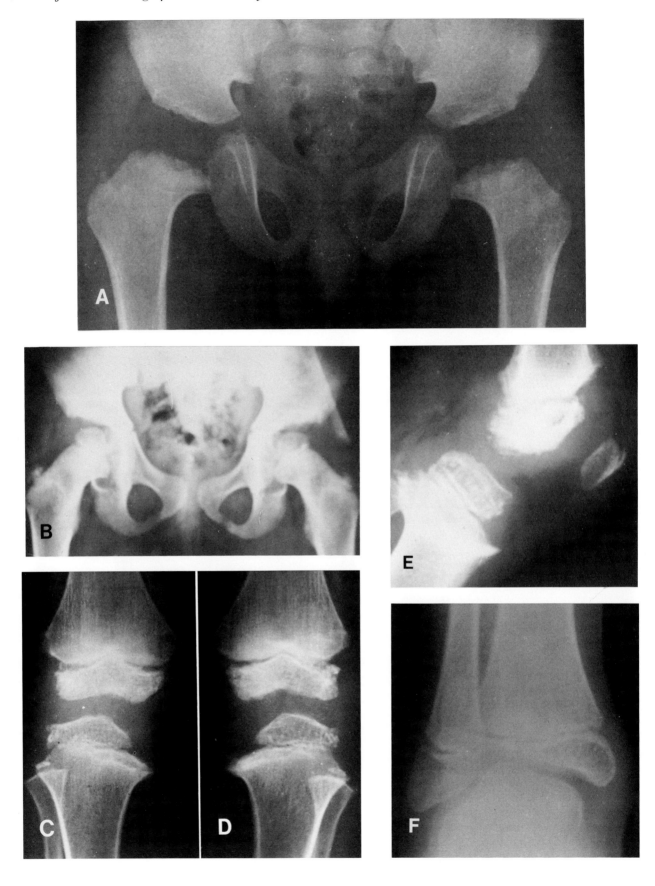

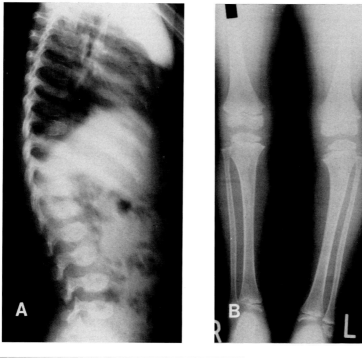

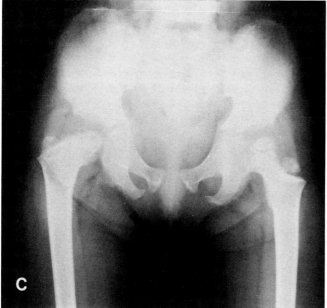

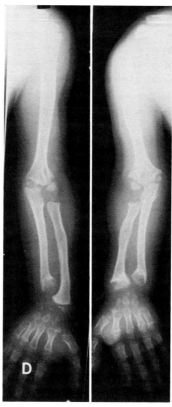

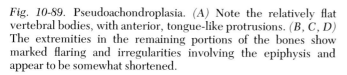

Fig. 10-89. Pseudoachondroplasia. *(A)* Note the relatively flat vertebral bodies, with anterior, tongue-like protrusions. *(B, C, D)* The extremities in the remaining portions of the bones show marked flaring and irregularities involving the epiphysis and appear to be somewhat shortened.

←

Fig. 10-88. Epiphyseal dysplasia. *(A)* Pelvis. The femoral capital epiphyses have not yet ossified despite this patient's relatively advanced age. *(B)* In an older individual, small, underdeveloped epiphyses are present. *(C, D)* The epiphyses in the knees are stippled and irregular. The proximal tibial epiphysis is also underdeveloped and somewhat flat along its medial surface. *(E)* A lateral projection of the knee in another patient again manifests distinct irregular and stippled epiphyses. *(F)* The ankle mortise is notably slanted. This is a characteristic finding.

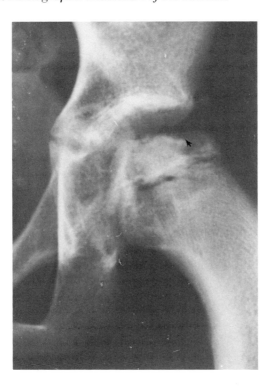

Fig. 10-90. Legg-Calvé-Perthes disease. The femoral capital epiphysis is markedly irregular, sclerotic, and flattened. A crescentic radiolucency located in the immediate subchondral area represents evidence of a fracture *(arrow)*.

notch on the superior and inferior surface. In Ollier's disease, the epiphyses are usually normal in childhood, but later, areas of irregular density and mottling can occur.

Osteochondrosis is a term describing a group of scattered lesions occurring within the growing skelton. Radiographically, compression fractures and compression of the provisional zones of calcification are evident. These lesions were originally considered to be the result of vascular ischemia. However, they are more likely related to trauma, with impairment of the local blood supply. Some forms of osteochondrosis are well known, such as Osgood-Schlatter disease and Legg-Calvé-Perthes disease. Others such as Köhler's bone disease and, Freiberg's disease, are not common. Legg-Calvé-Perthes disease however, is a fairly common, acquired lesion that is associated with a high incidence of disabling osteoarthritis that occasionally arises years latter. The disease develops between the ages of 3 and 12 years, with a maximum incidence between 6 to 8 years of age. Boys are affected approximately 4 times as frequently as girls, and the disease is bilateral in one out of ten patients. The presenting clinical signs usually include a limp and pain, with associated limited motion of the corresponding hip. Unfortunately, the radiographic pre-

sentation is well advanced by the time the clinical symptoms are manifested. The radiographic findings depend upon the phase of development. The earliest phase consists of a mild dislocation of the femoral head and is demonstrated as lateral displacement of the femur (Waldenström's sign). This is followed by a marginal fracture that is detectable by a radiolucent crescent paralleling the subchondral surface in the anterior outer quadrant of the ossification center. The fracture is best visualized in the frog position. Surface irregularity and beginning collapse of the osseous nucleus is the next stage, and the epiphysis becomes dense, fragmented, and flat (Fig. 10-90). As the lesion heals the epiphysis produces new bone in a reconstructive response. This also adds to the increased radiodensity. Alterations also occur in the metaphysis; the femoral neck becomes broad, short, and angles more anteriorly. The acetabulum subsequently undergoes corresponding changes to accommodate the abnormal hip. The findings may require months or years to occur and are sometimes followed by osteoarthritis.

Osgood-Schlatter disease is frequently encountered in active children between the ages of 10 and 15 years. The disease is clinically manifested by swelling and tenderness

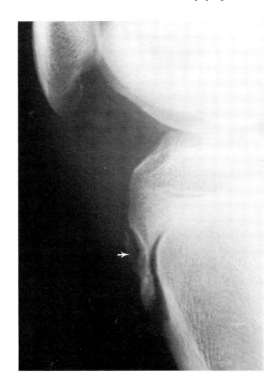

Fig. 10-91. Osgood-Schlatter disease. There is a distinct irregularity and fragmentation involving the tibial apophysis *(arrow).* An associated soft-tissue swelling is also present but is not well-defined here.

over the tibial tubercle. As a result, the radiographic findings are fragmentation of the tubercle and swelling of the overlying soft tissues (Fig. 10-91). Irregularity of the tubercle alone is insufficient radiographic evidence for the diagnosis, since this finding is common in normal children.

Gaucher's disease and sickle cell disease also present with varying degrees of aseptic necrosis which leads to fragmentation and irregular sclerosis of some epiphyses. The femoral heads are most frequently affected, although the heads of the humeri are also involved in sickle cell disease (Fig. 10-92).

Blunt trauma to the abdomen in some instances produces an acute pancreatitis with bone changes similar to osteonecrosis. This finding is being reported with increasing incidence in cases of child abuse. A similar process occurs in familial forms of hyperlipidemia.

The patella alone demonstrates an irregular spotty pattern of calcification in the cerebrohepato-renal syndrome (Zellweger's syndrome). This is the only significant radiographic finding in this rare condition. The syndrome consists of multiple renal cysts, liver disease that shows fibrosis and hemosiderosis, and cerebral abnormalities that include lissencephaly and sudanophilic leukodystroy-

phy. Clinically, the patient demonstrates an abnormal facies, marked hypotonia, and flexion contractures.

Discussion

Although the femoral capital epiphyses are well formed in infants with Morquio's syndrome, they suddenly become irregular between 3 to 6 years of age. Irregularities may persist until adolescence or early adulthood, at which time they disappear completely.

Although many conditions comprise the disease known as chondrodystrophia calcificans congenita, two main types predominate. The lethal rhizomelic type is transmitted by an autosomal recessive trait, and most patients expire in the 1st year of life. It is accompanied by gross shortening of the extremities, metaphyseal widening, epiphyseal stippling of the femurs and humeri, and coronal clefts of the vertebral bodies (Fig. 10-87C, D).

The Conradi-Hunermann type has a wide range of clinical and radiographic appearances as well as an excellent prognosis. The lesion is transmitted by a dominant trait. There is mild asymmetric shortening of the tubular bones, with asymmetric dysplastic epiphyses and intact metaphyses. The vertebral bodies may also be deformed. In general, however, the majority of cases regress, leaving no sequelae or deformities. In some cases persistent and progressive deformities have been noted, although the calcifications tend to regress. Recent observations have shown that the Conradi-Hunermann type also follows the maternal ingestion of anticonvulsive or anticoagulant (warfarin) medication during pregnancy. Some unusual prenatal infections, such as listerosis, have also been implicated as a possible cause of this abnormality.

Multiple epiphyseal dysplasia is a common skeletal dysplasia in which little or no vertebral changes occur. The patients are only mildly short in stature. It is clearly of autosomal dominant inheritance and effects either sex equally. In some cases, a form of chondrodystrophia calcificans may be the initial manifestation in the neonatal period. Most often the disorder is not apparent at birth or before the age of 2 years or more. The major complication is the development of an early and crippling osteoarthritis. It is still not clear whether this disease is a simple entity or another closely related collection of disorders.

A LACK OF OR DELAYED EPIPHYSEAL OSSIFICATION

Only a few epiphyses are evident at birth, such as the distal femur and the proximal tibia, which are the most apparent and are therefore excellent indicators of fetal maturity. In general, epiphyseal ossification follows a distinct, chronologic pattern, and any alteration in this time schedule indicates some insult to the fetus or growing infant.

Differential Diagnosis

Hypothyroidism is a disease that is mainly characterized radiographically by delayed ossification of the epiphysis. Insufficient amounts of circulating thyroid hormone result in reduction of bone formation and a delay in bone maturation (Fig. 10-93). The ossification centers eventually appear after an interval of months or even years and look like multiple distinct islands. The epiphysis is then basically stippled, irregular, and fragmented. In general, the bones show an overall increase in cortical thickening and a narrow medullary cavity. Some patients present with diffuse bone sclerosis, a phenome-

Disease Entities

Newborns
  Hypothyroidism
  Asexual pituitary dwarfism
  Thanatophoric dwarfism
  Achondrogenesis
  Multiple epiphyseal dysplasia
  Spondyloepiphyseal dysplasia congenita
  Mucopolysaccharidosis
  Cleidocranial dysplasia
  Nail-patella syndrome
  Diastrophic dwarfism
  Parastremmatic dwarfism
  Turner's syndrome
Infants and Children
  Constitutional disease
  Malnutrition
  Juvenile diabetes mellitus
  Rickets
  Steroids
  Morquio's syndrome
    (mucopolysacharridosis IV)

non perhaps related to increased calcium absorption with resultant hypercalcemia. Metastatic calcification and renal calculi have also been encountered. Most of the radiographic findings in hypothyroidism, however, are related to delayed ossification. For example, delayed closure of the fontanelles is common. The vertebral bodies at L1 and L2 are small and manifest some degree of developmental failure in the anterosuperior surface (Fig. 10-93B). The vertebral bodies are hook-shaped. Such an appearance is also noted in many forms of mucopolysaccharidosis. The clinical presentation consists of an apathetic, sluggish, and hypotonic child with a thick tongue and a protruding abdomen. These features are easily recognized in older infants, but they are seldom apparent in newborns. Therefore, the radiographic findings are important. Detection and treatment within the first 2 years minimizes the amount of mental retardation associated with this abnormality and therefore influences the ultimate clinical development of these infants.

In asexual pituitary dwarfism, the bone age is severely retarded. In the absence of replacement therapy, the epiphyseal plates may remain open until late in the 3rd decade or longer. The overall skeletal structure is normal, although small.

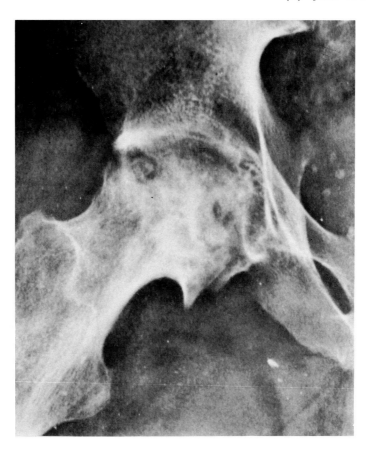

Fig. 10-92. Aseptic necrosis in sickle cell disease (adult). The right femoral capital epiphysis is enlarged, irregular, and sclerotic. Cystic changes are also apparent.

Lipoid storage diseases, cleidocranial dysostosis, and epiphyseal and spondyloepiphyseal dysplasia are all associated with some degree of retarded epiphyseal development (Fig. 10-88A). Small, irregular carpal bones are noted in mucopolysaccharidosis. These disorders are also associated with delayed ossification, but patients are surprisingly normal up to 1 year of age.

Multiple epiphyseal and spondyloepiphyseal dysplasia both demonstrate ossification centers that appear late and are small and mottled (Fig. 10-88A). However, spondylepiphyseal dysplasia is characterized by flat vertebral bodies that also manifest an oval or pear-shaped appearance on the lateral view. Hypoplasia and delayed ossification of the odontoid process is a common but unfortunate occurrence in spondyloepiphyseal dysplasia and is associated with severe instability of the C1—C2 area (Fig. 10-94B). The hands and feet are only minimally involved. The overall effect is a type of dwarfism associated with a short trunk and platyspondyisis and gross disorganization of the upper femurs, with deep acetabulae (Fig. 10-94C).

The findings are often confused with other forms of dysplasia effecting similar structures, such as Morquio's syndrome. The latter, however, occurs at a later age and produces a pelvis of distinctive configuration.

Thanatophoric dwarfism and achondrogenesis are two forms of lethal, short-limbed dwarfism which are manifested in newborns by a complete lack of epiphyses, along with other distinctive radiographic abnormalities. Both diseases resemble or have been confused with achondroplasia, although distinguishing radiographic bone changes are apparent. In thanatophoric dwarfism, the trunk is normal in length and the thorax narrow in all dimensions. The ribs are short and rarely extend beyond the axillary line. The vertebral bodies, in contrast to those of achondroplasia, are remarkably flat with wide intervertebral disc spaces. The extremities are noticeably short and demonstrate a characteristic curvature, with wide and irregular metaphyses (Fig. 10-95). However, both the trunk and limbs are short in achondrogenesis, and the thorax is not quite as nar-

(Text continued on p. 464.)

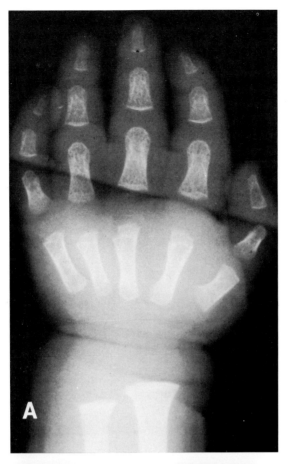

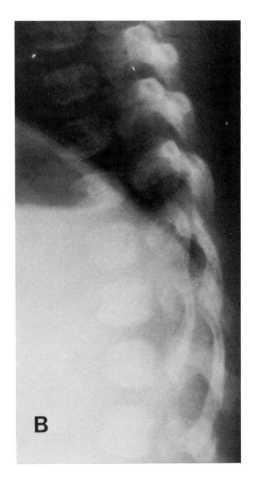

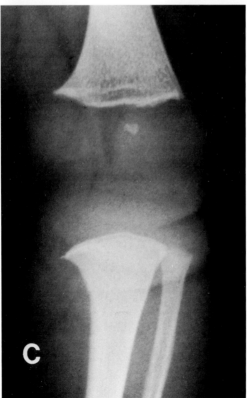

Fig. 10-93. Hypothyroidism. *(A)* In a 3-year-old there is no evidence of epiphyseal centers within the hand. *(B)* The lateral spine of the same patient reveals hypoplasia of the first lumbar vertebral body. *(C)* The knee reveals only a single, small, distal epiphysis.

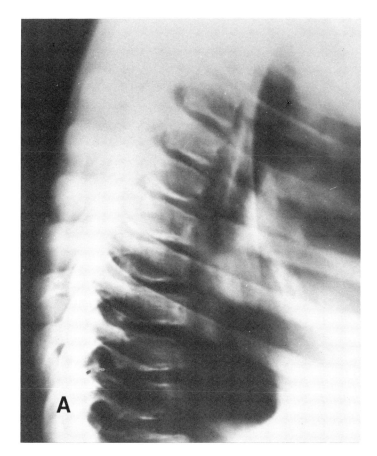
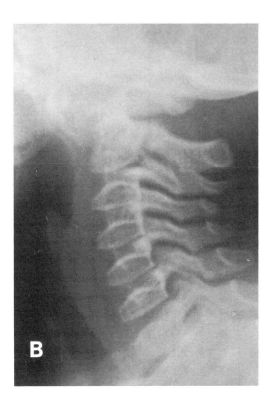
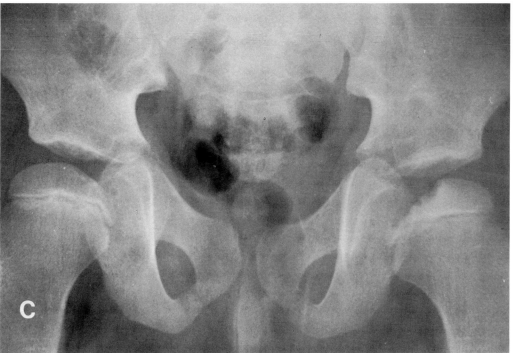

Fig. 10-94. Spondyloepiphyseal dysplasia. *(A)* The dorsal spine is flat, with a suggestive oval configuration. *(B)* Anterior dislocation at C1—C2 is present. Note again the flat oval configuration of the vertebral bodies. *(C)* The femoral capital epiphyses are irregular and somewhat flat. Findings resemble those of Legg-Calvé-Perthes disease.

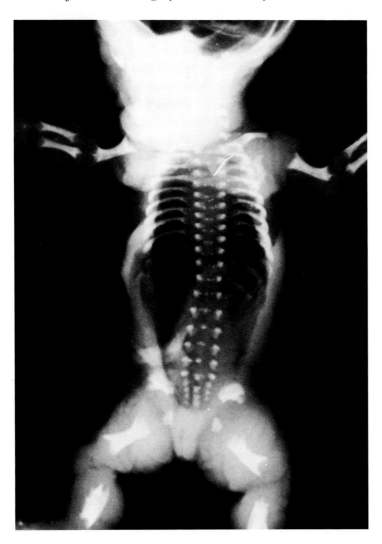

Fig. 10-95. Thanatophoric dwarfism. Note the short limbs, with a rather distinctive, curved appearance. The metaphyses are irregular, and there is complete absence of the epiphyses. Another distinctive feature of this form of dwarfism is the absolutely flat vertebral bodies.

row. The most obvious feature is diffuse, poor ossification of the entire skeleton, such that the bones in the lumbar, sacral, and pubic areas are almost completely indistinguishable. The prognosis is poor for patients with either thanatophoric dwarfism or achondrogenesis.

Diastrophic dwarfism, also characterized by short limbs, produces delayed epiphysial ossification in the long bones. The epiphyses, when they develop, are flat and distorted. The most important findings are severe scoliosis and contractures of most of the joints. The metaphyses are also slightly flared (Fig. 10-96). The hands and feet are broad, and the first metacarpal is short, resulting in a thumb that is located too far proximally

(hitch-hiker's thumb). The hip joints are severely affected, and the bones in the knee demonstrate flattened, upper tibial and lower femoral epiphyses that seem to be shifted medially.

Cleidocranial dysplasia is a generalized bone disease affecting mainly the skull and clavicles, although other bones such as the scapula, pelvis, and vertebrae can be involved. Ossification is retarded in certain areas and accounts for many of the abnormalities described. The ossification centers in the clavicles are partially or completely absent (Fig. 10-97A). Imperfect ossification with delayed fusion is a frequent finding, and the sutures remain open and membranous for a long period of time. Wormian bones de-

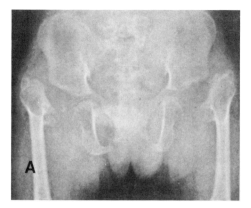

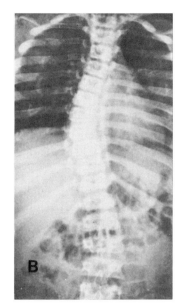

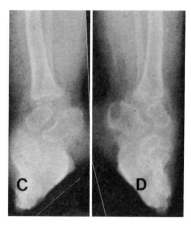

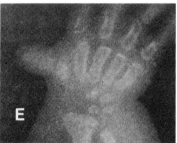

Fig. 10-96. Diastrophic dwarfism. *(A)* A radiograph of the pelvis reveals bilateral hip dislocation. The femoral heads are absent. *(B)* Severe scoliosis is present. *(C, D)* The lower extremities manifest severe joint contractures and deformities (talipes equinovarus). *(E)* The hand reveals the typically low articulating thumb, as well as other deformities within the wrist. (Courtesy of Holt, J. F., and Neuhauser, E. B. D., *In* Rubin, P.: Dynamic Classification of Bone Dysplasias. Chicago, Year Book Medical Publishers, 1964.)

velop as the cranial vault finally begins to ossify at multiple, separate ossification centers. Changes are also noted in the vertebral bodies, and in the femoral head, producing a degree of coxa vara. The pubic bones also ossify late and therefore appear to be open (Fig. 10-97D).

The nail-patella syndrome is rare but well recognized with a hypoplastic or absent patella and small dysplastic nails. Other associated radiographic findings include hypoplasia of the lateral femoral condyle and head of the fibula. Iliac horns are occasionally present (Fig. 10-98). Subluxation of the radial head has also been described. Although the bone changes are dramatic, they account for little disability or morbidity. However, one-third of the patients with this syndrome do have associated renal dysfunction, proteinuria, and subsequent renal failure. This is the result of hyaline thickening of the glomerular basement membrane and accounts for the renal abnormalities.

The capital femoral epiphyses are small and late in appearing in parastremmatic dwarfism. However, the distorted, twisted

appearance in the metaphysis is far more characteristic of this disease.

Many diseases may in some way impede overall growth and maturity. Those persisting over a longer period cause more obvious changes in epiphyseal development than does an acute process.

By contrast, inflammatory lesions affecting the joint and associated with hypervascularity cause early ossification and increased maturation of the epiphyseal centers. This has been observed frequently in juvenile rheumatoid arthritis and hemophilia.

CONE-SHAPED EPIPHYSES

Cone-shaped epiphyses in the phalanges are found in approximately 4 per cent of normal children. These are commonly noted in the foot, especially in females. The morphologic appearance of cone-shaped epiphyses varies considerably, and attempts have been made to categorize specific forms of bone dysplasia on the basis of these variations. Basically, cone-shaped epiphyses in the hand are nonspecific findings, although

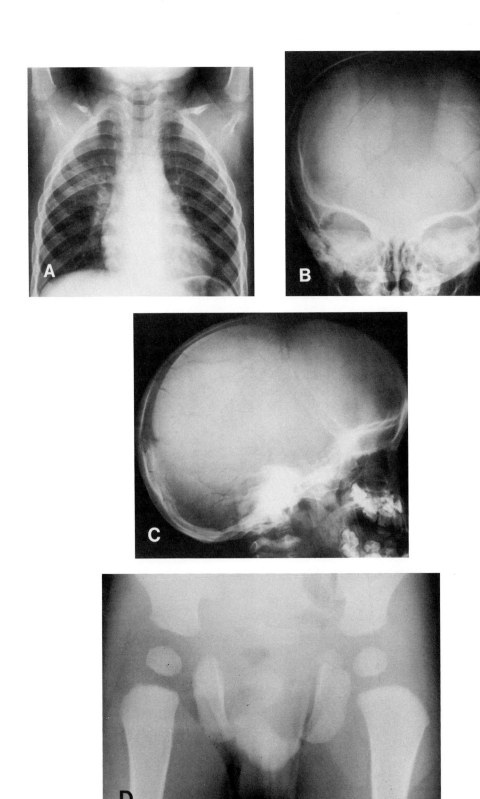

Fig. 10-97. Cleidocranial dysostosis. (*A*) Examination of the chest reveals severely hypoplastic and abnormally formed clavicles. This is best seen on the right where two ossifications centers are seen. The lateral ossification on the left is missing. Note also the stippled left humeral epiphysis. (*B, C*) Examination of the skull reveals markedly widened sutures. Multiple wormian bones are visualized. (*D*) The pubic bones are unossified.

they are prominent in the tricho-rhino-phalangeal syndrome and peripheral dysostosis.

Disease Entities

Tricho-rhino-phalangeal syndrome
Peripheral dysostosis
Ellis-van Creveld syndrome (chondroecto-dermal dysplasia)
Dyggve-Melchior-Claussen syndrome
Pseudohypoparathyroidism
Asphyxiating thoracic dystrophy
Parastremmatic dwarfism
Cleidocranial dysplasia
Oto-palato-digital syndrome
Larsen's disease
Achondroplasia
Pituitary dwarfism

Differential Diagnosis

Cone-shaped epiphyses in the hands are characteristic radiographic findings in the tricho-rhino-phalangeal syndrome (Fig. 10-99). The patients are short, with fine, sparse hair and unusually thin nails. The most prominent features of the face are a pear-shaped nose and increased nasolabial distance. Two main types seem to predominate. Type I characteristically demonstrates brachydactyly, large middle phalangeal joints, and ulnar deviation of the fingers (Fig. 10-99).

Patients with Type II manifest evidence of microcephaly and mental retardation. The joint are lax and the bones show multiple exostosis, which, associated with cone-shaped epiphyses, is diagnostic, but appears only after the 3rd year of life. Changes similar to those of Legg-Calvè-Perthes disease may occur in the capital femoral epiphyses.

Peripheral dysostosis is characterized essentially by short stature, small phalanges, and cone-shaped epiphyses in the proximal middle and distal phalanges. In addition to this, the proximal phalanges also assume different configurations. Frequently, they have a heart or a V-shaped notch. The cardinal findings are shortening of the metacarpals and metatarsals (Fig. 10-100).

The hands of patients with the Dyggve-Melchior-Claussen syndrome also show cone-shaped epiphyses in the phalanges. However, the disorder is extremely rare and becomes apparent during infancy and early childhood. The vertebral bodies are flat and have a characteristic notch on their inferior and superior surface, which has caused confusion with Morquio's syndrome. Irregular metaphyseal and epiphyseal ossification is also present, and the pelvis is short and broad. The capital femoral epiphysis appears late and manifests a characteristic spur on the medial aspect of the neck. The disease differs from Morquio's syndrome; no mucopolysaccharides are traceable in the urine, and affected children are mentally retarded.

The Ellis-van Creveld syndrome is a form of short-limbed dwarfism associated with postaxial polydactyly and disordered growth of nails, hair, and teeth. In the older child, cone-shaped epiphyses may be seen in the middle and terminal phalanges (Fig. 10-101A). In contrast to patients with achondroplasia, the distal part of the extremities are short. Polydactyly occurs only in the hand and on the side of the little finger. The borders of the metaphysis are rounded, and the humerus and femur may be broad and thick. The pelvis is short and a characteristic hook-like projection extends down the medial or sometimes lateral aspect of the acetabular roof (Fig. 10-101E). The upper tibial epiphysis is displaced medially, resulting in genu valgum. Other radiographic findings include a dislocated radial head and fused capitate and hamate bones.

In some cases of pseudohypoparathyroidism, cone-shaped epiphyses may appear following premature fusion of the epiphyses. The latter feature results in short third and fourth metacarpals and some of the phalanges (Fig. 10-102). The most characteristic finding is calcification of the basal ganglion.

The oto-palato-digital syndrome is a hereditary disorder which includes certain characteristic facial and digital abnormalties. The facial features include prominent supraorbital ridges, a depressed nasal bridge, maxillary and malar flattening, and a cleft palate. The thumbs are small and broad, and there is usually a large, conical epiphysis that disappears with age. The second metacarpal is undertubulated. There is a curious medial deviation of the fingers, best observed in the fifth finger (Fig. 10-103).

(Text continued on p. 470.)

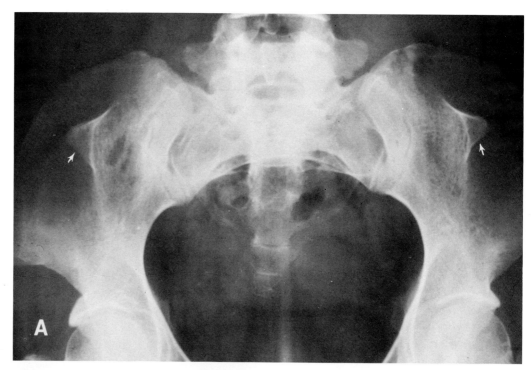

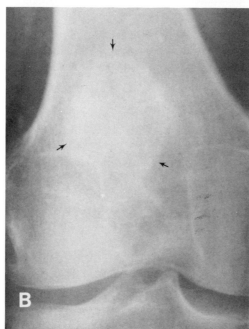

Fig. 10-98. Nail-patella syndrome. *(A)* Iliac horns.
Note the bony projections arising posteriorly from
both iliac bones. *(B)* A small patella is also present
in the same patient.

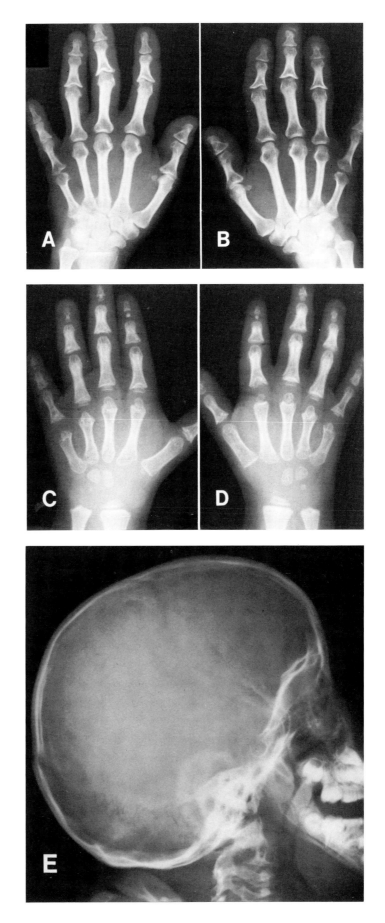

Fig. 10-99. Tricho-rhino-pha-langeal syndrome. The hands in a mother *(A, B)* and child *(C, D)* both reveal cone-shaped epiphyses involving most of the phalanges. The middle phan-geal joints are large and are as-sociated with ulnar deviation of the phalanges. *(E)* The skull of the child shows increased nasolabial distance. This was also noted in the mother.

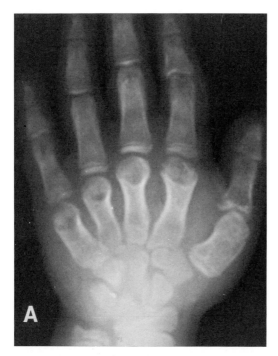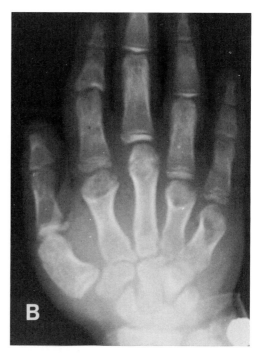

Fig. 10-100. Peripheral dysostosis. *(A, B)* Gross abnormalities involve the metacarpals, which are remarkably short. The distal ends of most of the bones are cone-shaped.

There is nothing radiographically distinctive about the pituitary dwarf. The bones are proportionately small in all dimensions but structurally normal. Cone-shaped epiphyses are unusually common in the hand.

Discussion

Many of the disorders associated with cone-shaped epiphyses are rare. Tricho-rhino-phalangeal dysplasia is associated with fine hair, a prominent nose, and a long philtrum. The two types described seem to be based on different genetic backgrounds. Type I is probably transmitted by an autosomal dominant trait, and the genetics of Type II still remains unknown.

Ellis-van Creveld syndrome is transmitted by an autosomal recessive trait. The disease has a high incidence among the Amish population. Congenital heart defects, such as a single atrium, frequently accompany the gross skeletal and other deformities.

Pseudohypoparathyroidism is basically due to an unresponsiveness of the renal tubules to parathyroid hormone. As a result, the hematologic changes are those of hypoparathyroidism, with hypocalcemia and hyperphosphatemia. The mode of inheritance is still not completely clear, although an X-linked domi-

nance may prevail. The patients are short, obese, and demonstrate a characteristic round face. Psuedopsuedohypoparathyroidism is no longer considered a separate entity but is believed to represent a variant of psuedohypoparathyroidism, with normal blood chemistry. In some instances, the parathyroids become hyperplastic, and secondary hyperparathyroidism with evidence of subperiostial absorption develops.

RINGED EPIPHYSES

Disease Entities

Scurvy
Osteopetrosis

Differential Diagnosis

The diagnosis in either scurvy or osteopetrosis is not difficult, since each has characteristic features. In addition, the appearance of the epiphyses are contrasting. For example, in scurvy, the epiphyseal ring is a thin sclerotic edge of bone surrounding a severely osteoporotic center (Fig. 10-63); in osteopetrosis, particularly in cases with fluctuating activity, a dense center is surrounded by a halo of less dense bone.

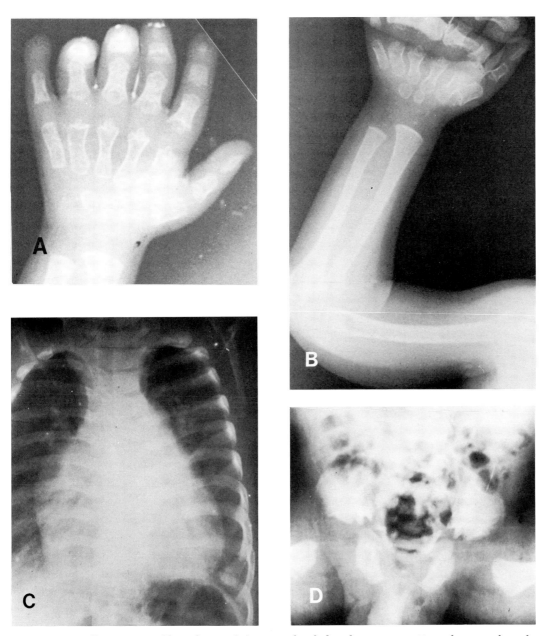

Fig. 10-101. Ellis-van Creveld syndrome. *(A)* Postaxial polydactyly is present. Irregular metaphyseal cupping and cone-shaped epiphyses are noted within the hands. *(B)* Examination of the forearm reveals a foreshortened extremity that begins within the forearm and the hand. *(C)* Examination of the heart reveals severe cardiac enlargement that is due to the presence of a single atrium. *(D)* The pelvis shows an irregular, trident acetabulum. The angle is horizontal.

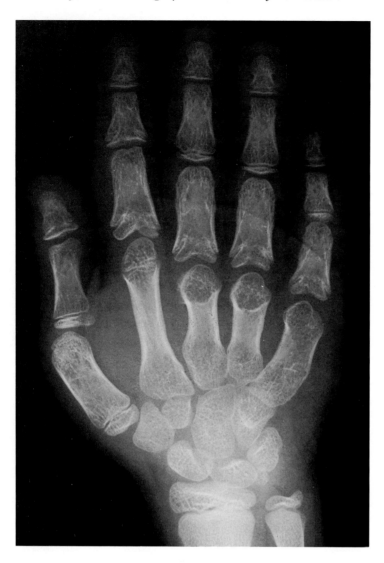

Fig. 10-102. Pseudohypoparathyroidism. Note the shortened third, fourth, and fifth metacarpals and associated cone-shaped epiphyses.

IVORY EPIPHYSES

Ivory epiphyses are dense but look normal otherwise. In general, such epiphyses have a typical shape but appear solid, with no visible trabecular structure.

Disease Entities

Ivory epiphyses in normal children
Tricho-rhino-phalangeal syndrome
Cockayne's syndrome
Epiphyseal dysplasia
Kirner's deformity
Renal osteodystrophy
Morquio's syndrome
Trisomy 18
Mucolipidosis III
Infantile idiopathic hypercalcemia

Differential Diagnosis

Distinguishing each disease entity by epiphyseal manifestations is not feasible. However, in a study of relatively normal children, the presence of ivory epiphyses was frequently associated with some degree of retarded maturation in the hand. Ivory epiphyses may be found in the distal phalanges of digits two to five in the tricho-rhino-phalangeal syndrome. Cone-shaped epiphyses, however, predominate in the rest. The association of these two unusual manifestations in a hand is therefore a strong indication of this disease. By contrast, Cockayne's syndrome frequently produces accelerated maturation of the hand with ivory epiphyses.

The additional diseases listed have demonstrated only rare association with ivory epiphyses.

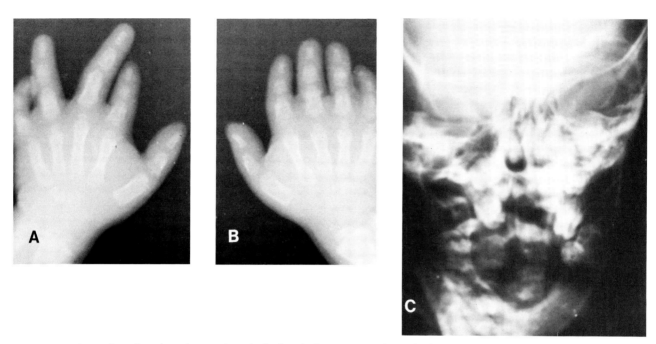

Fig. 10-103. Oto-palato-digital syndrome. *(A, B)* The hands demonstrate short, thick thumbs and an over-tubulated second metacarpal. Note the extreme medial deviation of the fifth finger. *(C)* Severe cleft palate is present.

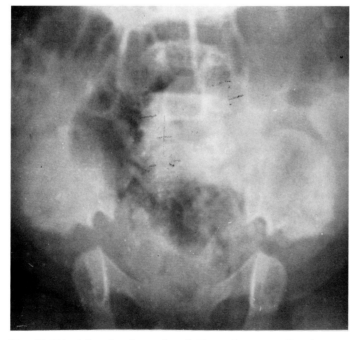

Fig. 10-104. Achondroplastic dwarf. The pelvis is small and squat, and the acetabular angle is horizontal. The interpediculate spaces are not well-defined but look narrow in the lower lumbar region.

SHORT BONES AND DWARFISM

Height less than just slightly below the third percentile signifies the presence of dwarfism. In general, two main conditions affect the ultimate growth of the skeleton: disease that primarily involves the skeleton, and systemic disease that secondarily retards growth. It is obvious that systemic disease, with the exception of cretinism, rickets, and Pott's disease, affects the overall growth pattern relatively uniformly. However, bodily proportions are usually abnormal in primary skeletal disease, which is divided into two broad groups: diseases with a known pathogenesis and diseases with an unknown pathogenesis. The first group includes the chromosomal aberrations and certain primary metabolic abnormalities, such as mucopolysaccharidosis and mucolipidosis; the second group consists of forms of osteochondrodysplasia (abnormalities of cartilage and/or bone growth development) and dysostosis (malformation of individual bones, simple or in combination). Osteochondrodysplasia can be divided into disease involving growth of tubular bones or the spine, or both (hence the terms short-limbed and short-trunk dwarf), disease characterized by disorganized development of cartilage and fibrous components of the skeleton, and disease characterized by abnormalities of bone density or the diaphyseal cortex, or abnormalities of metaphyseal modelling. Diseases affecting tubular growth or the spine are categorized by the extremity involved; proximal shortening or disproportionate shortening of the humerus and femur is known as *rhizomelic dwarfism;* shortening of the bones of the leg or forearm is known as *mesomelic dwarfism;* and shortening of small distal parts is known as *acromelic dwarfism.*

The age of the patient at the time of presentation (e.g., newborn, infant, child, or adult) is important in categorizing and analyzing the abnormalities resulting in dwarfism.

RHIZOMELIC DWARFISM

Disease Entities

Newborns
    Achondroplasia
    Chondrodysplasia punctata
Infants and Children
    Hypochondroplasia
    Pseudoachondroplasia

Differential Diagnosis

In rhizomelic dwarfism, the proximal part of the extremity is proportionately shorter than the remainder of the extremity. Achondroplasia is the classic example of rhizomelic dwarfism. The majority of cases of achondroplasia are due to spontaneous mutations, although the disease is transmitted by an autosomal dominant trait. In this disease, enchondral bone growth is abnormal although still organized. Since appositional bone growth proceeds normally, short bones of normal width are produced (Fig. 10-85). Platyspondylisis is not a feature of achondroplasia. The intervertebral disc spaces are, however, larger than normal, and the overall length of the spine is shorter. The vertebral bodies become taller as they grow, although the anteroposterior dimension of the body remains proportionately narrow. The pedicles of the lumbar spine remain short, and the neural canal is narrowed on the lateral radiograph. The interpediculate spaces also fail to widen in the lower lumbar spine (Fig. 10-104). The sacrum is narrow and articulates low on the ilium. The iliac bones are short and squat, and the sacrosciatic notches are narrow. The acetabular angle is horizontal, and the superior surface of the acetabulum is irregular in infancy. The skull is large, but the base of the skull, including the foramen magnum, is small because of the distorted enchondral bone growth. As a result, varying degrees of macrencephaly or hydrocephalus are present.

The extremities are short, and in newborns a wide and an obliquely orientated slant along the lateral margin of the distal femur is noted (Fig. 10-85). The proximal end of the femur, however, is rounded or square. In older children, the configuration of the distal metaphyses change. They become flared and produce a ball and socket appearance. This is especially noted in the distal femur (Fig. 10-85). The fibula is generally longer in length than the tibia. The ribs are short, with an overall decrease in the ventrodorsal diameter of the thorax.

It is not difficult to differentiate achondroplasia from most other forms of dwarfism in infancy such as achondrogenesis and thanatophoric dwarfism, which result in infant death and are both characterized by generalized micromelia. Achondrogenesis also demonstrates unossified or partially ossified vertebral bodies.

Asphyxiating thoracic dysplasia has also been confused with achondroplasia in newborns, although the extremities are not quite as short in the former. The pelvis resembles that of the achondroplastic dwarf, except for the absence of the squared ilia. However, the pelvis becomes normal with age, and the interpediculate spaces are normal. Asphyxiating thoracic dysplasia is accompanied by respiratory distress in the neonatal period and repeated pulmonary infections in infancy and childhood.

The rhizomelic form of chondrodysplasia punctata is not difficult to recognize. The structural abnormality of the extremities is overshadowed by the large and irregularly ossified epiphyses in all the extremities. These children rarely survive the neonatal period.

In older children, hypochondroplasia is occasionally difficult to distinguish from achondroplasia. The main difference is the apparent degree of skeletal abnormality, since the changes are not severe in hypochondroplasia. In fact, the patients are often mistaken for being constitutionally short. They do nevertheless, manifest some degree of narrowing of the interpediculate spaces, cranial frontal bossing (the skull is, nevertheless, usually normal), and abnormally narrow sciatic notches (Fig. 10-105). They also have an exaggerated lumbar lordosis, abdominal protuberance, and short limbs. Many physicians feel that hypochondroplasia is probably more common than anticipated. The disease becomes clinically obvious as the child matures.

Pseudoachrondroplasia is a form of short-limbed dwarfism, with bodily proportions resembling those of achondroplasia. However, pseudoachondroplasia is usually not evident until after the 1st year of life, and the face and skull are always normal. The vertebral bodies in pseudoachondroplasia are characteristically flattened and irregular and demonstrate an exaggerated, tongue-like protrusion in the central portion of the body (Fig. 10-89). These findings, surprisingly, become normal in adolescence. The pelvis of the pseudoachondroplastic dwarf shows irregular ossification of the ischial and pubic bones. The interpediculate spaces usually do not taper caudally. The metaphyses of the long tubular bones are angular, irregular, and cupped. As a result, the zones of provisional calcification are irregularly ossified. Valgus deformity occurs readily. This amount of ir-

regularity and disorganization of the extremities is never encountered in the achondroplastic dwarf.

Differentiating epiphyseal dysplasia congenita from pseudoachondroplasia may be a real problem. The epiphyseal centers in the hand are smaller and more irregular in epiphyseal centers in the hand are smaller and more irregular in epiphyseal dysplasia. This amount of irregularity and disorganization of the extremities is never encountered in achondroplasia.

MESOMELIC DWARFISM

Disease Entities

Dyschondrosteosis
Chondroectodermal dysplasia
Robinow-Silverman dwarfism
Acromesomelic dwarfism
Mesomelic dwarfism
Cornelia de Lange syndrome

Differential Diagnosis

One of the best known forms of mesomelic dysplasia is dyschondrosteosis of Leri-Weil. This autosomal dominant disease usually presents later in childhood, with short stature and a characteristically abnormal wrist called Madelung's deformity. The abnormality is usually bilateral, and the legs and forearms appear disporportionately shortened. The degree of involvement varies, resulting in different degrees of dwarfism and mesomelic abnormalities.

The carpal angle is decreased in Madelung's deformity, and the articular surfaces of the radius and ulna are angled toward each other, producing a V-shaped space between them (Fig. 10-106). The lunate bone is displaced proximally into the deep recess created between the articular margins of the distal radius and ulna. The radius is bowed laterally, exaggerating the interosseous space, and the distal end of the ulna shows subluxation dorsally. Proximally, the radius may be flared at its articulation with the capitellum.

Most forms of mesomelic dwarfism are not difficult to distinguish from each other because of characteristic patterns. Differentiation from other forms of dwarfism, however, may not be as simple.

Pseudoachondroplasia can be easily distinguished from dychondrosteosis; mesomelia is not a predominant feature of pseudoachon-

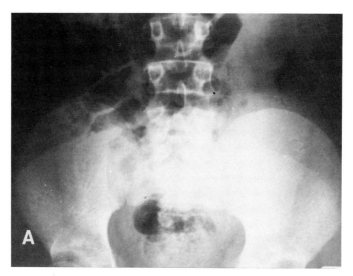

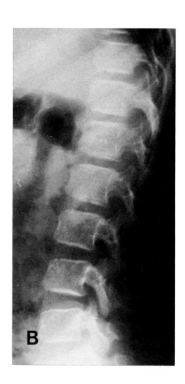

Fig. 10-105. Hypochondroplasia. (A) The pelvis is small, although the acetabula appear normal. Note the narrowed interpediculate spaces within the lower lumbar region. (B) The lumbar spine has an abnormal configuration. The anteroposterior diameter appears smaller than usual, and distinct cupping is noted posteriorly. (C, D, E, F) The distal metaphyses show evidence of cupping and flaring.

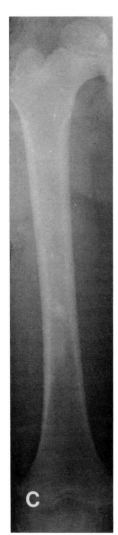

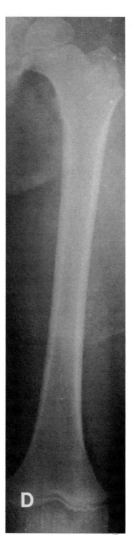

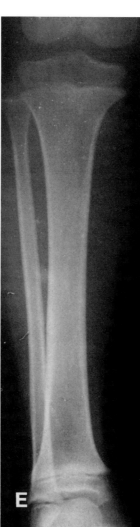

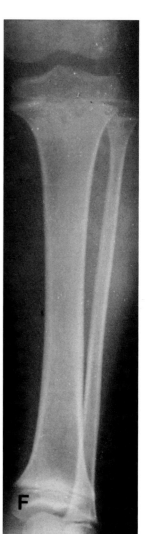

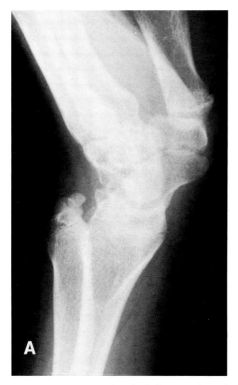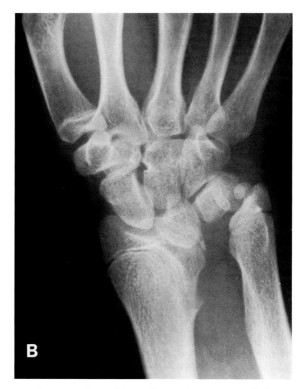

Fig. 10-106. Madelung's deformity. *(A, B)* The articulating surface of the radius and ulna are angled toward each other, producing a V-shaped notch between them, into which the lunate bone is displaced.

droplasia, and dysplasia of the metaphyses and involvement of the spine are characteristic. Mesomelia is a prominent feature in the acromesomelic form of dwarfism. However, acromelia is also present and is severe enough to overshadow any form of brachydactyly that may be seen in dyschondrosteosis. Unlike dyschondrosteosis, acromesomelic dwarfs have an ulna shorter than the radius, and the radial head is dislocated dorsally. All the bones of the extremities are shortened in acromesomelic dwarfism. However, the epiphyses and metaphyses are usually normal.

There are two distinct forms of mesomelic dwarfism that occur early in infancy, and they are easily distinguishable from dyschondrosteosis. The Nievergelt form is an autosomal dominant disease. Affected patients present at birth with a deformed leg. The striking feature of this disease is the short, triangular, or rhomboid, hatchet-head appearance of the tibia. Shortening of the fibula is also present. Radioulnar synostosis and tarsal synostosis may be present. As in acromesomelic dwarfism, there may be dorsal dislocation of the radial head.

In the Langer form, there is shortening of all of the long bones. This is most evident in the forearms and legs. A distinguishing feature is hypoplasia of the proximal fibula and distal ulna. The tibia and radius are markedly shortened. The radius is also severely bowed. The ribs, spine, and pelvis are normal in both forms of mesomelic dwarfism, as they are in dyschondrosteosis.

Hypoplasia of the fibula and ulna can be seen in the Reinhardt-Pfeiffer type of ulno-fibular dysplasia, but these patients are not as severely effected as patients with the Langer form of mesomelic dwarfism. However, there has been some question that ulno-fibular dysplasia may be related to Nievergelt's syndrome.

The Ellis-van Creveld syndrome is a form of short-limbed dwarfism characterized by progressive distal shortening of the extremities (Fig. 10-101). Other important radiographic findings are postaxial hexadactyly, thoracic dystrophy, dental abnormalities, and cardiac defects such as a single atrium. The pelvis is squat and the base of the iliac bones are low and hook downward, producing a trident configuration in the acetabular region. Genu valgus is a characteristic, with inadequate development of the lat-

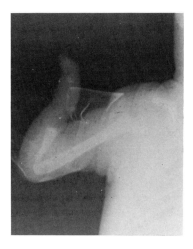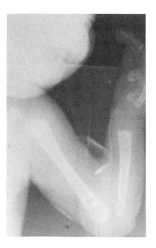

Fig. 10-107. Cornelia de Lange syndrome. Examination of the upper extremities of a patient with Cornelia de Lange syndrome reveals complete absence of the ulna. The residual radii are hypoplastic. This is best visualized on the right. Many phalanges are absent and symphalangism is present.

eral aspect of the tibial epiphysis and lateral drop-off of the proximal tibial metaphysis. Micromelia is present, and the metaphysis have a dumbbell shape due to flaring of their lower ends. These manifestations help to distinguish this syndrome from asphyxiating thoracic dysplasia. Both manifest a small thorax with short ribs, abnormal pelvis, polydactyly, and short legs below the knee. However, ectodermal dysplasia, cardiac defects, tibial defects, and fusion of hamate and capitate bones are not encountered in asphyxiating thoracic dysplasia. Mesomelic brachymelia is also a part of the Robinow-Silverman syndrome, which is characterized by short but otherwise normally formed leg and forearm bones, hypertelorism, macrocephaly, hemivertebra, and other less frequent abnormalities. Grossly, aside from the relatively normal bones, the patient resembles an achrondroplastic dwarf.

The Cornelia de Lange syndrome is discussed here because of the not uncommon association with ulnar hypoplasia or aplasia (Fig. 10-107). This deformity is far less frequent than absence of the radius and is therefore almost pathognomonic of this syndrome. Other skeletal anomalies are a lack of phalanges and a small skull. When all the phalanges are present, the first metacarpal and the middle phalange of the second and fifth digits are short. The physical features are typical and are easily recognized. In general, the infants are short, mentally retarded, and have a characteristic hirsutism.

Seckel's syndrome (bird-headed dwarfism) has also been associated with proximal hypoplasia of the radius and fibula, a lack of

epiphyses in the hand, and clinodactyly. Affected infants manifest mental retardation and a small neurocranium, in which the sutures close prematurely.

MESOMELIA AND POLYDACTYLY

Disease Entities
Ellis-van Creveld syndrome
Asphyxiating thoracic dystrophy
Short rib polydactyly (Saldino-Noonan form)
Short rib polydactyly (Majewski type)

Differential Diagnosis

These syndromes are all characterized by short limbs and postaxial polydactyly. The asphyxiating thoracic dystrophy and the Ellis-van Creveld syndromes are more common and bear striking resemblances to each other. There are, nevertheless, some distinguishing changes. In the neonatal period, the dysplastic nails and abnormalities of the upper limb are more common in chrondoectodermal dysplasia. Radiographic differences, however, may be more difficult to recognize in this period, since the changes relating to the epiphyses and the thorax are similar. However, the accessory digit in the Ellis-van Creveld syndrome is usually present on the side of the little finger, whereas in asphyxiating thoracic dystrophy, it is located on the thumb side. The bones, in general, appear to be more normal in length in the asphyxiating thoracic dystrophy syndrome. In later childhood, the short-limbed segments are more characteristic in the Ellis-van Creveld syn-

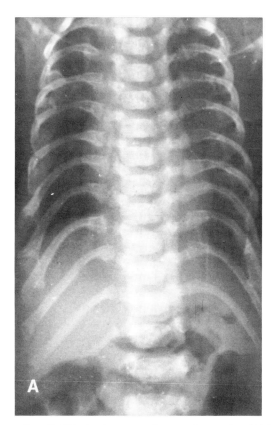 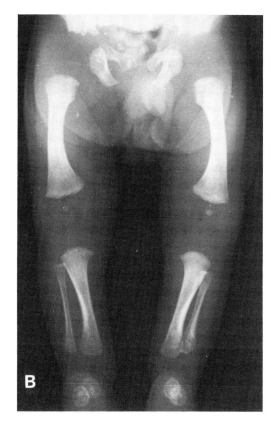

Fig. 10-108. Asphyxiating thoracic dystrophy. *(A)* Examination of the chest reveals a long, narrow thorax with relatively short ribs. *(B)* The pelvis is somewhat irregular and resembles the that of Ellis-van Creveld syndrome. Note also the shortened extremities.

drome, in which the deformity of the upper tibia and the fused hamate bones are quite characteristic. The Majewski and Saldino-Noonan types are distinct but exceptionally rare varieties of short-limbed dwarfism. The cardiovascular and renal anomalies are common in the Saldino-Noonan syndrome. In addition, the radiographic changes consisting of short, ragged ends of the long bones differ from the smooth and rounded configuration noted in the Majewski syndrome.

GENERALIZED MICROMELIC DWARFISM

Disease Entities

Thanatophoric dwarfism
Achrondrogenesis
Short rib polydactyly
Kniest dwarfism
Metatrophic dwarfism
Diastrophic dwarfism
Camptomelic dwarfism
Asphyxiating thoracic dystrophy

Differential Diagnosis

Many of the disease entities listed have already been discussed in this chapter. Although at one time some of these were considered to be variations of achrondroplasia, each shows characteristic manifestations. Micromelia in the thanatophoric dwarf is associated with curved femurs (Fig. 10-95); the ribs are short and the vertebral bodies flat. Achondrogenesis, by definition, is characterized by a poorly ossified skeleton and a large skull. The chief feature in asphyxiating thoracic dystrophy is the narrow cylindrical thorax with flared ribs (Fig. 10-108). The limbs are not remarkably short but postaxial polydactyly is an important feature. The disease is manifested at birth, but the deformities become less severe with growth. Unfortunately, there is a high incidence of renal disease in this syndrome, which becomes more severe with growth and results in progressive renal failure and death. The forms of short rib polydactyly also result in shortened limbs. The Saldino-Noonan form demonstrates short, irregular long bones in compar-

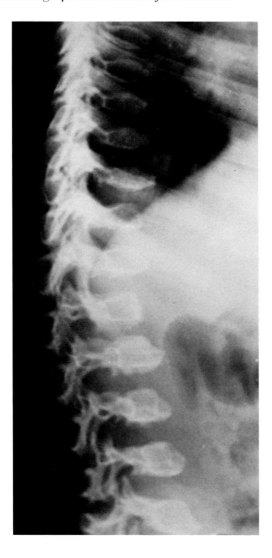

Fig. 10-109. Hurler's syndrome. The vertebral bodies in the lower lumbar region demonstrate a characteristic hook along their inferior margins. This abnormal configuration produces a suggestively small vertebral body. Note the flattened dorsal vertebrae.

ison to the smoothly rounded ends of the long bones in the Majewski type.

Metatrophic and Kniest dwarfs both have wide, flared, irregular metaphyses that distinguish them from other micromelic dwarfs. However, the thorax is narrow in the metatrophic dwarf and broad in the Kniest dwarf (Figs. 10-79, 10-80). In addition, the Kniest dwarf shows facial changes consisting of hypertelorism, cleft palate, and a depressed nasal bridge.

Diastrophic dwarfs have short limbs and severe skeletal deformities, such as scoliosis, talipes equinovarus, and joint contractures. The hands and feet are quite broad, and the thumb is placed too far proximally (Fig. 10-96A).

Comptomelic dwarfism is discussed here because of the apparent shortening of the limbs due to extreme bowing of the tubular bones of the lower extremity. The femurs and radii are often hypoplastic. Craniofacial abnormalities are also present that include a flat face, hypertelorism, micrognathia, and a cleft palate. In addition, a calcaneo-valgus deformity is often present. Many captomelic dwarfs die in the neonatal period.

LETHAL SHORT-LIMBED DWARFISM

Disease Entities
Thanatophoric dwarfism
Achondrogenesis
Asphyxiating thoracic dystrophy
Short Rib Polydactyly
Camptomelic dwarfism

Differential Diagnosis

Most of these disease entities are discussed elsewhere. They are grouped together here simply because they all indicate a poor prognosis in the majority of cases.

PLATYSPONDYLISIS

Disease Entities

Cephaloskeletal dysplasia
Kniest dwarfism
Metatropic dwarfism
Mucopolysaccharidosis
Osteogenesis imperfecta congenita
Parastremmatic dwarfism
Spondyloepiphyseal dysplasia congenita
Spondylometaphyseal dysplasia
Thanatophoric dwarfism
Dyggve-Melchoir-Claussen syndrome
Brachyolmia

Differential Diagnosis

Spondyloepiphyseal dysplasia congenita is an excellent example of dwarfism resulting in a shortened trunk. This autosomal dominant disease presents at birth, with radiographic findings of retarded skeletal maturation and platyspondylisis. In neonates, the vertebral bodies are of diminished vertical dimension, with posterior portions of the body being smaller than anterior portions, particularly in the dorsal spine (Fig. 10-94A). Such asymmetry may be apparent to a lesser degree in normal subjects, but as the patient with spondyloepiphyseal dysplasia grows, the vertebral bodies in the upper lumbar and lower thoracic spine develop a pointed appearance. Children with the Kozlowski type do not present at birth. The vertebrae are remarkably flattened, and in infancy and childhood they have a more rectangular appearance as growth and development proceed. The distinguishing feature is the irregular metaphyses in the long bones, which are most marked in the proximal femurs.

The vertebral bodies manifest impressive changes in both mucopolysaccharidosis and mucolipidosis. Most demonstrate an underdeveloped anterosuperior portion; the inferior part of the vertebral body projects forward and produces a broad, hook-like appearance (Fig. 10-109). This configuration occurs mainly in the last thoracic and first lumbar vertebrae and is associated with kyphosis. The severity of the vertebral deformity is variable in most of such storage diseases. Frequently, however, it is not observed in mucopolysaccharidosis Type V (Scheie's syndrome) and is poorly developed in Type III (Sanfillippo's syndrome). In Type IV (Morquio's syndrome), these vertebral changes may be noted in infancy. However, little subsequent increase in height of the vertebral body develops, and the ultimate configuration is platyspondylisis with a central, protruding tongue (Fig. 10-110). Morquio's syndrome is distinguished from the other forms of mucopolysaccharidosis and mucolipidosis by the presence of a poorly developed odontoid process and a pelvis that shows flared iliac wings, oblique acetabular roofs, and loss of the femoral neck angle. The flared iliac wings are greatest just above the anterior iliac spines, in contrast to the typical pelvis in Hurler's syndrome (Fig. 10-111). The joints in Morquio's syndrome are lax in comparision to the stiff joints in other types of storage diseases. This accounts for the genu valgum noted in this disease. Pectus carinatum is another major radiographic finding.

The Dyggve-Melchoir-Claussen syndrome has been confused with Morquio's syndrome because both deonstrate flat vertebral bodies that have a characteristic notch on the inferior and superior surface.

Typical features of Hurler's syndrome include a scaphocephalic skull, with thickened diploë and an enlarged, J-shaped sella turcica. The facial bones are small and the madibular condyles are hypoplastic or absent. The thorax is typical and manifests widened ribs anteriorly. The clavicles are short, thick, and may be hypoplastic or aplastic distally. The heart is enlarged (Fig. 10-112A). The long bones are thick and in the hands the phalanges and metacarpals show a thick shaft and a lack of diaphyseal modelling. The proximal ends are pointed (Fig. 10-112B).

In the neonate and young infant, thanatophoric, metatropic, and Kniest dwarfs present with platyspondylisis. The portion of the flat vertebral bodies in thanatophoric dwarfs is different from that of other neonatal dwarfs. The bodies are more biconcave and in the lumber region are bulbous anteriorly or are angular. The ribs are very short. Early death is the rule.

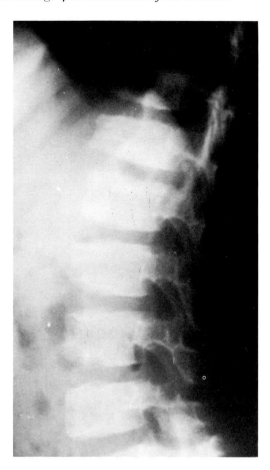

Fig. 10-110. Morquio's syndrome. A patient with Morquio's syndrome demonstrates flattened vertebral bodies, with a central protuding tongue.

Severe platyspondylisis is characteristic of the metatropic dwarf, although the shape is altogether different. The vertebrae are biconvex and more angular, sometimes demonstrating a diamond configuration (Fig. 10-113). Later, anterior wedging occurs and progressive kyphoscoliosis develops. The spine then becomes disproportionately short in comparison to the extremities, and a short trunk is the ultimate result.

The spine of Kniest dwarfs also demonstrates anterior wedging, but posterior deficiency is not present, as in metatropic dwarfism. The degree of platyspondylisis is, therefore, not as severe in the Kniest syndrome. A distinctive feature is the presence of cleft vertebral bodies, which are not evident in metatropic dwarfs. The extremities are similar in both but distinguishable.

Brachyolmia is of little clinicial importance and is characterized only by vertebral body flattening.

Discussion

Mucopolysaccharidosis and mucolipidosis are a group of storage diseases caused by enzymatic deficiences. They all have distinctive clinicial biochemical differences but demonstrate strikingly similar radiographic manifestations. In mucopolysaccharidosis Type IV the abnormal mucopolysaccharide is keratin sulphate. Dermatan sulphate or heparin sulphate, or a combination of both, are the abnormal polysaccharides in the other forms of mucopolysacchridosis. In mucolipidosis, there is no mucopolysacchariduria; mucopolysaccharides, glycolipid, and sphingolipids are stored in the tissue. This suggests that forms of mucolipidosis are related to both mucopolysaccharidosis and lipidosis. Lipidosis is an inborn error of metabolism in which a specific alteration in the lipid content of tissue occurs. The anatomic landmark in forms of lipidosis is the formation of a foam cell. Gaucher's dis-

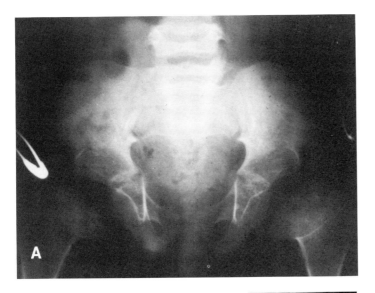

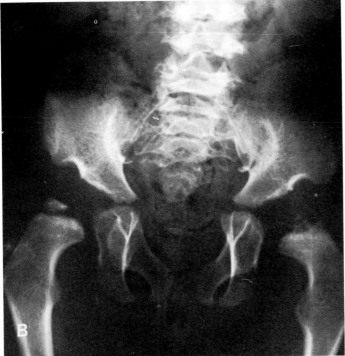

Fig. 10-111. Mucopolysaccharidosis. (A) Morquio's syndrome. The pelvis is somewhat short and broad. There is flaring of the iliac wings just above the acetabulum. Coxa vara is obvious. Note that there are no femoral capital epiphyses. (B) Hurler's syndrome. The pelvis is characteristic, showing a distinct irregularity of the acetabulum, as well as a coxa valga.

Table 10-1. Features of Storage Diseases

Disease	Onset	Clinical Features	Mucopolysaccharide in Urine	Defective Enzyme	Inheritance
Mucopolysaccharidosis					
Type I (Hurler's syndrome)	Early	Dwarfism, mental retardation, death at 10–15 years	Dermatan and heparin sulphate	L-Iduronidase	Autosomal recessive
Type II (Hunter's syndrome)	Age 6–12 months	Similar to those of Type I; affects males only	Dermatan and heparin sulphate	Sulphoiduronate sulphatase	X-linked recessive
Type III (Sanfilippo's syndrome)	Childhood	Mental retardation; may have no radiographic findings	Heparin sulphate	Acetyl-glucosaminidase	Autosomal recessive
Type IV (Morquio's syndrome)	Age 2–4 years	Dwarfism; normal intelligence	Keratin sulphate	?	Autosomal recessive
Type V (Scheie's syndrome)	Late childhood	Little skeletal changes; normal intelligence	Dermatan sulphate	L-Iduronidase	Autosomal recessive
Type VI (Maroteaux-Lamy syndrome)	Childhood	Skeletal changes similar to those of Type I	Dermatan sulphate	N-Ac-Gal-4-sulfatase	Autosomal recessive
Mucolipodosis					
Mucolipidosis I	Birth	Same as Hunter's syndrome		β-galactosidase	Autosomal recessive
Mucolipidosis II (I-cells)	Early infancy	Same as Hunter's syndrome			Autosomal recessive
Mucolipidosis III	Age 2–3 years	Same as Hunter's syndrome with claw hand and carpal tunnel syndrome			Autosomal recessive
Mannosidosis	Early	Same as Hurler's syndrome; no bone changes			Autosomal recessive

(Wynne-Davies, R., and Fairbank, T. J.: Fairbank's Atlas of General Affections of the Skeleton. ed. 2. Edinburgh, Churchill Livingstone, 1976.)

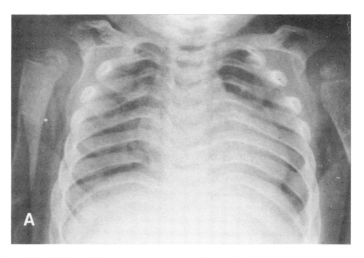

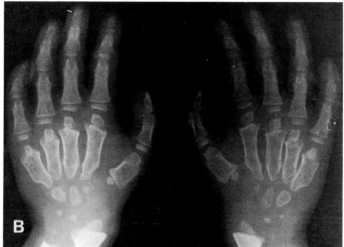

Fig. 10-112. Hurler's syndrome. *(A)* The chest radiograph is characteristic. The ribs are markedly widened anteriorly, producing a spatula shape. Similar widening is also noted in the extremities as well as the clavicles. The cardiac silhouette is also enlarged. *(B)* The same patient demonstrates widening of the shaft of the metacarpals, with a triangular configuration along the proximal margins.

ease, Neimann-Pick disease, and Tay-Sachs disease are included in this group of diseases.

Extra-skeletal disorders (e.g., endocrine, renal, gastrointestinal, cardiopulmonary) may result in short stature. Pituitary dwarfism is characterized by normal bodily proportions. However, a variety of types exist that are categorized by the deficient hormone. Basically, pituitary dwarfs are divided into two groups according to sexual maturity. Bone age can be severely retarded in the asexual pituitary dwarf. The role of the radiologist is to exclude recognizable organic lesions. Diencephalic tumors cause poor growth and weight gain, despite the presence of a voracious appetite. This combination is known as the diencephalic syndrome.

A common cause of transient dwarfism in children in constitutionally delayed growth, in which both puberty and its attendant growth spurt are delayed. When puberty arrives, growth may be agonizingly slow or rapid, and the child eventually attains a height commensurate with his genetic predisposition.

A relatively important and not too uncommon cause of growth failure is neglect and abuse. This form of psychosocial dwarfism is the result of inadequate mothering and emotional support at home. A change in environment quickly reverses this syndrome. One should be aware that once these children start to improve, they may have abnormally wide calvarial sutures.

Other causes of poor growth are chromosomal abnormalities, primordial dwarfism (caused by unknown factors), intrauterine growth retardation, progeria, liprachaunism, Cockayne's syndrome, and Bloom's syndrome.

RADIAL DYSPLASIA

The severity of radial dysplasia ranges from slight hypoplasia to aplasia. Since alteration of the radius is associated with first ray abnormalities (anomalies of the thumbs and first metacarpals), particularly severe hypoplasia or absence of the first thumb and its associated metacarpal are manifested. The resulting radiographic picture is a shortened forearm due to a correspondingly severe curvature involving the ulna. The wrist is flexed and a J- or L-shaped configuration of the extremity is produced (Fig. 10-114).

Disease Entities
Idiopathic radial dysplasia
Thrombocytopenia with radial aplasia
Trisomy 18
Esophageal atresia
Fanconi's anemia
Holt-Oram syndrome
Phocomelia
Mesomelic dwarfism (Langer type)

Differential Diagnosis

Radial dysplasia is an interesting anomaly and occurs frequently as an isolated finding. However, newborns with Fanconi's anemia may present with this anomaly and with little other obvious disease. Radial dysplasia is an integral and prominant feature of the disease. Aside from the changes involving the thumbs, first metacarpal, and radii, which are variable, syndactyly, clubfoot, and congenital dislocation of the hip and various soft-tissue deformities may be visible. Soft-tissue changes consist of patchy brown pigmentation of the skin due to deposition of melanin. Dwarfism, hypogenitalism, cryptorchidism, mental retardation, and renal abnormalities may also be present. The hematologic abnormalities in this syndrome are not usually apparent until the patients are several years old, although they have been seen as early as 15 months. Consequently, the bone and soft-tissue changes are of vital importance in making a prognosis. Fanconi's anemia resembles thrombocytopenia with radial aplasia, although they differ in the time of onset and the nature of the hematologic disorder. Thrombocytopenia is usually present at birth in the latter and tends to regress as the child matures.

Radial dysplasia has also been associated with esophageal atresia. Trisomy 18 occasionally presents with radial dysplasia, and in a few cases is also accompanied by esophageal atresia and thromobocytopenia (Fig. 10-60). This association of embryologic events suggests that all of these basic defects may be related somehow to chromosome 18. Other radiographic findings associated with Trisomy 18 are small thin bones, cardiac disease (ventricular septal defect), and a small pelvis with an antimongoloid slant of the iliac bones (Fig. 10-115). The skull looks dolichocephalic, with a fairly large, protruding posterior fossa.

The Holt-Oram syndrome is a familial disorder consisting basically of cardiac and skeletal abnormalities (Fig. 10-116). The skeletal deformities are mainly limited to the upper limb, and more specifically the thumb and wrist. Hypoplasia, aplasia, or a finger-like (triphalangial) appearance of the thumb may occur. In addition, an interdigital skin fold is present between the first and second fingers. The first metacarpal and radius are frequently hypoplastic or aplastic, and in severe cases phocomelia is also present. Less frequently described skeletal abnormalities include dislocation of the shoulder, coracoclavicular joints, and cervical ribs. The cardiac abnormality consists basically of an atrial septal defect. A ventricular septal defect has also been described.

The Langer type of mesomelic dwarfism is a rare abnormality and is associated with hypoplasia of the radius and absence of the proximal portion of the ulna.

The forearm changes in the Cornelia de Lange syndrome have been mistaken for radial dysplasia, but the ulna is actually hypoplastic or aplastic. This ulnar anomaly is almost pathognomonic of this syndrome, since it is far less common than radial dysplasia (Fig. 10-117).

BODY ASYMMETRY

The term asymmetry is used here en lieu of hypertrophy to designate unequal body growth, since the changes are often too subtle to distinguish the abnormal side. Selective enlargement is variable in extent and severity. An entire side (hemihypertrophy), a section, or only a single structure may be in-

(Text continued on p. 490.)

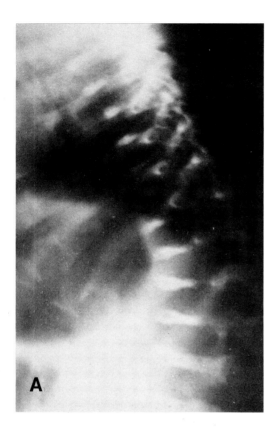

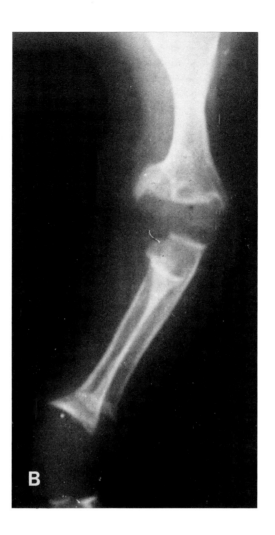

Fig. 10-113. Metatropic dwarf. (A) The vertebral bodies are biconvex and more angular, suggesting a diamond configuration. (B) The upper extremity is short, with characteristic bulbous flaring at the metaphyseal ends.

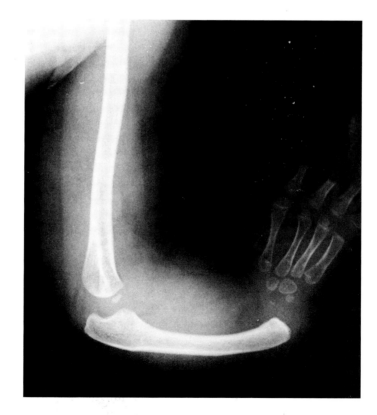

Fig. 10-114. Radial dysplasia in Fanconi's anemia. The characteristic J-shaped configuration involves the upper extremity. The entire radius is missing, and the ulna is somewhat foreshortened and curved. Severe hypoplasia of the first thumb and its associated metacarpal is present.

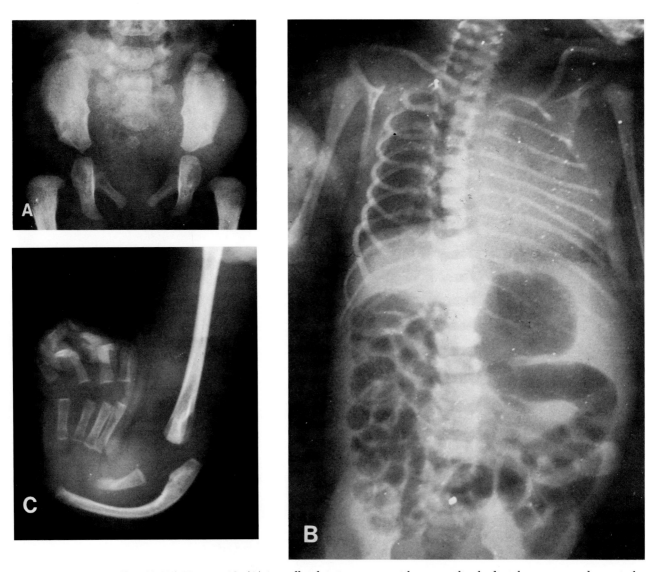

Fig. 10-115. Trisomy 18. *(A)* A small pelvis is present, with narrow iliac bodies that are rotated anteriorly, an anti-monogloid pelvis. *(B)* The chest and abdomen in a patient with Trisomy 18 reveal cardiac enlargement due to an intraventricular septal defect. The bones are thin and gracile. Malrotation is seen in the abdomen. Note the colon on the left and the small bowel on the right. *(C)* The radius is hypoplastic and the first metacarpal and phalange are absent. The ulna is severely bowed, and the extremity has a J-shaped configuration.

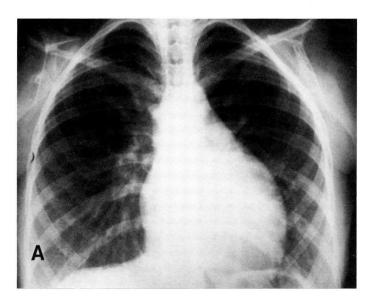

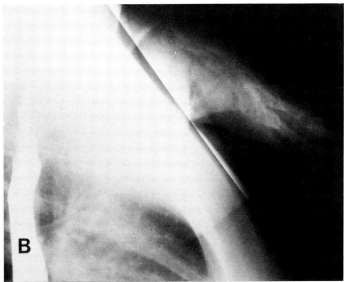

Fig. 10-116. Holt-Oram syndrome. *(A)* A young female in her teens showed cardiac enlargement and increased vascularity, with an atrial septal defect. Note the small humeri articulating with the scapulas. *(B)* Phocomelia is present in a sibling of the patient in *A*. The extremity consists only of parts of the hand that hang, as an appendage, from the upper portion of the patient's thorax.

volved (Fig. 10-118). In general, the gross structures as well as the basic tissue elements are involved in the hypertrophied region. Underdevelopment also produces asymmetry and can be congenital or acquired.

Disease Entities

Overgrowth
  Regional asymmetry
    Neurocutaneous syndromes
    Skin and vascular malformations
    Beckwith-Wiedemann syndrome
  Hemihypertrophy
    Idiopathic hemihypertrophy
    Beckwith-Wiedemann syndrome
    Wilms' tumor
    Adrenal tumors
Undergrowth
  Hemiatrophy
    Neurologic disorders
  Hemidystrophy
    Russel-Silver syndrome
    Chromosomal aberrations
    Cerebral palsy
    Hemifacial microsomia

Differential Diagnosis

The presence of hemihypertrophy without benefit of additional radiographic or clinical findings is not distinctive. At present, there is no explanation for the appearance of body asymmetry, and the difference between the sides tends to become less apparent as the patient ages. The incidence of associated malignancy, particularly Wilm's tumor, and occasionally hepatoblastomas and adrenal tumors in patients with congenital asymmetry, is high. As a result, patients with hemihypertrophy should be frequently evaluated for abdominal masses. The adrenal lesions more commonly arise in the cortex and are therefore endocrinologically active. Patients with body asymmetry associated with neoplasm also manifest an increased incidence of aniridia, polydactyly, and hypospadias. Abnormalities other than tumors also frequently occur in congenital asymmetry, including medullary sponge kidney, nephromegaly, or adrenomgaly. These must be distinguished from enlargement due to tumor. In the kidney, calyceal distortion is always present and well pronounced.

Regional hypertrophy can be encountered in neurofibromatosis, as well as in other forms of neurocutaneous diseases, such as Sturge-Weber, von Hippel-Lindau disease, and tuberous sclerosis. The diagnosis of neurofibromatosis is obvious if the external manifestations, such as fibromas and café au lait spots, are well developed. Von Hippel-Lindau disease is characterized by cystic disease of the liver, kidney, and pancreas, as well as vascular tumors in the brain. Hypernephromas also occur in this lesion.

Hemangiomas, arteriovenous fistulas, lymphangiomas, and other vascular malformations such as the Klippel-Trenaunay syndrome are mostly manifestations of regional enlargement and are not difficult to recognize. The majority of these malformations manifest typical external cutaneous abnormalities or characteristic angiographic findings. The Klippel-Trenaunay syndrome consists of a venous angiomatous malformation, with overgrowth of the involved extremity. Some lesions which cause asymmetry may be acquired (e.g., arteriovenous malformation). Although hemihypertrophy occurs in the Beckwith-Wiedemann syndrome, this syndrome is more commonly associated with gigantism and organomegaly, as well as macroglossia and hypoglycemia.

Hemiatrophy is a term used to describe acquired loss of body structures. Hemiatrophy is usually associated with neurologic disorders and is therefore easy to recognize. Radiographically, the changes demonstrate a marked decrease in size and volume of bone, muscle, and subcutaneous tissues.

Somatic underdevelopment of one side of the body is referred to as hemidystrophy. Silver's syndrome is a type of fetal dwarfism and is representative of this category; the term *asymmetrical dwarf* has been used to designate this abnormality. It is associated with café au lait spots, elevated serum level of gonadotropins, and a variety of anomalies of sexual development. Despite the elevated level of gonadotropins, a definite delay in bone maturation is present.

FRACTURES IN THE NEWBORN

Fractures are not often seen in the neonatal period. When they are present, the physician must determine if they are the result of trauma or congenital disease. The frac-

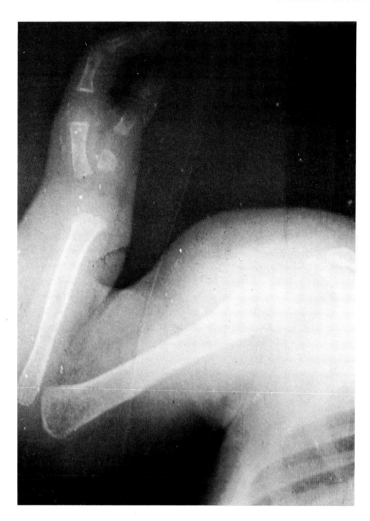

Fig. 10-117. Brachmann-de Lange syndrome. Note the complete absence of the ulna. The residual radius is hypoplastic. Some phalanges are also absent.

ture must be considered in terms of the type of bone affected, the number of bones involved, and the position of the fracture site within the bone (i.e., the metaphysis or diaphysis).

Disease Entities

Clavicle fracture
Rib fracture
Leg fracture
Metaphyseal fracture
Multiple fracture

Differential Diagnosis

Several different bones may be fractured as a result of birth trauma; a fracture of the clavicle is the most common. It occurs as the result of a difficult cephalic delivery. The diagnosis is often made by palpation. This form of birth trauma is often associated with other clinical findings, such as brachial plexus injuries and diaphragmatic paralysis due to phrenic nerve injury.

Rib fractures may also be the result of birth trauma and are normally only an incidental finding on the chest radiograph. If several ribs are injured, repiratory distress may be present.

Breech deliveries may be the cause of fracture of a lower extremity. The fracture is usually metaphyseal and closely resembles the findings seen in battered child syndrome. A fracture must also be suspected after birth if the neonate demonstrates spastic limbs, as in the caudal regression syndrome. Even normal obstetrical handling of a resistant limb can result in fracture.

A fracture may also be the result of rough handling while the neonate is in the hospital nursery. Insertion of a catheter into an arm

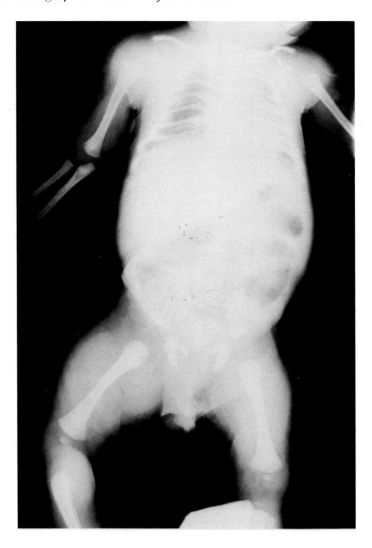

Fig. 10-118. Idiopathic hemi-hypertrophy. A newborn shows right-sided hemihypertrophy. Note the difference in size of the bone and of the soft-tissue structures.

may necessitate manipulation to such an extent that metaphyseal fracture results.

Congenital pseudarthrosis should be considered in cases where a fracture of the tibia (and occasionally the fibula) is present. Pseudarthrosis undergoes a specific sequential development and should be fairly easy to distinguish from a traumatic fracture. Pseudarthrosis is accompanied by extensive bowing of the extremity, with segmental narrowing at the potential site of fracture (Fig. 10-119). Pseudarthrosis may be observed at the first examination, since the fragments are more smooth and tapered than those of a traumatic fracture.

Multiple fractures in newborns have an entirely different, though limited number of possible causes. In premature infants, occasionally metaphyseal fractures with demineralization and fragmentation may be

seen. Osteogenesis inperfecta demonstrates fractures involving all bones in various stages of development (Fig. 10-120). In addition, marked demineralization is also an important feature. Very rarely, an extremely traumatic delivery results in multiple fractures.

Discussion

A clavicular fracture should be relatively easy to diagnose. However, occasionally the S-curved clavicle is radiographed somewhat obliquely, and this results in foreshortening and apparent overriding of the bone, which may be confused with a fracture. In addition, an abnormally developed clavicle in cleido-cranial dysostosis may cause confusion. Although absence of a clavicle may occur in cleidocranial disostosis, partial development is quite common. The presence of other associated deformities, such as a poorly

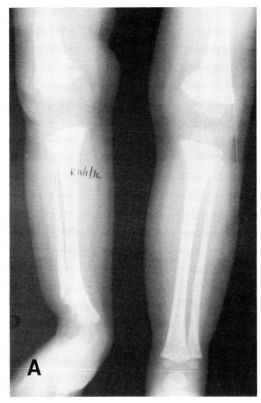
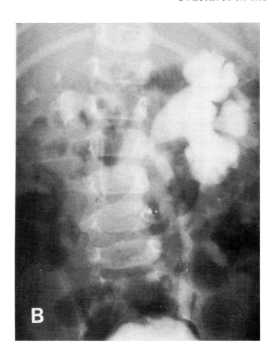

Fig. 10-119. Rothmund-Thomson syndrome. *(A)* Pseudoarthrosis of the lower distal fibula is very apparent, with changes beginning in the tibia. Note the extreme curvature and changes of the soft tissues. Some bone defects are also noted within the distal femoral metaphyses. *(B)* An intravenous pyelogram reveals obstructive uropathy of the left collecting systems.

mineralized calvarium, should clarify the diagnosis.

Pseudarthrosis is not a well-defined entity. The fracture normally occurs through a segment of bone containing fibrous dysplastic tissue. Approximately half the cases reveal some evidence of neurofibromatosis, such as cafe au lait spots, which are the most common. Physicians have suggested that congenital bands, local ischemia, or constriction caused by pushing an extremity through the amniotic sac may result in pseudarthrosis. The etiology should be obvious in such cases, since associated soft-tissue constriction would be present. Diseases like the Rothmund-Thompsom syndrome also present with pseudarthrosis. This syndrome is basically a cutaneous disease characterized by poikiloderma, ectodermal dysplasia, and cataracts. Visceral changes, however, also occur.

The bowed deformity of pseudarthrosis must be distinguished from prenatal bowed tibias. No intrinsic defect is encountered in the latter, and obviously there is a better prognosis.

Rickets in premature infants is not well-defined. Radiographically, many premature infants demonstrate radiolucent metaphyseal zones in the long bones. These look very similar to the metaphyseal radiolucencies seen in children with leukemia. They have been attributed to poor mineral retention related to immature kidneys and also to rapid growth. Rickets resolves without further sequelae in most of these patients. For reasons yet to be explained, it occasionally progresses to severe fragmentation and demineralization and some periosteal proliferation. Further research is needed to determine whether this is a severe manifestation of rickets in premature infants or an added complication.

Osteogenesis imperfecta is a diaphyseal problem. The epiphyses are unaffected, as osteoblastic activity appears altered. The severe cases develop multiple fractures in

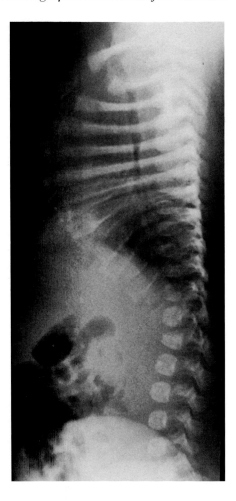

Fig. 10-120. Osteogenesis imperfecta. A lateral film of the rib cage demonstrates multiple fractures throughout.

utero and carry an increased mortality. During the neonatal period further fractures occur (Figs. 10-58, 10-120), and callus formation is very prominent. The fractures are characteristically of the shaft, and there should be no difficulty in distinguishing them from metaphyseal fractures of rickets, birth trauma, or rough handling. The bones of patients with osteogenesis imperfecta have thin cortices and flared metaphyses. As the extensive fracturing heals, gross deformities and atypical angulations result. Less severe forms of osteogenesis imperfecta may not manifest fractures for months or years after birth, and all show significant improvement at puberty.

REFERENCES

Periosteal Reaction

1. Caffey, J.: Infantile cortical hyperostosis. J. Pediatr., 29:541, 1946.

2. Capitano, M. A., and Kirkpatrick, J.: Early roentgenobservations in acute osteomyletis. Am. J. Roentgenol. Radium Ther. Nucl. Med., 108:488, 1970.
3. Stanley, P. H., Gwinn, J. L., and Sutcliffe, J.,: Osseous abnormalities in Menke's syndrome. Ann. Radiol., 19:167, 1976.
4. Waldvogel, F. A., Medoff, G., and Swartz, M. N.: Osteomyletis: a review of clinical features, therapeutic considerations and unusual aspects. N. Engl. J. Med.,

Solitary Osteolytic Lesions

5. Arcamono, J. P., et al.: Histiocytosis X. Am. J. Roentgenol. Radium Ther. Nucl. Med., 85:663, 1961.
6. Flaherty, R. A., et al.: Osteoid osteoma. Am J. Roentgenol. Radium Ther. Nucl. Med., 76:1041, 1956.
7. Lodwick, G. S.: Juvenile unicameral bone cyst. Am. J. Roentgenol. Radium Ther. Nucl. Med., 80:495, 1958.
8. Reynolds, J.: Fallen fragment sign in diag-

nosis of unicameral bone cysts. Radiology, 92:949, 1969.

9. Sherman, R. S., and Vzel, A. R.: Benign chondroblastoma of bone. Am. J. Roentgenol. Radium Ther. Nucl. Med., 76:1132, 1956.

Solitary Sclerotic Lesions of Bone

10. Cabenela, M. E., Sim, F. H., Beabout, J. W., and Dahlin, D. C.: Osteomyelitis appearing as neoplasms Arch. Surg., 109:72, 1974.

11. Lichtenstein, L.: Fibrous dysplasia of bone. *In* Diseases of Bone and Joints. St. Louis, C. V. Mosby, 1975.

12. McLeod, D. A., Dahlin, D. C., and Beabout, J. W.: The spectrum of osteoblastoma. Am. J. Roentgenol. Radium Ther. Nucl. Med., 126:321, 1976.

13. Price, C. M. G., et al.: Osteosarcoma in children. A study of 125 cases. J. Bone Joint Surg., 57-B:341, 1975.

14. Pritchard, D. J., Dahlin, D. C., Douphine, R. T., Taylor, W. F., and Beabout, J. W. Ewing's sarcoma. A clinicopathological and statistical analysis of patients surviving five years or longer. J. Bone Joint Surg., 57-A: 10, 1975.

15. Simmons, R. C., Horle, T. S., and Singleton, E. B.: The osseus manifestations of leukemia in children. Radiol. Clin. North Am., 6:115, 1968.

16. Snarr, J. W., Abell, M. R., and Martel, W.: Lympho-follicular synovitis with osteoid osteoma. Radiology, 106:557, 1973.

17. Sweet, D. E., and Allman, D. M.: Stress fracture. Radiology, 99:687, 1971.

18. Twersky, J., Kassner, G. E., Tenner, M. S., and Camera, A.: Vertebral and coastal osteochondromas, causing spinal cord compression., Am. J. Roentgenol. Radium Ther. Nucl. Med., 124:124, 1975.

Multiple Osteolytic Lesions

19. Bell, D., and Cockshott, W. P.: Tuberculosis of the vertebral pedicles. Radiology, 99:43, 1971.

20. Brunner, S., Gudbjerg, C. C., and Iverson, R.: Skeletal lesions in leukemia in children. Acta. Radiol., 49:419, 1958.

21. Caffey, J., and Anderson, D.: Metastatic embryonal rhabdomyosarcoma in the growing skeleton. Am. J. Dis. Child., 95:581, 1958.

22. Cheyne, C.: Histocytosis X. J. Bone Joint Surg., 53-B: 366, 1971.

23. Ennis, J. T., Whitehouse, G., Ross, F. G. M., et al.: The radiology of bone changes in histiocytosis. Clin. Radiol., 24:212, 1973.

24. Gehweiler, J. A., Capp, M. P., and Chick, E. W.: Observations on the roentgen pattern in blastomycosis of bone. Am. J. Roentgenol. Radium Ther. Nucl. Med., 108:497, 1970.

25. Gilmour, W. N.: Acute hematogenous osteomyelitis. J. Bone Joint Surg., 44-B:841, 1962.

26. Gorham, L. W., Sholtz, J. H., and Maxon, S. C.: Disappearing bone. A Form of acroosteolysis. Am. J. Med., 17:674, 1954.

27. Hodgson, J. R., Kennedy, R. L. J., and Coups, J. D.: Reticuloendotheliosis. Radiology., 57:642, 1951.

28. Kinhaid, O. W., Hodgson, J. R., and Dockeryy, M. D.: Neuroblastoma. A roentgenologic and pathologic study. Am. J. Roentgenol. Radium Ther. Nucl. Med., 78:420, 1957.

29. Lichtenstein, L.: Diseases of Bones and Joints. St. Louis, C. V. Mosby, 1975.

30. Merriam, G. R., Jr.: Retinoblastoma: analysis of 17 cases. Acta. Ophthalmol., 44:71, 1950.

31. Pear, B. L.: Skeletal manifestations of the lymphomas and leukemias. Semin. Roentgenol, IX:219, 1975.

32. Sechler, S. G., Rubin, H., and Rabinowitz, J. G.: Systemic cystic angiomatosis. Am. J. Med., 37:976, 1964.

33. Wolfson, J. J., Kane, W. J., et al.: Bone findings in chronic granulomatous disease of childhood. A genetic abnormality of leukocyte cyte function. J. Bone Joint Surg., 51-A:1572, 1969.

34. Wolstein, D., Rabinowitz, J. G., and Twersky, J.: Tuberculosis of the Rib. J. Can. Assoc. Radiol., 25:307, 1974.

Multiple Sclerotic Lesions

35. Beighton, P., Durr, L., and Hamersma, H.: Clinical features of sclerosteosis. Ann. Int. Med., 84:393, 1976.

36. Bloor, D. U.: A case of osteopathia striata. J. Bone Joint Surg., 36-B:261, 1954.

37. Campbell, C. J., et al.: Melorheostosis. A report of the clinical, roentgenographic and pathological findings in fourteen cases. J. Bone Joint Surg., 50-A:128, 1968.

38. Curth, H. O.: Dermato Fibrosis and Osteopoikilosis. Arch. Dermatol., 30:552, 1934.

39. Elmore, S.: Pyknodysostosis: a review. J. Bone Joint Surg., 49-A:153, 1967.

40. Engelfeldt, B., et al.: Studies in osteopetrosis. Roentgenological anatomical investigations on some of the bone changes. Arch. Pediatr., 49:391, 1960.

41. Girdany, B. R.: Engelmann's disease (progressive diaphyseal dysplasia). A nonprogressive familial form of muscular dystrophy with characteristic bone changes. Clin. Orthop., 14:102, 1959.

42. Gorlin, R. J., et al.: Pyle's disease (familial metaphyseal dysplasia). A preseutoliar of two cases and an argument for its separation from crainometaphyseal dysplasia. J. Bone Joint Surg., 52-A:347, 1970.

43. Green, A. E., Ellswood, W., and Collins, J. R.: Melorheostosis and osteopoikilosis.

Am. J. Roentgenol. Radium Ther. Nucl. Med., *87*:1096, 1962.

44. Hinkel, C. L., and Beiler, D. D.: Osteopetrosis in adults. Am. J. Roentgenol, Radium Ther. Nucl. Med., *74*:46, 1955.

45. Moseley, J. E.: Bone changes in Hematologic Disorders. New York, Grune and Stratton, 1963.

46. Pease, C. N., and Newton, M. D.: Metaphyseal dysplasia due to lead poisoning in children. Radiology, *79*:233, 1962.

47. Pyle, E.: A cause of unusual bone development. J. Bone Joint Surg., *13*:874, 1931.

Osteopenia

48. Arnstein, A. R.: Regional osteoporosis. Orthop. Clin. North Am., *3*:585, 1972.

49. DeLuca, H. F.: Recent advances in the metabolism and function of vitamin D. Fed. Proc., *28*:1678, 1969.

50. ———: The kidney as an endocrine organ involved in the function of vitamin D. Am. J. Med., *58*:39, 1975.

51. ———: Vitamin D endocrinology. Ann. Int. Med., *85*:367, 1976.

52. Dent, C. E., Friedman, M., and Watson, L.: Hereditary pseudo vitamin D deficiency rickets. J. Bone Joint Surg., *50-B*:708, 1968.

53. Dent, C. E., Richens, A., Rone, D. J. F., and Stamp, T. C. B.: Osteomalacia with long term anticonvulsant therapy in epilepsy. Br. Med. J., *4*:69, 1970.

54. Dent, C. E., and Stamp, T. C. B.: Hypophosphatemic osteomalacia presenting in adults. Q. J. Med., *40*:303, 1971.

55. Friedlander, H. L., et al.: Arthrogyposis multiplex congenita: a review of forty-five cases. J. Bone Joint Surg., *50-A*:89, 1968.

56. Garn, S. M.: The course of bone gain and phases of bone loss. Orthop. Clin. North Am., *3*:503, 1972.

57. Hunter, J., Maxwell, D. J., Stewart, D. A., Parsons, V., and Williams, R.: Altered calcium metabolism in epileptic children on anticonvulsants. Br. Med. J., *4*:202, 1971.

58. James, A. E., J., et al.: Trisomy 18. Radiology, *92*:37, 1969.

59. Jaworski, Z. F. G.: Pathophysiology, diagnosis and treatment of osteomalacia. Orthop. Clin. North Am., *3*:601, 1972.

60. Kirkwood, J. R., Ozonoff, M. B., and Steinbach, H. L.: Epiphyseal displacement after metaphyseal fracture in renal osteodystrophy. Am. J. Roentgenol. Radium Ther. Nucl. Med., *115*:547, 1972.

61. McKusick, V. A.: Heritable Disorders of Connective Tissue. ed. 3. St. Louis, C. V. Mosby, 1966.

62. Newton, J. H., and Carpenter, M. E.:

Ehlers-Danlos syndrome with acroosteolysis. Br. J. Radiol., *32*:739, 1959.

63. Parfitt, A. M.: Hypophosphatemic vitamin D refractory rickets and osteomalacia. Orthop. Clin. North Am., *3*:653, 1972.

64. ———: Renal osteodystrophy. Orthop. Clin. North Am., *3*:681, 1972.

65. ———: Soft tissue calcification in uremia. Arch. Int. Med., *124*:544, 1969.

66. Park, E. A., et al.: The recognition of scurvy with special reference to the early x-ray changes. Arch. Dis. Child., *10*:265, 1935.

67. Rabinowitz, J. G., et al.: Trisomy 18, esophageal atresia, anomalies of the radius, and congenital hypoplastic thrombocytopenia. Radiology, *89*:488, 1967.

68. Rarien, V. A., and Duri, M.: Trisomy 17-18 syndrome: report of a case with diffuse myocardial fibrosis and review of cardiovascular abnormalities. Am. J. Cardiol., *21*:431, 1968.

69. Reynolds, W. A., and Karo, J. J.: Radiologic diagnosis of metabolic bone disease. Orthop. Clin. North Am., *3*:521, 1972.

70. Salassa, R. M., Jowsey, J., and Arnaus, C. D.: Hypophosphatemia osteomalacia associated with "nonendocrine" tumors. N. Engl. J. Med., *283*:65, 1970.

71. Shea, D., and Mankin, H. J.: Slipped capital femoral epiphysis in renal rickets. Report of three cases. J. Bone Joint Surg., *48-A*:349, 1966.

72. Smith, R. M. A.: The pathophysiology and management of rickets, Orthop. Clin. North Am., *3*:601, 1972.

73. Steinback, H. L.: The roentgen appearance osteoporosis, Radiol. Clin. *2*:191, 1964.

74. Steinbach, H. L., and Noetzeli, M.: Roentgen appearance of the skeleton in osteomalacia and rickets. Am. J. Roentgenol. Radium Ther. Nucl. Med., *91*:955, 1964.

Metaphyseal Abnormalities

75. Al-Rashid, R. A., and Spauger, J.: Neonatal copper deficiency. N. Engl. J. Med., *285*:841, 1971.

76. Caffey, J.: Congenital stenosis of medullary spaces in tabular bones and cavaria in two proportionate dwarfs. Am. J. Roentgenol. Radium Ther. Nucl. Med., *100*:1, 1967.

77. ———: Traumatic cupping of the metaphysis of growing bones. Am. J. Roentgenol. Radium Ther. Nucl. Med., *108*:451, 1967.

78. Carlson, D. H., and Harris, G. B. C.: Craniometaphyseal dysplasia. Radiology, *103*:147, 1972.

79. Cavallino, R., and Grossman, H.: Wilson's disease presenting with rickets. Radiology, *90*:493, 1968.

80. Clipps, B. E., et al.: Single bone involvement in congenital syphilis. Pediatr. Radiol., 5:50, 1976.
81. Condon, V. R., and Allen, R. P.: Congenital generalized fibromatosis. Am. J. Roentgenol. Radium Ther. Nucl. Med., 76:444, 1961.
82. Cremin, B. J., and Fisher, R. M.: The Lesions of Congenital Syphilis. Br. J. Radiol., 43:333, 1970.
83. Gorlin, R. J., et al.: Pyle's disease. J. Bone Joint Surg., 52-A:347, 1970.
84. Graham, C. B., et al.: Rubella-like bone changes in congenital cytomegalic inclusion disease. Radiology, 94:39, 1970.
85. Griscom, N. T., et al.: Systemic bone disease developing in small premature infants. Pediatrics, 48:883, 1971.
86. Kozlowski, K., et al.: Hypophosphatasia. Pediatr. Radiol., 5:103, 1976.
87. Levin, E. J.: Healing in congenital osseous syphilis. Am. J. Roentgenol. Radium Ther. Nucl. Med., 110:591, 1970.
88. Merten, D. F., and Gooding, C. A.: Skeletal manifestations of congenital cytomegalic inclusion disease. Radiology, 95:333, 1970.
89. Mindelzun, R.: Skeletal changes in Wilson's disease. Radiology, 94:127, 1970.
90. Morreels, C. L., et al.: The roentgenographic features of homocystinuria. Radiology, and 90:1150, 1968.
91. Padfield, E., and Hiclsen, P.: Cortical hyperostosis in infants. Br. J. Radiol., 43:231, 1970.
92. Pease, C. N., and Newton, G. G.: Metaphyseal dysplasia due to lead poisoning in children. Radiology, 79:233, 1962.
93. Poznanski, A. L., and LaRowe, P. C.: Radiographic manifestations of the arthrogryposis syndrome. Radiology, 95:353, 1970.
94. Rabinowitz, J. G., et al.: Osseous changes in rubella embryopathy. Am. J. Roentgenol. Radium Ther. Nucl. Med., 85:494, 1965.
95. Saldino, R. M.: Lethal lettral short limbed dwarfism. Am. J. Roentgenol. Radium Ther. Nucl. Med., 112:185, 1971.
96. Schwarz, E.: Roentgen findings in progeria. Am. J. Roentgenol. Radium Ther. Nucl. Med., 79:411, 1962.
97. Siegelman, S. S., et al.: Congenital indifference to pain. Am. J. Roentgenol. Radium Ther. Nucl. Med., 97:242, 1966.
98. Silverman, F. N., Bilden, J. J.: Congenital Insensitivity to Pain. Am. J. Roentgenol. Radium Ther. Nucl. Med., 72:176, 1959.
99. Soloman, A., and Rosen, E.: The aspect of trauma in the bone changes of congenital lues. Pediatr. Radiol., 3:176, 1975.
100. Spranger, J.: The bio-chemical basis of bone dysplasia. Progress in Pediatric Radiology, 4:29. Basel, S. Karger, 1973.
101. Taybi, H.: Generalized skeletal dysplasia with miltiple anomalies. Am. J. Roentgenol. Radium Ther. Nucl. Med., 88:450, 1962.
102. Thomas, P. S., and Nevin, N. C.: Spondylometaphyseal dysplasia. Am. J. Roentgenol. Radium Ther. Nucl. Med., 128:89, 1977.
103. Wesenberg, R. L., et al.: Radiologic findings in the kinky-hair syndrome. Radiology, 92:500, 1969.
104. Whalen, J. P., et al.: Growing Bone—The Race of Internal Resorption and its Control. In Kaufman, H. (ed.): Progress in Pediatric Radiology, 4:45. Basel, S. Karger, 1973.
105. Winchester, P. H., et al.: a new mucopolysaccharidosis with skeletal deformities simulating rheumatoid arthritis. Am. J. Roentgenol. Radium Ther. Nucl. Med., 106:121, 1969.

Epiphyseal Abnormalities

106. Becker, M. H., Genilser, N. B., Finegold, M., and Miranda, D.: Chondrodysplasia punctata: is maternal warfarin therapy a factor? Am. J. Dis. Child., 129: 356, 1975.
107. Gorlin, R., Cohen, M. M., and Wolfson, J.: Tricho-rhino-phalangeal syndrome. Am. J. Dis. Child., 118:595, 1969.
108. Kuhns, L. R., Poznanski, A. K., Harper, H., and Garn, S. M.: Ivory epiphysis of the hands. Radiology, 109:643, 1973.
109. Mason, R. C., and Kozlowski, F.: Chondrodysplasia punctata. Radiology, 109:145, 1973.
110. Poznanski, A. K., Nosanchuk, J., Baublis, J., and Holt, J.: The cerebro-hepato-renal syndrome (CHRS): Zellweger's syndrome. Am. J. Roentgenol. Radium Ther. Nucl. Med., 109:313, 1970.
111. Poznanski, A. K., et al.: The hand in oto-palato-digital syndrome. Acta Radiol., 16:203, 1973.
112. Saldina, R. M., and Mainzor, F.: Cone-shaped epiphysis in siblings with hereditary renal disease and retinitis pigmentosa. Radiology, 98:39, 1971.

Short Bones and Dwarfism

113. Cremin, B. J., and Beighton, P.: Dwarfism in the newborn; the nonemclature, radiological features and genetic significnace. Br. J. Radiol., 47:77, 1974.
114. Dorst, J. P., Scott, C. I., and Hall, J. G.: The radiologic assessment of short stature—dwarfism Radiol. Clin. North Am., 10:393, 1972.
115. Capitanio, M. A., and Kirkpatrick, S. A.: Widening of the cranial sutures. A roentgen observation during periods of accelerated

growth in patients treated for deprivation dwarfism. Radiology, 92:53, 1969.

116. Wynne-Davies, R., and Fairbank, T. J.: Fairbank's Atlas of General Affections of the Skeleton. ed. 2. Edinburgh, Churchill-Livingston, 1976.

Radial Dysplasia

117. Mosely, J. T.: Bone changes in Hematologic Disorders. New York, Grune and Stratton, 1963.
118. Rabinowitz, J. G., Camera, A., and Oran, D.: Holt-Oram associated with carcinoma. Clin. Radiol., 22:346, 1971.
119. Rabinowitz, J. G., Moseley, J. T., Mitty, H.

A., and Hirschhorn, K.: Trisomy 18, esophageal atresia, anomalies of the radius, and hypoplastic congenital thormobocytopenia. Radiology, 88:488, 1967.

Body Asymmetry

120. Kirks, D. R., and Shackelford, G. D.: Idiopathic congenital hemihypertrophy with associated ipsilateral benign nephromegaly. Radiology, 115:145, 1975.
121. Pfister, R. C., et al.: Congenital asymmetry (hemihypertrophy) and abdominal disease: radiologic features in 9 cases. Radiology, 716:685, 1975.

Index

Numbers in *italics* indicate a figure; "t" following a page number indicates a table.

499